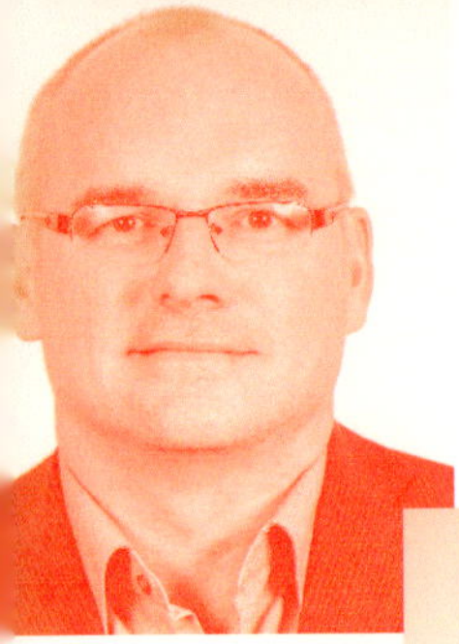
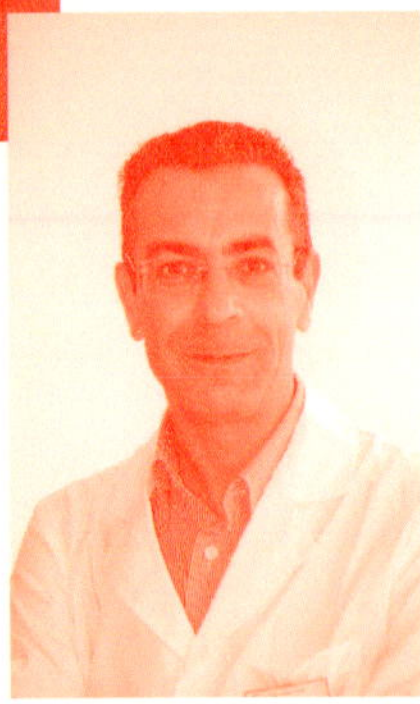
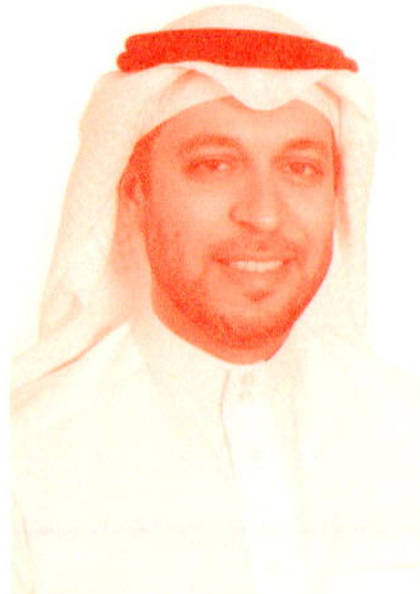
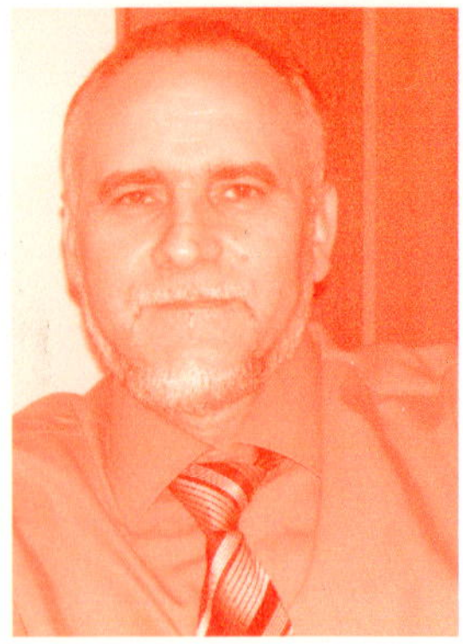
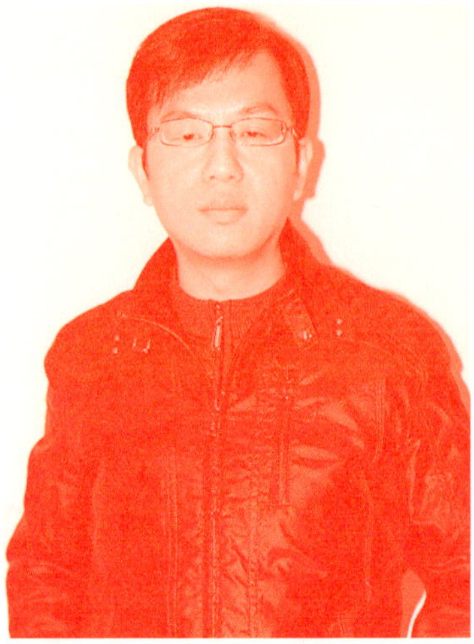
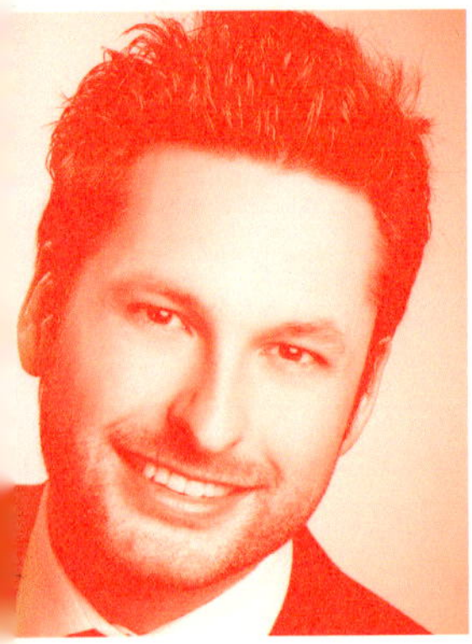
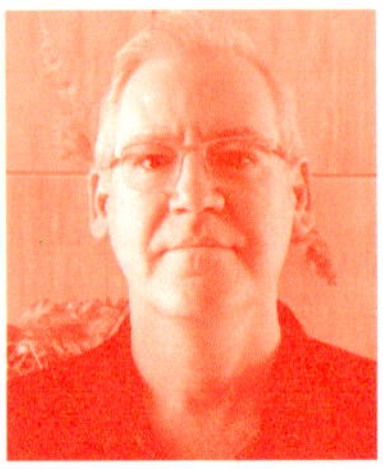

IntechOpen

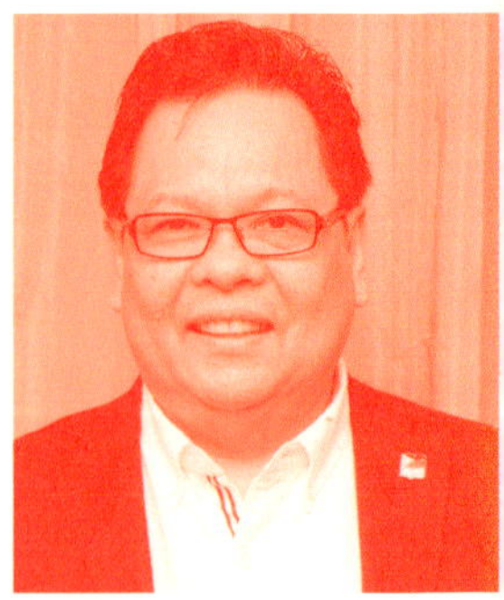
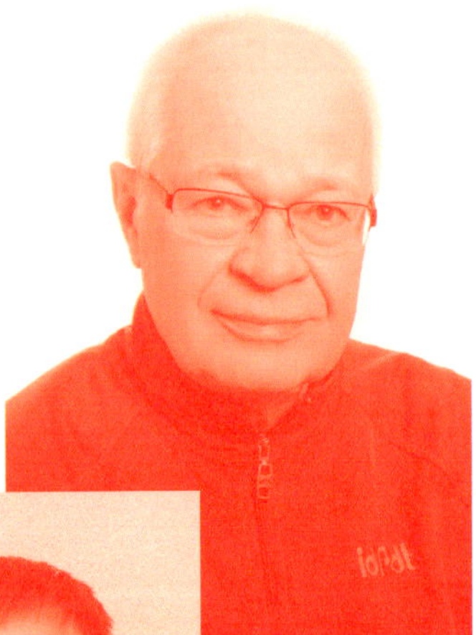
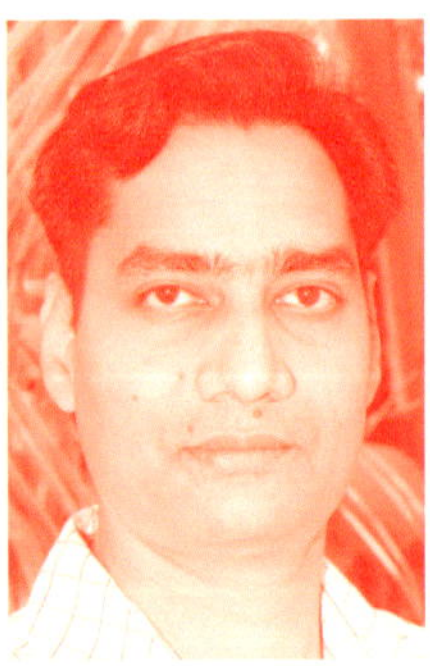
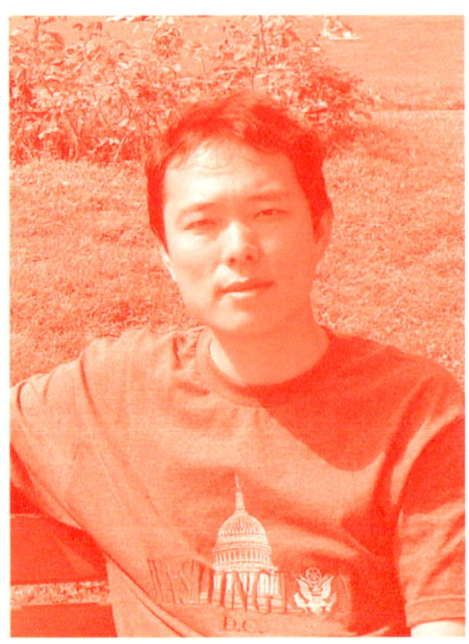
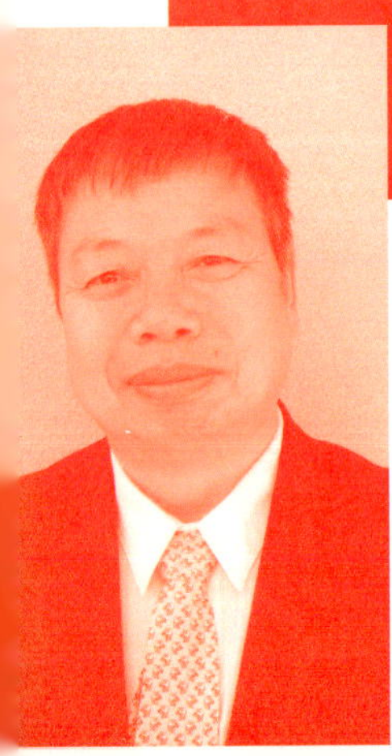
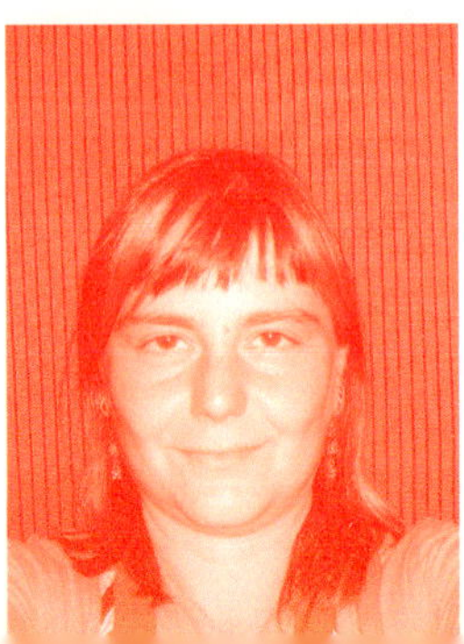

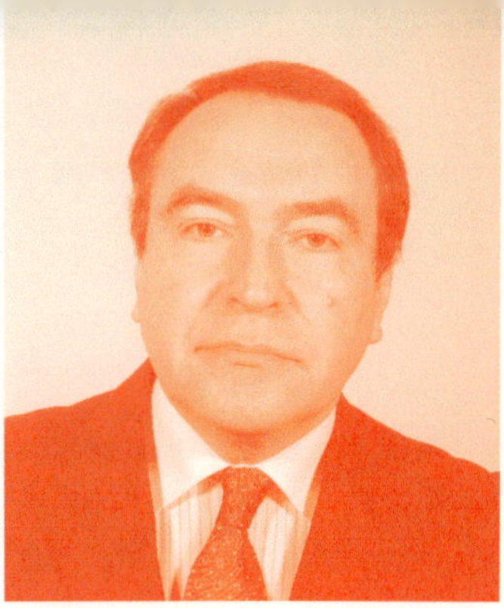
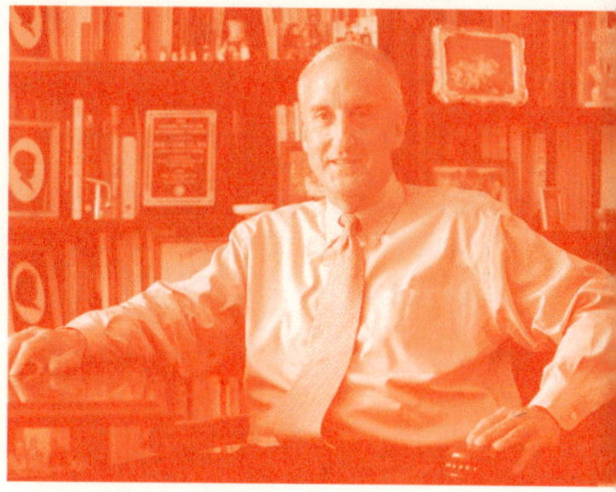
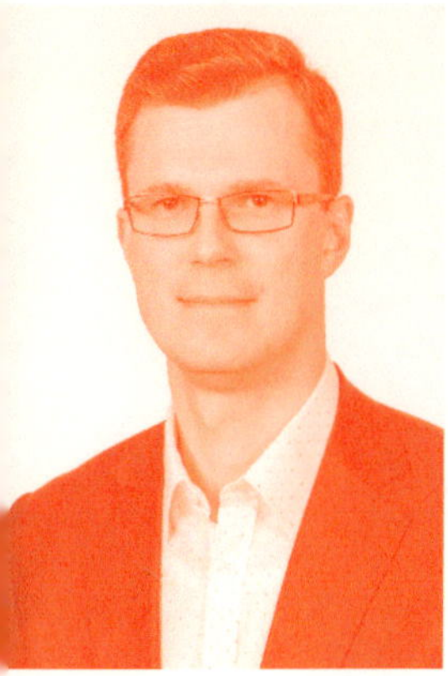
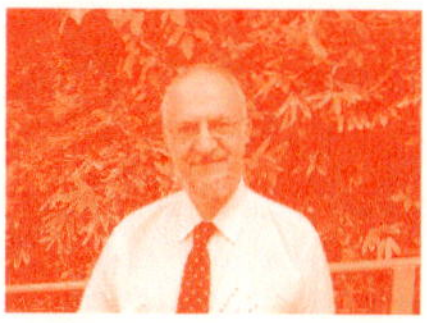
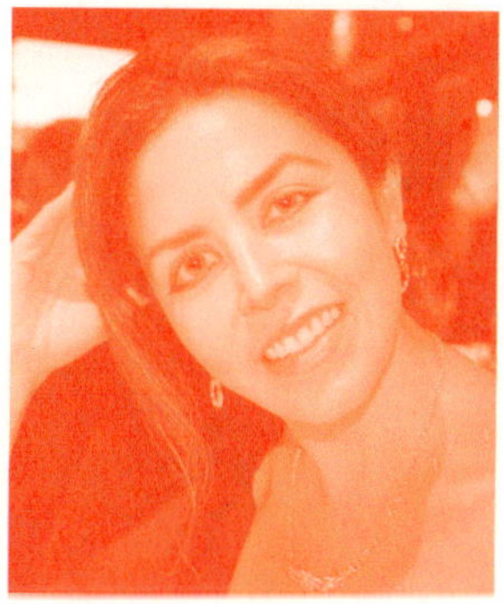

Supporting open minds since 2005

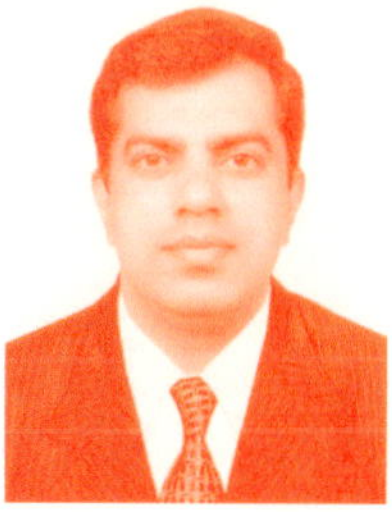
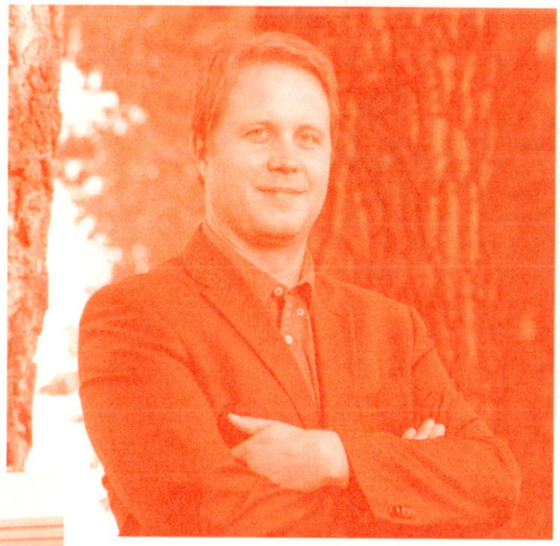
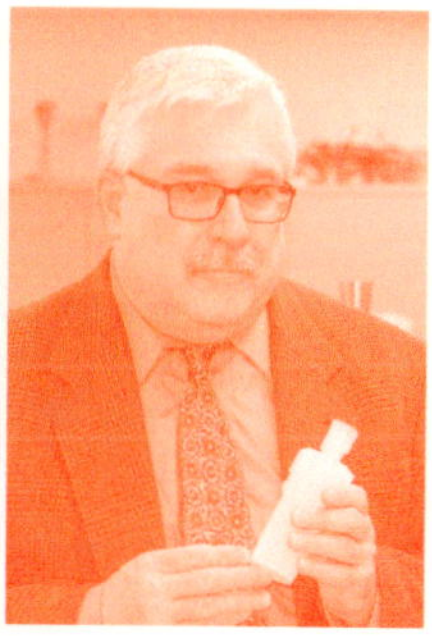
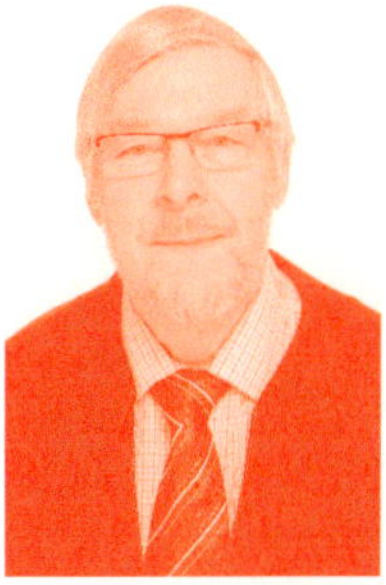
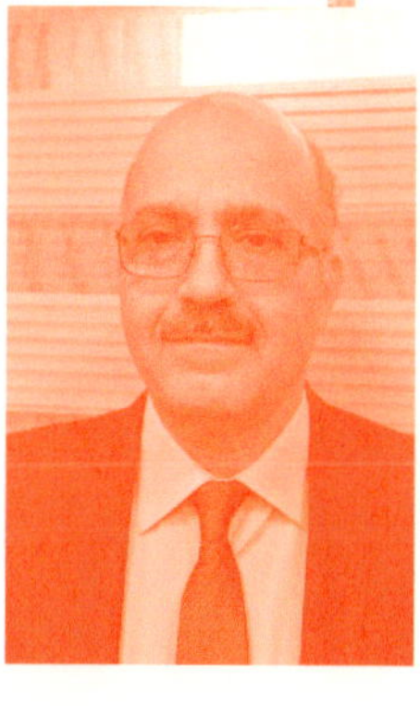
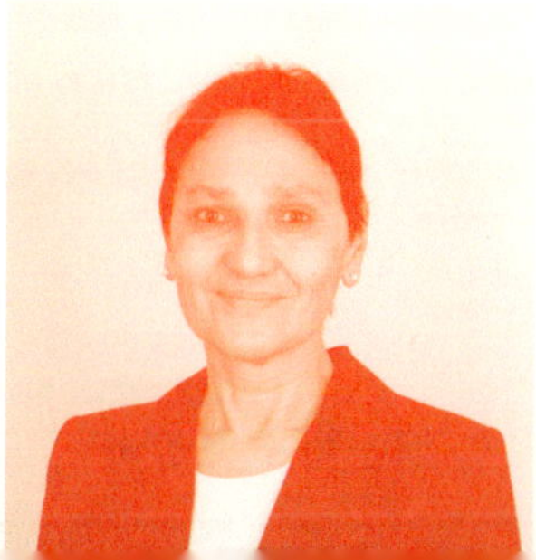
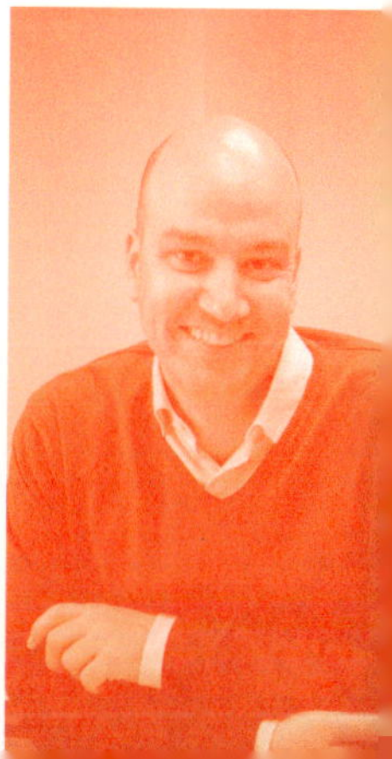

Antioxidants - Benefits, Sources, Mechanisms of Action
http://dx.doi.org/10.5772/intechopen.92918
Edited by Viduranga Waisundara

Contributors
Cheryl A. Frye, Vincent F. Lembo, Christophe Hano, Samantha Drouet, Huda Mahmood Alfatal, Andrei Florin Danet, Atika Eddaikra, Naouel Eddaikra, Vijay Laxmi Trivedi, Mohan Chandra Nautiyal, Mauricio Homem-de-Mello, Giulia Oliveira Timo, Adriana Françozo de Melo, Manju Singh Makhaik, Raosaheb Kale, Arvind K. Shakya, Paolo Bellavite, Perçin Karakol, Emin Kapi, Oluyomi Adeyemi, Musbau Akanji, Damilare Rotimi, Lawrence Boluwatife Afolabi, Heritage Demilade Fatinikun, Sung-Jae Lee, Chanjae Lee, Min K. Bae, Md Sanaullah Biswas, Masuma Zahan Akhi, Md. Manjurul Haque, Cenk Aydin, Nilay Seyidoglu, Loknath Deshmukh, Rajendra Singh, Sardul Singh Sandhu, Ziad Moussa, Mohammed Ali Al-Mamary, Christian Cortes-Rojo, Rocío Montoya - Pérez, Alfredo Saavedra-Molina, Alain Raimundo Rodriguez-Orozco, Manjury Jatziry Hernández-Esparza, Claudia Guadalupe Flores-Ledesma, Elizabeth Calderon-Cortes, Amala Reddy, Thendarl Selvam, Pavithra Muthukumar, Varuna Suresh, Hideo Yamasaki, Yasuko Sakihama, Pedro Ferreira Ferreira-Santos, José António Teixeira, Claudia Manuela Da Cunha Ferreira Botelho, Cristina Rocha, Zlatina Genisheva, Donovan McGrowder, Fabian Miller, Chukwuemeka Nwokocha, Cameil Wilson-Clarke, Lennox Anderson-Jackson, Lowen Williams, Melisa Anderson, Betül Çalişkan, Ali Cengiz Çalişkan, Mohamad Eid Hammadeh, Houda Amor, Nyaz Shelko, Peter Michael Jankowski, Massooma Mohsammed, Wassim Guermazi, Sana Gammoudi, Ines Dahmen-Ben Moussa, Habib Ayadi, Neila Annabi-Trabelsi, Banashree Nath, Hirok Roy, Abdulkerim Eroglu, Emilio Balbuena, Junrui Cheng, Isao Yumoto, Isao Hara, Yoshiko Hanaoka, Pinakin Gunvant Gunvant Davey, Drake W. Lem, Dennis L. Gierhart, Viduranga Waisundara, Asel Chandula Weerasekara, Kanchana Priyadarshani Samarasinghe, Heethaka Krishantha Sameera Krishantha Sameera de Zoysa, Thushara Chathuranga Bamunuarachchige

First published in London, United Kingdom, 2021 by IntechOpen
IntechOpen is the global imprint of INTECHOPEN LIMITED, registered in England and Wales, registration number: 11086078, 5 Princes Gate Court, London, SW7 2QJ, United Kingdom
Printed in Croatia

British Library Cataloguing-in-Publication Data
A catalogue record for this book is available from the British Library

Additional hard and PDF copies can be obtained from orders@intechopen.com

Antioxidants - Benefits, Sources, Mechanisms of Action
Edited by Viduranga Waisundara
p. cm.
Print ISBN 978-1-83968-864-5
Online ISBN 978-1-83968-865-2
eBook (PDF) ISBN 978-1-83968-866-9

Meet the editor

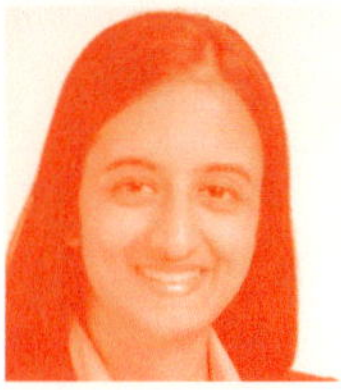

Dr. Viduranga Waisundara obtained her Ph.D. in Food Science & Technology from the Department of Chemistry, the National University of Singapore in 2010. She was a lecturer at the Temasek Polytechnic, Singapore, from July 2009 to March 2013. She relocated to her motherland of Sri Lanka and spearheaded the Functional Food Product Development Project at the National Institute of Fundamental Studies from April 2013 to October 2016. She was a senior lecturer on a temporary basis, at the Department of Food Technology, Faculty of Technology, Rajarata University of Sri Lanka. She is currently the deputy principal of the Australian College of Business & Technology – Kandy Campus, in Kandy, Sri Lanka. She is also the present Global Harmonization Initiative (GHI) ambassador to Sri Lanka.

Contents

Preface

Antioxidants have become a household name ever since their potency against many non-communicable diseases was demonstrated several decades ago. It is one of the most sought-after and active areas of research where the velocity of scientific discovery has remained at a steady increase. Not only among the scientific community, but even among consumers, the term "antioxidants" is a familiar matter. With an increasing number of consumers looking toward health and wellness, this group of biological compounds has gained much popularity, where incorporation of the word itself has been known to boost product sales.

The intention of this book is to provide an overview of antioxidants, their pathways of action, the mechanisms of antioxidant assays, and their potential sources. While most of these areas might appear mundane and therefore, already reviewed, it is without a doubt that the knowledge along these aspects keep getting renewed on a daily basis. There are several chapters of interest for readers who are from a nonscientific background, especially when it comes to identifying potent sources of antioxidants.

At the same time, almost all the contents of this book are positioned in the form of an update, where new discoveries and novel perspectives are provided. The authors contributing to this book span over various scientific backgrounds throughout several countries; therefore, the variety adds more color and value to its content.

I would like to take this opportunity to extend my appreciation to the authors who have contributed so many wonderful chapters to this book as well as my heartfelt appreciation to the IntechOpen Publisher with whom I have worked on several publications. Last, but not least, my appreciation goes to Mr. Josip Knapić - the Author Service Manager assigned to this book, who has rendered his fullest support in putting the material together.

Dr. (Mrs.) Viduranga Waisundara
Australian College of Business and Technology,
Kandy Campus, Sri Lanka

Section 1

Antioxidants and Prevention of Diseases

Chapter 1

Antioxidants: Pharmacothearapeutic Boon for Diabetes

Varuna Suresh, Amala Reddy, Pavithra Muthukumar and Thendarl Selvam

Abstract

Glucose-induced oxidative stress can be found related to "glucose variability" and "glucose memory". The irregular low and elevated glucose conditions cause damage to endothelial cell function than a steady, constant rise in level of glucose. Activation of PKC, NADPH oxidases, and mitochondrial oxidants are some of the pathways exhibited as a result of this aggravated cellular response. Regarding glucose memory, long after the normalization elevated level of glucose in the endothelial cells of diabetic rats and culture, a existance or 'memory' of induced basement membrane mRNA is expressed. This demonstrates that glucose causes dangerous long-term effects beyond the hyperglycemia period. Oxidative stress give rise to glucotoxicity and lipotoxicity which are phenomena's related to diabetes. Following the pathogenesis of diabetes, hyperglycemia and hyperlipidemia exerts a supplementary toxic effect on the beta-cells. So, hyperglycemia can be considered as a requirement for the destructive effects of lipotoxicity. Thus glucolipotoxicity can be considered as a substitute for lipotoxicity which relates the detrimental correlation between lipids and beta-cell function. Generally, the antioxidant pharmacotherapy can be coupled with drugs to boost the natural cellular defense mechanisms as the naturally existing antioxidant components, which neutralizes free radical damage. This considers antioxidant a boon tool for pharmacotherapeutic agent.

Keywords: Hyperglycaemia, Glucose, Pharmaco therapeutic, Antioxidants

1. Introduction

Diabetes is a metabolic disorder which is characterized based on the blood glucose level over a certain interval of time. It can also be termed as a condition that impairs the ability of the body to process blood sugar. This disorder has now been a common problem irrespective of age and gender [1]. As per the statistical surveys reported the count of people effected by diabetes is increasing over the world in a quite faster rate [2]. Diabetes are of two type in which type-1 is a chronic condition in which pancreas produces very little insulin, this may be due to loss of beta cells [3]. Beta cells dysfunction results from prolonged exposure of high level of glucose. Type-2 is a condition were that affects the way the body processes blood sugar [4]. Diabetes can lead to many complications that can show severe negative impact on different organs, mainly nerves, heart, kidney, eyes and blood vessels [5].

Diabetes can cause oxidative stress which can be caused by imbalance between production and accumulation of reactive oxygen species, which can damage DNA, lipid, protein beside these it can triggers the activation of different cellular pathways. When these molecules which are having notable regulatory effects in the body if deregulated it can lead to several diabetic complication [6–8].

When there is higher concentration of reactive oxygen species in the body with a minimal amount of anti-oxidant enzymes it can cause oxidative stress [9]. Whenever an external stimuli enters the body it can lead to reduction of the amount of anti-oxidant enzymes in the body and can cause inflammation [10].

Free radicles contain unpaired electrons and therefore lack stability which in turn search for another electron to stabilize themselves resulting in process that damages DNA and other parts of human cell [11]. Antioxidants are substances that can prevent the cells from damages that can be caused by free radicles. The antioxidants which is produced by the body is called endogenous antioxidants and those which is taken from outside is called exogenous [12].

There are many health benefits for anti-oxidants and this work pay attention on the benefits shown by antioxidants against oxidative stress, how it helps to reduce the formation of reactive species and thus in preventing or treating of diabetes and related complications that is the pharmacotherapy of antioxidants in treating diabetes [13]. Pharmacotherapy can be the therapy utilizing a drug that can cause relief to a particular disease. This work focuses on the characteristics of antioxidants and the use of same in prevention of diabetes [14].

2. Effect of BETA cell dysfunction and oxidative stress on hyperglycemia and lipotoxicity

Impaired glucose utilization can lead to hyperglycaemia. Beta cell dysfunction may be due to pancreatic diseases, drugs, surgery, tumors [15]. It may result from the long duration of exposure to high glucose, beta cells are meant to be sensitive towards reactive oxygen species because they are low at antioxidant enzymes such as catalase, SOD, GPx. Thus this end up in damaging mitochondria and blunt insulin secretion [16].

There are several studies that states the negative effect of oxidative stress on cell and tissues that finally leads to the damage of the same when there is an over production of reactive species that can lead to toxic effect and can cause cytostatic effects leads to membrane damage and can initiate cell death pathway [17]. If the pancreatic beta cells are healthy they can respond to nutrients and other insulin resistance via hyper secretion of insulin. This is done to maintain the energy level but this is a long process that requires a extended time period. The beta cell cannot withstand a response that can be compensatory which results in dysfunction of beta cell and death of beta cells [18].

There are also several studies that point out the impairment in beta cells can be due to the exposure of beta cell to the high glucose, which can cause glycolytic flux and thus producing reactive oxygen species including hydrogen peroxide, hydroxyl radicles and superoxide [19]. Hydrogen peroxide can be formed form superoxide this can be catalase and GPX. Many studies including in vitro and in vivo stated the over expression of superoxide production during diabetes [20].

There are many metabolic pathway which are activated during superoxide production which include advanced glycation and products (AGEs), polyol pathway activation of protein kinase c (PKC) [21]. Conversion of glucose to sorbitol is done during hyperglycemia that can further leads to the reduction of nicotinamide adenine dinucleotide phosphate (NADPH) and glycothione and this is the reason behind the reduction in the amount of antioxidants which in then can cause oxidative which in then can cause oxidative stress [22, 23].

In case of AGEs, adduct is formed by the reaction of amino group with glucose, which can interfere with cell integrity, and can lead to the production of reactive oxygen species [24]. During hyperglycermia there will be production of advanced glycation end product, which enhance PKC and hexosamine pathway which can lead to oxidative stress. Excess reactive oxygen species can react with nitric oxide radicle firming peroxy nitriate anion and cause tissue damage [25]. The other way of beta cell dysfunction may be due to the high glucose along with the free fatty acid whose origin can be utra-abdoman fat stores. Although the exact cause for the beta cell dysfunction is not known there are many hypothesis that have stated mitochondrial dysfunction, endoplasmic stress, and oxidative stress as the cause for the improper functioning of beta cell [26].

Other studies has pointed out that the free fatty acid can cause negative effect on functions of mitochondria leading to oxidative phosphorylation uncoupling and generation of reactive oxygen species [27]. Therefore dysfunction of mitochondria and oxidative stress can be reason for impairment of endogenous antioxidant defense. To add more to this point free fatty acid can generate reactive oxygen species and can cause fragmentation of DNA. Recent experimental studies suggest that lipotoxicity induced beta cell death may be due to the formation of hydrogen peroxide in peroxisomes [28].

Free fatty acid can activate nucleus factor kappa-β (NFK β), which allows the translocation of some into nucleus and produce cellular effect. In the case it can lead to the production of cytokines and can produce nitric acid through inducible NO synthase (iNOS) expression [29]. By this way over production of NO by iNOS takes place which can react with suoeroxide and leads to production of toxic substance peroxynitrite [30]. Thus free fatty acid can up-regulate the expression of iNOS, therefore increasing the production of NO simultaneously reducing the output insulin. Therefore all these can be brought to a conclusion that reactive oxygen species. Reactive oxygen species can increase in oxidative stress can play critical role in diabetes development [31].

3. Antioxidant and their role IN diabetes

The substances that can delay or inhibit the oxidation of other molecules are termed as antioxidants. Recently therapy using antioxidants has gained more importance in the field of medicine and can be used in treatment of several diseases including diabetes [32]. Diabetes complications can be reduced to a greater extend with the help of antioxidants is studied in many experimental works. Antioxidants can be used as a drug substrate, combined drug in the treatment focused in their antioxidant activity are also utilized in the treatment of diabetes [33].

The function of beta cell can be secured by antioxidants by fighting against oxidative stress, which tries to defend the beta cells. Thus it can diminish diabetes related complications and helps in recovering of insuli9n sensitivity. Dietary antioxidant intake can also be considered as a tool in treatment of diabetes [34]. There are several antioxidants which are present naturally and whose intake can reduce the risk of this disease. Vitamin E, vitamin C, alpha lipoic acid, selenium fall under this category. The role played by these antioxidants at a prescribed quantity will aim at reducing the risk of diabetes [35].

4. Vitamin E

It is a lipophilic antioxidant that are found in tocopherol and tocotrienol form. Vitamin E is a naturally occurring antioxidant and can help in defending the cells against oxidative stress [36]. Many studies focused on the ability of vitamin E in reducing the risk of hyperglycemia and their effect in using it as a combined drug in therapy for diabetes [37]. Hepatic lipid peroxide level is decreased in streptozotocin induced diabetes by vitamin E is shown in many experimental model studies [38].

The increase in the level of lipid peroxide can be due to the change in status of antioxidant level. Administration of vitamin E can be significantly decreased when supplemented by vitamin E. During diabetes the antioxidant enzyme such as SOD, CAT and GPX decrease [39]. Therefore the oral administration of vitamin E (440 mg/kg of body weight) once in a week for one month has shown positive results in increasing the activity of antioxidant enzyme and decreasing hyper oxide level [40].

Glucose in high concentration will get attached to hemoglobin forming glycosylated hemoglobin, which is a important marker for diabetes can be prevented using vitamin E it can also reduce HbA1C level by oxidative stress inhibition [41]. The exact way by which the glucose level is reduced using antioxidants is not so clear but it reduces the plasma glucose while increasing the metabolic of glucose in peripheral tissues. Thus antioxidants can reduce the risk of several disease including diabetes and cancer. The antioxidant activity of vitamin E which helps in curing hyperglycemia can reduce the micro-vascular and macro-vascular complications in people affected with diabetes [42].

5. Vitamin C

It is a powerful antioxidant scavengering free radicals in aqueous compartment. In aqueous state, vitamin C is a chain breaking antioxidant. The stability of cell membrane can be increased by vitamin C [43]. On a statistical survey taken from the study done in diabetic research centre, Iran, a total of 84 patients was supplemented with 500 mg or 100 mg of ascorbic acid for 6 weeks among which the patients provided with 100 mg of vitamin C shown significant reduce in blood glucose and lipid level where as the ones treated with 500 mg did not show any significant response [44]. There studies carried out showed that when vitamin C was provided in a high dose it reduced the fasting glucose level, improved hBA1 and glycemia control [45].

The risk of type-2 diabetes is found to be reduced by continuous intake of vitamin C as a dietary source in a population based study. The correct or prescribed dose (as per weight of the body) of vitamin C and vitamin E can reduce the level of blood glucose [46]. However no further increase in SOD is found when treated with vitamin C. Some studies stated that decrease in plasma vitamin C and vitamin E during diabetes can be due to increased oxidative stress [47]. Vitamin C play major role in ameliorating insulin resistance of diabetic patients and can decrease or diminish the micro albuminuria, erythrocyte sorbitol level. All these are turned to be possible by vitamin C due to their antioxidant property [48].

6. Alpha lipoic acid

The injuries in cells which is caused by free radical triggering can be treated using alpha lipoic acid. It has the ability to restore other antioxidants such as vitamin C, vitamin E glutathione. Thus can be very useful in the effective treatment of disease related to liver, cardiovascular disease and diabetes [49].

Alpha lipoic acid is known for improving glucose metabolism in diabetes patients. This can be achieved by activating threonine, tyrosine lipid kinase in target cell which is responsible for stimulating glucose uptake. The translocation of GLUT1 and GLUT4 to plasmid membrane of adipocyte and skeletal muscle is done by alpha lipoic acid is stated in many invitro studies [50]. This can help in increasing the activity of protein in insulin signaling pathway intake of this antioxidant can reduce the glucose and cholesterol level. During diabetes it can regenerate other antioxidant including vitamin C, vitamin E and SOD. An increase of insulin stimulated glucose disposal is seen in diabetic patients when administrated with 500 mg ALA for about 10 days but no change is seen in fasting plasma glucose level. Insulin resistance can be accured by intake of this antioxidant. Plasma insulin sensitivity can be raised by the oral supplementation of ALA. ALA has the ability to scavenge the reactive oxygen species which are produced during peroxidation of lipid thus saving the cells from damage. Continuous supplementation of ALA helps in reducing hyperglycemia as well as diabetic complication including diabetic nephropathy [51].

7. Selenium

This is an antioxidant which is commonly seen in several food it exist in both organic and inorganic form, in which organic form include selenocysteine and selenomethionine and selenite and selenate falls under inorganic form. This antioxidant has major role in immune function. There are several clinical studies that proved the efficacy of selenium to treat several diseases and this power of selenium is due to its antioxidant activity [52]. Earlier selenium was considered as toxic as it caused poisoning in both human and animal but later studies proved that deficiency of the same can create numerous problems in both animal and humans. Glucose metabolism can be maintained using small concentration of selenium as it can mimic insulin action, but the exact mechanism of this mimicking is not understood, reports depicts that activation of protein which is responsible for insulin signaling cascade can be done by selenuium [53].

By activating kinases, sodium selenate and sodium selenite which are inorganic selenium are involved in insulin signaling cascade. Selenate can increase glucose uptake and are involved in insulin receptor phosporylation. Insulin like activity cab be shown by selenium is because of their glucose tolerance anf their ability to alter the gluconeogenic activity. There are studies which shows the combined treatment of selenium along with vitamin C, vitamin E and alpha lipoic acid which are studied to be useful in the management of diabetes. Therefore for the curing of diseases antioxidant based formation are commonly used now a days [54].

8. Resveratrol

It is known as polyphenolic phytoalexin that is developed in significant amounts in grapevines as a secondary metabolite in response to fungal infections and has been shown to lower the risk of cardiovascular disease. Resveratrol has been shown to have positive benefits on the onset and progression of atherosclerosis, including control of vasodilator and vasoconstrictor production, and inhibition of anti-platelet aggregation and low density lipo protein [55]. In addition, previous research has shown that resveratrol supplementation reduces plaque development in animal brains and other neurodegenerative diseases. Oral resveratrol significantly reduced brain plaque in the hypothalamus (−90%), striatum (−89%), and medial cortex (−48%) of mice [56].

Oral doses of resveratrol in humans are thought to minimize beta amyloid plaque, which is linked to aging changes in the brain. Researchers believe that resveratrol's ability to chelate Cu++ is one mechanism for plaque eradication. It appears to be a promising bioactive natural molecule with possible applications in phytotherapy or pharmacology, based on current knowledge [57]. Moreover, diabetic rats given resveratrol (5 mg kg1 b.w. d1) orally for 30 days had significantly lower blood glucose, blood urea, serum uric acid, serum creatinine, glycosylated hemoglobin, and reduced functions of pathophysiological enzymes including aspartate transaminase (AST), alkaline phosphatase (ALP) and alanine transaminase (ALT). The antihyperglycemic properties of resveratrol are also demonstrated by improvements in plasma insulin and hemoglobin levels. According to recent studies, resveratrol can be an important therapeutic agent used to treat diabetes [58].

9. Cyanidins

They are primarily found in red-blue colored fruits, tomatoes, rice, potatoes, beans, and red wines, implying that we consume substantial quantities of these compounds on a regular basis from plant-based diets [59]. This anthocyanin was isolated from black rice, which contains high levels of cyanidin 3-glucoside, and its protective effect on insulin sensitivity was tested in cultured adypocytic cells which were exposed to tumor necrosis factor alpha (TNF-α) [60].

Adipocyte dysfunction is closely linked to the development of obesity and insulin resistance. The control of kinase expression by adypocites cells is an essential target for obesity prevention and insulin sensitivity improvement [61]. The effects of cyanidin 3-glucoside on hydrogen peroxide or TNF-induced insulin resistance were found to be dose-dependent. The intracellular development of ROS and the activation of Jun N-terminal kinases were reduced when adipocytes cells were pretreated with cyanidin 3-glucoside [62].

By controlling the glucose transporter 4 (GLUT-4) and retinol binding protein 4 systems, cyanidin 3-glucoside increases insulin sensitivity. Since retinol binding protein 4 expression is reduced in diabetic mice, cyanidin 3-glucoside lowers blood glucose levels and increases insulin sensitivity. Eventually, cyanidin 3-glucoside has been shown to protect rat brains fed ochratoxin A in a recent study [63].

Adipocyte glucose uptake and GLUT4 membrane translocation were increased by cyanidin-3-glucoside and its key intestinal metabolite protocatechuic acid, according to a study conducted [64]. There were also huge rise in nuclear PPAR activity, as well as adiponectin and GLUT4 output.It's important to note that PPAR inhibition reversed the polyphenol-induced increases in adiponectin and GLUT4, implying that PPAR is directly involved in this phase. As a result of PPAR activation, cyanidin-3-glycoside and protocatechuic acid, its key intestinal metabolite, can exert insulin-like activities, indicating a causal relationship between this transcription factor and adiponectin and GLUT4 upregulation [65].

10. Antioxidant response against oxidative stress

Beta cell dysfunction which can be caused by oxidative stress which can lead to diabetic condition is mainly due to the poor or in efficient antioxidant defense mechanism. There should be a proper balance between oxidants and antioxidant which is required for survival of cells and thus a healthy life. The degree to which component of cells that persist in oxidative state define the redox states, whereby oxidative stress can be prevented by a reducing environment. Therefore such a reducing environment should be maintained and this can be done by antioxidant enzymes such as SOD and catalase that can be useful in removing reactive oxygen species which gives more strength to the statement that endogenous antioxidant enzymes can stand against the negative role played by reactive oxygen species. Main antioxidant enzyme that helps in minimizing the oxidative stress are SOD, catalase and GPX [66].

The antioxidant enzymes including SOD and catalase can reduce the susceptibility of pancreatic islet to oxidative stress. Catalase can protect against the expression of pro-inflammatory cytokines. Thus can also protect the pancreatic islet against hydrogen peroxide and streptozotocin and cytokine toxicity [67]. It is also noted that difference in level of mitochondrial enzyme and increment in production of beta cells can alter susceptibility to dysfunction and development of diabetes. Antioxidant such as vitamin C, alpha-lipoic acid can act as cofactor in metabolic mitochondrial energy and can reduce the level of reactive oxygen species and reactive nitrogen species in pancreatic islet cells [68].

Alpha lipoic acid can reduce oxidizing forms of antioxidant including vitamin E and vitamin C and can increase the levels of GSH by increasing cysteine uptake resulting positive therapeutic advantage in diabetes. It can also improve glucose disposal that helps in reducing body weight that will be beneficial for diabetic obese patients. Lipoic acid can reduce ubiquinone which is an important component of mitochondrial respiratory complex [69]. There are also several plants derived flavonoids that has a broad spectrum of bioactivity. They show biochemical and pharmacological characteristics which matches antioxidant properties. Some of these include quercetin ginseng, curcumin. The above mentioned flavonoid can limit the production of reactive oxygen species, regulation of cell signaling which is then can result in reducing oxidative stress and controlling diabetes [70].

Vegetables and fruits hold a very high nutritional value and there are several studies that talk about the foods that are rich in antioxidants. There are evidences that states that antioxidant rich fruits and vegetables intake can reduce the risk of type-2 diabetes. As these fruits and vegetables are rich in the antioxidant content they can contribute to the reduction of oxidative stress. Fruits and vegetables are good source of alphalinolenic acid nd omega 3 poly unsaturated fatty acid [71].

These are several medicinal plants which has been used for the treatment of type 2 diabetes for past years. There are more than 800 plants which shows antioxidant properties and thus have been using for the treatment of diabetes [72]. With the advancement in the technologies there has been a rapid increment in researching on anti-diabetic plants. Which came out with new herbs and their principles activity working in their anti-diabetic properties. There are plants by products that show anti-diabetic characteristics. Lignans, flavanoids, terpenoids are some among them [73].

11. Conclusion

Diabetes is a metabolic disorder which is caused due to impaired insulin secretion. When the beta cells are normal they respond to nutrients and insulin resistance by secretion of insulin in a higher mode which can balance the glucose intolerance. Type-2 diabetes is due to the deleterious effect of beta cells. There are many evidences which states that high level of glucose can lead to the generation of reactive oxygen species which can intern cause oxidative stress.

Therefore beta cells become worse with respect to insulin secretion. In addition to that the production of reactive oxygen species can lead to the activation of several signaling pathway. Thus low antioxidant defense can lead to oxidative stress and beta cell dysfunction. Antioxidant treatment can increase the defense capacity to fight against oxidative stress. Hydrogen peroxide molecules play roles in insulin secretion.

This paper focused on antioxidant as a therapy for the treatment of diabetes. As there is no clear evidence on how the antioxidant work on curing the disease, but all the possible mechanisms are discussed here. Evidences from the experiments shows that oxidative stress can lead to dysfunction of beta cells. Redox status change and depletion in antioxidant occur during this stress and lead to reactive oxygen species production.

Author details

Varuna Suresh, Amala Reddy*, Pavithra Muthukumar and Thendarl Selvam
Animal Cell Culture Laboratory, Department of Biotechnology, SRM Institute of Science and Technology, Chennai, Tamilnadu, India

*Address all correspondence to: amalar@srmist.edu.in

References

[1] Mellitus D. Diagnosis and classification of diabetes mellitus. Diabetes care. 2005 Jan 1;28 (S37):S5-10.

[2] Mellitus DI. Diagnosis and classification of diabetes mellitus. Diabetes care. 2006 Jan 1;29:S43.

[3] Bastaki A. Diabetes mellitus and its treatment. International journal of Diabetes and Metabolism. 2005 Jan 1;13(3):111.

[4] Nathan DM. Long-term complications of diabetes mellitus. New England Journal of Medicine. 1993 Jun 10;328(23):1676-85.

[5] Power AC. Diabetes mellitus. Harrison's principles of internal medicine, 16th ed. Mc Graw-Hill Medical pub. 2005:2152-80.

[6] Asmat U, Abad K, Ismail K. Diabetes mellitus and oxidative stress—A concise review. Saudi pharmaceutical journal. 2016 Sep 1;24(5):547-53

[7] Yang H, Jin X, Lam CW, Yan SK. Oxidative stress and diabetes mellitus. Clinical chemistry and laboratory medicine. 2011 Nov 1;49(11):1773-82.

[8] Maiese K, Chong ZZ, Shang YC. Mechanistic insights into diabetes mellitus and oxidative stress. Current medicinal chemistry. 2007 Jul 1;14(16):1729-38.

[9] CHANDRA K, SINGH P, DWIVEDI S, Jain SK. Diabetes Mellitus and Oxidative Stress: A Co-relative and Therapeutic Approach. Journal of Clinical & Diagnostic Research. 2019 May 1;13(5).

[10] Tabak O, Gelisgen R, Erman H, Erdenen F, Muderrisoglu C, Aral H, Uzun H. Oxidative lipid, protein, and DNA damage as oxidative stress markers in vascular complications of diabetes mellitus. Clinical and Investigative Medicine. 2011 Jun 1:E163-71.

[11] Fang YZ, Yang S, Wu G. Free radicals, antioxidants, and nutrition. Nutrition. 2002 Oct 1;18(10):872-9.

[12] Halliwell B, Aeschbach R, Löliger J, Aruoma OI. The characterization of antioxidants. Food and Chemical Toxicology. 1995 Jul 1;33(7):601-17

[13] Rahimi R, Nikfar S, Larijani B, Abdollahi M. A review on the role of antioxidants in the management of diabetes and its complications. Biomedicine & Pharmacotherapy. 2005 Aug 1;59(7):365-73.

[14] Johansen JS, Harris AK, Rychly DJ, Ergul A. Oxidative stress and the use of antioxidants in diabetes: linking basic science to clinical practice. Cardiovascular diabetology. 2005 Dec;4(1):1-1.

[15] Mooradian AD. Antioxidants and diabetes. Nutritional Management of Diabetes Mellitus and Dysmetabolic Syndrome. 2006;11:107-25.

[16] Golbidi S, Alireza Ebadi S, Laher I. Antioxidants in the treatment of diabetes. Current diabetes reviews. 2011 Mar 1;7(2):106-25.

[17] Scott JA, King GL. Oxidative stress and antioxidant treatment in diabetes. Annals of the New York Academy of Sciences. 2004 Dec;1031(1):204-13.

[18] A Haidara M, Z Yassin H, Zakula Z, P Mikhailidis D, R Isenovic E. Diabetes and antioxidants: myth or reality?. Current vascular pharmacology. 2010 Sep 1;8(5):661-72.

[19] Rosca MG, Mustata TG, Kinter MT, Ozdemir AM, Kern TS, Szweda LI, Brownlee M, Monnier VM, Weiss MF. Glycation of mitochondrial proteins

from diabetic rat kidney is associated with excess superoxide formation. American Journal of Physiology-Renal Physiology. 2005 Aug;289(2):F420-30.

[20] Hiramatsu K, Arimori S. Increased superoxide production by mononuclear cells of patients with hypertriglyceridemia and diabetes. Diabetes. 1988 Jun 1;37(6):832-7.

[21] Hotamisligil GS. Inflammatory pathways and insulin action. International Journal of Obesity. 2003 Dec;27(3):S53-5.

[22] Bierhaus A, Hofmann MA, Ziegler R, Nawroth PP. AGEs and their interaction with AGE-receptors in vascular disease and diabetes mellitus. I. The AGE concept. Cardiovascular research. 1998 Mar 1;37(3):586-600.

[23] Koya D, King GL. Protein kinase C activation and the development of diabetic complications. Diabetes. 1998 Jun 1;47(6):859-66.

[24] Peyroux J, Sternberg M. Advanced glycation endproducts (AGEs): pharmacological inhibition in diabetes. Pathologie Biologie. 2006 Sep 1;54(7):405-19.

[25] Bierhaus A, Hofmann MA, Ziegler R, Nawroth PP. AGEs and their interaction with AGE-receptors in vascular disease and diabetes mellitus. I. The AGE concept. Cardiovascular research. 1998 Mar 1;37(3):586-600.

[26] Talior I, Tennenbaum T, Kuroki T, Eldar-Finkelman H. PKC-δ-dependent activation of oxidative stress in adipocytes of obese and insulin-resistant mice: role for NADPH oxidase. American Journal of Physiology-Endocrinology and Metabolism. 2005 Feb;288(2):E405-11.

[27] Bergman RN, Ader M. Free fatty acids and pathogenesis of type 2 diabetes mellitus. Trends in Endocrinology & Metabolism. 2000 Nov 1;11(9):351-6.

[28] Kusminski CM, Shetty S, Orci L, Unger RH, Scherer PE. Diabetes and apoptosis: lipotoxicity. Apoptosis. 2009 Dec;14(12):1484-95.

[29] Evans JL, Goldfine ID, Maddux BA, Grodsky GM. Oxidative stress and stress-activated signaling pathways: a unifying hypothesis of type 2 diabetes. Endocrine reviews. 2002 Oct 1;23(5):599-622.

[30] Boden G, She P, Mozzoli M, Cheung P, Gumireddy K, Reddy P, Xiang X, Luo Z, Ruderman N. Free fatty acids produce insulin resistance and activate the proinflammatory nuclear factor-κB pathway in rat liver. Diabetes. 2005 Dec 1;54(12):3458-65.

[31] Boden G. Effects of free fatty acids (FFA) on glucose metabolism: significance for insulin resistance and type 2 diabetes. Experimental and clinical endocrinology & diabetes. 2003 Jun;111(03):121-4.

[32] Thakur P, Kumar A, Kumar A. Targeting oxidative stress through antioxidants in diabetes mellitus. Journal of drug targeting. 2018 Oct 21;26(9):766-76.

[33] Koya D, Hayashi K, Kitada M, Kashiwagi A, Kikkawa R, Haneda M. Effects of antioxidants in diabetes-induced oxidative stress in the glomeruli of diabetic rats. Journal of the American Society of Nephrology. 2003 Aug 1;14(suppl 3):S250-3.

[34] Marrazzo* G, Barbagallo* I, Galvano F, Malaguarnera M, Gazzolo D, Frigiola A, D'Orazio N, Li Volti G. Role of dietary and endogenous antioxidants in diabetes. Critical reviews in food science and nutrition. 2014 Dec 2;54(12):1599-616.

[35] Cao H, Xie Y, Chen X. Type 2 diabetes diminishes the benefits of

dietary antioxidants: Evidence from the different free radical scavenging potential. Food chemistry. 2015 Nov 1;186:106-12.

[36] Herrera E, Barbas C. Vitamin E: action, metabolism and perspectives. Journal of physiology and biochemistry. 2001 Mar;57(1):43-56.

[37] Brigelius-Flohé R, Traber MG. Vitamin E: function and metabolism. The FASEB Journal. 1999 Jul;13(10): 1145-55.

[38] Niki E, Traber MG. A history of vitamin E. Annals of Nutrition and Metabolism. 2012;61(3):207-12.

[39] Fardoun RZ. The use of vitamin E in type 2 diabetes mellitus. Clinical and Experimental Hypertension. 2007 Jan 1;29(3):135-48.

[40] Tuzcu M, Baydas G. Effect of melatonin and vitamin E on diabetes-induced learning and memory impairment in rats. European journal of pharmacology. 2006 May 10;537(1-3): 106-10.

[41] Upritchard JE, Sutherland WH, Mann JI. Effect of supplementation with tomato juice, vitamin E, and vitamin C on LDL oxidation and products of inflammatory activity in type 2 diabetes. Diabetes care. 2000 Jun 1;23(6):733-8.

[42] Lonn E, Yusuf S, Hoogwerf B, Pogue J, Yi Q, Zinman B, Bosch J, Dagenais G, Mann JF, Gerstein HC. Effects of vitamin E on cardiovascular and microvascular outcomes in high-risk patients with diabetes: results of the HOPE study and MICRO-HOPE substudy. Diabetes care. 2002 Nov 1;25(11):1919-27.

[43] Linster CL, Van Schaftingen E. Vitamin c. The FEBS journal. 2007 Jan 1;274(1):1-22.

[44] Will JC, Byers T. Does diabetes mellitus increase the requirement for vitamin C?. Nutrition reviews. 1996 Jul 1;54(7):193-202.

[45] Lee DH, Folsom AR, Harnack L, Halliwell B, Jacobs Jr DR. Does supplemental vitamin C increase cardiovascular disease risk in women with diabetes?. The American journal of clinical nutrition. 2004 Nov 1;80(5):1194-200.

[46] Som S, Basu S, Mukherjee D, Deb S, Choudhury PR, Mukherjee S, Chatterjee SN, Chatterjee IB. Ascorbic acid metabolism in diabetes mellitus. Metabolism. 1981 Jun 1;30(6):572-7.

[47] Gaede P, Poulsen HE, Parving HH, Pedersen O. Double-blind, randomised study of the effect of combined treatment with vitamin C and E on albuminuria in type 2 diabetic patients. Diabetic Medicine. 2001 Sep;18(9): 756-60.

[48] Young IS, Torney JJ, Trimble ER. The effect of ascorbate supplementation on oxidative stress in the streptozotocin diabetic rat. Free Radical Biology and Medicine. 1992 Jul 1;13(1):41-6.

[49] Packer L, Witt EH, Tritschler HJ. Alpha-lipoic acid as a biological antioxidant. Free radical biology and medicine. 1995 Aug 1;19(2):227-50.

[50] Budin SB, Othman F, Louis SR, Bakar MA, Radzi M, Osman K, Das S, Mohamed J. Effect of alpha lipoic acid on oxidative stress and vascular wall of diabetic rats. Rom J Morphol Embryol. 2009 Jan 1;50(1):23-30.

[51] Vallianou N, Evangelopoulos A, Koutalas P. Alpha-lipoic acid and diabetic neuropathy. The review of diabetic studies: RDS. 2009;6(4): 230.

[52] Dkhil MA, Zrieq R, Al-Quraishy S, Abdel Moneim AE. Selenium nanoparticles attenuate oxidative stress and testicular damage in

streptozotocin-induced diabetic rats. Molecules. 2016 Nov;21(11):1517.

[53] Reddi AS, Bollineni JS. Selenium-deficient diet induces renal oxidative stress and injury via TGF-β1 in normal and diabetic rats. Kidney international. 2001 Apr 1;59(4):1342-53.

[54] Asemi Z, Jamilian M, Mesdaghinia E, Esmaillzadeh A. Effects of selenium supplementation on glucose homeostasis, inflammation, and oxidative stress in gestational diabetes: Randomized, double-blind, placebo-controlled trial. Nutrition. 2015 Oct 1;31(10):1235-42.

[55] Truong VL, Jun M, Jeong WS. Role of resveratrol in regulation of cellular defense systems against oxidative stress. Biofactors. 2018 Jan;44(1):36-49.

[56] Tian X, Liu Y, Ren G, Yin L, Liang X, Geng T, Dang H, An R. Resveratrol limits diabetes-associated cognitive decline in rats by preventing oxidative stress and inflammation and modulating hippocampal structural synaptic plasticity. Brain research. 2016 Nov 1;1650:1-9.

[57] Zhang H, Zhang J, Ungvari Z, Zhang C. Resveratrol improves endothelial function: role of TNFα and vascular oxidative stress. Arteriosclerosis, thrombosis, and vascular biology. 2009 Aug 1;29(8):1164-71.

[58] Schmatz R, Perreira LB, Stefanello N, Mazzanti C, Spanevello R, Gutierres J, Bagatini M, Martins CC, Abdalla FH, da Silva Serres JD, Zanini D. Effects of resveratrol on biomarkers of oxidative stress and on the activity of delta aminolevulinic acid dehydratase in liver and kidney of streptozotocin-induced diabetic rats. Biochimie. 2012 Feb 1;94(2):374-83.

[59] Lee JS, Kim YR, Song IG, Ha SJ, Kim YE, Baek NI, Hong EK. Cyanidin-3-glucoside isolated from mulberry fruit protects pancreatic β-cells against oxidative stress-induced apoptosis. International Journal of Molecular Medicine. 2015 Feb 1;35(2):405-12.

[60] Suantawee T, Thilavech T, Cheng H, Adisakwattana S. Cyanidin Attenuates Methylglyoxal-Induced Oxidative Stress and Apoptosis in INS-1 Pancreatic β-Cells by Increasing Glyoxalase-1 Activity. Nutrients. 2020 May;12(5): 1319.

[61] Qi SS, He J, Yuan LP, Le Wu J, Zu YX, Zheng HX. Cyanidin-3-glucoside from black rice prevents renal dysfunction and renal fibrosis in streptozotocin-diabetic rats. Journal of Functional Foods. 2020 Sep 1;72: 104062.

[62] Rahman S, Mathew S, Nair P, Ramadan WS, Vazhappilly CG. Health benefits of cyanidin-3-glucoside as a potent modulator of Nrf2-mediated oxidative stress. Inflammo pharmacology. 2021 Mar 19:1-7.

[63] Speciale A, Canali R, Chirafisi J, Saija A, Virgili F, Cimino F. Cyanidin-3-O-glucoside protection against TNF-α-induced endothelial dysfunction: involvement of nuclear factor-κB signaling. Journal of agricultural and food chemistry. 2010 Nov 24;58(22):12048-54.

[64] Yu L, Zhang SD, Zhao XL, Ni HY, Song XR, Wang W, Yao LP, Zhao XH, Fu YJ. Cyanidin-3-glucoside protects liver from oxidative damage through AMPK/Nrf2 mediated signaling pathway in vivo and in vitro. Journal of Functional Foods. 2020 Oct 1;73:104148.

[65] Edirisinghe I, Burton-Freeman B. Anti-diabetic actions of Berry polyphenols–Review on proposed mechanisms of action. Journal of Berry Research. 2016 Jan 1;6(2):237-50.

[66] Pamplona R, Costantini D. Molecular and structural antioxidant defenses against oxidative stress in animals. American Journal of Physiology-Regulatory, Integrative and Comparative Physiology. 2011 Oct;301(4):R843-63.

[67] Djordjevic A, Spasic S, Jovanovic-Galovic A, Djordjevic R, Grubor-Lajsic G. Oxidative stress in diabetic pregnancy: SOD, CAT and GSH-Px activity and lipid peroxidation products. The Journal of Maternal-Fetal & Neonatal Medicine. 2004 Dec 1;16(6):367-72.

[68] Marangon K, Devaraj S, Tirosh O, Packer L, Jialal I. Comparison of the effect of α-lipoic acid and α-tocopherol supplementation on measures of oxidative stress. Free Radical Biology and Medicine. 1999 Nov 1;27(9-10):1114-21.

[69] Smith AR, Shenvi SV, Widlansky M, Suh JH, Hagen TM. Lipoic acid as a potential therapy for chronic diseases associated with oxidative stress. Current medicinal chemistry. 2004 May 1;11(9):1135-46.

[70] Goraca A, Piechota A, Huk-Kolega H. Effect of alpha--Lipoic acid on LPS-induced oxidative stress in the heart. Acta physiologica Polonica. 2009 Mar 1;60(1):61.

[71] Kaneto H, Kajimoto Y, Miyagawa JI, Matsuoka TA, Fujitani Y, Umayahara Y, Hanafusa T, Matsuzawa Y, Yamasaki Y, Hori M. Beneficial effects of antioxidants in diabetes: possible protection of pancreatic beta-cells against glucose toxicity. Diabetes. 1999 Dec 1;48(12):2398-406.

[72] Saleh NS, Allam TS, El-Rabeai RM, El-Sabbagh HS. Protective Effect of Some Egyptian Medicinal Plants Against Oxidative Stress in Rats. Alexandria Journal for Veterinary Sciences. 2018 Jul 1;58(1).

[73] Chandran R, Abrahamse H. Identifying plant-based natural medicine against oxidative stress and neurodegenerative disorders. Oxidative Medicine and Cellular Longevity. 2020 Sep 15;2020.

Chapter 2

Micronutrient Antioxidants in the Chemoprevention of Breast Cancer and Effect on Breast Cancer Outcomes

Donovan McGrowder, Fabian Miller, Chukwuemeka Nwokocha, Cameil Wilson-Clarke, Melisa Anderson, Lennox Anderson-Jackson and Lowen Williams

Abstract

Breast cancer remains one of the most frequent cancers affecting women globally. The incidence of breast cancer is rising due to improved screening and awareness, and there is epidemiological data signifying an interaction among environmental and biological risk factors in the development and progress of breast cancer. There is substantial experimental data of the protective effect of micronutrient antioxidants for breast cancer via alteration of many signaling pathways and molecular events including inducing apoptosis, and inhibition of breast cancer cell proliferation and invasion. The main focus of this review is to examine past and current epidemiological evidence that suggests that nutritional micronutrients with antioxidant properties in dietary or supplemental form may be beneficial in protecting women against breast cancer and affect outcomes.

Keywords: breast cancer, risk, antioxidants, micronutrients, mortality, recurrence, dietary, intake

1. Introduction: breast cancer

1.1 Etiology of breast cancer and role of oxidative stress

Breast cancer remains one of the most frequent cancers affecting women globally. In 2018, 2.1 million new cases were reported, accounting for approximately one in every four cases of cancer among women [1]. Breast cancer accounted for almost 15% of cancer-related deaths in women in 2018 [2]. It is more common in the developed world, with highest incidence in regions such as Europe and Northern America [1]. However, mortality rates are higher in developing regions such as Africa [1]. Breast cancer is linked to numerous risk factors including family history, gene mutations, obesity, hormonal therapy, and alcohol consumption [3] but a recognizable risk profile is not usually present in most women who develop the disease [4]. Even though curative therapy is promising following early detection, approximately 30% of cases diagnosed at early stages will progress to metastatic disease [5]. Furthermore, cases of disseminated disease are almost always untreatable and radical prophylactic mastectomy remains the only primary preventative measure [6]. These challenges have spawned a shift in the treatment paradigm of the disease, which has led to major treatment advancements and improved palliative care. However, drug resistance and adverse side effects are common nuisances of current therapy [7]. Therefore, new approaches to breast cancer management with treatments that have minimal harmful effects and can retard tumor progression are required.

To determine effective treatment approaches for breast cancer, it may be worthwhile to elucidate the complexity of the tumor microenvironment. It has been suggested that impaired mitochondrial metabolism may be a feature of tumor progression [8]. Additionally, it has been reported that a hallmark feature of mitochondrial dysfunction is the generation of reactive oxygen species (ROS) which may cause pro-tumorigenic outcomes such as DNA damage and genomic instability [8]. Reactive oxygen species include molecules such as superoxide anion, hydrogen peroxide, hydroxyl radical and singlet oxygen. They are involved in cell signaling through second messenger pathways in both cancer cells and their normal counterparts [9]. It was reported that various cancers are characterized by overproduction of ROS that can increase pro-tumorigenic signaling, cell survival and DNA aberrations [10]. Similarly, another study reported that elevated ROS levels is necessary to support and sustain metastasis [11].

Oxidative stress is widely considered to play a major role in the initiation and pathogenesis of breast cancer [12]. It refers to the imbalance between ROS production and clearance favoring decreased clearance and a pro-oxidant environment caused by either an overproduction of ROS or decreased antioxidant activity [13]. In breast cancer, a vast majority of stromal fibroblasts becomes activated following exposure to oxidative stress resulting in hydrogen peroxide production which triggers tumorigenic changes in breast epithelial cells [12]. A plethora of high energy nutrients and growth factors are also produced which fuels metastasis [12]. Congruently, it was reported that higher levels of oxidative stress biomarkers such as malondialdehyde and oxidized glutathione were found in breast cancer patients compared to control subjects [14]. The human body comprises an antioxidant defense system which exerts its function by generating antioxidants including the catalases, glutathione peroxidases and superoxide dismutase which offer protective effects by metabolizing and scavenging free radicals to inhibit and minimize tissue damage [15]. It is important to note that despite the presence of an endogenous antioxidant system, DNA damage ensues and accumulates throughout life and could considerably contribute to the initiation and progression of cancers [16]. Given the accumulation of evidence supporting the role of ROS in the pathogenesis of breast cancer, there is a possibility that dietary micronutrient antioxidants may be useful to counteract oxidative stress induced cancer. Moreover, it was reported that antioxidant supplement use among breast cancer patients was 45–80% [17].

This paper will review information in the literature on the relationship between dietary and supplement micronutrient antioxidants including vitamins C and E and their association with the risk of breast cancer as well as outcomes such as disease recurrence and mortality.

2. Method of article selection

A literature search was conducted for all English language literature published before December 2020. The search was conducted using the electronic databases, including PubMed, Embase, Web of Science, and Cochrane Library. The search strategy included keywords such as breast cancer, epidemiology, incidence, risk, recurrence, mortality, vitamin E, vitamin C, carotenoids, flavonoids and green tea. The authors include many interventional and observational studies that have reported findings of dietary and supplemental micronutrient antioxidants, breast cancer incidence, and progression. The majority of these studies focused on vitamins E and C, carotenoids, specifically beta- and alpha-carotene, lycopene as well as the flavonoids, flavonols and isoflavones.

3. Epidemiological evidence of vitamins as antioxidants

3.1 Vitamin C

3.1.1 Vitamin C and breast cancer risk

Vitamin C is a naturally occurring essential micronutrient that is soluble in water and its antioxidant properties involve neutralizing reactive oxygen species as well as other free radicals [18]. Investigational experiments and epidemiologic findings on vitamin C and breast cancer risk are still inconclusive and reviews of data have suggested both detrimental and protective effects on overall risk of breast cancer [19]. Prospective studies on vitamin C intake and breast cancer risk have yielded diverse findings [20–23]. A recent meta-analysis reported that dietary vitamin C but not supplements was associated with a lesser risk of breast cancer incidence (RR = 0.89; 95% CI: 0.82–0.96) [20]. In the European Prospective Investigation into Cancer and Nutrition Study of 7,502 primary invasive breast cancer cases with a median follow-up time of approximately 9 years, multivariate analyses showed that vitamin E and C were not related with breast cancer risk in postmenopausal and premenopausal women. However, high intake of vitamin C was associated with decreased breast cancer risk in postmenopausal women utilizing exogenous hormones [21]. Earlier, in the Netherlands Cohort Study comprising of 62,573 women with 650 incident breast cancer cases identified after a follow-up of 4.3 years, dietary Vitamin E and vitamin C supplement use did not influence breast cancer risk, but there a small reduction in risk with increasing dietary intake of vitamin C particularly at the highest quintile [22]. Correspondingly, findings from the Women's Health Initiative Observational Study which followed 84,805 women for approximately 8 years with 2,879 incident invasive cancer cases ascertained, showed a weak positive association of breast cancer risk with total and supplemental vitamin C particularly among postmenopausal women (**Table 1**) [23].

Other prospective studies showed increased breast cancer risk with dietary or supplemental vitamin C. Using a large cohort of 2,482 invasive breast cancer cases in 57,403 postmenopausal Women, Cadeau et al. examine the association between vitamin C supplement use and breast cancer risk while bearing in mind dietary vitamin C intake, and found no relation with the overall risk, but females in the fourth quartile of vitamin C intake from foods had a 32% increase in breast cancer risk [24]. Published in 2011, a meta-analysis of 51 studies comparing highest with the lowest vitamin C intake from supplements may be associated with higher breast cancer risk [25], but it was noted that the overall result was influenced by a single large study [23]. In this same meta-analysis, dietary and total vitamin E, and dietary vitamin A significantly decreased breast cancer risk for cohort studies, but the results became nonsignificant when case–controlled studies were pooled [25]. Notably, Sharhar et al. examined relations between oxidative stress and antioxidant status in 57 newly diagnosed breast cancer cases and found poor antioxidant status

Vitamin/ Micro-nutrient (antioxidant)	Reference	Study design	Population (Case, participants)	Exposure	Risk estimates (95% CI)	Outcome
Vitamin C and E	29	Case–control	297 breast cancer cases and 311 controls	Dietary vitamin C	Vitamin C: OR = 0.53 (0.33–0.86) Vitamin E: OR = 0.55 (0.34–0.88)	Reduction by 47% (mainly in premenopausal women) Reduction by 45%
Lycopene	150	Case–control	46 breast cancer cases and 63 controls	Lycopene in adipose tissue	OR = 0.32 (0.11–0.94)	Reduction by 68%
Vitamin E	29	Case–control	297 breast cancer cases and 311 controls	Dietary vitamin E	OR = 0.55 (0.34–0.88)	Reduction by 45%
Vitamin E	53	Population-based case–control	2,362 breast cancer cases and 2,462 controls	Vitamin E (supplement)	OR = 0.75 (0.58–0.97)	Reduction by 25%
Alpha-carotene and beta-carotene	90	Population-based case–control	5,707 women with incident invasive breast cancer	Alpha-carotene and beta-carotene (supplement)	Alpha-carotene OR = 0.82 (0.68–0.98; P_{trend} = 0.07) Beta-carotene OR = 0.81 (0.68–0.98; Ptrend = 0.009)	Reduction by 18% for premenopausal women Reduction by 19% for premenopausal women
Alpha-carotene and beta-carotene	23	Women's Health Initiative Observational Study	84,805 women followed for average 7.6 yrs.	Alpha-carotene and beta-carotene (supplement)	Alpha-carotene RR = 0.83 (0.70–0.99, P_{trend} = 0.019). Beta-carotene RR = 0.78 (0.66–0.94, P_{trend} = 0.021)	Reduction by 17% (highest vs. lowest quintile) Reduction by 22% (highest vs. lowest quintile)

Vitamin/ Micro-nutrient (antioxidant)	Reference	Study design	Population (Case, participants)	Exposure	Risk estimates (95% CI)	Outcome
Total flavonoids and flavonols	110	Case–control	1522 breast cancer cases and 1547 controls	Dietary total flavonoids and flavonols	Total flavonoids: OR = 0.66 (0.54–0.82) Flavonols: OR = 0.51 (0.41–0.63)	Reduction by 34% Reduction by 49%
Flavones and flavonols	112	Case–control	1,434 breast cancer cases and 1,440 controls	Dietary flavones and flavonols	Flavones: OR = 0.61, (0.45–0.83) Flavonols: OR = 0.54 (0.40–0.73)	Reduction by 39% Reduction by 46%
Soy isoflavones	129	The Shanghai Breast Cancer Survival Study (prospective)	4,139 stage 0 –III breast cancer patients and 1987 pre–/ perimenopausal and 2152 postmenopausal patients	Dietary soy isoflavones	HR = 0.22, (0.09–0.53)	Reduction by 78% in premenopausal women (high intake)
Lycopene and beta-carotene	93	Case–control	122 breast cancer cases and 632 healthy controls	Dietary lycopene and beta-carotene	Lycopene: Adjusted OR = 0.26, (0.14–0.46) Beta-carotene: Adjusted OR = 0.43 (0.23–0.82)	Reduction by 74% Reduction by 57%

Table 1.
Summary of selected studies that provide risk estimates of the associations between dietary and supplemental vitamins and micronutrients (antioxidants) and breast cancer risk.

as indicated by low plasma vitamin C which elevated by two to three times the breast cancer risk [26].

The findings of reduced breast cancer incidence with vitamin C consumption was more evident in case–control studies. In Nurses' Health Study involving a large cohort of 83,234 women where 2,697 incident cases of invasive breast cancer was identified after 14 years, the associations between vitamins A, C and E, fruit and vegetables, and specific carotenoids and breast cancer risk were examined. There was a weakly inverse association between dietary vitamin A and breast cancer risk in premenopausal women and strong inverse association with increasing quartiles of dietary vitamin C, alpha-carotene and beta-carotene among premenopausal women who had a positive family history of breast cancer [27]. Likewise, a case–control study conducted in Korea comprising 224 incident breast cancer cases and 250 matched controls establish that vitamin C and beta-carotene intake were associated with decreased breast cancer risk, thus possibly lowered incidence in Korean women [28]. Moreover, in an earlier case–control study of 297 breast cancer cases matched with 311 control subjects, there was a significant reduction in breast cancer risk with beta-carotene, alpha-tocopherol and vitamin C when the lowest quartile was used as reference and odds ratios adjusted for the highest quartile [29] (**Table 1**). Conversely, no evidence of association between dietary or total vitamin C intake and breast cancer risk in the UK Dietary Cohort Consortium pooled analysis involving a nested case–control study [30], nor between dietary and supplement vitamin C intake and breast cancer risk in a large prospective study of 89,494 women during eight years of follow-up [31].

3.1.2 Vitamin C and survival outcomes

Cancer chemoprevention in vitro studies have demonstrated that vitamin C in pharmacological concentrations is cytotoxic to numerous type of cancer cells including ovarian and pancreatic while not affecting normal cells [32].

Globally, there is increasing use of vitamins among cancer patients and in the UK Women's Cohort Study comprising 12,453 females, there was self-reported frequently high dose vitamin C supplement intake use among breast cancer patients [33]. Furthermore, a number of epidemiologic studies have investigated the association between dietary vitamin C, vitamin C supplements and survival outcomes subsequent to breast cancer diagnosis. In a meta-analysis of prospective studies, post-diagnosis vitamin C supplement use was associated with decreased risk for breast cancer-specific (RR = 0.85, 95%CI: 0.74–0.99) and total mortality (RR = 0.81, 95%CI: 0.72–0.91) while dietary intake was also statistically significant for these two survival outcomes [34]. It was noted that in the Swedish Mammography Cohort Study comprising of 3,405 females with invasive breast cancer there was a marginal significant association between dietary vitamin C intake and all-cause mortality, but no association between supplement use subsequent to diagnosis and breast cancer-specific mortality [35].

Nevertheless, the findings are not consistent with intake of dietary vitamin C stated to decrease mortality risk in some studies [36, 37], while no relation in other epidemiologic studies [38–40]. There are also other prospective studies, which have investigated the relationship between vitamin C supplement use and breast cancer survival [17, 41, 42], and recently there is a published meta-analysis of observational studies [20]. In this meta-analysis, pooled results from 69 studies, the hazard risk for all-cause mortality was 0.82 (95% CI: 0.74–0.91), breast cancer recurrence 0.81 (95% CI: 0.67–0.99) and breast cancer-specific mortality 0.78 (95% CI: 0.69–0.88) [20].

3.1.3 Vitamin C use during chemotherapy and radiation therapy

There are apprehensions that supplement use, mainly antioxidants might decrease the cytotoxicity of chemotherapy and make it less operative [43]. Dietary antioxidant supplementation with radiation treatment and conventional chemotherapy have yielded conflicting results and many randomized clinical trials have reported deceased therapy-related side effects [44, 45]. There is data that attest to the protective effect of tumor cells as well as healthy cells by antioxidants since they neutralize reactive oxygen species and other free radical generated by some forms of chemotherapy and radiotherapy, thus reducing efficacy and ultimately survival [46, 47]. In the Breast Cancer Enrolled in a Cooperative Group Clinical Trial (SWOG S0221), Ambrosone et al. assessed associations between dietary antioxidant supplement (vitamins C, E and A as well as coenzyme Q and carotenoids) before and during chemotherapy (doxorubicin, paclitaxel and cyclophosphamide) treatment and survival outcomes. The use of any of the dietary supplements such as vitamin C resulted in a 41% higher hazard of recurrence of marginal significance, with a comparative but lesser association with mortality [48]. The authors suggested that patients should exercise caution when contemplating the use of supplement vitamin C during chemotherapy [48].

Conversely, epidemiologic studies have demonstrated improved usefulness of numerous cancer therapeutic agents with less adverse side effects when administered concomitantly with antioxidants [49]. Interesting, in a recent study it was found that vitamin C increased the therapeutic window of bromodomain and extra-terminal inhibitors thereby improving their efficacy for treating patients with aggressive triple negative breast cancer [50].

3.2 Vitamin E

3.2.1 Vitamin E and breast cancer risk

The role of dietary and vitamin E supplements in preventing breast cancer still remains unclear [51]. Previous research have demonstrated that there is a lack of any consistent association between vitamin E and the risk of breast cancer [52]. In a large population-based case–control study conducted in Canada that examined antioxidants intakes from diet and supplements and their potential breast cancer risk, 10 years or more supplementation with vitamin E was associated with reduced breast cancer risk (OR = 0.75, 95% CI: 0.58–0.97). However, no significant effect of dietary vitamin E intake or from supplementation less than 10 years was observed [53] (**Table 1**). Likewise, Fulan et al. conducted a meta-analysis of 51 studies on vitamin E intake and found that dietary vitamin E significantly decreased breast cancer risk, but there was no significant dose–response relationship in the higher intake of vitamin E [25]. An earlier case–control study comprising 297 breast cancer cases and 311 control subjects conducted in the United States found a significant reduction in breast cancer risk associated with high intake of dietary vitamin E (OR = 0.55; 95% CI: 0.34–0.88). However, no association was observed between vitamin E supplement intake and breast cancer risk [29]. Notably, findings from the Shanghai Breast Cancer Study suggests that vitamin E supplements may confer safeguard against breast cancer (OR = 0.80; 95%CI, 0.60–1.00) among Chinese women who had low dietary intake [54]. In addition, there were other studies that corroborated these finding including an inverse association of dietary vitamin E with breast cancer risk in a hospital-based case–control study of Chinese women [55] and vitamin E significantly decreased breast cancer risk in a case–control study comprising Greek women [56].

However, there are a number of prospective and case–control studies that reported no association between dietary and/or supplement vitamin E intake and breast cancer risk [22, 31, 57]. Verhoeven et al. reported findings from the Netherlands Cohort Study, a large prospective cohort research that examined the relationships between various vitamins, vegetables and fruits with breast cancer risk and found no strong evidence of dietary vitamin E intake in the etiology of breast cancer [22]. An earlier large prospective study found that large intake of dietary vitamin E did not protect from breast cancer (OR = 0.99, 95%CI: 0.83–1.19) [31]. Results from other studies on dietary or supplemental vitamin E intake demonstrated similar null association [58, 59]. These include: a case–control by Wang et al. that did not find any meaningful association of dietary vitamin E intake with breast cancer risk [60], no association of higher dietary intake of vitamin E (in early adult life) among postmenopausal women in the Nurses' Health Study II [57], and meta-analysis of 26 studies that found no effect of vitamin E supplementation on breast cancer risk on reviewing data from five cohort and four case–control studies [61].

3.2.2 Vitamin E use during chemotherapy and radiation therapy

Over the last decade the use of antioxidant supplements after breast cancer diagnosis and during treatment significantly increased and has become quite common among survivors [53, 61]. In a review of the literature on non-herbal nutrition supplements use in relieving symptoms induced by chemotherapy or radiation treatment, Samuels et al. showed that a number of studies suggest that antioxidant supplements use comprising glutamine, vitamin E and acetyl-L-carnithine possibly might decrease the occurrence and severity of paclitaxel-induced neuropathy [62]. In a comprehensive review of the 22 prospective studies by Greenlee et al. in 2009 that examined the association between use of antioxidant supplements (vitamin E as well as multivitamins, vitamin C, antioxidant combinations, soy isoflavones, melatonin, glutathione, or glutamine) and patient outcomes, there were no single antioxidant supplement during conventional breast cancer therapy that had a significant effect on recurrence, tumor response, toxicities, or survival. The authors indicated that findings from limited studies proposed that vitamin E decrease the hot flashes in patients treated with hormonal therapy and glutamine for oral mucositis [17]. In a more recent study, Huang et al. assessed the associations of dietary intake of fish, fruit and vegetable supplemented with vitamins E and B, and post-therapy cognitive recovery in 1,047 patients with breast cancer enrolled in the Shanghai Breast Cancer Survival Study. Higher dietary intake and supplement use were associated with greater cognitive scores at 36 months post-diagnosis thus improvement in post-therapy mental recovery [63].

3.2.3 Vitamin E and survival outcomes

Globally, the consumption of dietary supplements including vitamins and multivitamins/multi-minerals is increasing more so among females than males [64, 65]. However, there are only few studies that have examined vitamin E supplementation and survival outcomes in breast cancer patients. A well-designed prospective population-based prospective cohort study comprised of 4,877 females diagnosed with invasive breast cancer in China reported that vitamin E as well as multivitamin use were beneficial in improving survival and mortality rates. There was a 22% decreased recurrence risk and 18% lower mortality risk in females who use vitamin E supplement within 6 months after breast cancer diagnosis [42] (**Table 2**). Likewise, in the Life After Cancer Epidemiology (LACE) Study comprising of 2,264 females with early-stage breast cancer, 81% use antioxidants post-diagnosis. The regular use of vitamin E was concomitant with reduced risk of disease recurrence (HR = 0.71, 95%CI: 0.54–0.94) and diminished risk for all-cause mortality (HR = 0.76, 95%CI: 0.58–1.00) [41] (**Table 2**). Similarly, data from the After Breast Cancer Pooling Project showed that vitamin E was associated with reduced risk of breast cancer recurrence (RR = 0.88; 95%CI 0.79–0.99) [66]. The findings of a case–control study comprising 385 post-menopausal breast cancer patients performed in the United States corroborated previous reports as the use of antioxidant supplement (vitamins E or C, selenium or β-carotene) was associated with decreased breast cancer-specific death [37]. While these results suggest that antioxidants supplement use may have a protective effect and improve breast cancer survival, there were concerns of recall bias and the legitimacy of the exposure assessment. Furthermore, a recent systematic review and meta-analysis comprising randomized clinical trials and observational studies showed that vitamin E significantly reduced total mortality (RR = 0.76, 95% CI: 0.64–0.90) and breast cancer recurrence (RR = 0.69, 95% CI: 0.55–0.85) [67] (**Table 3**).

3.3 Multivitamins

3.3.1 Multivitamins use during chemotherapy and radiation therapy

Despite over thirty years of research examining dietary antioxidant supplement use during radiation therapy and conservative chemotherapy, there are significant disagreements regarding the effectiveness of this complementary therapy [68, 69]. Encouraging results from many randomized control trials confirmed that the concomitant administration of supplementation antioxidants with radiation therapy and chemotherapy decreases side effects related to treatment [70]. However, some studies have suggested that antioxidant supplementation may guard malignant tumor cells from the pro-oxidant effects such as oxidative injury produced by chemotherapeutic agents and radiation treatment [71, 72].

The quality of life and performance of normal daily activities can be negatively impacted by chemotherapy-induced peripheral neuropathy [73]. Using data from the Diet, Exercise, Lifestyle, and Cancer Prognosis (DELCaP) study, Zirpoli et al. reported that the use of multivitamins prior to diagnosis was associated with decreased symptoms of chemotherapy-induced peripheral neuropathy while use during therapy was slightly related with this outcome [74]. However, in a recent study, Jung et al. reported findings from the population-based Mamma Carcinoma Risk Factor Investigation (MARIE) study and noted that pre and post-diagnosis supplement use among of 2,223 postmenopausal women diagnosed with non-metastatic breast cancer was 36% and 45% respectively. The use of antioxidants throughout radiation therapy and chemotherapy was associated with higher total mortality risk (HR = 1.64; 95% CI: 1.01–2.66) and exacerbated recurrence-free survival (HR = 1.84; 95% CI: 1.26–2.68) [75]. The was also no relations between post-diagnosis use of supplement and disease prognosis, and the authors suggests that breast cancer patients should not use antioxidants during radiation therapy and chemotherapy [75].

3.3.2 Multivitamins and survival outcomes

The natural activity of dietary and supplement antioxidants is due to a number of factors comprising the existing level of oxidative stress, collaborations of antioxidants, and the level of antioxidants present in cells [45]. The consumption of vitamin supplements among breast cancer patients post-diagnosis is quite common [76]. There are prospective studies that have demonstrated that multivitamin

Vitamin/ Micro-nutrient (antioxidant)	Reference	Study design	Population (Case, participants)	Exposure	Risk estimates (95% CI)	Outcome
Vitamin E, C and multivitamins	42	Population-based prospective cohort	4,877 women diagnosed with breast cancer (aged 20–75 yrs)	Vitamin E, C and multivitamins	HR = 0.82 (0.65–1.02) for mortality HR = 0.78 (0.63–0.95) for risk of breast recurrence	Reduction by 18% and 22% respectively
Vitamin E and C	41	Life After Cancer Epidemiology (LACE) cohort	2,264 women with early stage breast cancer	Vitamin E and C (supplement)	(i) Vitamin E: HR = 0.71 (0.54–0.94) for breast cancer recurrence and HR = 0.76 (0.58–1.00) for all-cause mortality Vitamin C: HR = 0.73 (0.55–0.97) for risk of breast cancer recurrence	Reduction by 29% and 24% respectively Reduction by 27%
Vitamin C and E	66	After Breast Cancer Pooling Project	Four cohorts of 12,019 breast cancer survivors	Vitamin C and E (supplement)	Vitamin C: RR = 0.81 (0.55–0.97) for all-cause mortality Vitamin E: RR = 0.88 (0.79–0.99) for risk of breast cancer recurrence	Reduction by 19% Reduction by 12%
Soy isoflavones or soy protein	143	The Shanghai Breast Cancer Survival Study (a large, population-based cohort	5,042 female breast cancer survivors	Soy isoflavones or soy protein intake	HR = 0.68 (0.64–0.87) for risk of breast cancer recurrence (HR = 0.71 (0.54–0.92) for all-cause mortality (ER+ or ER- women)	Reduction by 32% Reduction by 29%
Soy isoflavonones	144	Prospective	256 Chines women		Soy isoflavones: OR = 0.25 (0.09–0.54) for breast cancer mortality	Reduction by 75%

Table 2.
Summary of selected studies that provide risk estimates of the associations between dietary and supplemental vitamins and micronutrients (antioxidants) and breast cancer outcomes such as recurrence and mortality.

Vitamin/ Micro-nutrient (antioxidant)	Reference	Study design	Population (Case, participants)	Exposure	Risk estimates (95% CI)	Outcome
Vitamin C	20	Meta-analysis	69 studies relevant to breast cancer risk (54 studies) and survival (15 studies)	Dietary vitamin C	RR = 0.78 (0.69–0.88) for breast cancer-specific mortality; RR = 0.81 (0.67–0.99) for risk of breast cancer recurrence	Reduction by 22% and 19% respectively
Vitamin C	34	Meta-analysis	10 studies	Supplement vitamin C	RR = 0.81 (0.72–0.91) for total mortality & RR = 0.85 (0.74–0.99) for risk of breast cancer-specific mortality	Reduction by 19% and 15% respectively
Vitamin C and E	67	Meta-analysis	Observational studies and randomized clinical trials	Vitamin C and E (supplement)	Vitamin C: RR = 0.79 (0.68–0.92) for total mortality and RR = 0.76 (0.64–0.91) for risk of breast cancer recurrence Vitamin E: RR = 0.76 (0.64–0.90) for total mortality and RR = 0.69 (0.55–0.85) for risk of breast cancer recurrence	Reduction by 21% and 24% respectively Reduction by 24% and 31% respectively
Alpha carotene and beta-carotene	91	Meta-analysis	33 observational studies	Dietary alpha carotene and beta-carotene	Alpha-carotene: RR_{pooled} = 0.91 (0.85–0.8, P = 0.01) for breast cancer risk Beta-carotene RR_{pooled} = 0.94 (0.88–1.00, P = 0.05)for breast cancer risk	Reduction by 9% Reduction by 6%
Soy isoflavones	135	Meta-analysis	35	Soy flavones intake	Premenopausal: OR = 0.59 (0.48–0.69) for breast cancer risk Postmenopausal women: OR = 0.59, (0.44–0.74) for breast cancer risk particularly in Asian women	Reduction by 41% Reduction by 41%
Soy isoflavones	146	Meta-analysis	18 studies	Soy isoflavones intake	RR = 0.89 (0.79–0.99) for risk of breast cancer incidence RR = 0.84 (0.70–0. 99) for risk of breast cancer recurrence	Reduction by 11% Reduction by 16%

Vitamin/ Micro-nutrient (antioxidant)	Reference	Study design	Population (Case, participants)	Exposure	Risk estimates (95% CI)	Outcome
Lutein/zeaxanthin	151	Meta-analysis	8 cohort studies	Lutein/zeaxanthin	RR = 0.84 (0.70–1.01, P_{trend} = 0.05)	Reduction by 16%
Quercetin	116	Meta-analysis	12 studies (6 prospective cohort and 6 case controls)	Quercetin intake	RR = 0.88 (0.80–0.98)	Reduction by 12%

Table 3.
Summary of selected meta-analysis and systematic reviews that provide risk estimates of the associations between dietary and supplemental vitamins and micronutrients (antioxidants) and breast cancer risk.

consumption improve survival rates in breast cancer patients [66, 77]. In the After Breast Cancer Pooling Project, Poole et al. examined the associations between post-diagnosis supplement use (multivitamins, vitamin E, D, C and B) and survival outcomes such as breast cancer-specific mortality, total disease mortality and risk of breast cancer recurrence in four cohorts of 12,019 patients in China and the United States. Using multivariate models, antioxidant supplement use (multivitamins, vitamin E or, C) was associated with improved survival as there was a 16% reduced risk of total mortality but not related with disease recurrence [66]. The findings of the Life After Cancer Epidemiology study that comprised of 2,236 women diagnosed with early-stage breast cancer indicate that multivitamin use may be valuable in improving breast cancer outcomes as frequent use prior to and after diagnosis was associated with non-significant reduced death from any cause and disease recurrence. In addition, the protective effect was for only breast cancer survivors treated by both radiation and chemotherapy, and radiation only and those who ate more fruits and vegetable and engaged in physical exercise had improved overall survival [77]. Notably, a recent systematic review and meta-analysis comprising randomized clinical trials and observational studies reported that multivitamin use lower breast cancer recurrence, and these findings were mostly based on observational studies while more randomized clinical trials are required to justify any recommendation for the dietary supplement use [67].

Conversely, in a large retrospective cohort study of breast cancer patients belonging to the British Columbia Cancer Agency followed for 68 months, an administered regimen mega-dose vitamin/mineral supplements non-significantly increase the hazard ratios for disease-free survival and breast cancer-specific mortality. However, limitations include absence of critical information on use of over-the-counter vitamins, treatment compliance and possible selection bias [78]. Moreover, in a multicenter study of 3,081 early-stage breast cancer patients, although dietary supplement users had acceptable intakes of micronutrients, vitamin use and mineral intake was not concomitant with all-cause mortality.

4. Epidemiological evidence of carotenoids as antioxidants

4.1 Fruit, vegetables and breast cancer risk

Epidemiologic studies have suggested that increased fruit and vegetable intake is associated with lower risk of breast cancer [79]. Supporting evidence is provided by findings from a pooled analysis of eight prospective cohort studies where total fruit and vegetable intake was associated with decreased breast cancer risk (RR = 0.93, 95% CI: 0.86–1.00; P_{trend} = 0.12) when comparing the highest with the lowest quartiles [80]. Recent systemic review and meta-analysis indicated that high intakes of vegetables and fruits were associated with lower risks of breast cancer [81, 82], while a large-scale study demonstrated that the same may be related with improved overall survival among primary breast cancer patients [83]. However, a large prospective study such as the European Prospective Investigation into Cancer and Nutrition did not find a relationship between fruit and vegetable intake, and breast cancer risk [84].

4.2 Carotenoids

4.2.1 Alpha-carotene, beta-carotene intake and breast cancer risk

Carotenoids such as alpha-carotene, beta-carotene, lycopene and beta-cryptoxanthin are found in fruits and in dark green leafy vegetables as well as in yellow and orange vegetables [85]. The chemo-prevention and protective potential of carotenoids lies in their antioxidant, retinoic and anti-proliferative activities and obstructing estrogen signaling of 17β-estradiol, with subsequent weakening of the properties of malignancies such as breast cancer that are hormone-dependent [86]. There are a number of studies that have examined the relation of breast cancer risk with dietary and/or supplemental consumption of carotenoids [87–89]. In a large population-based case–control study consisting of 5,707 women with incident invasive breast cancer (3,516 postmenopausal women and 2,363 premenopausal women), there were inverse associations observed among premenopausal women for high levels of alpha-carotene (OR = 0.82, 95% CI: 0.68–0.98) and beta-carotene (OR = 0.81, 95% CI: 0.68–0.98) but not for postmenopausal women [90] (**Table 1**). Likewise, in the Women's Health Initiative Observational Study, high dietary beta-carotene intake (RR = 0.78; 95% CI: 0.66–0.94; P_{trend} = 0.021) and elevated alpha-carotene (RR = 0.83; 95% CI: = 0.70–0.99; P_{trend} = 0.019) were inversely related to risk of estrogen receptor (ER)-positive and progesterone receptor (PR)-positive breast cancer. However, supplemental or total beta-carotene were not related to breast cancers demarcated by PR and ER status [23]. In an earlier population-based case–control study conducted in Canada, Nkondjock et al. found decreased risk for beta-carotene for those who never used hormone replacement therapy [89] but increased breast cancer risk associated with significantly high serum levels of alpha-carotene (OR = 2.40; 95% CI: 0.90–6.41) in premenopausal women.

These findings were corroborated by a review study that systematically summarized the associations between beta-carotene and alpha-carotene, and breast cancer risk. In the meta-analysis that comprehensively review the associations between carotenoids and breast cancer, higher intakes of dietary beta-carotene significantly decreased breast cancer risk by 6.0% (RR_{pooled} = 0.94; 95% CI: 0.88–1.00) and dietary alpha-carotene lower the risk by 9.0% when the cohort studies were pooled. Furthermore, significant dose–response associations were seen in both the higher intake of dietary and total beta-carotene with decreased breast cancer risk when considering cohort studies and case–control studies [91] (**Table 3**). There are other observational studies that have confirmed an inverse relationship of dietary or supplemental alpha-carotene or beta-carotene with risk of breast cancer [27, 87, 92, 93].

However, there are few studies that have reported null association between the carotenoids and breast cancer risk [84, 88, 94]. Terry et al. found no clear association between alpha-carotene and beta-carotene, and breast cancer risk in a large cohort of women who were registered in the Canadian National Breast Screening Study [88]. In subsequently large prospective study of women enrolled in the European Prospective Investigation Into Cancer and Nutrition there was no association of dietary beta-carotene with breast cancer risk, although beta-carotene supplement demonstrated a protective effect against lobular breast cancer (IRR = 0.72; 95%CI: 0.57–0.91] [84]. This study also found no association between overall breast cancer and any micronutrients, while some effects were shown when stratifying by breast cancer subtypes [84]. Finally, there is another study that have reported null association between the carotenoids and breast cancer risk [95].

4.2.2 Serum and plasma levels of carotenoids (alpha-carotene, beta-carotene) and breast cancer risk

Blood vitamin intakes are regarded as biomarkers of the consumption of vegetables and fruits [96]. Plasma or serum levels of antioxidants such as vitamin E are thought to be related to breast cancer risk but results from prospective and case control studies remain inconclusive [97]. In a nested case–control study comprising

1,502 incident breast cancer cases and 1,502 controls within the European Prospective Investigation into Cancer and Nutrition cohort, plasma vitamin E level was not statistically associated with ER negative or ER positive breast cancer [98]. Epplein et al. earlier published a nested case–control study, a sub-cohort of the Multiethnic Cohort Study which demonstrated that multiethnic women with breast cancer were more likely to have lower levels of vitamin E than matched controls [99]. Notably, a meta-analysis of 40 studies by Hu et al. summarize the associations between plasma levels of vitamins A, C and E, and breast cancer risk and observed significant relationship between plasma vitamin E levels and breast cancer incidence (OR_{pooled} = 0.42, 95% CI: 0.25–0.72, p = 0.001). The authors suggested that severe vitamin E could increase breast cancer risk [100]. Furthermore, even though there was an association between serum vitamin E [biomarker of fruit and vegetable intake, (OR = 0.68, 95% CI: 0.41–1.10)] in the E3N-EPIC Study, it was not statistically significant (P_{trend} = 0.26) [101].

However, there are findings from studies that do not support plasma or serum levels of vitamin E being associated with reduced risk of breast cancer [54, 102]. In a nested case–control comprising of 365 incident breast cancer cases and 726 individually matched control women within the prospective population-based Shanghai Women's Health Study, there was no association between plasma levels of vitamin E and reduced breast cancer risk, although the authors noted that there may be protective effects among sub-groups of women [54]. Likewise, in an earlier case–control study nested in a prospective cohort from the Breast Cancer Serum Bank in Missouri, United States no evidence of the protective effect of vitamin E was observed for breast cancer, although carotenoids such as lycopene and beta-cryptoxanthin may protect against breast cancer [103]. There are other studies that have reported null findings in the relationship between serum or plasma levels of vitamin E and breast cancer risk [102, 104]. These include: no association between plasma vitamin E levels and breast cancer risk in the Nurses' Health Study [105] and no significant association of plasma vitamin E levels in a nested case-referent study conducted in Sweden [106].

5. Epidemiological evidence of flavonoids as antioxidants

5.1 Flavonols and breast cancer risk

Flavonoids are an assembly of naturally occurring phenolic compounds located in vegetables and fruits and are classified into 6 main sub-classes based on the complexity of their structure. They include flavanones, flavones, flavonols, flavan-3-ols, isoflavanones and anthocyanins [107]. Investigational studies have suggested that flavonoids such as flavonols, flavones and flavanones possess preventative biological activity on breast carcinogenesis and is protective against commencement and development of tumor [108]. Nevertheless, epidemiological data regarding the associations between these flavonoid biomarkers and risk of breast cancer is inadequate and is very much needed to evaluate the definite effects of flavonoids in humans [109].

There is epidemiological evidence determined by prospective cohort study and case-study designs that have suggested an associations between dietary and supplemental flavonoids intake and breast cancer risk [110, 111]. In a recent case–control study that examined the relationship between breast cancer risk and total and subclasses of flavonoids, higher dietary intakes of total flavonoids (OR = 0.66, 95% CI: 0.54–0.82), flavonols (OR = 0.51, 95% CI: 0.41–0.63) were inversely associated with breast cancer risk [110] (**Table 1**). No significant relationship was observed between the flavins, flavan-3-ol monomers and flavanols, and breast cancer risk [110]. These findings are compatible with those of a large case–control study conducted in Italy, where decreased breast cancer risk was found for flavonols (OR = 0.80, P_{trend} 0.06) and flavones (OR = 0.81, P_{trend} = 0.02), but not for flavan-3-ols, flavanones, isoflavones and anthocyanidins [111]. Similarly, in a subsequent case–control study of United States women reduced breast cancer risk was related with high dietary uptake of flavones (OR = 0.61, 95% CI: 0.45, 0.83), flavonols (OR = 0.54, 95% CI: 0.40–0.73) and flavan-3-ols in postmenopausal women. The authors suggested that consuming sufficient amount of these flavonoids could be beneficial to these women in the chemoprevention of breast cancer [112] (**Table 1**). Notably, in a recent hospital-based case–control, higher levels of serum flavonols (OR = 0.52, 95% CI 0.38–0.70) and flavanone (OR = 0.45, 95% CI: 0.34–0.60) were significantly associated with decreased breast cancer risk [113]. The outcomes of these studies corroborated those of other case–control studies [114, 115] which supported the protective influence of high dietary intake of flavonols and flavones against breast cancer particularly among postmenopausal females.

The findings from prospective cohort studies are not so favorable regarding the chemo-preventative actions of flavonoids. In a meta-analysis of epidemiologic studies comprising 6 prospective cohort and 6 case–control studies, higher dietary intake of flavones (RR = 0.83, 95% CI: 0.76–0.91), flavonols (RR = 0.88, 95% CI: 0.80–0.98) decreased breast cancer risk although there were no significant relation of flavanones, flavan-3-ols and anthocyanins particularly in post-menopausal women [116] (**Table 3**). However, The Nurses' Health Study II investigated the effect of dietary flavonols on breast cancer risk, and found a non-significant null association with a risk ratio of 0.94 (95% CI: 0.72–1.22, P_{trend} = 0.54) that was reported for flavonol-rich foods. Furthermore, dietary intakes of flavonol containing foods such as beans and lentils were inversely associated with breast cancer risk but this was not observed for onions, apples, blueberries tea, green pepper and broccoli [117]. There was also no association and thus no protective effects against breast cancer risk for increased intake of flavanones [118–120], flavanols [118, 119], flavonols [118–120], flavones [118], anthocyanidins [118] as well as total flavonoids [118–122].

5.2 Soy isoflavones and breast cancer risk

Isoflavones are a subclass of flavonoids and are found in legumes such as soybeans and soy products. These polyphenolic compounds are derived from plants and the three main isoflavones are daidzin, glycitin and genistin [123]. Globally the consumption of soy and soy products is increasing as the health benefits due to their biological actions including estrogenic and anti-estrogenic properties, inhibition of tumor proliferation, antioxidant, anti-inflammatory and lower risk for cardiovascular disease [124, 125]. Notwithstanding potential mechanisms from experimental studies, epidemiological evidence from case–control and prospective cohort studies regarding association of soy food and isoflavone, and breast cancer risk provide unreliable results [126–128].

In The Shanghai Breast Cancer Survival Study that assessed bone fracture incidence and its relationship with soy food consumption among breast cancer patients, high soy isoflavone intake was concomitant with decreased risk among both peri- and premenopausal subjects (HR = 0.22, 95% CI: 0.09–0.53) but no association for postmenopausal subjects [129] (**Table 1**). Similarly, a recent study that examined the relationship between isoflavone intake and hereditary breast cancer risk, reported that high intake of this flavonoid was inversely related with luminal A breast cancer hazard in women who are BRCA2 mutation carriers [130]. Conversely, in a large prospective study comprising women from the Epidemiologique aupres de Femmes de la Mutuelle Generale de l'Education Nationale (E3N) cohort, there was no relation between past consumption of soy isoflavones supplement and breast cancer risk (HR = 1.36, 95% CI: 0.95–1.93) particularly among premenopausal patients [131]. Furthermore, in this study, there were contrasting associations of soy supplements with estrogen receptor-positive (HR = 0.78, 95%CI: 0.60–0.99) and estrogen receptor-negative (HR = 2.01, 95%CI: 1.41–2.86) breast cancer risk [131]. In another contemporary study, null association was observed between breast cancer risk and soy products containing isoflavones in a large cohort study of North American women although greater dairy milk intakes were associated with increased breast cancer risk, after adjusted for consumption [132]. The authors suggested that caution should be exercised when viewing existing guidelines for dairy milk intake [132].

There are meta-analyses that have indicated that higher levels of soy products and isoflavones with lower incident breast cancer risk [133, 134]. In a meta-analysis of 35 studies soy isoflavone intake has a protective effect in that it is inversely associated with breast cancer for both pre- (OR = 0.59, 95%CI: 0.48–0.69 and post-menopausal women (OR = 0.59, 95%CI: 0.44–0.74) particularly in Asian women while no evidence of a relationship in Western women [135] (**Table 3**). Nonetheless, in a previous meta-analysis of prospective cohort studies, there was no significant association between high (versus low) intake of isoflavones (RR = 0.99, 95% CI: 0.91–1.09) and moderate (versus low) intake of isoflavones (RR = 0.99, 95% CI = 0.92–1.05) and breast cancer risk, indicating that women with high dietary intake of soy isoflavones may experience decreased breast cancer incidence [136]. Support for the null finding was observed in a large Multiethnic Cohort study of women with a wide range of soya intake level and who were followed for 13 years, where no statistically association was detected between overall breast cancer risk and high dietary isoflavone intake (HR = 0.96, 95% CI: 0.85–1.08). The authors posited that higher consumption may be protective for Japanese American, Latina and African American women [137]. Notably, a recent publication of the China Kadoorie Biobank (CKB) study which involved a dose–response meta-analysis of dietary data of soy intake over a follow-up period of 10 years, the relative risk for high soy isoflavones consumption was 1.00 (95% CI: 0.81–1.22) [138]. A 3% decreased breast cancer risk for each 10 mg/day increment of soy isoflavones was observed. The results suggests that soy isoflavone was not related with breast cancer risk though increased intake may be beneficial in preventing breast cancer [138].

There are not many case–control studies that investigated the relation between soy isoflavone intake and breast cancer risk. In a case–control study conducted in Japan, increasing intake of isoflavone significantly reduced breast cancer risk in premenopausal women (OR = 0.44; 95% CI: 0.22–0.89), while no significant association was observed among postmenopausal women [139]. This shows the need to conduct more case–control studies in order to afford a clearer picture on the relationship between soy products and breast cancer incidence.

5.3 Soy proteins and soy isoflavones and breast cancer outcomes

There are studies that have examined the association between soy products and isoflavones intake and breast cancer survival, however the results are not definitive [140–142]. There are prospective cohort and meta-analyses studies that have reported significant inversely association between soy protein and soy isoflavones and breast cancer survival outcomes. In looking at prospective studies, The Shanghai Breast Cancer Survival Study comprised of 5,033 surgically treated breast cancer patients that were followed for 3.9 years. High soy protein intake was inversely associated with breast cancer recurrence (HR = 0.68, 95%CI: 0.64–0.87) and all-cause mortality (HR = 0.71, 95%CI: 0.54–0.92) among women with either estrogen receptor-positive or -negative breast cancer [143] (**Table 2**). In an earlier prospective study of 256 Chinese women, elevated soy isoflavones intake was associated with reduced risk of breast cancer mortality (OR = 0.25, 95% CI: 0.09–0.54) and high soy protein was also concomitant with significant decreased breast cancer risk (OR = 0.38, 95% CI: 0.17–0.86) [144] (**Table 2**). In another study published in the same year involving 339 Korean women, dietary soy isoflavones was inversely related with breast cancer recurrence in HER2-positive breast cancer patients (HR = 0.23, 95%CI: 0.06–0.89) while no effect was observed with total soy intake [145].

The findings from systematic and meta-analysis of prospective cohort and case–control studies are also inconsistent. In a meta-analysis of protective studies, soy isoflavones intake was inversely linked with risk of breast cancer incidence (RR = 0.89, 95% CI: 0.79–0.99) and also inversely concomitant with risk of breast cancer recurrence (RR = 0.84, 95% CI: 0.70–0.99) [146] (**Table 3**). Likewise, Nachvak et al. conducted a systematic review and dose–response meta-analysis of 23 prospective cohort studies and reported that a 9% reduced risk of breast cancer-specific mortality for each 10 mg/day increase in soy isoflavones intake and a 12% decrease in the same survival outcome for each 5-g/day elevation of soy protein intake [147]. On the other hand, Qiu and Jiang conducted a systematic review and meta-analysis of 12 studies that explored the relationship between soy and isoflavones intake and breast cancer survival and recurrence. Pre- and post-diagnosis of soy and isoflavones intake were associated with minor reduction in risk of breast cancer recurrence (HR = 0.84 95% CI: 0.71–0.98) and breast cancer specific survival (HR = 0.89 95% CI: 0.74–1.07). Stratified analyses revealed no significant relationship between post-diagnosis soy and isoflavones consumption with overall survival (HR = 0.80, 95% CI: 0.62–1.04), and breast cancer specific survival (HR = 0.83, 95%CI: 0.64–1.07) [141].

5.4 Lycopene and breast cancer risk

The consumption of fruits and vegetables particularly those containing lycopene may offer protection against different types of cancers including breast cancer. There are a number of prospective and case–control studies that examined the relationship between dietary lycopene and breast cancer risk. In a case–control study conducted among Chinese women comprising of 122 primary breast cancer cases and 632 age-matched healthy females, high intake of dietary lycopene was statistically strongly associated with lower breast cancer risk (adjusted OR = 0.26, 95% CI: 0.14–0.46) [93] (**Table 1**). In the Women's Health Initiative Observational Study comprising 84 805 women with reported 2,879 incident breast cancer cases during a follow-up period of 7.6 years, high intake of dietary lycopene non-significantly reduced breast cancer risk by 15% (RR = 0.85; 95% CI: 0.73–1.00; P_{trend} = 0.064) in ER+ and PR+ breast cancer among post-menopausal women [23]. Also, a Swiss case–control study comprising 289 incident breast cancer cases and 442 controls reported a significant inverse association for lycopene with breast cancer risk (OR = 0.64) [148].

However, there are both prospective and case–control studies that have found null association between dietary lycopene and breast cancer risk. In a case–control study of Chinese women involving of 561 cases and 561 age-matched control high intake of lycopene was not associated with breast cancer risk (0.89, 95% CI: 0·61–1·30) [118]. Likewise, in another case–control study of non-Hispanic White and Hispanic women there was no association and therefore no protective effect of dietary lycopene on breast cancer risk [60]. Furthermore, there are other studies of dietary lycopene intake including prospective cohort [57, 88, 105, 146], case–control [149] and meta-analysis [91] that have found no association of lycopene with breast cancer risk.

Epidemiologic studies evaluating whether circulating lycopene is associated with breast cancer risk have yielded equivocal answers. A nested case–control study conducted comprising 295 breast cancer cases and 295 age- and race-matched controls demonstrated significantly strong inverse association of high levels of lycopene with the risk of developing breast cancer [97]. In another case–control study among women in the United States (46 breast cancer cases and 63 controls), there was a strong inverse association of lycopene (OR = 0.32, 95% CI: 0.11 -, 0.94) in breast adipose tissue and risk of breast cancer [150] (**Table 1**). Likewise, a pilot case–control study of Caucasian and African American women found a weak inverse relation between plasma lycopene concentration and risk of breast cancer (Simon et al., 2000). The findings of these study were in agreement with that of a comprehensive pooled analysis of 8 prospective cohort studies conducted by Eliassen and colleagues. They found serum or plasma levels of lycopene significantly lower the risk of breast cancer patients by 22% (RR = 0.78, 95% CI: 0.62–0.99, P_{trend} = 0.02) [151] (**Table 3**).

Others studies with findings in consonant with an inverse association between serum or plasma levels of lycopene and breast cancer risk include two case–control studies that showed deceased risk among females with elevated mammographic density [152] and blood donors [103] and a nested case–case control in the Nurses' Health Study [153]. Likewise, in a nested case–control study, stepwise increase in plasma lycopene levels were not associated (RR = 0.95, 1.15, 0.93, 1.00 (reference, P trend = 0.86) with decreased breast cancer risk in older and middle-aged females [154].

5.5 Lutein and zeaxanthin and breast cancer risk

There are a few epidemiologic studies that have investigate the protective effect of dietary lutein and zeaxanthin on breast cancer incidence [90, 119, 155]. A case–control study of Chinese women found that lutein/zeaxanthin reduced breast cancer risk by 51% (OR = 0·49, 95% CI: 0·34–0·71) particularly among premenopausal women and those exposed to second-hand smoke [119]. In an earlier large population-based case–control study of United States residents, an inverse association was shown for higher consumption of lutein/zeaxanthin (OR = 0.83, 95% CI 0.68–0.99, P_{trend} = 0.02) and breast cancer risk among postmenopausal women [90]. Likewise, Bae conducted a pooled analysis of eighteen prospective cohort studies and reported that lutein/zeaxanthin demonstrated protective effect on ER- and PR+ as well as ER-/PR- breast cancer [155].

However, a case–control study of Chinese women demonstrated that high dietary lutein/zeaxanthin were not inversely associated with breast cancer risk [93]. Similarly, in a large cohort study of Canadian women Terry et al. reported no clear association between dietary intake of lutein/zeaxanthin and risk of breast cancer [88]. In a later meta-analysis involving 33 studies, high dietary intake of lutein/+zeaxanthin offered no protective effect and thus no significant association with breast cancer risk [91].

In addition to epidemiological studies that have discovered the anti-cancer potential of dietary lutein/zeaxanthin, there are a few research that investigated the protective role of this circulating antioxidant. Serum or plasma levels of lutein/zeaxanthin are more suitable biological indicators of the amount of these flavonol available for chemo-preventative action [156]. In a case–control study conducted among Chinese women, there was a significantly strong inverse association of high serum levels of lutein/zeaxanthin with breast cancer risk (OR = 0·26, 95% CI: 0·17–0·38) [157]. Likewise, a nested case–control study comprising 604 incident breast cancer cases and 626 controls in the Nurses' Health Study found that circulating lycopene, alpha-carotene and beta-cryptoxanthin were concomitant with a significant 40% - 50% decrease in the risk of breast cancer ($P_{trend} < 0.05$) [152]. These findings were corroborated by a comprehensive analysis of 8 cohort studies where lutein/zeaxanthin was significantly inversely associated with breast cancer risk (RR = 0.84, 95% CI: 0.70–1.01, $P_{trend} = 0.05$) [151]. Interestingly, in a nested case–control study (270 breast cancer cases, 270 matched controls) the risk of breast cancer increased due to low blood levels (OR = 2.08, 95% CI: 1.11–3.90) [158].

However, In a nested case–control study (1502 breast cancer cases and 1502 individually matched controls) conducted within the European Prospective Investigation into Cancer and Nutrition cohort, there was no statistical association of plasma levels of lutein with of ER- breast tumors [98]. Supporting evidence was also observed in a case–control cohort (201 breast cancer cases and 290 referents) where plasma concentrations of lutein was significantly inversely related with breast cancer risk in premenopausal women [106].

5.6 Quercetin and breast cancer risk

The number of epidemiological research involving quercetin and potential relationship with breast cancer risk is lacking. In a linkage of multi-centered case–control studies conducted in Italy (comprising 10,000 incident breast cancer cases and 16,000 controls) high intake of flavonols including quercetin was inversely associated with breast cancer risk (OR = 0.80) [158]. Similarly, in an earlier large-case control study also conducted in Italy (2,569 incident breast cancer cases and 2,588 controls), increasing consumption of flavonols decreased breast cancer risk by 20% (OR = 0.80; $P_{trend,}$ 0.06) [111]. The findings of another large case–control study comprising Greek women was consistent with these two previous results where a strong significant inverse relationship of daily flavonols in fruit comprising quercetin with breast cancer risk [114]. Higher intake of quercetin reduced breast cancer risk by 38% (RR = 0.62, 95%CI: 0.37–1.03, P = 0.25) and the relation was stronger when modification was made in lieu of other dietary sources with a lower risk of 46% (RR = 0.54, 95%CI: 0.30–0.95, P = 0.14) [120]. Lastly, in a meta-analyses of 6 case–controls and 6 prospective cohort studies, breast cancer risk due to high intake (compared with low consumption) of flavonols such as quercetin declined by 12% in females (RR = 0.88, 95% CI: 0.80–0.98). It was also observed that further analyses of 3 case–control studies, high flavonol intake (compared with low consumption) was associated with decreased breast cancer risk in post-menopausal women [116].

6. Green tea

6.1 Green tea intake and breast cancer risk

Green tea is a product of dry tea leaves of the plant *Camellia sinensis*, and numerous pre-clinical and epidemiologic studies have been conducted examining the possible protective effect of green tea from various types of human cancers including breast carcinoma [159]. Epidemiologic studies have described a protecting effect of green tea consumption against the initiation and progression of breast cancer, although the results has not being conclusive. A case–control study (1009 incident breast cancer cases and 1009 age-matched controls) of regular green tea (dried green tea leaves per annum) consumption in a dose-dependent manner significantly reduced breast cancer risk [(OR = 0.87, 95% CI: 0.73–1.04) for 1–249 g; (OR = 0.68, 95% CI: 0.54–0.86) for 250–499 g and (OR = 0.59, 95 CI: 0.45–0.77) for 500–749 g, $P_{trend} < 0.001$) [160]. Likewise, in a population-based, case–control study of Asian women with breast cancer (501 breast cancer patients and 594 controls), there was a significant trend of reducing risk with cumulative amount of green tea consumption ([OR = 0.71, 95% CI: 0.51–0.99) and (OR = 0.53, 95% CI: 0.35–0.78) for 0–85.7 ml and > 85.7 ml of green tea per day respectively] [161]. These findings were corroborated by a population-based case–control study of Chinese women in which regular green tea mildly decreased breast cancer risk by 18% (OR = 0.88; 95% CI: 0.79–0.98). It was observed that a dose-dependent association existed with the quantity of green tea intake per month and catechol-O-methyltransferase rs4680 genotypes did not modify the relationship [162].

Two other nested case–control studies are consistent with the protective effect of green tea consumption. Yuan et al. piloted a nested case–control study (297 incident breast cancer cases and 665 controls) inside the Singapore Chinese Health Study and found that frequent green tea consumption significantly decreases breast cancer risk in women with high angiotensin-converting enzyme activity (OR = 0.33, 95%CI: 0.13–0.82, $P_{trend} = 0.039$) [163]. In an earlier nested case–control study (380 incident breast cancer cases and 662 controls) also within the Singapore Chinese Health Study, women with low folate intake and daily or weekly green tea consumption had a 55% reduced breast cancer risk (OR = 0.45, 95% CI: 0.26–0.79, $P_{interaction} = 0.02$). Green tea consumption was not associated with breast cancer risk at high folate intake and the authors suggested that inhibition of the folate intake may be a possible mechanism which account for the protective effect of green tea against breast carcinoma [164].

There are two meta-analyses that support the reduction of breast cancer incidence and recurrence due to green tea consumption. A meta-analysis of studies by Ogunleye et al. of breast cancer recurrence and risk comprising 5,617 cases showed that increased green tea intake (greater than 3 cups/day) was inversely related with breast cancer recurrence ($RR_{pooled} = 0.73$, 95%CI: 0.56–0.96 [165] (Ogunleye et al., 2010). An analysis of only case–control studies showed that the inverse relationship was preserved ($RR_{pooled} = 0.81$, 95%CI: 0.75–0.88) while there was no protective effect and therefore null association of breast cancer risk among prospective cohort studies [165]. There was additional supportive evidence in a more recent meta-analysis of 13 studies (5 case–control and 8 cohort studies comprising of 63,810 women) where a statistically significant inverse association existed between green tea consumption and breast cancer incidence with a 15% risk reduction ($OR_{pooled} = 0.85$, 95% CI: 0.80–0.92, p = 0.0001) [166]. Analysis of only case–control studies also showed a significant inverse relationship with a 19% decrease in the risk of breast cancer (ORpooled = 0.81, 95%CI: 0.74–0.88, p = 0.000) [166].

The results of prospective cohort studies demonstrating a protective effects against breast cancer were less conclusive with some of the studies reporting null association. In a prospective cohort study of the Hospital-based Epidemiologic Research Program in Japan, there was reduced breast cancer recurrence among subjects who consumed 3 or more cups of green tea (HR = 0.69, 95%CI: 0.47–1.00), particularly in stage I disease (HR = 0.43, 95%CI: 0.22–0.84) [167]. In the Shanghai Women's Health Study, a large population based study comprising 74,942 Chinese females, subjects who began drinking green tea less than or at 25 years of age were less likely to develop breast cancer (HR = 0.69, 95% CI: 0.41–1.17) [168]. However, in a later population-based prospective cohort study also conducted in Japan, there was no association of breast cancer risk and green tea consumption (> 5 or more cups/day; HR = 1.12, 95%CI: 0.81–1.56; P_{trend} = 0.60) [169]. Green tea intake was not associated with a reduced breast cancer risk in another prospective study conducted in Japan [170] and in 2 prospective studies piloted among 35,004 Japanese women (RR = 0.84, 95%CI: 0.57–1.24; > 5 cups/day) [171].

6.1.1 Epigallocatechin-3-gallate intake and breast cancer risk

Epigallocatechin-3-gallate is a natural antioxidant and it has been reported to be more efficient at arresting reactive oxygen species and other radical than vitamin C and E [172]. Experimental studies have demonstrated that epigallocatechin-3-gallate, the biologically active and most abundant tea catechins displays anticancer and chemotherapeutic effects against breast cancer [173]. Epidemiologic studies relating to epigallocatechin-3-gallate are lacking. In a nested case–control study (144 incident breast cancer cases and 288 age-matched controls) in the Japan Public Health Center-based Prospective Study, elevated plasma levels of epigallocatechin-3-gallate along with epicatechin-3-gallate, epicatechin and epigallocatechin were not associated with reduced breast cancer risk [epigallocatechin-3-gallate (OR = 1.21, 95%CI: 0.52–2.80; P_{trend} = 0.53)] [169]. In another study published three years ago, green tea extract capsules comprising 843 mg epigallocatechin-3-gallate administered for 1 year decreased mammographic density in healthy postmenopausal women [174]. Interesting, epigallocatechin-3-gallate (400 mg capsules, 3 times/day for 2–8 weeks) orally administered to breast cancer subjects undergoing radiotherapy potentiate the effectiveness of the treatment as evident by decreased metalloproteinase-9 and metalloproteinase-2 activities and elevated serum concentration of vascular endothelial growth factor [175].

The few reports of epidemiologic evidence of epigallocatechin-3-gallate and inconclusive findings in prospective studies suggests that further exploration of its probable chemo-preventative.

7. Discussion and conclusion

The epidemiological evidence shown by a number of case–control, prospective cohort studies as well as meta-analysis and systematic reviews presented does support the view that nutritional micronutrients with antioxidant properties in dietary or supplemental form may be beneficial in protecting women against breast cancer. However, there are studies that have demonstrated null association between the dietary and supplemental micronutrients, and the risk or survival outcomes of breast cancer. Thus overall the findings are inconsistent and epidemiological data on some of the antioxidants as it relates to breast cancer outcomes such as recurrence, and breast cancer-specific and all-cause mortality is inadequate.

Notably, there is substantial evidence which is well documented in the literature of the protective action and modification of many signaling pathways and molecular events by these antioxidants inducing apoptosis, inhibition of breast cancer cell proliferation and invasion, and preventing angiogenesis and metastasis. However, the findings of epidemiological results are somewhat disappointing and are not concurrent with experimental results for most of these natural antioxidants. There are limiting factors which negatively impact epidemiological association studies such as genetic, confounding lifestyle, samples sizes, possible selection bias in case–control studies, the length of intervention, possible recall bias in retrospective studies, not accurately measuring dietary intake in prospective studies, interaction among different micronutrients which may nullify individual effect among others.

Nevertheless, despite the inconsistencies, the findings of the chemo-preventative effects of vitamins, flavonoids and green tea presented in this review are encouraging. There need to be more large-scale and randomized controlled studies to investigate the association of these antioxidants and outcomes such as breast cancer recurrence, and breast cancer-specific mortality. More studies investigating the dietary intake of these antioxidants with sub-types of breast cancer, namely ER and PR status among both premenopausal and postmenopausal women is warranted. The elucidation of the mechanism of action by which these antioxidants decrease breast cancer risk may be helpful in recognizing sub-groups who could benefit from the consumption of these antioxidants with better dietary endorsements for the prevention of breast cancer.

Furthermore, the finding that the inhibition of folate intake may be a possible mechanism which account for the protective effect of green tea against breast cancer is noted. Large prospective randomized control trials are warranted as they could provide definitive information on the beneficial or harmful effects of green tea intake on breast cancer development.

Author details

Donovan McGrowder[1*], Fabian Miller[2,5], Chukwuemeka Nwokocha[3], Cameil Wilson-Clarke[3], Melisa Anderson[4], Lennox Anderson-Jackson[1] and Lowen Williams[5]

1 Department of Pathology, Faculty of Medical Sciences, The University of the West Indies, Jamaica, West Indies

2 Department of Physical Education, Faculty of Education, The Mico University College, Jamaica, West Indies

3 Department of Basic Medical Sciences, Faculty of Medical Sciences, The University of the West Indies, Jamaica, West Indies

4 School of Allied Health and Wellness, College of Health Sciences, University of Technology, Jamaica, West Indies

5 Department of Biotechnology, Faculty of Science and Technology, The University of the West Indies, Jamaica, West Indies

*Address all correspondence to: dmcgrowd@yahoo.com

References

[1] Bray F, Ferlay J, Soerjomataram I, Siegel RL, Torre LA, Jemal A. Global cancer statistics 2018: GLOBOCAN estimates of incidence and mortality worldwide for 36 cancers in 185 countries. CA: A Cancer Journal for Clinicians. 2018;**68**(6):394-424

[2] World Health Organization. Breast Cancer. 2020. https://www.who.int/cancer/prevention/diagnosis-screening/breast-cancer/en/

[3] Majeed W, Aslam B, Javed I, Khaliq T, Muhammaf F, Ali A, Raza A. Breast Cancer: Major risk factors and recent developments in treatment. Asian Pacific Journal Cancer Prevention. 2014;**15**(8):3353-3358

[4] Ben-Chioma A, Obunwo C, Ebirien–Agana B, Ndokiari B. Evaluation of heavy metal levels in the serum of breast cancer patients in Port Harcourt, Nigeria. International Journal of Contemporary Medical Research. 2018;**4**(12):1-5

[5] Lee C. Delay in breast cancer: Implications for stage at diagnosis and survival. Frontiers in Public Health. 2014;**2**:87. doi: 10.3389/fpubh.2014.00087

[6] Kennecke H, Yerushalmi RR, Woods, et al. Metastatic behavior of breast cancer subtypes. Journal of Clinical Oncology. 2010;**28**(20):3271-3277

[7] Cherny NI, Paluch-Shimon S, Berner-Wygoda Y. Palliative care: Needs of advanced breast cancer patients. Breast Cancer (Dove Medical Press), 2018;**10**, 231-243. doi.org/10.2147/BCTT.S160462

[8] Sarmiento-Salinas LF, Delgado-Magallón A, Montes-Alvarado JB, Ramírez-Ramírez D, Flores-Alonso J, Cortés-Hernández P, Reyes-Leyva J, Herrera-Camacho I, et al. Breast cancer subtypes present a differential production of reactive oxygen species (ROS) and susceptibility to antioxidant treatment. Frontiers in Oncology. 2019;**9**:480. doi: 10.3389/fonc.2019.00480

[9] Chio IIC, Tuveson DA. ROS in cancer: the burning question. Trends in Molecular Medicine. 2017;**23**:411-429

[10] Moloney JN, Cotter TG. ROS signalling in the biology of cancer. Seminars in Cell and Developmental Biology. 2018;**80**:50-64. doi: 10.1016/j.semcdb.2017.05.023

[11] Piskounova E, Agathocleous M, Murphy MM, Hu Z, Huddlestun SE, Zhao Z, Leitch AM, Johnson TM, DeBerardinis RJ, Morrison SJ. Oxidative stress inhibits distant metastasis by human melanoma cells Nature. 2015;**527**:186-191

[12] Jezierska-Drutel A, Rosenzweig SA, Neumann CA. A Role of oxidative stress and the microenvironment in breast cancer development and progression. Advance Cancer Research. 2013;**119**:107-125. doi: 10.1016/B978-0-12-407190-2.00003-4

[13] Hecht F, Pessoa CF, Gentile LB, Rosenthal D, Carvalho DP, Fortunato RS. The role of oxidative stress on breast cancer development and therapy. Tumor Biology. 2016;**37**(4):4281-4291

[14] Hewala TI, Ramadan Abo El-soud. The clinical significance of serum oxidative stress biomarkers in breast cancer females. Medical Research Journal 2019;**4**(1):1-7

[15] Adwas AA, Elsayed ASI, Azab AE, Quwaydir FA. Oxidative stress and antioxidant mechanisms in human

body. Journal of Applied Biotechnology & Bioengineering. 2019;**6**(1):43-47. doiI: 10.15406/jabb.2019.06.00173

[16] Pham-Huy LA, He H, Pham-Huy C. Free radicals, antioxidants in disease and health. International Journal of Biomedical Science. 2008;**4**(2):89-96

[17] Greenlee H, Hershman DL, Jacobson JS. Use of antioxidant supplements during breast cancer treatment: a comprehensive review. Breast Cancer Res. Treat. 2009;**115**(3):437-452

[18] Willcox JK, Ash SL, Catignani GL. Antioxidants and prevention of chronic disease. Critical Reviews in Food Science and Nutrition. 2004;**44**(4):275-295

[19] Traber MG, Stevens JF. Vitamins C and E: beneficial effects from a mechanistic perspective. Free Radic Biol Med. 2011;**51**:1000-1013

[20] Zhang D, Xu P, Li Y, Wei B, Yang S, Zheng Y, Lyu L, Deng Y, Zhai Z, Li N, Wang N, Lyu J, Dai Z. Association of vitamin C intake with breast cancer risk and mortality: a meta-analysis of observational studies. Aging (Albany NY). 2020;**12**(18):18415-18435

[21] Nagel G, Linseisen J, van Gils CH, Peeters PH, Boutron-Ruault MC, Clavel-Chapelon F, Romieu I, Tjønneland A, Olsen A et al. Dietary beta-carotene, vitamin C and E intake and breast cancer risk in the European Prospective Investigation into Cancer and Nutrition (EPIC). Breast Cancer Res Treat. 2010;**119**(3):753-765

[22] Verhoeven DT, Assen N, Goldbohm RA, Dorant E, van 't Veer P, Sturmans F, Hermus RJ, van den Brandt PA. Vitamins C and E, retinol, beta-carotene and dietary fibre in relation to breast cancer risk: a prospective cohort study. Br J Cancer. 1997;**75**(1):149-155

[23] Cui Y, Shikany JM, Liu S, Shagufta Y, Rohan TE. Selected antioxidants and risk of hormone receptor-defined invasive breast cancers among postmenopausal women in the Women's Health Initiative Observational Study. Am J Clin Nutr. 2008;**87**(4):1009-1018

[24] Cadeau C, Fournier A, Mesrine S, Clavel-Chapelon F, Fagherazzi G, Boutron-Ruault MC. Vitamin C supplement intake and postmenopausal breast cancer risk: interaction with dietary vitamin C. Am J Clin Nutr. 2016;**104**(1):228-234

[25] Fulan H, Changxing J, Baina WY, Wencui Z, Chunqing L, Fan W, Dandan L, Dianjun S, Tong W, Da P, et al. Retinol, vitamins A, C, and E and breast cancer risk: a meta-analysis and meta-regression. Cancer Causes Control. 2011;**22**:1383-1396

[26] Sharhar S, Normah H, Fatimah A, Fadilah RN, Rohi GA, Amin I, Cham BG, Rizal RM, Fairulnizal MN. Antioxidant intake and status, and oxidative stress in relation to breast cancer risk: a case-control study. Asian Pac J Cancer Prev. 2008;**9**(2):343-349

[27] Zhang S, Hunter DJ, Forman MR, Rosner BA, Speizer FE, Colditz GA, Manson JE, Hankinson SE, Willett WC. Dietary carotenoids and vitamins A, C, and E and risk of breast cancer. J Natl Cancer Inst. 1999;**91**(6):547-556

[28] Do MH, Lee SS, Jung PJ, Lee MH. Intake of dietary fat and vitamin in relation to breast cancer risk in Korean women: a case-control study. Journal of Korean Medical Science. 2003;**18**(4):534-540

[29] Freudenheim JL, Marshall JR, Vena JE, Laughlin R, Brasure JR, Swanson MK, Nemoto T, Graham S. Premenopausal breast cancer risk and

intake of vegetables, fruits, and related nutrients. J Natl Cancer Inst. 1996;**88**(6):340-348

[30] Hutchinson J, Lentjes MA, Greenwood DC, Burley VJ, Cade JE, Cleghorn CL, Threapleton DE, Key TJ, Cairns BJ, Keogh RH, et al. Vitamin C intake from diary recordings and risk of breast cancer in the UK Dietary Cohort Consortium. Eur J Clin Nutr. 2012;**66**(5):561-568

[31] Hunter DJ, Manson JE, Colditz GA, Stampfer MJ, Rosner B, Hennekens CH, Speizer FE, Willett WC. A prospective study of the intake of vitamins C, E, and A and the risk of breast cancer. N Engl J Med. 1993;**329**(4):234-240

[32] Ullah M, Khan H, Zubair H, Shamim U, Hadi S. The antioxidant ascorbic acid mobilizes nuclear copper leading to a prooxidant breakage of cellular DNA: implications for chemotherapeutic action against cancer. Cancer Chemother Pharmacol. 2011;**67**(1):103-110

[33] Hutchinson J, Burley VJ, Greenwood DC, Thomas JD, Cade JE. High-dose vitamin C supplement use is associated with self-reported histories of breast cancer and other illnesses in the UK Women's Cohort Study. Public Health Nutr. 2011;**14**(5):768-777

[34] Harris HR, Orsini N, Wolk A. Vitamin C and survival among women with breast cancer: a meta-analysis. Eur J Cancer. 2014;**50**(7):1223-1231

[35] Harris HR, Bergkvist L, Wolk A. Vitamin C intake and breast cancer mortality in a cohort of Swedish women. Br J Cancer. 2013;**109**(1):257-264

[36] McEligot A, Largent J, Ziogas A, Peel D, Anton-Culver H. Dietary fat, fiber, vegetable, and micronutrients are associated with overall survival in postmenopausal women diagnosed with breast cancer. Nutr Cancer. 2006;**55**(2):132-140

[37] Fleischauer AT, Simonsen N, Arab L. Antioxidant supplements and risk of breast cancer recurrence and breast cancer-related mortality among postmenopausal women. Nutr Cancer. 2003;**46**(1):15-22

[38] Saquib J, Rock CL, Natarajan L, Saquib N, Newman VA, Patterson RE, Thomson CA, Al-Delaimy WK, Pierce JP. Dietary intake, supplement use, and survival among women diagnosed with early-stage breast cancer. Nutr Cancer. 2011;**63**(3):327-333

[39] Holmes MD, Stampfer MJ, Colditz GA, Rosner B, Hunter DJ, Willett WC. Dietary factors and the survival of women with breast carcinoma. Cancer. 1999;**86**(5):826-835

[40] Saxe GA, Rock CL, Wicha MS, Schottenfeld D. Diet and risk for breast cancer recurrence and survival. Breast Cancer Res Treat. 1999;**53**(3):241-253

[41] Greenlee H, Kwan ML, Kushi LH, Song J, Castillo A, Weltzien E, Quesenberry CP Jr, Caan BJ. Antioxidant supplement use after breast cancer diagnosis and mortality in the Life After Cancer Epidemiology (LACE) cohort. Cancer. 2012;**118**(8):2048-2058

[42] Nechuta S, Lu W, Chen Z, Zheng Y, Gu K, Cai H, Zheng W, Shu XO. Vitamin supplement use during breast cancer treatment and survival: a prospective cohort study. Cancer Epidemiol Biomarkers Prev. 2011;**20**(2):262-271

[43] Zirpoli GR, Brennan PM, Hong CC, McCann SE, Ciupak G, Davis W, Unger JM, Budd GT et al. Supplement use during an intergroup clinical trial for breast cancer (S0221). Breast Cancer Res Treat. 2013;**137**(3):903-913

[44] Lamson DW, Brignall MS. Antioxidants in cancer therapy; their

actions and interactions with oncologic therapies. Altern Med Rev. 1999;**4**(5):304-329

[45] Lawenda BD, Kelly KM, Ladas EJ, Sagar SM, Vickers A, Blumberg JB. Should supplemental antioxidant administration be avoided during chemotherapy and radiation therapy? J Natl Cancer Inst. 2008;**100**(11):773-783

[46] Fuchs-Tarlovsky V. Role of antioxidants in cancer therapy. Nutrition. 2013;**29**(1):15-21

[47] Salganik, RI. The benefits and hazards of antioxidants: controlling apoptosis and other protective mechanisms in cancer patients and the human population. J Am Coll Nutrition 2001;**20**(5 Suppl.) 464S–467S.

[48] Ambrosone CB, Zirpoli GR, Hutson AD, McCann WE, McCann SE, Barlow WE, Kelly KM, Cannioto R, et al. Dietary supplement use during chemotherapy and survival outcomes of patients with breast cancer enrolled in a Cooperative Group Clinical Trial (SWOG S0221). J Clin Oncol. 2020;**38**(8):804-814

[49] Singh K, Bhori M, Kasu YA, Bhat G, Marar, T. Antioxidants as precision weapons in war against cancer chemotherapy induced toxicity - Exploring the armoury of obscurity. Saudi Pharmaceutical Journal, 2018;**26**(2);177-190

[50] Roa FJ, Peña E, Gatica M, Escobar-Acuña K, Saavedra P, MaldonadoM,CuevasME,Moraga-CidG, RivasCI,Muñoz-MontesinoC.Therapeutic use of vitamin C in cancer: Physiological considerations. Front Pharmacol. 2020;**11**:211. doi: 10.3389/fphar.2020.00211

[51] Kimmick GG, Bell RA, Bostick RM. Vitamin E and breast cancer: a review. Nutr Cancer. 1997;**27**(2):109-117.

[52] Ronco AL, Stefani ED, Mendoza B, Vazquez A, Abbona E, Sanchez G, Rosa AD. Mate and tea intake, Dietary antioxidants and risk of breast cancer: a case-control study. Asian Pac J Cancer Prev. 2016;**17**(6):2923-2933

[53] Pan SY, Zhou J, Gibbons L, Morrison H, Wen SW; Canadian Cancer Registries Epidemiology Research Group [CCRERG]. Antioxidants and breast cancer risk- a population-based case-control study in Canada. BMC Cancer. 2011;**24**(11):372. doi: 10.1186/1471-2407-11-372

[54] Dorjgochoo T, Shrubsole MJ, Shu XO, Lu W, Ruan Z, Zheng Y, Cai H, Dai Q, Gu K, Gao YT, Zheng W. Vitamin supplement use and risk for breast cancer: the Shanghai Breast Cancer Study. Breast Cancer Res Treat. 2008;**111**(2):269-278

[55] Zhang C, Ho SC, Lin F, Cheng S, Fu J, Chen Y. Soy product and isoflavone intake and breast cancer risk defined by hormone receptor status. Cancer Science. 2010;**101**(2):501-507

[56] BohlkeK,SpiegelmanD,TrichopoulouA, Katsouyanni K, Trichopoulos D. Vitamins A, C and E and the risk of breast cancer: results from a case-control study in Greece. British Journal of Cancer. 1999;**79**(1):23-29

[57] Cho E, Spiegelman D, Hunter DJ, Chen WY, Zhang SM, Colditz GA, Willett WC. Premenopausal intakes of vitamins A, C, and E, folate, and carotenoids, and risk of breast cancer. Cancer Epidemiol Biomarkers Prev. 2003;**12**(8):713-720

[58] Rohan TE, Hiller JE, McMichael AJ. Dietary factors and survival from breast cancer. Nutr Cancer. 1993;**20**:167-177

[59] Shibata A, Paganini-Hill A, Ross RK, Henderson BE. Intake of vegetables, fruits, beta-carotene, vitamin C and vitamin supplements

and cancer incidence among the elderly: a prospective study. Br J Cancer. 1992;**66**:673-679

[60] Wang C, Baumgartner RN, Yang D, Slattery ML, Murtaugh MA, Byers T, Hines LM, Giuliano AR, Baumgartner KB. No evidence of association between breast cancer risk and dietary carotenoids, retinols, vitamin C and tocopherols in Southwestern Hispanic and non-Hispanic White women. Breast Cancer Res Treat. 2009;**114**(1):1371-45

[61] Misotti AM, Gnagnarella P. Vitamin supplement consumption and breast cancer risk: a review. Ecancer Medical Science. 2013;7:365. doi: 10.3332/ecancer.2013.365

[62] Samuels N, Schiff E, Ben-Arye E. Non-herbal nutritional supplements for symptom relief in adjuvant breast cancer: creating a doctor-patient dialogue. BMJ Support Palliat Care. 2014;**4**(3):e1. doi: 10.1136/bmjspcare-2013-000463

[63] Huang Z, Shi Y, Bao P, Cai H, Hong Z, Ding D, Jackson J, Shu XO, Dai Q. Associations of dietary intake and supplement use with post-therapy cognitive recovery in breast cancer survivors. Breast Cancer Res Treat. 2018;**171**(1):189-198

[64] Meulepas JM, Newcombe PA, Burnett-Hartman AN, Hampton JM, Trentham-Dietz A. Multivitamin supplement use and risk of invasive breast cancer. Public Health Nutr. 2010;**13**(10):1540-1545

[65] Gahche J, Bailey R, Burt V, Hughes J, Yetley E, Dwyer J, Picciano MF, McDowell M, Sempos C. Dietary supplement use among U.S. adults has increased since NHANES III (1988-1994) NCHS Data Brief. 2011;**61**:1-8

[66] Poole EM, Shu X, Caan BJ, Flatt SW, Holmes MD, Lu W, Kwan ML, Nechuta SJ, Pierce JP, Chen WY. Post-diagnosis supplement use and breast cancer prognosis in the After Breast Cancer Pooling Project. Breast Cancer Res Treat. 2013;**139**(2):529-537

[67] Kanellopoulou A, Riza E, Samoli E, Benetou V. Dietary supplement use after cancer diagnosis in relation to total mortality, cancer mortality and recurrence: A systematic review and meta-analysis. Nutr Cancer. 2020;**9**:1-15

[68] Simone CB 2nd, Simone NL, Simone V, Simone CB. Antioxidants and other nutrients do not interfere with chemotherapy or radiation therapy and can increase kill and increase survival, part 1. Altern Ther Health Med. 2007;**13**(1):22-28

[69] Moss RW. Should patients undergoing chemotherapy and radiotherapy be prescribed antioxidants? Integr Cancer Ther. 2006;**5**(1):63-82

[70] Yasueda, A, Urushima, H, Ito, T. Efficacy and interaction of antioxidant supplements as adjuvant therapy in cancer treatment: A systematic review. Integrative Cancer Therapies. 2016;**15**(1):17-39

[71] Conklin KA. Dietary antioxidants during cancer chemotherapy: impact on chemotherapeutic effectiveness and development of side effects. Nutr Cancer. 2000;**37**(1):1-18

[72] Block K, Koch A, Mead M, Newman RA, Gyllenhaal C. Re: Should supplemental antioxidant administration be avoided during chemotherapy and radiation therapy? J Natl Cancer Inst. 2009;**101**(2):124-125

[73] Beijers A, Mols F, Dercksen W, Driessen C, Vreugdenhil G. Chemotherapy-induced peripheral neuropathy and impact on quality of life 6 months after treatment with

chemotherapy. J Community Support Oncol. 2014;**12**(11):401-406

[74] Zirpoli GR, McCann SE, Sucheston-Campbell LE, et al. Supplement use and chemotherapy-induced peripheral neuropathy in a cooperative group trial (S0221): The DELCaP study. J Natl Cancer Inst. 2017;**109**:djx098. doi: 10.1093/jnci/djx098

[75] Jung AY, Cai X, Thoene K, Obi N, Jaskulski S, Behrens S, Flesch-Janys D, Chang-Claude J. Antioxidant supplementation and breast cancer prognosis in postmenopausal women undergoing chemotherapy and radiation therapy. Am J Clin Nutr. 2019;**109**(1):69-78

[76] Greenlee, H., Kwan, M.L., Ergas, I.J. et al. Changes in vitamin and mineral supplement use after breast cancer diagnosis in the Pathways Study: a prospective cohort study. BMC Cancer 2014;**14**:382. doi.org/10.1186/1471-2407-14-382

[77] Kwan ML, Greenlee H, Lee VS, Castillo A, Gunderson EP, Habel LA, Kushi LH, Sweeney C, Tam EK, Caan BJ. Multivitamin use and breast cancer outcomes in women with early-stage breast cancer: the Life After Cancer Epidemiology study. Breast Cancer Res Treat. 2011;**130**(1):195-205

[78] Lesperance ML, Olivotto IA, Forde N, Zhao Y, Speers C, Foster H, Tsao M, MacPherson N, Hoffer A. Mega-dose vitamins and minerals in the treatment of non-metastatic breast cancer: an historical cohort study. Breast Cancer Res Treat. 2002;**76**(2):137-143

[79] Kooshki A, Moghaddam M Y, Akbarzadeh R. Study of fruit and vegetable intake in breast cancer patients in the city of Sabzevar. Electronic Physician. 2016;**8**(9):3011-3014.

[80] Smith-Warner SA, Spiegelman D, Yaun SS, Adami HO, Beeson WL, van den Brandt PA, Folsom AR, Fraser GE, et al. Intake of fruits and vegetables and risk of breast cancer: a pooled analysis of cohort studies. JAMA. 2001;**285**(6):769-776

[81] Kazemi A, Barati-Boldaji R, Soltani S, Mohammadipoor N, Esmaeilinezhad Z, Clark CCT, Babajafari S, Akbarzadeh M. Intake of various food groups and risk of breast cancer: A systematic review and dose-response meta-analysis of prospective studies. Advances in Nutrition (Bethesda, Md.). 2020. doi: 10.1093/advances/nmaa147

[82] Farvid MS, Holmes MD, Chen WY, Rosner BA, Tamimi RM, Willett WC, Eliassen AH. Post-diagnostic fruit and vegetable consumption and breast cancer survival: Prospective analyses in the Nurses' Health Studies. Cancer Res. 2020; **80**(22):5134-5143.

[83] Buja A, Pierbon M, Lago L, Grotto G, Baldo V. Breast cancer primary prevention and diet: An umbrella review. Int J Environ Res Public Health. 2020;17(13):4731. doi: 10.3390/ijerph17134731

[84] van Gils CH, Peeters PH, Bueno-de-Mesquita HB, Boshuizen HC, Lahmann PH, Clavel-Chapelon F, Thiébaut A, Kesse E et al. Consumption of vegetables and fruits and risk of breast cancer. JAMA. 2005 293(2):183-193

[85] Steinmetz KA, Potter JD. Vegetables, fruit, and cancer. II. Mechanisms. Cancer Causes Control. 1991;**2**:427-442

[86] Hirsch K, Atzmon A, Danilenko M, Levy J, Sharoni Y. Lycopene and other carotenoids inhibit estrogenic activity of 17beta-estradiol and genistein in cancer cells. Breast Cancer Res Treat. 2007;**104**:221-230

[87] Gaudet MM, Britton JA, Kabat GC, Steck-Scott S, Eng SM, Teitelbaum SL, Terry MB, Neugut AI, Gammon MD. Fruits, vegetables, and micronutrients in relation to breast cancer modified by menopause and hormone receptor status. Cancer Epidemiol Biomarkers Prev. 2004;**13**:1485-1494

[88] Terry P, Jain M, Miller AB, Howe GR, Rohan TE. Dietary carotenoids and risk of breast cancer. Am J Clin Nutr. 2002;**76**:883-888

[89] Nkondjock A, Ghadirian P. Intake of specific carotenoids and essential fatty acids and breast cancer risk in Montreal, Canada. Am J Clin Nutr. 2004;**79**(5):857-864

[90] Mignone L I, Giovannucci E, Newcomb P A, Titus-Ernstoff L, Trentham-Dietz A, Hampton J. M, Willett W C, Egan K M. Dietary carotenoids and the risk of invasive breast cancer. International Journal of Cancer. 2009;**124**(12):2929-2937

[91] Hu F, Wang Yi B, Zhang W, Liang J, Lin C, Li D, Wang F, Pang D, Zhao Y. Carotenoids and breast cancer risk: a meta-analysis and meta-regression. Breast Cancer Res Treat. 2012;**131**(1):239-253

[92] Larsson SC, Bergkvist L, Wolk A. Dietary carotenoids and risk of hormone receptor-defined breast cancer in a prospective cohort of Swedish women. Eur J Cancer. 2010;**46**(6):1079-1085

[93] Huang JP, Zhang M, Holman CD, Xie X. Dietary carotenoids and risk of breast cancer in Chinese women. Asia Pac J Clin Nutr. 2007;16(Suppl 1):437-442

[94] Baena Ruiz R, Salinas Hernández P. Cancer chemoprevention by dietary phytochemicals: Epidemiological evidence. Maturitas. 2016;**94**:13-19.

[95] Rohan TE, Jain M, Howe GR, Miller AB. A cohort study of dietary carotenoids and lung cancer risk in women (Canada). Cancer Causes Control. 2002;**13**(3):231-237.

[96] Duthie S J, Duthie G G, Russell W R, Kyle J, Macdiarmid J I, Rungapamestry V, Stephen S, Megias-Baeza C, et al. Effect of increasing fruit and vegetable intake by dietary intervention on nutritional biomarkers and attitudes to dietary change: a randomized trial. European Journal of Nutrition. 2018;**57**(5):1855-1872

[97] Sato R, Helzlsouer KJ, Alberg AJ, Hoffman SC, Norkus EP, Comstock GW. Prospective study of carotenoids, tocopherols, and retinoid concentrations and the risk of breast cancer. Cancer Epidemiol Biomarkers Prev. 2002;**11**(5):451-457

[98] Bakker MF, Peeters PH, Klaasen VM, Bueno-de-Mesquita HB, Jansen EH, Ros MM, Travier N, Olsen A, Tjønneland A et al. Plasma carotenoids, vitamin C, tocopherols, and retinol and the risk of breast cancer in the European Prospective Investigation into Cancer and Nutrition cohort. Am J Clin Nutr. 2016; **103**(2):454-464

[99] Epplein M, Shvetsov YB, Wilkens LR, Franke AA, Cooney RV, Le Marchand L, Henderson BE, Kolonel LN, Goodman MT. Plasma carotenoids, retinol, and tocopherols and postmenopausal breast cancer risk in the Multiethnic Cohort Study: a nested case-control study. Breast Cancer Res. 2009;**11**(4):R49. doi:10.1186/bcr2338

[100] Hu F, Wu Z, Li G, Teng C, Liu Y, Wang F, Zhao Y, Pang D. The plasma level of retinol, vitamins A, C and α-tocopherol could reduce breast cancer risk? A meta-analysis and meta-regression. J Cancer Res Clin Oncol. 2015;**141**(4):601-614

[101] Maillard V et al. Serum carotenoid, tocopherol and retinol concentrations and breast cancer risk in the E3N-EPIC study. Int J Cancer. 2009;**127**:1188-1196

[102] Kabat GC, Kim M, Adams-Campbell LL, Caan BJ, Chlebowski RT, Neuhouser ML, Shikany JM, Rohan TE; WHI Investigators. Longitudinal study of serum carotenoid, retinol, and tocopherol concentrations in relation to breast cancer risk among postmenopausal women. Am J Clin Nutr. 2009; **90**(1):162-169

[103] Dorgan JF, Sowell A, Swanson CA, Potischman N, Miller R, Schussler N, Stephenson HE Jr. Relationships of serum carotenoids, retinol, alpha-tocopherol, and selenium with breast cancer risk: results from a prospective study in Columbia, Missouri (United States). Cancer Causes Control. 1998;**9**(1):89-97

[104] Riboli E, van Gils CH. Plasma carotenoids, vitamin C, tocopherols, and retinol and the risk of breast cancer in the European Prospective Investigation into Cancer and Nutrition cohort. Am J Clin Nutr. 2016;**103**(2):454-464

[105] Tamimi RM, Hankinson SE, Campos H, Spiegelman D, Zhang S, Colditz GA, Willett WC, Hunter DJ. Plasma carotenoids, retinol, and tocopherols and risk of breast cancer. Am J Epidemiol. 2005;**161**(2):153-160

[106] Hultén K, Van Kappel AL, Winkvist A, Kaaks R, Hallmans G, Lenner P, Riboli E. Carotenoids, alpha-tocopherols, and retinol in plasma and breast cancer risk in northern Sweden. Cancer Causes Control. 2001;**12**(6):529-537

[107] Panche A N, Diwan A D, Chandra SR. Flavonoids: an overview. Journal of Nutritional Science, 5, e47. doi.org/10.1017/jns.2016.41

[108] Batra P, Sharma AK. Anti-cancer potential of flavonoids: recent trends and future perspectives. Biotech. 2013;**3**:439-459

[109] Sak K. Epidemiological evidences on dietary flavonoids and breast cancer risk: A narrative review. Asian Pacific Journal of Cancer Prevention. 2017;**18**(9):2309-2328.

[110] Feng XL, Ho SC, Mo XF, Lin FY, Zhang NQ, Luo H, Zhang X, Zhang CX. Association between flavonoids, flavonoid subclasses intake and breast cancer risk: a case-control study in China. Eur J Cancer Prev. 2020 **29**(6):493-500

[111] Bosetti C, Spertini L, Parpinel M, Gnagnarella P, Lagiou P, Negri E, Franceschi S, Montella M, Peterson J, Dwyer J, Giacosa A, La Vecchia C. Flavonoids and breast cancer risk in Italy. Cancer Epidemiol Biomarkers Prev. 2005, **14**(4):805-808

[112] Fink BN, Steck SE, Wolff MS, et al. Dietary flavonoid intake and breast cancer risk among women on Long Island. Am J Epidemiol. 2007;**165**:514-523

[113] Feng XL, Zhan XX, Zuo LS, Mo XF, Zhang X, Liu KY, Li L, Zhang CX. Associations between serum concentration of flavonoids and breast cancer risk among Chinese women. Eur J Nutr. 2020. doi: 10.1007/s00394-020-02331-z

[114] Peterson J, Lagiou P, Samoli E, et al. Flavonoid intake and breast cancer risk: a case-control study in Greece. Br J Cancer. 2003;**89**:1255-1229

[115] Torres-Sanchez L, Galvan-Portillo M, Wolff MS, Lopez-Carrillo L. Dietary consumption of phytochemicals and breast cancer risk in Mexican women. Public Health Nutr. 2009;**12**:825-831

[116] Hui C, Qi X, Qianyong Z, Xiaoli P, Jundong Z, Mantian M. Flavonoids, flavonoid subclasses and breast cancer risk: a meta-analysis of epidemiologic studies. PLoS One. 2013;**8**(1):e54318. doi: 10.1371/journal.pone.0054318

[117] Adebamowo CA, Cho E, Sampson L, Katan MB, Spiegelman D, Willett WC, Holmes MD. Dietary flavonols and flavonol-rich foods intake and the risk of breast cancer. Int J Cancer. 2005;**114**:628-633

[118] Zamora-Ros R, Ferrari P, Gonzalez CA, et al. Dietary flavonoid and lignan intake and breast cancer risk according to menopause and hormone receptor status in the European prospective investigation into cancer and nutrition (EPIC) Study. Breast Cancer Res Treat. 2013;**139**:163-176

[119] Wang Y, Gapstur SM, Gaudet MM, et al. Evidence for an association of dietary flavonoid intake with breast cancer risk by estrogen receptor status is limited. J Nutr. 2014;**144**:1603-1611

[120] Knekt P, Kumpulainen J, Järvinen R, et al. Flavonoid intake and risk of chronic diseases. Am J Clin Nutr. 2002;**76**:560-568

[121] Pantavos A, Ruiter R, Feskens EF, et al. Total dietary antioxidant capacity, individual antioxidant intake and breast cancer risk: the Rotterdam study. Int J Cancer. 2015;**136**:2178-2186

[122] Goldbohm RA, Hertog MG, Brants HA, van Poppel G, van den Brandt PA. Intake of flavonoids and cancer risk:a prospective cohort study. In: Armado R, Andersson H, Bardocz S, Serra F, editors. In 'Polyphenols in food'. Luxembourg: Office for Official Publications of the European Communities; 1998;159-166

[123] Křížová L, Dadáková K, KašparovskáJ, KašparovskýT. Isoflavones. Molecules (Basel, Switzerland), 2019;**24**(6):1076. doi.org/10.3390/molecules24061076

[124] Sacks FM, Lichtenstein A, Van Horn L, et al. Soy protein, isoflavones, and cardiovascular health - An American heart association science advisory for professionals from the nutrition committee. Circulation. 2006;**113**:10341044

[125] Xiao CW. Health effects of soy protein and isoflavones in humans. J Nutrition. 2008;138:1244S–1249S.

[126] Wu Y.C. Meta-analysis of studies on breast cancer risk and diet in Chinese women. Int J Clin Exp Med. 2015;**8**(1):73-85

[127] Nechuta S.J. Soy food intake after diagnosis of breast cancer and survival: an in-depth analysis of combined evidence from cohort studies of US and Chinese women. Am J Clin Nutr 2012;**96**(1):123-132

[128] Zhong X., Zhang C. Soy food intake and breast cancer risk: a meta-analysis. Wei Sheng Yan Jiu. 2012;**41**(4):670-676

[129] Zheng N, Hsieh E, Cai H, Shi L, Gu K, Zheng Y, Bao PP, Shu XO. Soy food consumption, exercise, and body mass index and osteoporotic fracture risk among breast cancer survivors: The Shanghai Breast Cancer Survival Study. JNCI Cancer Spectr. 2019;**3**(2):pkz017. doi: 10.1093/jncics/pkz017

[130] Sim EJ, Ko KP, Ahn C, Park SM, Surh YJ, An S, Kim SW, Lee MH, Lee JW, Lee JE, Kim KS, Yom CK, Kim HA, Park SK. Isoflavone intake on the risk of overall breast cancer and molecular subtypes in women at high risk for hereditary breast cancer. Breast Cancer Res Treat. 2020;**184**(2):615-626.

[131] Touillaud M, Gelot A, Mesrine S, Bennetau-Pelissero C, Clavel-Chapelon F, Arveux P, Bonnet F, Gunter M,

Boutron-Ruault MC, Fournier A. Use of dietary supplements containing soy isoflavones and breast cancer risk among women aged >50 y: a prospective study. Am J Clin Nutr. 2019;**109**(3):597-605

[132] Fraser GE, Jaceldo-Siegl K, Orlich M, Mashchak A, Sirirat R, Knutsen S. Dairy, soy, and risk of breast cancer: those confounded milks. Int J Epidemiol. 2020. dyaa007. doi: 10.1093/ije/dyaa007

[133] Dong JY, Qin LQ. Soy isoflavones consumption and risk of breast cancer incidence or recurrence: a meta-analysis of prospective studies. Breast Cancer Res Treat. 2011;**125**(2):315-323.

[134] Xie Q, Chen ML, Qin Y, Zhang QY, Xu HX, Zhou Y, et al. Isoflavone consumption and risk of breast cancer: a dose-response meta-analysis of observational studies. Asia Pac J Clin Nutr. 2013;**22**(1):118-127.

[135] Chen M, Rao Y, Zheng Y, Wei S, Li Y, Guo T, et al. Association between soy isoflavone intake and breast cancer risk for pre- and post-menopausal women: a meta-analysis of epidemiological studies. PLoS ONE. 2014;**9**(2):e89288. doi: 10.1371/journal.pone.0089288

[136] Zhao TT, Jin F, Li JG, Xu YY, Dong HT, Liu Q, Xing P, Zhu GL, Xu H, Miao ZF. Dietary isoflavones or isoflavone-rich food intake and breast cancer risk: A meta-analysis of prospective cohort studies. Clin Nutr. 2019;**38**(1):136-145

[137] Morimoto Y, Maskarinec G, Park SY, Ettienne R, Matsuno RK, Long C, Steffen AD, Henderson BE, Kolonel LN, Le Marchand L, Wilkens LR. Dietary isoflavone intake is not statistically significantly associated with breast cancer risk in the Multiethnic Cohort. Br J Nutr. 2014;**112**(6):976-983

[138] Wei Y, Lv J, Guo Y, Bian Z, Gao M, Du H, Yang L, Chen Y, Zhang X, Wang T, Chen J, Chen Z, Yu C, Huo D, Li L; China Kadoorie Biobank Collaborative Group. Soy intake and breast cancer risk: a prospective study of 300,000 Chinese women and a dose-response meta-analysis. Eur J Epidemiol. 2020;**35**(6):567-578

[139] Hirose K, Imaeda N, Tokudome Y, Goto C, Wakai K, Matsuo K, Ito H, Toyama T, Iwata H, Tokudome S, Tajima K. Soybean products and reduction of breast cancer risk: a case-control study in Japan. Br J Cancer. 2005;**93**(1):15-22

[140] Messina M. Soy and health update: Evaluation of the clinical and epidemiologic literature. Nutrients. 2016;**8**(12):754. doi.org/10.3390/nu8120754

[141] Qiu S, Jiang C. Soy and isoflavones consumption and breast cancer survival and recurrence: a systematic review and meta-analysis. Eur J Nutr. 2019;**58**(8):3079-3090

[142] Guha N, Kwan ML, Quesenberry CP Jr, Weltzien EK, Castillo AL, Caan BJ. Soy isoflavones and risk of cancer recurrence in a cohort of breast cancer survivors: the Life After Cancer Epidemiology study. Breast Cancer Res Treat. 2009;**118**(2):395-405

[143] Shu XO, Zheng Y, Cai H, Gu K, Chen Z, Zheng W, Lu W. Soy food intake and breast cancer survival. JAMA. 2009;**302**(22):2437-2443

[144] Kang HB, Zhang YF, Yang JD, Lu KL. Study on soy isoflavone consumption and risk of breast cancer and survival. Asian Pac J Cancer Prev. 2012;**13**(3):995-998

[145] Woo HD, Park KS, Ro J, Kim J. Differential influence of dietary soy intake on the risk of breast cancer

recurrence related to HER2 status. Nutr Cancer. 2012;**64**(2):198-205

[146] Dong JY, Qin LQ. Soy isoflavones consumption and risk of breast cancer incidence or recurrence: a meta-analysis of prospective studies. Breast Cancer Res Treat. 2011;**125**(2):315-323

[147] Nachvak SM, Moradi S, Anjom-Shoae J, Rahmani J, Nasiri M, Maleki V, Sadeghi O. Soy, Soy isoflavones, and protein intake in relation to mortality from all causes, cancers, and cardiovascular diseases: A Systematic Review and Dose-Response Meta-Analysis of Prospective Cohort Studies. J Acad Nutr Diet. 2019;**119**(9):1483-1500

[148] Levi F, Pasche C, Lucchini F, La Vecchia C. Dietary intake of selected micronutrients and breast-cancer risk. Int J Cancer. 2001;**15**;91(2):260-263

[149] Freudenheim JL, Marshall JR, Vena JE, Laughlin R, Brasure JR, Swanson MK, Nemoto T, Graham S. Premenopausal breast cancer risk and intake of vegetables, fruits, and related nutrients. J Natl Cancer Inst. 1996;**88**(6):340-348

[150] Zhang S, Tang G, Russell RM, Mayzel KA, Stampfer MJ, Willett WC, Hunter DJ. Measurement of retinoids and carotenoids in breast adipose tissue and a comparison of concentrations in breast cancer cases and control subjects. Am J Clin Nutr. 1997;**66**(3):626-632

[151] Eliassen AH, Hendrickson SJ, Brinton LA, Buring JE, Campos H, Dai Q, Dorgan JF, Franke AA et al. Circulating carotenoids and risk of breast cancer: pooled analysis of eight prospective studies. J Natl Cancer Inst. 2012;**104**(24):1905-1916

[152] Tamimi RM, Colditz GA, Hankinson SE. Circulating carotenoids, mammographic density, and subsequent risk of breast cancer. Cancer Res. 2009;**69**(24):9323-9329

[153] Eliassen AH, Liao X, Rosner B, Tamimi RM, Tworoger SS, Hankinson SE. Plasma carotenoids and risk of breast cancer over 20 y of follow-up. Am J Clin Nutr. 2015;**101**(6):1197-1205

[154] Sesso HD, Buring JE, Zhang SM, Norkus EP, Gaziano JM. Dietary and plasma lycopene and the risk of breast cancer. Cancer Epidemiol Biomarkers Prev. 2005;**14**(5):1074-1081

[155] Bae JM, Kim EH. Breast density and risk of breast cancer in Asian Women: A Meta-analysis of observational studies. J Prev Med Public Health. 2016;**49**(6):367-375

[156] Ribaya-Mercado JD, Blumberg JB. Lutein and zeaxanthin and their potential roles in disease prevention. J Am Coll Nutr. 2004;**23**(6 Suppl):567S–587S

[157] Yan B, Lu MS, Wang L, Mo XF, Luo WP, Du YF, Zhang CX. Specific serum carotenoids are inversely associated with breast cancer risk among Chinese women: a case-control study. Br J Nutr. 2016;115(1):129-137.

[158] Toniolo P, Van Kappel AL, Akhmedkhanov A, et al. Serum carotenoids and breast cancer. Am J Epidemiol. 2001;**153**:1142-1147

[159] Rossi M, Bosetti C, Negri E, Lagiou P, La Vecchia C. Flavonoids, proanthocyanidins, and cancer risk: A network of case-control studies from Italy. Nutr Cancer. 2010;**62**(7):871-877

[160] Zhang M, Holman CD, Huang JP, Xie X. Green tea and the prevention of breast cancer: a case-control study in Southeast China. Carcinogenesis. 2007;**28**:1074-1078

[161] Wu AH, Yu MC, Tseng CC, Hankin J, Pike MC. Green tea and risk of

breast cancer in Asian Americans. Int J Cancer. 2003;**106**:574-579

[162] Shrubsole MJ, Lu W, Chen Z, Shu XO, et al. Drinking green tea modestly reduces breast cancer risk. J Nutr. 2009;**139**:310-316

[163] Yuan JM, Koh WP, Sun CL, Lee HP, Yu MC. Green tea intake, ACE gene polymorphism and breast cancer risk among Chinese women in Singapore. Carcinogenesis. 2005;**26**:1389-1394

[164] Inoue M, Robien K, Wang R, Van Den Berg DJ, et al. Green tea intake, MTHFR/TYMS genotype and breast cancer risk: the Singapore Chinese Health Study. Carcinogenesis. 2008;**29**:1967-1972

[165] Ogunleye AA, Xue F, Michels KB. Green tea consumption and breast cancer risk or recurrence: a meta-analysis. Breast Cancer Res Treat. 2010;**119**(2):477-484

[166] Gianfredi V, Nucci D, Abalsamo A, Acito M, Villarini M, Moretti M, Realdon S. Green tea consumption and risk of breast cancer and recurrence-A systematic review and meta-analysis of observational studies. Nutrients. 2018;10(12):1886-1886

[167] Inoue M, Tajima K, Mizutani M, Iwata H, et al. Regular consumption of green tea and the risk of breast cancer recurrence: follow-up study from the Hospital-based Epidemiologic Research Program at Aichi Cancer Center (HERPACC), Japan. Cancer Lett. 2001;**167**:175-182

[168] Dai Q, Shu XO, Li H, Yang G, et al. Is green tea drinking associated with a later onset of breast cancer? Ann Epidemiol. 2010;**20**:74-81

[169] Iwasaki M, Inoue M, Sasazuki S, Sawada N, et al. Green tea drinking and subsequent risk of breast cancer in a population to based cohort of Japanese women. Breast Cancer Res. 2010;12:R88. doi: 10.1186/bcr2756

[170] Nagano J, Kono S, Preston DL, Mabuchi K. A prospective study of green tea consumption and cancer incidence, Hiroshima and Nagasaki (Japan) Cancer Causes Control. 2001;**12**:501-508

[171] Suzuki Y, Tsubono Y, Nakaya N, Koizumi Y, Tsuji I. Green tea and the risk of breast cancer: pooled analysis of two prospective studies in Japan. Br J Cancer. 2004;90:1361-1363

[172] Musial, C., Kuban-Jankowska, A., & Gorska-Ponikowska, M. (2020). Beneficial Properties of Green Tea Catechins. International Journal of Molecular Sciences, 2020;**21**(5):1744. https://doi.org/10.3390/ijms21051744

[173] Singh, BN, Shankar S, Srivastava RK. Green tea catechin, epigallocatechin-3-gallate (EGCG): mechanisms, perspectives and clinical applications. Biochemical Pharmacology, 2001;**82**(12): 1807-1821. https://doi.org/10.1016/j.bcp.2011.07.093

[174] Samavat H, Ursin G, Emory TH, Lee E, Wang R, Torkelson CJ, Dostal AM, Swenson K, Le CT, Yang CS, Yu MC, Yee D, Wu AH, Yuan JM, Kurzer MS. A randomized controlled trial of green tea extract supplementation and mammographic density in postmenopausal women at increased risk of breast cancer. Cancer Prev Res (Phila). 2017;**10**(12):710-718

[175] Zhang G, Wang Y, Zhang Y, Wan X, Li J, Liu K, Wang F, Liu K, Liu Q, Yang C, Yu P, Huang Y, Wang S, Jiang P, Qu Z, Luan J, Duan H, Zhang L, Hou A, Jin S, Hsieh TC, Wu E. Anti-cancer activities of tea epigallocatechin-3-gallate in breast cancer patients under radiotherapy. Curr Mol Med. 2012;**12**(2):163-176

Chapter 3

Role of Antioxidants Supplementation in the Treatment of Male Infertility

Houda Amor, Nyaz Shelko, Massooma Mohammed, Peter Michael Jankowski and Mohamad Eid Hammadeh

Abstract

Nutritional utilization of antioxidants, such as vitamins C, E, ß-Carotene and micronutrients, such as folate and zinc, have been shown to be critically essential for normal semen quality and reproductive function. However, it is still, a large knowledge gap exists concerning the role of antioxidants on semen parameters and the role in treatment of male subfertility. Therefore, the current review article designed to find out the positive effect of antioxidants on semen quality, alterations in physiological functions of spermatozoa and infertility treatment It is advisable that patients with oxidative DNA disruption should be asked to take a simple course of antioxidants prior to undertaking assisted reproduction treatment (ART). In conclusion, antioxidant may be employed as a potent antioxidant and may improve infertility treatment outcomes with ART.

Keywords: antioxidants, male infertility, semen quality, ART

1. Introduction: The impact of oxidative stress on spermatozoa

ROS include a broad category of species including: a) Oxygen free radicals, such as superoxide anion (O_2), hydroxyl radical (OH) and hyperoxyl radical (HOO). b) Non radical species, such as hypochlorous acid (HOCl) and hydrogen peroxide (H_2O_2). c) Reactive nitrogen species and free nitrogen radicals such as nitroxylion, nitrous oxide, peroxynitrite, etc. [1–3]. These ROS are generated during normal aerobic metabolism and their level increases under stress which reflects a basic health danger. Mitochondrion is the primary cell organelle involved in ROS production. Besides, several endogenous cells and cellular components contribute towards the initiation and propagation of ROS [4, 5].

Overproduction of ROS or the deficiency of antioxidants provokes an imbalance between the per-oxidation and the anti-oxidation in the normal human body. This phenomenon is termed as Oxidative stress [6–8].

Subsequently, it leads to alterationsin peroxidation of lipid membranes of sperm, disrupting the structure of membrane receptors, enzymes, transport proteins, and causes an increase in the level of DNA fragmentation of sperm [9] (**Figure 1**).

ROS have a significant effect on the sperm plasma membrane and subsequent functional integrity of the sperm resulting in a loss of acrosome reaction [11],

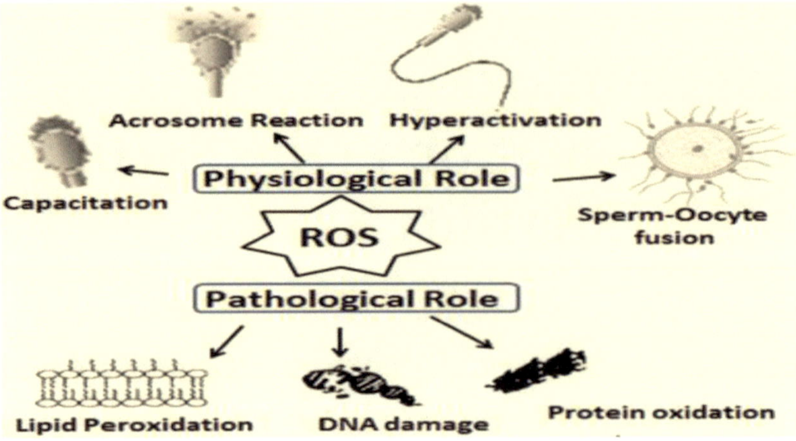

Figure 1.
Role of reactive oxygen species in male reproduction [10].

the sperm potential for fertilization [12], sperm motility and vitality [13, 14] as well as impair the sperm capacitation [15] (**Figure 1**).

Both seminal plasma and spermatozoa contain antioxidant systems able to detoxify the harmful effects of ROS. The imbalance between total antioxidant capacity and ROS generationin seminal fluid presents oxidative stress and is strongly correlated with male infertility [16].

In addition, insufficient penetration of the sperm into the oocyte in oligospermia men with elevated levels of ROS has been identified [7]. Moreover, ROS concentrations are considerably elevated in semen samples from infertile men as compared with those of healthy controls, which has suggests that infertile men may benefit highly from antioxidant supplementation [17].

Several lifestyle, stress, and environmental factors encourage excessive free radical generation and oxidative stress, including: Air pollution, cigarette smoke, alcohol intake, toxins, bacterial, fungal, or viral infections, radiation, including extensive sun bathing, intense and lengthy exercise, which provoke tissue damage, antioxidant deficiency and finally enormous intake of antioxidants, such as vitamins C and E etc.

Hammadeh presented that the oxidative stress and smoking markers, (ROS), malondialdehyde, 8-Hydroxyguanosine (8-OHdG) and cotinine were significantly higher ($P < 0.010$) in smokers as compared to non-smokers [18].

In a second study, both fertile and infertile smokers presented elevated seminal ROS level [19].

Alcohol, known as ethyl alcohol or ethanol; EtOH, promotes ROS. These ROS ultimately interact with macromolecules, among them membrane lipids, generating aldehydes such as 4-Hydroxynonenal (4-HNE) and Malondialdehyde (MDA). It is also known that aldehydes and ROS can directly interact with both proteins and DNA, ultimately leading to transcription-repression of concrete genes. In fact, the impactof ROS and aldehydes seems to serve as key factor for these alterations, partially affirmed by the fact that intake of antioxidants prevents these EtOH-induced cellular alterations [20].

The effect of oxidative stress on sperm quality has been studied extensively and estimated to be the problem in 25–87% of male infertility cases [21]. Another major driving hypothesis states that these conditions, by increasing reactive oxygen species (ROS) and nitrogen species (RONS), are capable of altering the balance of the redox status of both the steroidogenic cell population and the germ line cell populations, causing the disruption of the hypothalamic–pituitary–testicular axis and the impairment of sperm quality [22].

Therefore, the human body has developed a very concise defense system in which antioxidants play a very important role. Antioxidants are capable of decreasing the generation of free radicals, slowing or inhibiting the oxidation and repairing the damage [23]. Mirończuk-Chodakowska also presented that ROS can serveas mediators and regulators of cell metabolism and apoptosis [23].

2. Antioxidants and the sperm quality (count, motility and morphology) and function

Sperms are especially susceptible to oxidative damages due to the presence of excessive amounts of polyunsaturated fatty acids in the plasma membrane, making them highly vulnerable for lipid peroxidation by ROS, causing decreased flexibility of the sperm membrane and decreased tail motion [24]. Besides, the cytoplasm is extracted during the final stages of spermatogenesis, leaving behind the spermatozoa alone without these important enzymes to protect them from ROS altering the sperm DNA [24].

A Significant positive correlation has also been described between levels of reactive oxygen species (ROS) and percentage of spermatozoa with several types of abnormalities such as, abnormal heads, acrosome abnormalities, mid piece anomalies, cytoplasmic droplets and tail defects [25].

In previous studies, it has been demonstrated that the generation of reactive oxygen species has been linked with loss of motility and a reduced capacity for sperm–oocyte fusion [26].

In addition, seminal oxidative stress is rather negatively correlated with sperm count, function, and motility, adversely interfering with fusion required for successful fertilization [27].

Prospective studies have indicated that men with elevated levels of ROS have seven times less chance of fertilizing in comparison with men with low ROS levels. Moreover, ROS results in sperm cell damage and its high values have a negative correlation with sperm number and motility [28].

Other studies reveal that sperm exposed to elevated levels of ROS show reduction in viability and motility as confirmed through both conventional assessment and the utilization of computer-assisted sperm motility analysis [29, 30].

Antioxidant supplements are commercially available to assist treat male infertility, but research on its impact on semen quality and rates of pregnancy and live birth are rather very limited and controversial.

The male reproductive condition can be enhanced by supplementation of beneficial elements such as zinc or selenium which provide positive changes in sperm count and motility [31]. Melatonin, beta-carotene, or luteine also maintain high semen quality [32, 33]. Several studies have affirmed that higher intake of vitamin E, vitamin C, and beta –cartotine, is linked with improved sperm count motility, in both fertile and infertile men [34, 35].

Also, spermatozoa are dependent on antioxidants which already present in seminal plasma as ascorbic acid (vitamin C), α-tocopherol (vitamin E), glutathione (GSH), amino acids (taurine and hypotaurine), albumin, carnitine and carotenoids [36].

A clinical trial on the impact of antioxidants on male factor infertility enrolled a population of 171 couples. The male partner presented at least one abnormal reading concentration, mobility, morphology and DNA quality; the female partners presented normal fertility test results. Men received a placebo or an antioxidant supplement comprising of vitamins C, E, D, selenium, L-carnitine, zinc, folic acid and lycopene from three to six months [37].

In this study, no statistically significant differences in sperm concentration, mobility, morphologically normal sperm and DNA quality between the placebo and antioxidant groups after three months have been observed. Moreover, live birth rates did not differ at six months between the antioxidant (15%) and placebo (24%) groups.

3. Antioxidants and sperm DNA fragmentation and apoptosis

Spermatozoa chromatin is relatively tightly packed due to the positively charged protamine unlike histone in somatic cells [38]. This highly dense and stable structure decreases the capability of DNA disruption. Unfortunately, as spermatozoa have only a few repair mechanisms, DNA damage is generally encountered in human spermatozoa, even within the fertile donor population [39].

It has been presented that almost 40% of men searching for a fertility treatment are fertile and free of sperm oxidative DNA damage [40].

In fact, this topic was discussed in several studies. Mark et al. described that spermatozoa are especially prone to oxidative stress due to the elevated ROS level can provokea break down of sperm phospholipids and fatty acids [41].

Others have been illustrated that an increase degeneration of ROS by morphologically abnormal spermatozoa and/or decreased antioxidant capacity of seminal plasma are possible reasons of DNA damage in these patients [42, 43].

Hammadeh et al., demonstrated that the ROS level in subfertile patients was significantly higher compared with normal subjects [18].

Besides, 8-hydroxydeoxyguanosine (8OHdG) is considered to be an important sensitive oxidative biomarker for evaluating oxidative sperm DNA damage, and its levels were found be significantly higher in infertile patients compared with normal ones [18, 44].

Defective spermatozoa are also postulated to retain high residual cytoplasm, allowing them to produce excessive reactive oxygen species (ROS), which, provided their incomplete chromatin packaging, causes DNA damage [45]. Therefore, DNA damage in spermatozoa is primarily related to oxidative stress [45].

Sperm DNA damage could be testicular or post-testicular [46]. These damages may include disruptions in spermatogenesis (e.g., genetic or developmental abnormalities) and testicular or post-testicular damage (e.g., gonadotoxins, hyperthermia, oxidants, and endocrine abnormalities). It has been postulated that protamine deficiency (with subsequent aberrant chromatin remodeling), reactive oxygen species and abortive apoptosis may be associated with sperm DNA damage [18, 47].

WalczakJędrzejowska described the damaging impact of oxidative stress on sperm cells including a reduction in activity of anti-oxidative mechanisms, disruption of DNA and accelerated apoptosis [48].

Another study demonstrated that oxidative parameters in the semen of infertile men were significantly rather higher than in fertile men, and a very high correlation was observed between oxidative parameters, sperm ROS generation, and DNA fragmentation level [49].

Since sperm DNA disruption can be associated by oxidative and non-oxidative stress (caused by incomplete sperm protamination or aberrant apoptosis), the utilization of DNA fragmentation tests may not be the perfect procedure for identifying individuals with high sperm DNA damage related to oxidative stress.

Therefore, the most ideal parameters to assess DNA damage might not be DNA fragmentation but sperm-oxidation level which indirectly interferes with DNA disruptions [50, 51].

Antioxidants utilized as dietary supplements removed free radicals and decrease the degree of oxidative insult by improving the cellular redox equilibrium [52].

Several studies demonstrated positive results in the therapy of patients with moderate DNA damage exploiting oral antioxidants [42, 53, 54].

Greco and colleagues reportedan enhancement in DNA damage in 76% of patients with moderate DNA damage (≥15%) after oral intake with vitamins [53].

The beneficial impact of raised antioxidant consumption on sperm concentration and motility in the infertile patient population with no effect on sperm DNA integrity has also been observed [55].

The advantages of antioxidant therapy in male infertility are rather inconclusive with both a positive effect [53, 54] and no significant effect reported [56]. Also, Silver analyzed a cohort of fertile men and did not report any relationships between dietary antioxidant consumption (vitamins C, E or ß-carotene) and sperm DNA damage [56].

Treatment with antioxidant supplements is generally related with decreased levels of sperm DNA integrity and/or increased fertility potential [57].

The impactof these antioxidants in prohibiting sperm from endogenous ROS, gentle sperm processing and cryopreservation has yet not been established [58].

It is advisable that patients with oxidative DNA disruption should be asked to take a simple course of antioxidants prior to under taking assisted reproduction treatment. The utilization of antioxidants in decreasing sperm oxidative stress has been the topic of some 20 clinical trials over the last decade for a review [59].

Systematic review involving 29 studies evaluated the impact of oral antioxidant therapy on fertility outcomes and affirmed an overall positive effect of antioxidant supplementation on basic semen parameters, advanced sperm function, results of assisted reproductive therapy (ART), and live birth rate [60].

Oral supplementation of a either a single antioxidant or a combination of antioxidants such as L-carnitine, L-acetyl carnitine, N-acetyl-cysteine, Coenzyme Q10, selenium, vitamin C, vitamin E, and lycopene has been reported to enhance semen parameters and sperm DNA integrity in idiopathic infertile men [61].

4. Types of antioxidants

Seminal plasma comprises of a number of antioxidant enzymes, such as, superoxide dismutase, glutathione peroxidase, glutathione reductase, and catalase, and also include non-enzyme antioxidants, such as vitamin C, vitamin E, beta carotenes, carotenoids, flavonoids and metal binding proteins such as albumin, ferritin, coenzyme Q10 and myoglobin, which serve as antioxidant by inactivating pro-oxidant transition metal ions (**Figure 2**) [62–64].

The non- enzymatic antioxidants may protect the spermatozoa from oxidative DNA and membrane disruption by decreasing the singlet oxygen and the detrimental effect of lipid peroxidation on sperm [65].

4.1 Enzymatic natural antioxidants

The male reproductive system has an endogenous antioxidant for shielding spermatozoa from oxidative insult and these are categorized into enzymatic and non-enzymatic [1]. The enzyme system includes ssuperoxide dismutase (SOD), glutathione peroxidase/reductase and catalase acting as a defense against lipid peroxidation in mammalian sperm. The malfunction of these enzyme activities could lead to a loss of the cell function [66].

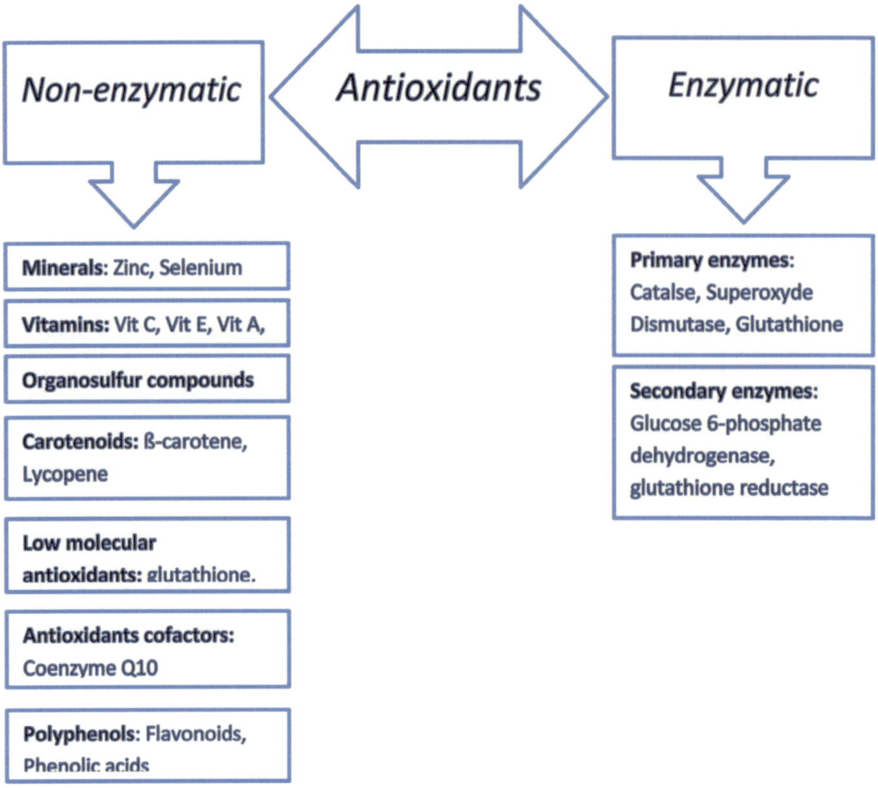

Figure 2.
Enzymatic and non-enzymatic antioxidants.

These enzymes catalytically eliminate reactive oxygen species from biological systems. Sperm themselves predominantly channel this enzymatic antioxidant [66]. Spermatozoa comprising of low intracellular antioxidant activity include superoxide dismutase (SOD), nuclear glutathione peroxidase (GPx), peroxiredoxin (PRDX), thioredoxin (TRX), and thioredoxin reductase (TRD) [67].

4.1.1 N-acetyl-cystein (NAC)

NAC serves as a precursor of glutathione (GSH) and has thus been employed as an antioxidant in many studies and trials.

The most important studies which demonstrate positive impact with varying doses in vitro are those reported by Baker et al., Oedaet al., and Lopes et al., [68–70].

Baker et al., witnessed decreased ROS generation and enhanced motility with doses ranging from 1 to 10 mmol [68]. Oeda et al. reported preserved motility with doses from 0.1 to 15 mg/ml [69] and Lopes et al. reported decreased DNA damage with 0.1 mmol of NAC [70]. The three most relevant in vivo studies provided conflicting outcomes: Comhaire et al., did not find any enhancement in sperm parameters after 3 months' administration of NAC (600 mg for 21 days) [71]; whilst the same dosage seemed to enhance sperm motility, volume, viscosity and oxidative status according to Ciftci et al., [72]. In another trial conducted on 468 patients with idiopathic OAT treated for 6 months with 600 mg/day of NAC or 200 mg/day of selenium or both, an enhancement in sperm count, motility and morphology was observed, with additive beneficial impact when both therapies were dispensed [73].

4.1.2 Glutathione peroxidase (GPx4)

Like peroxidase, Gpx4 is a member of the large family of peroxide reducing enzymes that employs glutathione as electron donor [74].

GPX4 exploits thiols in nuclear protein to reduce glutathione and may function as a redox regulation of sperm motility activation [75].

Sakai et al., found a correlation between undue production of glutathione peroxidase (GPx4) and infertility due to inhibition of ROS generation. GPx4 is not only an essential antioxidant enzyme required for sperm motility; it also plays a key role prior to capacitation [76]. However, while GPx4 shields sperm apoptosis, it decreases ROS which is an important factor for capacitation. Naturally occurring mutations in the human GPX4 gene have been related to the pathogenesis of oligoasthenozoospermia [77].

4.1.3 L-Glutathion (GSH)

GSH is one of the most essential endogenous antioxidant, implicated in sustaining the antioxidant balance in human tissues and directly engaged in the removal of ROS [78].

Due to its widely recognized antioxidant characteristics, GSH has been explored as a possible therapy for infertile patients. In vitro studies performed by Griveau and Le Lannou and by Lopes et al. have demonstrated a protective impact of 10 mmol of GSH against DNA damage caused by ROS [70, 79].

In vivo studies, two trials performed by (Lenzi et al.; Lenzi et al.,) revealed that GSH exerted a positive, statistically significant impact on sperm parameters [80, 81]. The first, Lenzi et al., discovered that 600 mg of GSH dispensed every other day for 2 months increased the motility and morphology in 21 men treated with varicocele or male accessory gland infection [82]. The second, performed the following year on 10 infertile men with the same attributes, led to similar outcomes, although a significant upsurge in sperm concentration was also observed [80, 81].

Tail-beat frequency and the shielding effect of 5–10 and 1–10 mmol GSH in vitro against the disruption of sperm motility by activated polymorphonuclear leukocytes has been reported [68, 83].

Parinaud et al., investigated the impact of Sperm-Fit, an antioxidant solution comprising of glucose and GSH, on sperm motility and showed that motility was well-preserved in leukocyte spermic samples, thus enhancing the possibility of recovering motile sperm after liquefaction and centrifugation [84].

Raijmakers et al., reported the presence of substantial amounts of GSH in the seminal plasma of both fertile and subfertile men. However, the median GSH concentrations were remarkable higher in fertile men in comparison with subfertile men. Furthermore, the concentrations of GSH in seminal plasma were directly correlated with sperm motility and inversely correlated with sperm morphology [85].

4.1.4 Superoxide dismutase (SOD)

There is some consensus on the helpful impacts of SOD on lipid peroxidation in vitro. A plethora of studies, published in last two decades of 20th century i.e. between 1991 and 1998, (for a review Lombardo et al.,) described enhanced motility and decreased lipid peroxidation in samples dosed with between 87.7 and 500 IU ml of SOD [86]. Similarly, Kovalski et al. reportedthat the incorporation of 1 mg of SOD conserved motility [87].

In the contrary, other found no decreasein lipid peroxidation after the in corporation of between 100 and 500 IU ml SOD [88]. Besides, some investigators could not affirm the impact of SOD on semen quality and sperm fertilizing potential [89]. However, the amount of endogenous antioxidants such as superoxide dismutase and catalase were also observed to be lower in smokers in comparison with fertile non-smokers [19, 90].

A direct correlation between the SOD activity and sperm damage and sperm motility was endorsed by several researchers [7].

4.1.5 Catalase (CAT)

Catalase represents one of the most effective natural enzymes which catalyzes the conversion of H_2O_2 into H_2O and O_2. CAT could play an essential role in male fertility and could turn out to be an excellent target for male infertility diagnosis.

In vitro investigations confirmed the positive impact of catalase in doses ranging from 0.008 to 0.1 mg/ml or from 50 to 2000 IU/ml on motility, peroxidation and DNA disruption [70, 79, 87].

However, Twigg et al., reported that the addition of 250, 500 or 2000 IU/ml of catalase to sperm samples did not provide any effect on lipid peroxidation. In the same study, no enhancement was observed in lipid peroxidation after the supplementation of albumin at a dose of 0.3–10% [88].

Other researcherse valuated the effects produced by different types of antioxidant therapies on semen quality in infertile males via measurement of CAT activity on seminal plasma through exogenous H_2O_2 degeneration. The results revealed that catalase activity improved after the administration of antioxidant treatments when compared to control samples without antioxidant administration [91–93].

Moreover, Catalase has also been shown to play a crucial role in male fertility. Its antioxidant activity prevents the upsurge of oxidative stress which can cause damage in sperm level, and accordingly, to reduced fertility. However, even though consensus prevails among most authors on the correlation of this scavenger with male fertility, it has only been investigated to a very limited degree of extent in this field [94].

4.1.6 Coenzyme Q10

A very strong relationship has been described to occur between sperm count, motility, and ubiquinol concentration in seminal fluid [95].

Lewin and Lavon employed coenzyme Q10 both in vivo and in vitro and revealed that the incorporation of 50 mmol in vitro caused a significant improvement in motility, whilst in vivo incorporation of 60 mg/day for almost four months resulted in an enhancement in the fertilization rate but did not provide any impact on motility, morphology or concentration in 17 patients with decreased fertilization rates after in vitro fertilization with intracytoplasmic sperm injection for male factor infertility [96].

A stimulating in vivo study conducted on 60 patients with idiopathic asthenozoospermia who were provided with either placebo or 200 mg daily of coenzyme Q10 showed a remarkable advancement in motility after 6 months of treatment; this enhancement was markedly decreased after a period of 3 months in treated subjects [97].

The exogenous incorporation of CoQ10 enhances both ubiquinone and ubiquinol levels in semen and can be useful in increasing sperm kinetic features in patients suffering from idiopathic asthenozoospermia [97].

CoQ10 biosynthesis is highly active in the testes and elevated levels of ubiquinol are found in sperm [98, 99]. Gvozdjakova et al., revealed a direct relationship between seminal plasma CoQ10 total concentration and sperm motility [100].

4.2 Non-enzymatic/synthetic/dietary supplements

4.2.1 Vitamin A

The name vitamin A includes both preformed vitamin A (retinol and its esters) and pro vitamin A carotenoids (mostly α-carotene, β-carotene, and β-cryptoxanthin). Retinol can be oxidized to retinal in a reversible manner, which provides all of the biological implications of retinol; or even further oxidized to retinoic acid, which represents the primary active metabolite of vitamin A [101].

Pro-vitamin A carotenoids can be endogenously transformed into retinoic acid whilst other carotenoids, including lutein, zeaxanthin, and lycopene, are not precursors of vitamin A but contain antioxidant capacity. Carotenoids are naturally found in fruits and vegetable. They impart the yellow, red and orange pigment in plant [102].

The most important phytochemical in the carotenoid family is lycopene which among the carotenoids, ranks as one of the most highest quencher of singlet oxygen. A combination of carotenoids, however, is highly potent as compared to individual compounds [103].

In in vitro models, β-carotene may act both as an antioxidant or a prooxidant, depending upon the redox status of the biological environment in which it acts [104].

Comhaire et al., investigated the impact of a combination therapy of 180 mg day vitamin E and 30 mg day b-carotene on a group of 27 infertile men: ROS generation decreased significantly, although no significant enhancement in semen parameters was observed [71].

Zareba et al., evaluated the effect of regular carotenoid intake on the enhancement of sperm quality in 189 young, healthy men. They evaluated semen volume, total sperm count, motility, and morphology after a period on antioxidant rich diet and observed that beta-carotene and lutein utilization elevated sperm motility [33]. However, high exploitation of some vitamins, such as vitamin A, may cause adverse reproductive outcomes [105].

4.2.1.1 Lycopene

Lycopene is one of the several constituents of the carotenoid family. Provitamin A carotenoids can be endogenously transformed into retinoic acid whilst other carotenoids, including lutein, zeaxanthin, and lycopene, which are not the precursors of vitamin A but contain antioxidant capacity. Lycopene exhibits good antioxidant activity includes singlet oxygen and free radical scavenging [106].

The presence of lycopene in human semen has been confirmed and its quantity can be enhanced after dietary intake with a natural source of Lycopene [107]. Also, very little is known about the efficacy of carotenoids, particularly that of lycopene—a potent antioxidant and singlet oxygen quencher [108].

Zini et al., preincubated washed sperm suspensions with and without lycopene followed by incubation with H_2O_2 and presented a significant decrease in sperm mobility and significant elevation of sperm DNA defragmentation in lycopne untreated samples whilst the treated samples showed a significant decrease in sperm DNA defragmentation [109].

Ghyasvand et al., performed another study to evaluate the levels of lycopene, beta-carotene and retinol in serum and their relationship with sperm DNA disruption and lipid peroxidation in infertile and normo-spermic males, and concluded that lycopene, beta-carotene, and retinol can decrease sperm DNA fragmentation and lipid peroxidation via their antioxidant effect [110].

4.2.1.2 Lutein and zeaxanthin

Comhaire et al., conducted a study involving 30 subfertile men which were treated with 16 mg a day of astaxanthin, a carotenoid which is not transformed into vitamin A in humans, for 3 months and did not find any, significant enhancement in concentration, motility, morphology or volume in the 11 treated men compared with the 19 control patients [111].

Intriguingly, Ming-Chieh Li, et al., found an unusual and unexpected inverse relationship of β-carotene administration from foods and of lutein and zeaxanthin administration with live birth rates. Within the observed administration ranges, total consumption of vitamins A, C and E before initiating infertility treatment with ART was not correlated with live birth rates [112].

4.2.2 Vitamin B (folic acid)

Folic Acid is a B-vitamin which is necessary for the synthesis of DNA and transfer of RNA.

The micronutrients folate and zinc are closely related with semen quality. Blood plasma and seminal plasma levels of folate are positively related with sperm concentration and count [113, 114].

Moreover, folic acid, the synthetic form of folate, effectively scavenges oxidizing free radicals and inhibits lipid peroxidation [115].

The evidence on the impact of folate on fertility is unclear. Wong et al., reported that in vivo utilization of folic acid, alone or combined with zinc sulphate (5 and 66 mg day respectively), enhanced sperm concentration and count in their formerly discussed controlled trial. The results were, however, significant only for the 103 infertile men involved in the study, whilst the 107 fertile men did not present any enhancement in sperm parameters [116].

Also, nutritional utilization of antioxidants, such as vitamins C and E, and β-carotene, and micronutrients, such as folate and zinc, have been shown to be critically essential for normal semen quality and reproductive function as confirmed by a large number of studies in both animals and humans [55].

Ebisch et al., showed that administration of zinc and folic acid enhancesnot only sperm quality but also the outcome of varicocelectomy [117].

Other researchers have revealed that a low folate concentration in seminal plasma is correlated with increased sperm DNA damage in infertile men [118].

Schisterman et al., designed and conducted a trial involving 2,370 couples planning infertility treatments. The men were assigned arbitrarily and received either a placebo or a daily supplement comprising of 5 milligrams of folic acid and 30 milligrams of zinc. The results indicated that the live births did not alter significantly among the two groups: 404 (34%) in the supplement group and 416 (35%) in the placebo group. Similarly, the groups did not show difference among various semen parameters, such as sperm motility, morphology and total count. However, the fraction of sperm DNA fragmentation was elevated in the supplement group (29.7%), when compared to the placebo group (27.2%). Men in the supplement group also presented an elevated proportion of gastrointestinal symptoms, when compared to the placebo group: abdominal discomfort (6% vs. 3%), nausea (4% vs. 2%) and vomiting (3% vs. 1%). The authors reported that these dietary supplements have a very little to no impact on fertility and may even provoke mild gastrointestinal symptoms [119].

4.2.3 Vitamin C

Ascorbic acid represents the main natural water-soluble antioxidant and is an essential dietary nutriment. This water-soluble antioxidant is an essential dietary nutrient.

Beside, its high potency for scavenging ROS [120], Vit-C serves as an excellent source of electrons, providing an electron to free radicals such as superoxides and hydroxyls radicals, which decreases their reactivity and damages [121].

Ascorbic acid exhibits both antioxidant and prooxidant properties depending upon the amount [122]. As an exogenous antioxidant in semen, ascorbic acid played a very crucial role in controlling the oxidative stress [47].

In an extensive study comprising of 30 infertile but healthy men, daily intake of 200 mg and 100 mg vitamin C enhanced sperm count by 112 and 140 percent respectively. Intriguingly the concentration of ascorbic acid in the seminal plasma is 10-fold higher than the serum [123].

The concentration of ascorbic acid in the seminal plasma was observed to be negatively correlated with reactive oxygen species activity in sperm of infertile men, and the reduced ascorbic acid intake was correlated with an elevated oxidative damage in the sperm of healthy men [124].

Hughes et al., reported the significance of vitamins C (300-600 mmol/l) and E (30–60 mmol/l) in protecting sperm DNA integrity in Percoll preparations; however, this combination has generated contrasting outcomes with excessive DNA damage, which is likely associated to pro-oxidant effects [125].

Donnelly et al. reported decreased H_2O_2-induced ROS production and DNA damage after the utilization of both vitamin C (300 and 600 mmol/l) and vitamin E (40 and 60 mmol/l) to normozoospermic and asthenozoospermic samples [126].

Vitamin C acts as a cofactor for various key enzymes. It assists in the metabolic processes of folic acid, tyrosine and tryptophan [127]. In cells, ascorbic acid interacts with glutathione in maintaining the reduced form of tocopherol [128].

Kini et al., reported a significant increase in the testicular GSH and SOD level but a reduction in testicular MDA level after pre-treatment of rats with Vitamin-C before cadmium chloride exposure [129]. Similar outcomes were observed by Behairy et al. [130]. In addition, vitamin C is vital in protecting from oxidative damage to the sperm and steroid cells of the Leydig cells and in the sperm chamber [131].

A potent and combined action of vitamin C and E has been observed to protect the spermatozoa against peroxidative insult and DNA fragmentation [132].

Vitamin C reduces the inter chain disulphide bridges in protamines opening the cysteine net and subsequently causing DNA decondensation in spermatozoa [54, 133, 134].

4.2.4 Vitamin D

Vitamin D plays a significant role in regulating both male and female fertility [135]. The quality of spermatozoa strongly dependen upon vitamin D [136]. Vitamin D is also responsible for retaining sperm motility [137]. Low fertility rates have also been credited to low vitamin D levels in the serum of males [138]. Vitamin D deficiency, in contrast, decreases the probabilities of success when undergoing assisted reproductive technology [139–141]. Islamian et al. investigated the combined effect of vitamin D complement and docosahexaenoic acid on oxidative stress indices of semen in asthenospermic men. The outcome showed that the combined treatment with fatty acid complement, docosahexaenoic acid and vitamin E in asthenospermic men decreased oxidative stress in seminal plasma [142].

4.2.5 Vitamin E (α-tocopherol)

Vitamin E represents a fat-soluble antioxidant molecule which serves as a major chain breaking antioxidant in membranes.

Numerous studies were conducted on vitamin E. The first clinical trials showed that vitamin E supplementation increase the fertilization rates by decreasing lipid peroxidation potential [143]. Kodama et al., reported elevated sperm concentration and decreased DNA damage in 36 infertile patients who underwent 2 months of therapy with vitamin E (200 mg day), vitamin C (200 mg day) and glutathione (GSH; 400 mg day), with no significant enhancement in motility or morphology [144].

Similarly, in another study in which a co-administration of vitamin E and selenium for six months resulted in a significant increase in sperm motility and a decreased percentage of defective spermatozoa in comparison with pre-supplementation period [145, 146]. Besides, it has also been reported that vitamin E decreases the oxvidative damage resulting an increase in the fertilization rate [71].

A plethora of research has been dedicated to show that antioxidants such as vitamins E and C and carnitines assist in reducing oxidative stress by quenching free radicals [42]. Greco et al. showed a significant enhancement in 38 men with increased sperm DNA fragmentation after 2 months of combined therapy comprising of 1 g of vitamin C and 1 g of vitamin E daily: clinical pregnancy and implantation rates presented a remarkable increase after the second attempt in comparison with an initial failed intracytoplasmic sperm injection attempt before treatment [53].

Also, vitamin E as an antioxidant may directly quench free radicals and together with CoQ10 shield lipid membranes from peroxidative insult [147].

Moslemi et al., showed that supplementation of vitamin E can significantly decrease lipid peroxidation in seminal plasma, enhance sperm motility and boost pregnancy occurrence [148].

However, in a Meta-analysis, four studies confirmed that it had a very little or no impact on semen parameters, whilst beneficial effects were shown in the remaining 18 studies [86].

4.2.6 Carnitine

The antioxidant activity of carnitines shields against lipid peroxidation of cells membrane, stimulating a large number of in vivo trials examining their impact on sperm parameters.

In the trial conducted by Costa and colleagues [149], 3 g day of L-carnitine was provided to 100 asthenozoospermic men. After 4 months of treatment, a significant enhancement in sperm concentration, motility and morphology was observed.

Balercia et al., evaluated various doses of L-carnitine and acetyl-L-carnitine (3 g of L-carnitine, 3 g of acetyl-L-carnitine, or 2 g L carnitine and 1 g acetyl-L-carnitine daily), showing enhanced sperm motility in asthenozoospermic subjects [150].

Also, Carnitine supplementation has been reported to enhance sperm concentration, mobility, viability, morphology, and total antioxidative capacity [151].

In contrast, Sigman et al., did not find any enhancements in semen parameters in 26 men diagnosed with asthenozoospermia and underwent 6 months of therapy with L-carnitine and L-acetyl-carnitine with 2 and 1 g day, respectively [152].

Gvozdjáková et al., demonstrated a beneficial impact of treatment with a combination of different antioxidants (carnitine with ubiquinol, vitamins E and C) on sperm density, which improved by 39.8% after 3 months of therapy and by 78.0% after 6 months of therapy and sperm motility was enhanced. Sperm pathology reduced in 25.8% after 3-month treatment [153].

4.2.7 Flavonoids

Flavonoids comprise of a very large heterogeneous group of benzopyran derivatives found naturally in fruits, vegetables, and herbs. This group of plant antioxidants has many beneficial health effects.

Flavonoids exhibit a positive health effect in cancer and neurodegenerative diseases, owing to their innate free radical-scavenging activities [154].

These flavonoid glycosides serve as extremely potent free radical scavengers [155, 156]. Some of the most popular and well-known antioxidant flavonoids also serve as prooxidants even when a transition metal is available [157].

Quercetinis one of the most abundant natural flavonoids found in a large variety of fruits and vegetables [158, 159].

The pentahydroxy flavone protect from oxidative injury and cell death by scavenging free radicals, donating hydrogen compound, quenching singlet oxygen, and shielding lipid peroxidation or chelating metal ions [160].

4.2.8 Selenium

Selenium is a very important trace mineral which is highly essential for the human body, including the immune system, cognitive function, and male and female fertility.

According to the United States Office of Dietary Supplements, it participates in the metabolism of thyroid hormone and DNA synthesis, and protects against infection and oxidative damage.

Selenium significantly contributes in the construction of the mitochondrial protective shield in sperm cells and interferes with the condition and function of sperm, and is potent in the treatment of impaired fertility [161].

Searching for a concrete proof of the advantages of in vivo selenium therapy is problematic, since various studies with a range of dosages have resulted in conflicting results.

Iwanier and Zachara did not find any positive impact after 3 months of therapy with selenium at a dose of 200 mg day in 33 subfertile men [162].

In 1998, Scott and his colleagues executed a trial on a group of 64 men (comprising of 46 men diagnosed with OAT and 16 classified as subfertile), dispensing selenium alone or in combination with vitamins A, C and E at daily doses of 100 mg, 1 mg, 10 mg and 15 mg respectively. No significant enhancement was observed in sperm concentration even after 3 months, although motility was increased in treated subjects [163].

However, most of the other studies have claimed enhancements in several parameters after several months of combined therapy with selenium and other antioxidants.

Vezina et al., reported that combination of selenium and vitamin E enhanced the sperm motility, morphology and viability, and the concentration, however, did not alter significantly, as previously discussed [145].

Keskes-Ammar et al., and Safarinejad employed a combination therapy—selenium and vitamin E in the former and selenium and NAC in the latter—which enhanced the motility in both studies and improved the sperm count and morphology in the latter [73, 164].

Besides, it has been demonstrated that Selenium is a fundamental element for semen quality and plays an important function in keeping reproductive condition [31, 48].

4.2.9 Zinc

Zinc is an important micronutrient which also serves as a multifunctional co-factor for more than 80 metallo enzymes involved in DNA transcription and protein synthesis [117]. Moreover, zinc finger proteins are extensively involved in the genetic expression of steroid hormone receptors [165], and it also has antioxidant [166] and anti-apoptotic properties [167].

An interesting correlation was also revealed between the level of Zn in serum and semen in oligozoospermic infertile men, with significantly decreased levels of Zn in serum and semen of men with fertility problems [168]. Zinc levels in seminal plasma have also been positively correlated with sperm concentration and motility in the literature [169, 170].

The Zinc in seminal plasma also serves as antioxidant and anti-bacterial agent which shields the semen from heavy metals accumulation [171].

Two studies were published in which $ZnSO_4$ was utilized: in the first, 500 mg/day of Zinc sulphate ($ZnSO_4$) was dispensed to 100 asthenozoospermic men for 3 months, and a significant upturn in sperm count, motility and membrane integrity was observed [172]. The second study, published 10 years later, employed a combination of drugs and Zinc sulphate ($ZnSO_4$) has been postulated as an infertility treatment, although only a few studies have shown its impact on semen parameters when applied in vivo [173].

Wong et al. observed an elevated sperm count and enhanced semen concentration in a controlled trial with 103 infertile and 107 fertile men who had consumed 5 mg folic acid and 66 mg $ZnSO_4$ per day for 6 months, either alone or in combination but no enhancements in any of the sperm parameters, most notably concentration were observed [116].

Due to its key role in the processes of DNA compaction, administration of this micronutrient i.e. Zn was very successful in enhancing sperm morphology and DNA integrity in patients suffering from prostate abnormalities [174, 175].

High seminal Zn levels may provide harmful effect on the spermatozoa-zona pellucida-induced acrosome reaction in normozoospermic men [176].

Zinc, is extensively involved in processes of reproduction, not only in the hormone metabolism but also in sperm formation and in the regulation of sperm viability and motility [31].

4.2.10 Manganese (Mn)

Manganese (Mn2+) is one of the most abundant element which is widely distributed in soil, air, water, and food [177].

It is known by its ability to quench the superoxide anions and hydroxyl radicals and due to its chain breaking capacity [178].

The structural flexibility induced by Mn2+ is also vital for enzyme dynamics, since Mn is crucial for RNA polymerization [179].

Therefore, Manganese is an essential metal which serves as a co-factor for several enzymes and plays several important biological functions [180]. Mn2+ may stimulate the enzymes of glutathione cycle and interact with the total thiols (TSH), glutathione reduced (GSH), glutathione oxidized (GSSG) contents in human spermatozoa. It reduces the generation of thiobarbituric acid reactive substances. In several organisms, elevated intracellular manganese shields against oxidative damage via unknown pathways [181].

Few studies have evaluated the impact of Mn exposure on male reproductive health. Lafond et al., showed that decreased Mn levels in seminal plasma from men with diminished sperm densities [182]. Besides, Mn2+ is a very potent stimulator of sperm motility through the stimulation of adenylate cyclase activity [183].

In addition, Manganese accelerates the progressive motility of human washed sperm in a time and dose dependent manner [184]. Moreover, it is proposed that anti-oxidative activity of Mn2+ stabilizes the plasma membrane, thereby sustaining the membrane integrity and viability [185].

Also, Mn is a necessary element for humans, but although it has several crucial functions for normal reproductive health, overexposure to Mn2 may be harmful to reproductive health [176, 186].

4.2.11 Pentoxyfilline (PTX)

PTX is a derivative of xanthine and a methylxanthine, it is a vasodilating compound which increases red blood cell deformability, prevents from inflammatory reactions and decreases blood viscosity by avoiding platelet aggregation [187].

Pentoxifylline serves as a phosphodiesterase inhibitor and shields the cells from lipid peroxidation by H_2O_2, therefore it may be helpful to minimize H_2O_2 induced embryo damage and improve IVF outcome [188].

Controversial outcomes were presented in various studies. Some studies reported that the pentoxifylline exerts a beneficial effect on sperm parameters, by decreasing the superoxide anion generation [189–191] or by minimizing lipid peroxidation [191, 192]. However, Twigg et al., did not find any enhancement in lipid peroxidation after the utilization of 3.6 mmol/l of pentoxifylline [88].

Safarinejad carried out a randomized controlled trial on a population comprising of men with idiopathic Oligoasthenoteratozoospermie (OAT). He investigated the response of semen parameters to supplementation with 400 mg of PTX twice daily for a 24-week therapy phase followed by a 12-week therapy-free period. The outcomes of that study revealed a significant enhancement in seminal parameters such as concentration, motility, and morphology [91].

It was also reported that PTX exhibited a positive impact on ICSI outcomes, including fertilization, embryo quality, and pregnancy rates, in asthenozoospermic patients [187].

In conclusion, antioxidants intake separately or combined for at least three monthes is advisable for patients who planning to undergoing ART therapy.

Conflict of interest

The authors declare that they have no conflict of interest.

Author details

Houda Amor[1], Nyaz Shelko[1,2], Massooma Mohammed[3], Peter Michael Jankowski[1] and Mohamad Eid Hammadeh[1*]

1 Department of Obstetrics and Reproductive Medicine, University of Saarland, Homburg/Saar, Germany

2 Community Health Departments, Technical College of Health, Sulaimani Polytechnic University, Kurdustan, Iraq

3 Gynecology and Obstetrics, Medicall College, University of Sulaimani, Kurdustan, Iraq

*Address all correspondence to: mehammadeh@yahoo.de; mohamad.eid.hammadeh@uks.eu

References

[1] S.C Sika, "Relative impact of oxidative stress on male reproductive functions." Curr. Med. Chem., 2001. Volume 8, Number 7, 2001, pp. 851-862(12), doi: https://doi.org/10.2174/0929867013373039

[2] V. Darley-Usmar, H. Wiseman, and B. Halliwell, "Nitric oxide and oxygen radicals: a question of balance," FEBS Letters. 1995, doi: 10.1016/0014-5793(95)00764-Z.

[3] A. R. Talebi, Sperm nuclear maturation: A basic and clinical approach. 2011.

[4] Y. Liu, G. Fiskum, and D. Schubert, "Generation of reactive oxygen species by the mitochondrial electron transport chain," J. Neurochem., 2002, doi: 10.1046/j.0022-3042.2002.00744.x.

[5] M. Inoue et al., "Mitochondrial Generation of Reactive Oxygen Species and its Role in Aerobic Life," Curr. Med. Chem., 2005, doi: 10.2174/0929867033456477.

[6] A. Agarwal, A. Hamada, and S. C. Esteves, "Insight into oxidative stress in varicocele-associated male infertility: Part 1," Nature Reviews Urology. 2012, doi: 10.1038/nrurol.2012.197.

[7] A. Agarwal, G. Virk, C. Ong, and S. S. du Plessis, "Effect of Oxidative Stress on Male Reproduction," World J. Mens. Health, 2014, doi: 10.5534/wjmh.2014.32.1.1.

[8] P. P. Mathur and S. C. D'Cruz, "The effect of environmental contaminants on testicular function," Asian Journal of Andrology. 2011, doi: 10.1038/aja.2011.40.

[9] P. Gałecka, E.; Mrowicka, M.; Malinowska, K.; Gałecki, "Role of free radicals in the physiological processes," Woln. Rod. tlenu i azotu w Fizjol. Pol. Merk. Lek, pp. 24, 446-448., 2008.

[10] *S. Fatima*, "Role of Reactive Oxygen Species in Male Reproduction," in Novel Prospects in Oxidative and Nitrosative Stress, 2018.

[11] T. Ichikawa, T. Oeda, H. Ohmori, and W. B. Schill, "Reactive oxygen species influence the acrosome reaction but not acrosin activity in human spermatozoa," Int. J. Androl., 1999, doi: 10.1046/j.1365-2605.1999.00145.x.

[12] J. G. ALVAREZ, J. C. TOUCHSTONE, L. BLASCO, and B. T. STOREY, "Spontaneous Lipid Peroxidation and Production of Hydrogen Peroxide and Superoxide in Human Spermatozoa Superoxide Dismutase as Major Enzyme Protectant Against Oxygen Toxicity," J. Androl., 1987, doi: 10.1002/j.1939-4640.1987.tb00973.x.

[13] K. Tremellen, "Oxidative stress and male infertility - A clinical perspective," Human Reproduction Update. 2008, doi: 10.1093/humupd/dmn004.

[14] R. Mahfouz et al., "Semen characteristics and sperm DNA fragmentation in infertile men with low and high levels of seminal reactive oxygen species," Fertil. Steril., 2010, doi: 10.1016/j.fertnstert.2009.12.030.

[15] R. J. Aitken and B. J. Curry, "Redox regulation of human sperm function: From the physiological control of sperm capacitation to the etiology of infertility and DNA damage in the germ line," Antioxidants Redox Signal., 2011, doi: 10.1089/ars.2010.3186.

[16] R. K. Sharma, F. F. Pasqualotto, D. R. Nelson, A. J. Thomas, and A. Agarwal, "The reactive oxygen species - Total antioxidant capacity score is a new measure of oxidative stress to predict male infertility," Hum. Reprod., 1999, doi: 10.1093/humrep/14.11.2801.

[17] A. Agarwal, G. Ahmad, and R. Sharma, "Reference values of reactive oxygen species in seminal ejaculates using chemiluminescence assay," J. Assist. Reprod. Genet., 2015, doi: 10.1007/s10815-015-0584-1.

[18] M. E. Hammadeh, M. F. Hamad, M. Montenarh, and C. Fischer-Hammadeh, "Protamine contents and P1/P2 ratio in human spermatozoa from smokers and non-smokers," Hum. Reprod., 2010, doi: 10.1093/humrep/deq226.

[19] E. A. Taha, A. M. Ez-Aldin, S. K. Sayed, N. M. Ghandour, and T. Mostafa, "Effect of smoking on sperm vitality, DNA integrity, seminal oxidative stress, zinc in fertile men," Urology, 2012, doi: 10.1016/j.urology.2012.07.002.

[20] H. H. Byung. et al., "Contribution of reactive oxygen species to cerebral amyloid angiopathy, vasomotor dysfunction, and microhemorrhage in aged Tg2576 mice," Proc. Natl. Acad. Sci. U. S. A., 2015.

[21] R. Smits, K. D'Hauwers, J. Inthout, Di. Braat, and K. Fleischer, "Impact of a nutritional supplement (Impryl) on male fertility: Study protocol of a multicentre, randomised, double-blind, placebo-controlled clinical trial (SUppleMent Male fERtility, SUMMER trial)," BMJ Open, 2020, doi: 10.1136/bmjopen-2019-035069.

[22] A. Ferlin and C. Foresta, "New genetic markers for male infertility," Current Opinion in Obstetrics and Gynecology. 2014, doi: 10.1097/GCO.0000000000000061.

[23] I. Mirończuk-Chodakowska, A. M. Witkowska, and M. E. Zujko, "Endogenous non-enzymatic antioxidants in the human body," Advances in Medical Sciences. 2018, doi: 10.1016/j.advms.2017.05.005.

[24] *C. Lewis* and A. T. Ford, "Infertility in male aquatic invertebrates: A review," Aquatic Toxicology. 2012, doi: 10.1016/j.aquatox.2012.05.002.

[25] C. I. Kobayashi and T. Suda, "Regulation of reactive oxygen species in stem cells and cancer stem cells," Journal of Cellular Physiology. 2012, doi: 10.1002/jcp.22764.

[26] A. Agarwal, R. A. Saleh, and M. A. Bedaiwy, "Role of reactive oxygen species in the pathophysiology of human reproduction," Fertility and Sterility. 2003, doi: 10.1016/S0015-0282(02)04948-8.

[27] S. L, "Human Physiology from Cell to Systems. 6th ed," Cengage Learn. Boston, MA, USA, 2011.

[28] A. Mehrotra, D. K. Katiyar, A. Agarwal, V. Das, and K. K. Pant, "Role of total antioxidant capacity and lipid peroxidation in fertile and infertile men," Biomed. Res., 2013.

[29] T. Y. Shi et al., "Effects of reactive oxygen species from activated leucocytes on human sperm motility, viability and morphology," Andrologia, 2012, doi: 10.1111/j.1439-0272.2011.01252.x.

[30] L. S. De Castro et al., "Sperm oxidative stress is detrimental to embryo development: A dose-dependent study model and a new and more sensitive oxidative status evaluation," Oxid. Med. Cell. Longev., 2016, doi: 10.1155/2016/8213071.

[31] F. Atig, M. Raffa, B. A. Habib, A. Kerkeni, A. Saad, and M. Ajina, "Impact of seminal trace element and glutathione levels on semen quality of Tunisian infertile men," BMC Urol., 2012, doi: 10.1186/1471-2490-12-6.

[32] R. J. Aitken and S. D. Roman, "Antioxidant systems and oxidative stress in the testes.," Oxidative medicine and cellular longevity. 2008, doi: 10.4161/oxim.1.1.6843.

[33] P. Zareba et al., "Semen quality in relation to antioxidant intake in a healthy male population," Fertil. Steril., 2013, doi: 10.1016/j.fertnstert.2013.08.032.

[34] M. Akmal, J. Q. Qadri, N. S. Al-Waili, S. Thangal, A. Haq, and K. Y. Saloom, "Improvement in human semen quality after oral supplementation of vitamin C," J. Med. Food, 2006, doi: 10.1089/jmf.2006.9.440.

[35] D. P. D. A. F. Braga, G. Halpern, R. D. C. S. Figueira, A. S. Setti, A. Iaconelli, and E. Borges, "Food intake and social habits in male patients and its relationship to intracytoplasmic sperm injection outcomes," Fertil. Steril., 2012, doi: 10.1016/j.fertnstert.2011.10.011.

[36] S. E. M. Lewis et al., "The impact of sperm DNA damage in assisted conception and beyond: Recent advances in diagnosis and treatment," Reproductive BioMedicine Online. 2013, doi: 10.1016/j.rbmo.2013.06.014.

[37] A. Z. Steiner et al., "The effect of antioxidants on male factor infertility: the Males, Antioxidants, and Infertility (MOXI) randomized clinical trial," Fertil. Steril., 2020, doi: 10.1016/j.fertnstert.2019.11.008.

[38] S. Sepaniak, T. Forges, H. Gerard, B. Foliguet, M. C. Bene, and P. Monnier-Barbarino, "The influence of cigarette smoking on human sperm quality and DNA fragmentation," Toxicology, 2006, doi: 10.1016/j.tox.2006.03.001.

[39] L. Simon, G. Brunborg, M. Stevenson, D. Lutton, J. McManus, and S. E. M. Lewis, "Clinical significance of sperm DNA damage in assisted reproduction outcome," Hum. Reprod., 2010, doi: 10.1093/humrep/deq103.

[40] P. Cohen-Bacrie, S. Belloc, Y. J. R. Ménézo, P. Clement, J. Hamidi, and M. Benkhalifa, "Correlation between DNA damage and sperm parameters: a prospective study of 1,633 patients," Fertil. Steril., 2009, doi: 10.1016/j.fertnstert.2008.01.086.

[41] V. Mak, K. Jarvi, M. Buckspan, M. Freeman, S. Hechter, and A. Zini, "Smoking is associated with the retention of cytoplasm by human spermatozoa," Urology, 2000, doi: 10.1016/S0090-4295(00)00700-7.

[42] A. Agarwal, K. P. Nallella, S. S. R. Allamaneni, and T. M. Said, "Role of antioxidants in treatment of male infertility: An overview of the literature," Reproductive BioMedicine Online. 2004, doi: 10.1016/S1472-6483(10)61641-0.

[43] S. I. Moskovtsev, J. Willis, A. Azad, and J. B. M. Mullen, "Sperm DNA integrity: Correlation with sperm plasma membrane integrity in semen evaluated for male infertility," Arch. Androl., 2005, doi: 10.1080/014850190512770.

[44] S. Loft et al., "Oxidative DNA damage in human sperm influences time to pregnancy," Hum. Reprod., 2003, doi: 10.1093/humrep/deg202.

[45] R. J. Aitken and G. N. De Iuliis, "On the possible origins of DNA damage in human spermatozoa," Molecular Human Reproduction. 2009, doi: 10.1093/molehr/gap059.

[46] F. D. Henkel RR, "Sperm DNA fragmentation: origin and impact on human reproduction.," J Reprod Biotech Fertil., pp. 2: 88-108., 2011.

[47] A. Zini, O. Albert, and B. Robaire, "Assessing sperm chromatin and DNA damage: Clinical importance and development of standards," Andrology. 2014, doi: 10.1111/j.2047-2927.2014.00193.x.

[48] R. Walczak-Jedrzejowska, J. K. Wolski, and J. Slowikowska-Hilczer, "The role of oxidative stress and

antioxidants in male fertility," Cent. Eur. J. Urol., 2013, doi: 10.5173/ceju.2013.01.art19.

[49] G. Aktan, S. Doğru-Abbasoğlu, C. Küçükgergin, A. Kadioğlu, G. Özdemirler-Erata, and N. Koçak-Toker, "Mystery of idiopathic male infertility: Is oxidative stress an actual risk?," Fertil. Steril., 2013, doi: 10.1016/j.fertnstert.2012.11.045.

[50] A. Noblanc et al., "DNA oxidative damage in mammalian spermatozoa: Where and why is the male nucleus affected?," Free Radic. Biol. Med., 2013, doi: 10.1016/j.freeradbiomed.2013.07.044.

[51] S. Vorilhon et al., "Accuracy of human sperm DNA oxidation quantification and threshold determination using an 8-OHdG immuno-detection assay," Hum. Reprod., 2018, doi: 10.1093/humrep/dey038.

[52] W. Y. Wong, C. M. G. Thomas, J. M. W. M. Merkus, G. A. Zielhuis, and R. P. M. Steegers-Theunissen, "Male factor subfertility: Possible causes and the impact of nutritional factors," Fertility and Sterility. 2000, doi: 10.1016/S0015-0282(99)00551-8.

[53] E. Greco, M. Iacobelli, L. Rienzi, F. Ubaldi, S. Ferrero, and J. Tesarik, "Reduction of the incidence of sperm DNA fragmentation by oral antioxidant treatment," J. Androl., 2005, doi: 10.2164/jandrol.04146.

[54] Y. J. R. Ménézo et al., "Antioxidants to reduce sperm DNA fragmentation: An unexpected adverse effect," Reprod. Biomed. Online, 2007, doi: 10.1016/S1472-6483(10)60887-5.

[55] B. Eskenazi, S. A. Kidd, A. R. Marks, E. Sloter, G. Block, and A. J. Wyrobek, "Antioxidant intake is associated with semen quality in healthy men," Hum. Reprod., 2005, doi: 10.1093/humrep/deh725.

[56] E. W. Silver, B. Eskenazi, D. P. Evenson, G. Block, S. Young, and A. J. Wyrobek, "Effect of antioxidant intake on sperm chromatin stability in healthy nonsmoking men," J. Androl., 2005, doi: 10.2164/jandrol.04165.

[57] P. Piomboni, L. Gambera, F. Serafini, G. Campanella, G. Morgante, and V. De Leo, "Sperm quality improvement after natural anti-oxidant treatment of asthenoteratospermic men with leukocytospermia," Asian J. Androl., 2008, doi: 10.1111/j.1745-7262.2008.00356.x.

[58] A. Zini, M. San Gabriel, and A. Baazeem, "Antioxidants and sperm DNA damage: A clinical perspective," Journal of Assisted Reproduction and Genetics. 2009, doi: 10.1007/s10815-009-9343-5.

[59] P. Gharagozloo and R. J. Aitken, "The role of sperm oxidative stress in male infertility and the significance of oral antioxidant therapy," Human Reproduction. 2011, doi: 10.1093/humrep/der132.

[60] A. Majzoub and A. Agarwal, "Systematic review of antioxidant types and doses in male infertility: Benefits on semen parameters, advanced sperm function, assisted reproduction and live-birth rate," Arab J. Urol., 2018, doi: 10.1016/j.aju.2017.11.013.

[61] M. Arafa et al., "Efficacy of antioxidant supplementation on conventional and advanced sperm function tests in patients with idiopathic male infertility," Antioxidants, 2020, doi: 10.3390/antiox9030219.

[62] M. G. GERMAN, J. B., & TRABER, "Nutrients and oxidation: Actions, transport, and metabolism of dietary antioxidants.," Handb. Vitamins. 3rd Ed, Rucker RB, JW Suttie, DB McCormick,

LJ Machlin (Eds), Marcel Dekker Inc., New York, USA, pp. 569-588., 2001.

[63] L. C. GM, . "Potential for *Ginkgo biloba* as a functional food," Dr. Diss., 2004.

[64] S. Jube and D. Borthakur, "Recent Advances in Food Biotechnology Research," in Food Biochemistry and Food Processing, 2007.

[65] S. E. M. Lewis, E. S. L. Sterling, I. S. Young, and W. Thompson, "Comparison of individual antioxidants of sperm and seminal plasma in fertile and infertile men," Fertil. Steril., 1997, doi: 10.1016/S0015-0282(97)81871-7.

[66] N. Sheikh, I. Amiri, M. Farimani, R. Najafi, and J. Hedeie, "Correlation between sperm parameters and sperm DNA fragmentation in fertile and infertile men," Iran. J. Reprod. Med., 2008.

[67] C. O'flaherty, "Peroxiredoxin 6: The protector of male fertility," Antioxidants. 2018, doi: 10.3390/antiox7120173.

[68] H. W. G. Baker, J. Brindle, D. S. Irvine, and R. J. Aitken, "Protective effect of antioxidants on the impairment of sperm motility by activated polymorphonuclear leukocytes," Fertil. Steril., 1996, doi: 10.1016/s0015-0282(16)58109-6.

[69] T. Oeda, R. Henkel, H. Ohmori, and W. B. Schill, "Scavenging effect of N-acetyl-L-cysteine against reactive oxygen species in human semen: A possible therapeutic modality for male factor infertility?," Andrologia, 1997, doi: 10.1111/j.1439-0272.1997.tb00305.x.

[70] S. Lopes, A. Jurisicova, J. G. Sun, and R. F. Casper, "Reactive oxygen species: Potential cause for DNA fragmentation in human spermatozoa," Hum. Reprod., 1998, doi: 10.1093/humrep/13.4.896.

[71] F. H. Comhaire, A. B. Christophe, A. A. Zalata, W. S. Dhooge, A. M. A. Mahmoud, and C. E. Depuydt, "The effects of combined conventional treatment, oral antioxidants and essential fatty acids on sperm biology in subfertile men," Prostaglandins Leukot. Essent. Fat. Acids, 2000, doi: 10.1054/plef.2000.0174.

[72] H. Ciftci, A. Verit, M. Savas, E. Yeni, and O. Erel, "Effects of N-acetylcysteine on Semen Parameters and Oxidative/Antioxidant Status," Urology, 2009, doi: 10.1016/j.urology.2009.02.034.

[73] M. R. Safarinejad and S. Safarinejad, "Efficacy of Selenium and/or N-Acetyl-Cysteine for Improving Semen Parameters in Infertile Men: A Double-Blind, Placebo Controlled, Randomized Study," J. Urol., 2009, doi: 10.1016/j.juro.2008.10.015.

[74] L. Flohé and F. Ursini, "Peroxidase: A term of many meanings," Antioxidants and Redox Signaling. 2008, doi: 10.1089/ars.2008.2059.

[75] R. J. Aitken, "Possible redox regulation of sperm motility activation," Journal of Andrology. 2000, doi: 10.1002/j.1939-4640.2000.tb02113.x.

[76] S. O., U. T., I. H., U. T., and A. S., "Role of glutathione peroxidase 4 in conjunctival epithelial cells," Investig. Ophthalmol. Vis. Sci., 2015.

[77] M. Diaconu et al., "Failure of phospholipid hydroperoxide glutathione peroxidase expression in oligoasthenozoospermia and mutations in the PHGPx gene," Andrologia, 2006, doi: 10.1111/j.1439-0272.2006.00729.x.

[78] X. Shan, T. Y. Aw, and D. P. Jones, "Glutathione-dependent projection against oxidative injury," Pharmacology and Therapeutics. 1990, doi: 10.1016/0163-7258(90)90045-4.

[79] J. E. GRIVEAU and D. LE LANNOU, "Effects of antioxidants on human sperm preparationtechniques," Int. J. Androl., 1994, doi: 10.1111/j.1365-2605.1994.tb01247.x.

[80] *A. lenzi*, F. Culasso, L. Gandini, F. Lombardo, and F. Dondero, "Andrology: Placebo-controlled, double-blind, cross-over trial of glutathione therapy in male infertility," Hum. Reprod., 1993, doi: 10.1093/oxfordjournals.humrep.a137909.

[81] *A. lenzi* et al., "Andrology: Glutathione treatment of dyspermia: Effect on the lipoperoxidation process," Hum. Reprod., 1994, doi: 10.1093/oxfordjournals.humrep.a138391.

[82] L. A., C. F., G. L., L. F., and D. F., "Placebo-controlled, double-blind, cross-over trial of glutathione therapy in male infertility," Hum. Reprod., 1993.

[83] C. Y. Hong, M. F. Lee, L. J. Lai, and C. P. Wang, "Effect of lipid peroxidation on beating frequency of human sperm tail," Andrologia, 1994, doi: 10.1111/j.1439-0272.1994.tb00757.x.

[84] J. Parinaud, D. Le Lannou, G. Vieitez, J. F. Griveau, P. Milhet, and G. Richoilley, "Enhancement of motility by treating spermatozoa with an antioxidant solution (Sperm-Fit®) following ejaculation," Hum. Reprod., 1997, doi: 10.1093/humrep/12.11.2434.

[85] M. T. M. Raijmakers et al., "Glutathione and glutathione S-transferases A1-1 and P1-1 in seminal plasma may play a role in protecting against oxidative damage to spermatozoa," Fertil. Steril., 2003, doi: 10.1016/S0015-0282(02)04404-7.

[86] F. Lombardo, A. Sansone, F. Romanelli, D. Paoli, L. Gandini, and *A. lenzi*, "The role of antioxidant therapy in the treatment of male infertility: An overview," Asian Journal of Andrology. 2011, doi: 10.1038/aja.2010.183.

[87] N. N. Kovalski, E. De Lamirande, and C. Gagnon, "Reactive oxygen species generated by human neutrophils inhibit sperm motility: Protective effect of seminal plasma and scavengers," Fertil. Steril., 1992, doi: 10.1016/s0015-0282(16)55332-1.

[88] J. Twigg, N. Fulton, E. Gomez, D. Stewart Irvine, and R. John Aitken, "Analysis of the impact of intracellular reactive oxygen species generation on the structural and functional integrity of human spermatozoa: Lipid peroxidation, DNA fragmentation and effectiveness of antioxidants," Hum. Reprod., 1998, doi: 10.1093/humrep/13.6.1429.

[89] Y. Y. Hsieh, Y. L. Sun, C. C. Chang, Y. S. Lee, H. Der Tsai, and C. S. Lin, "Superoxide dismutase activities of spermatozoa and seminal plasma are not correlated with male infertility," J. Clin. Lab. Anal., 2002, doi: 10.1002/jcla.10029.

[90] M. F. Elshal, I. H. El-Sayed, M. A. Elsaied, S. A. El-Masry, and T. A. Kumosani, "Sperm head defects and disturbances in spermatozoal chromatin and DNA integrities in idiopathic infertile subjects: Association with cigarette smoking," Clin. Biochem., 2009, doi: 10.1016/j.clinbiochem.2008.11.012.

[91] M. R. Safarinejad, "Effect of pentoxifylline on semen parameters, reproductive hormones, and seminal plasma antioxidant capacity in men with idiopathic infertility: A randomized double-blind placebo-controlled study," Int. Urol. Nephrol., 2011, doi: 10.1007/s11255-010-9826-4.

[92] A. Nadjarzadeh et al., "Effect of Coenzyme Q10 supplementation on antioxidant enzymes activity and oxidative stress of seminal plasma: A double-blind randomised clinical trial," Andrologia, 2014, doi: 10.1111/and.12062.

[93] B. Tartibian and B. H. Maleki, "The effects of honey supplementation on seminal plasma cytokines, oxidative stress biomarkers, and antioxidants during 8 weeks of intensive cycling training," J. Androl., 2012, doi: 10.2164/jandrol.110.012815.

[94] N. Rubio-Riquelme, N. Huerta-Retamal, M. J. Gómez-Torres, and R. M. Martínez-Espinosa, "Catalase as a molecular target for male infertility diagnosis and monitoring: An overview," Antioxidants. 2020, doi: 10.3390/antiox9010078.

[95] R. Alleva, A. Scararmucci, F. Mantero, S. Bompadre, *L. Leoni*, and G. P. Littarru, "The protective role of ubiquinol-10 against formation of lipid hydroperoxides in human seminal fluid," 1997, doi: 10.1016/S0098-2997(97)00040-X.

[96] A. Lewin and H. Lavon, "The effect of coenzyme Q10 on sperm motility and function," 1997, doi: 10.1016/S0098-2997(97)00036-8.

[97] G. Balercia et al., "Coenzyme Q10 and male infertility," Journal of Endocrinological Investigation. 2009, doi: 10.3275/6301.

[98] A. Mancini, G. Conte, D. Milardi, L. De Marinis, and G. P. Littarru, "Relationship between sperm cell ubiquinone and seminal parameters in subjects with and without varicocele," Andrologia, 1998, doi: 10.1111/j.1439-0272.1998.tb01374.x.

[99] G. P. Littarru and L. Tiano, "Clinical aspects of coenzyme Q10 in relationship with its bioenergetic and antioxidant properties," in Mitochondrial Medicine: Mitochondrial Metabolism, Diseases, Diagnosis and Therapy, 2008.

[100] A. Gvozdjakova et al., "Importance of the assessment of coenzyme Q10, alpha-tocopherol and oxidative stress for the diagnosis and therapy of infertility in men," Bratislava Med. J., 2013, doi: 10.4149/BLL_2013_129.

[101] S. NW, "Vitamin A In: Erdman JWMI, Zeisel SH, ed. Present Knowledge in Nutrition. 10th Edition ed," John Wiley Sons Ltd, pp. 149-184, 2012.

[102] A. V. Rao, M. R. Ray, and L. G. Rao, "Lycopene," Advances in Food and Nutrition Research. 2006, doi: 10.1016/S1043-4526(06)51002-2.

[103] A. V. Rao and S. Agarwal, "Role of lycopene as antioxidant carotenoid in the prevention of chronic diseases: A review," Nutrition Research. 1999, doi: 10.1016/S0271-5317(98)00193-6.

[104] P. Palozza, S. Serini, F. Di Nicuolo, E. Piccioni, and G. Calviello, "Prooxidant effects of β-carotene in cultured cells," Molecular Aspects of Medicine. 2003, doi: 10.1016/S0098-2997(03)00031-1.

[105] K. J. Rothman, L. L. Moore, M. R. Singer, U.-S. D. T. Nguyen, S. Mannino, and A. Milunsky, "Teratogenicity of High Vitamin A Intake," N. Engl. J. Med., 1995, doi: 10.1056/nejm199511233332101.

[106] E. J. Johnson, "The role of carotenoids in human health.," Nutrition in clinical care : an official publication of Tufts University. 2002, doi: 10.1046/j.1523-5408.2002.00004.x.

[107] A. Goyal, M. Chopra, B. A. Lwaleed, B. Birch, and A. J. Cooper, "The effects of dietary lycopene supplementation on human seminal plasma," BJU Int., 2007, doi: 10.1111/j.1464-410X.2007.06804.x.

[108] A. V. Rao and L. G. Rao, "Carotenoids and human health," Pharmacological Research. 2007, doi: 10.1016/j.phrs.2007.01.012.

[109] A. Zini, M. San Gabriel, and J. Libman, "Lycopene supplementation in vitro can protect human sperm deoxyribonucleic acid from oxidative damage," Fertil. Steril., 2010, doi: 10.1016/j.fertnstert.2009.04.004.

[110] T. Ghyasvand, M. T. Goodarzi, I. Amiri, J. Karimi, and M. Ghorbani, "Serum levels of Lycopene, beta-carotene, and retinol and their correlation with sperm DNA damage in Normospermic and infertile men," Iran. J. Reprod. Med., 2015, doi: 10.29252/ijrm.13.12.787.

[111] F. H. Comhaire, Y. El Garem, A. Mahmoud, F. Eertmans, and F. Schoonjans, "Combined conventional/antioxidant 'Astaxanthin' treatment for male infertility: A double blind, randomized trial," Asian J. Androl., 2005, doi: 10.1111/j.1745-7262.2005.00047.x.

[112] L. M.-C. et al., "Men's Intake of Vitamin C and β-Carotene Is Positively Related to Fertilization Rate but Not to Live Birth Rate in Couples Undergoing Infertility Treatment," J. Nutr., 2019.

[113] L. M. Wallock, T. Tamura, C. A. Mayr, K. E. Johnston, B. N. Ames, and R. A. Jacob, "Low seminal plasma folate concentrations are associated with low sperm density and count in male smokers and nonsmokers," Fertil. Steril., 2001, doi: 10.1016/S0015-0282(00)01697-6.

[114] J. R. Wallock L, Tamura T, Ames B, Johnston K, Gretz D, "Improvements in folate indices in blood and seminal plasma following vitamin supplementation in smokers and nonsmokers [abstract].," FASEB J, p. 13:A890., 1999.

[115] R. Joshi, S. Adhikari, B. S. Patro, S. Chattopadhyay, and T. Mukherjee, "Free radical scavenging behavior of folic acid: Evidence for possible antioxidant activity," Free Radic. Biol. Med., 2001, doi: 10.1016/S0891-5849(01)00543-3.

[116] W. Y. Wong, H. M. W. M. Merkus, C. M. G. Thomas, R. Menkveld, G. A. Zielhuis, and R. P. M. Steegers-Theunissen, "Effects of folic acid and zinc sulfate on male factor subfertility: A double-blind, randomized, placebo-controlled trial," Fertil. Steril., 2002, doi: 10.1016/S0015-0282(01)03229-0.

[117] I. M. W. Ebisch, C. M. G. Thomas, W. H. M. Peters, D. D. M. Braat, and R. P. M. Steegers-Theunissen, "The importance of folate, zinc and antioxidants in the pathogenesis and prevention of subfertility," Human Reproduction Update. 2007, doi: 10.1093/humupd/dml054.

[118] J. C. Boxmeer et al., "Low folate in seminal plasma is associated with increased sperm DNA damage," Fertil. Steril., 2009, doi: 10.1016/j.fertnstert.2008.06.010.

[119] E. F. Schisterman et al., "Effect of Folic Acid and Zinc Supplementation in Men on Semen Quality and Live Birth among Couples Undergoing Infertility Treatment: A Randomized Clinical Trial," JAMA - J. Am. Med. Assoc., 2020, doi: 10.1001/jama.2019.18714.

[120] T. Brzozowski et al., "Comparison of nitric oxide-releasing NSAID and vitamin C with classic NSAID in healing of chronic gastric ulcers; involvement of reactive oxygen species," Med. Sci. Monit., 2001.

[121] E. Levine M., Ebenuwa I., Violet P.-C.Chapter 17—Vitamin C. In: Prasad A.S., Brewer G.J., "Essential and Toxic Trace Elements and Vitamins in Human Health," Acad. Press. Cambridge, MA, USA, pp. 241-262, 2020.

[122] M. Y. Seo and S. M. Lee, "Protective effect of low dose of ascorbic acid on hepatobiliary function

in hepatic ischemia/reperfusion in rats," J. Hepatol., 2002, doi: 10.1016/S0168-8278(01)00236-7.

[123] R. A. Jacob, F. S. Pianalto, and R. E. Agee, "Cellular ascorbate depletion in healthy men," J. Nutr., 1992, doi: 10.1093/jn/122.5.1111.

[124] C. G. Fraga, P. A. Motchnik, M. K. Shigenaga, H. J. Helbock, R. A. Jacob, and B. N. Ames, "Ascorbic acid protects against endogenous oxidative DNA damage in human sperm," Proc. Natl. Acad. Sci. U. S. A., 1991, doi: 10.1073/pnas.88.24.11003.

[125] C. M. Hughes, S. E. M. Lewis, V. J. McKelvey-Martin, and W. Thompson, "The effects of antioxidant supplementation during Percoll preparation on human sperm DNA integrity," Hum. Reprod., 1998, doi: 10.1093/humrep/13.5.1240.

[126] E. T. Donnelly, N. McClure, and S. E. M. Lewis, "The effect of ascorbate and α-tocopherol supplementation in vitro on DNA integrity and hydrogen peroxide-induced DNA damage in human spermatozoa," Mutagenesis, 1999, doi: 10.1093/mutage/14.5.505.

[127] K. Iqbal, A. Khan, and M. Muzaffar Ali Khan Khattak, "Biological Significance of Ascorbic Acid (Vitamin C) in Human Health-A Review," 2004.

[128] A. E. Wagner et al., "Free radical scavenging and antioxidant activity of ascorbigen versus ascorbic acid: Studies in vitro and in cultured human keratinocytes," J. Agric. Food Chem., 2008, doi: 10.1021/jf802403d.

[129] K. P. . Kini R.D., Tripathi Y.B., Raghuveer C.V., Pai S., Ramaswamy C., "Role of vitamin C as an antioxidant in cadmium chloride induced testicular damage," Int. J. Appl. Biol. Pharm, pp. 2: 484-488, 2011.

[130] A. Behairy et al., "The modulatory role of vitamin C in boldenone undecylenate induced testicular oxidative damage and androgen receptor dysregulation in adult male rats," Antioxidants, 2020, doi: 10.3390/antiox9111053.

[131] E. Mangoli et al., "Vitamin C attenuates negative effects of vitrification on sperm parameters, chromatin quality, apoptosis and acrosome reaction in neat and prepared normozoospermic samples," Taiwan. J. Obstet. Gynecol., 2018, doi: 10.1016/j.tjog.2018.02.006.

[132] U. R. Acharya, M. Mishra, J. Patro, and M. K. Panda, "Effect of vitamins C and E on spermatogenesis in mice exposed to cadmium," Reprod. Toxicol., 2008, doi: 10.1016/j.reprotox.2007.10.004.

[133] D. Giustarini, I. Dalle-Donne, R. Colombo, A. Milzani, and R. Rossi, "Is ascorbate able to reduce disulfide bridges? A cautionary note," Nitric Oxide - Biol. Chem., 2008, doi: 10.1016/j.niox.2008.07.003.

[134] E. T. Donnelly, N. McClure, and S. E. M. Lewis, "Antioxidant supplementation in vitro does not improve human sperm motility," Fertil. Steril., 1999, doi: 10.1016/S0015-0282(99)00267-8.

[135] M. J. Berridge, "Vitamin d deficiency: Infertility and neurodevelopmental diseases (attention deficit hyperactivity disorder, autism, and schizophrenia)," American Journal of Physiology - Cell Physiology. 2018, doi: 10.1152/ajpcell.00188.2017.

[136] I. M. Boisen, L. Bøllehuus Hansen, L. J. Mortensen, B. Lanske, A. Juul, and M. Blomberg Jensen, "Possible influence of vitamin D on male reproduction," Journal of Steroid Biochemistry and Molecular Biology. 2017, doi: 10.1016/j.jsbmb.2016.09.023.

[137] M. B. Jensen et al., "Vitamin D deficiency and low ionized calcium are linked with semen quality and sex steroid levels in infertile men," Hum. Reprod., 2016, doi: 10.1093/humrep/dew152.

[138] M. Tartagni et al., "Males with low serum levels of vitamin D have lower pregnancy rates when ovulation induction and timed intercourse are used as a treatment for infertile couples: Results from a pilot study," Reprod. Biol. Endocrinol., 2015, doi: 10.1186/s12958-015-0126-9.

[139] S. Ozkan et al., "Replete vitamin D stores predict reproductive success following in vitro fertilization," Fertil. Steril., 2010, doi: 10.1016/j.fertnstert.2009.05.019.

[140] M. M. Pacis, C. N. Fortin, S. M. Zarek, S. L. Mumford, and J. H. Segars, "Vitamin D and assisted reproduction: should vitamin D be routinely screened and repleted prior to ART? A systematic review," J. Assist. Reprod. Genet., 2015, doi: 10.1007/s10815-014-0407-9.

[141] P. Skowrońska et al., "The role of vitamin D in reproductive dysfunction in women – a systematic review," Ann. Agric. Environ. Med., 2016, doi: 10.5604/12321966.1226865.

[142] J. P. Islamian and H. Mehrali, "Lycopene as a carotenoid provides radioprotectant and antioxidant effects by quenching radiation-induced free radical singlet oxygen: An overview," Cell Journal. 2015, doi: 10.22074/cellj.2015.485.

[143] E. Geva, B. Bartoov, N. Zabludovsky, J. B. Lessing, L. Lerner-Geva, and A. Amit, "The effect of antioxidant treatment on human spermatozoa and fertilization rate in an in vitro fertilization program," Fertil. Steril., 1996, doi: 10.1016/S0015-0282(16)58514-8.

[144] H. Kodama, H. Kasai, R. Yamaguchi, T. Tanaka, and J. Fukuda, "Increased oxidative deoxyribonucleic acid damage in the spermatozoa of infertile male patients," Fertil. Steril., 1997, doi: 10.1016/S0015-0282(97)00236-7.

[145] D. Vézina, F. Mauffette, K. D. Roberts, and G. Bleau, "Selenium-vitamin E supplementation in infertile men: Effects on semen parameters and micronutrient levels and distribution," Biol. Trace Elem. Res., 1996, doi: 10.1007/BF02784546.

[146] S. Sinclair, "Male infertility: Nutritional and environmental considerations," Alternative Medicine Review. 2000.

[147] C. Ross et al., "A systematic review of the effect of oral antioxidants on male infertility," Reproductive BioMedicine Online. 2010, doi: 10.1016/j.rbmo.2010.03.008.

[148] M. K. Moslemi and S. Tavanbakhsh, "Selenium-vitamin E supplementation in infertile men: Effects on semen parameters and pregnancy rate," Int. J. Gen. Med., 2011, doi: 10.2147/IJGM.S16275.

[149] M. Costa, D. Canale, M. Filicori, S. D'lddio, and *A. lenzi*, "L- carnitine in idiopathic asthenozoospermia: a multicenter study," Andrologia, 1994, doi: 10.1111/j.1439-0272.1994.tb00780.x.

[150] G. Balercia, F. Regoli, T. Armeni, A. Koverech, F. Mantero, and M. Boscaro, "Placebo-controlled double-blind randomized trial on the use of L-carnitine, L-acetylcarnitine, or combined L-carnitine and L-acetylcarnitine in men with idiopathic asthenozoospermia," Fertil. Steril., 2005, doi: 10.1016/j.fertnstert.2005.03.064.

[151] X. Zhou, F. Liu, and S. Zhai, "Effect of L-carnitine and/or L-acetyl-carnitine

in nutrition treatment for male infertility: A systematic review," 2007, doi: 10.6133/apjcn.2007.16.s1.70.

[152] M. Sigman, S. Glass, J. Campagnone, and J. L. Pryor, "Carnitine for the treatment of idiopathic asthenospermia: a randomized, double-blind, placebo-controlled trial," Fertil. Steril., 2006, doi: 10.1016/j.fertnstert.2005.10.055.

[153] A. Gvozdjáková, J. Kucharská, J. Dubravicky, V. Mojto, and R. B. Singh, "Coenzyme Q10, α-tocopherol, and oxidative stress could be important metabolic biomarkers of male infertility," Dis. Markers, 2015, doi: 10.1155/2015/827941.

[154] C. A. Rice-evans, N. J. Miller, P. G. Bolwell, P. M. Bramley, and J. B. Pridham, "The relative antioxidant activities of plant-derived polyphenolic flavonoids," Free Radic. Res., 1995, doi: 10.3109/10715769509145649.

[155] K. C. Huang, "The Pharmacology of Chinese Herbs, Second Edition By K. C. Huang (University of Louisville). CRC Press, Inc., Boca Raton, FL. 1998. xxi + 512 pp. 17.5 × 25 cm. $129.00. ISBN 0-8493-1665-0," J. Nat. Prod., 1998, doi: 10.1021/np980247y.

[156] Y. C. S. Attele A.S., Wu J.A., "Multiple constituents and multiple actions.," Biochem. Pharm., 1999.

[157] B. Halliwell, "Are polyphenols antioxidants or pro-oxidants? What do we learn from cell culture and in vivo studies?," Archives of Biochemistry and Biophysics. 2008, doi: 10.1016/j.abb.2008.01.028.

[158] and T. A. Ahmad AH; Rahal A, "Optimising drug potential of plants," Proc. Symp. Recent Trends Dev. Herb. Drugs Challenges Oppor. 6th Annu. Conf. ISVPT, pp. 23-25, 2006.

[159] Mahima et al., "Immunomodulatory and therapeutic potentials of herbal, traditional/indigenous and ethnoveterinary medicines," Pakistan J. Biol. Sci., 2012, doi: 10.3923/pjbs.2012.754.774.

[160] J. Lee, E. R. Hahm, and S. V. Singh, "Withaferin A inhibits activation of signal transducer and activator of transcription 3 in human breast cancer cells," Carcinogenesis, 2010, doi: 10.1093/carcin/bgq175.

[161] V. Badmaev, M. Majeed, and R. A. Passwater, "Selenium: a quest for better understanding [published erratum appears in Altern Ther Health Med 1996 Sep;2(5):101]," Altern Ther Heal. Med, 1996.

[162] K. IWANIER and B. A. ZACHARA, "Selenium Supplementation Enhances the Element Concentration in Blood and Seminal Fluid But Does Not Change the Spermatozoal Quality Characteristics in Subfertile Men," J. Androl., 1995, doi: 10.1002/j.1939-4640.1995.tb00561.x.

[163] R. Scott, A. Macpherson, R. W. S. Yatest, B. Hussain, and J. Dixon, "The effect of oral selenium supplementation on human sperm motility," Br. J. Urol., 1998, doi: 10.1046/j.1464-410X.1998.00683.x.

[164] L. Keskes-Ammar et al., "Sperm oxidative stress and the effect of an oral vitamin E and selenium supplement on semen quality in infertile men," Arch. Androl., 2003, doi: 10.1080/01485010390129269.

[165] A. E. Favier, "The role of zinc in reproduction - Hormonal mechanisms," Biol. Trace Elem. Res., 1992, doi: 10.1007/BF02784623.

[166] M. P. Zago and P. I. Oteiza, "The antioxidant properties of zinc: Interactions with iron and antioxidants," Free Radic. Biol. Med., 2001, doi: 10.1016/S0891-5849(01)00583-4.

[167] F. Chimienti, M. Aouffen, A. Favier, and M. Seve, "Zinc

Homeostasis-regulating Proteins: New Drug Targets for Triggering Cell Fate," Curr. Drug Targets, 2005, doi: 10.2174/1389450033491082.

[168] H. Mohan, J. Verma, I. Singh, P. Mohan, S. Marwah, and P. Singh, "Inter-relationship of Zinc Levels in Serum and Semen in Oligospermic Infertile Patients and Fertile Males," Indian J. Pathol. Microbiol., 1997.

[169] H. Fuse, T. Kazama, S. Ohta, and Y. Fujiuchi, "Relationship between zinc concentrations in seminal plasma and various sperm parameters," Int. Urol. Nephrol., 1999, doi: 10.1023/A:1007190506587.

[170] S. E. Chia, C. N. Ong, L. H. Chua, L. M. Ho, and S. K. Tay, "Comparison of zinc concentrations in blood and seminal plasma and the various sperm parameters between fertile and infertile men," J. Androl., 2000, doi: 10.1002/j.1939-4640.2000.tb03275.x.

[171] N. Batra, B. Nehru, and M. P. Bansal, "Influence of lead and zinc on rat male reproduction at 'biochemical and histopathological levels,'" J. Appl. Toxicol., 2001, doi: 10.1002/jat.796.

[172] A. E. Omu, H. Dashti, and S. Al-Othman, "Treatment of asthenozoospermia with zinc sulphate: Andrological, immunological and obstetric outcome," Eur. J. Obstet. Gynecol. Reprod. Biol., 1998, doi: 10.1016/S0301-2115(97)00262-5.

[173] A. E. Omu, M. K. Al-Azemi, E. O. Kehinde, J. T. Anim, M. A. Oriowo, and T. C. Mathew, "Indications of the mechanisms involved in improved sperm parameters by zinc therapy," Med. Princ. Pract., 2008, doi: 10.1159/000112963.

[174] C. Foresta et al., "Role of zinc trafficking in male fertility: From germ to sperm," Hum. Reprod., 2014, doi: 10.1093/humrep/deu075.

[175] A. Fallah, A. Mohammad-Hasani, and A. H. Colagar, "Zinc is an essential element for male fertility: A review of zn roles in men's health, germination, sperm quality, and fertilization," Journal of Reproduction and Infertility. 2018.

[176] D. Y. Liu, B. S. Sie, M. L. Liu, F. Agresta, and H. W. G. Baker, "Relationship between seminal plasma zinc concentration and spermatozoa-zona pellucida binding and the ZP-induced acrosome reaction in subfertile men," Asian J. Androl., 2009, doi: 10.1038/aja.2009.23.

[177] D. GB, "Manganese Clin. Toxicol," pp. 37: 293-307, 1999.

[178] R. K. Anand and U. Kanwar, "Role of some trace metal ions in placental membrane lipid peroxidation," Biol. Trace Elem. Res., 2001, doi: 10.1385/bter:82:1-3:061.

[179] M. M. Poranen et al., "Structural explanation for the role of Mn2+ in the activity of φ6 RNA-dependent RNA polymerase," Nucleic Acids Res., 2008, doi: 10.1093/nar/gkn632.

[180] J. P. Prestifilippo et al., "Acute effect of manganese on hypothalamic luteinizing hormone releasing hormone secretion in adult male rats: Involvement of specific neurotransmitter systems," Toxicol. Sci., 2008, doi: 10.1093/toxsci/kfn135.

[181] A. R. Reddi et al., "The overlapping roles of manganese and Cu/Zn SOD in oxidative stress protection," Free Radic. Biol. Med., 2009, doi: 10.1016/j.freeradbiomed.2008.09.032.

[182] J. L. Lafond, B. Sele, and A. Favier, "Concentration of selected metals in normal and pathological human seminal plasma.," J. Trace Elem. Electrolytes Health Dis., 1988.

[183] S. Lapointe, I. Ahmad, M. M. Buhr, and M. A. Sirard, "Modulation of

Postthaw Motility, Survival, Calcium Uptake, and Fertility of Bovine Sperm by Magnesium and Manganese," J. Dairy Sci., 1996, doi: 10.3168/jds.S0022-0302(96)76592-X.

[184] Magnus, I. Brekke, T. Åbyholm, and K. Purvis, "Effects of manganese and other divalent cations on progressive motility of human sperm," Syst. Biol. Reprod. Med., 1990, doi: 10.3109/01485019008986875.

[185] A. Bansal and G. Bilaspuri, "Effect of manganese on bovine sperm motility, viability, and lipid peroxidation in vitro," Anim. Reprod., 2008.

[186] J. G. Anderson, P. T. Cooney, and K. M. Erikson, "Inhibition of DAT function attenuates manganese accumulation in the globus pallidus," Environ. Toxicol. Pharmacol., 2007, doi: 10.1016/j.etap.2006.08.006.

[187] A. Ghasemzadeh, F. Karkon-Shayan, S. Yousefzadeh, M. Naghavi-Behzad, and K. Hamdi, "Study of pentoxifylline effects on motility and viability of spermatozoa from infertile asthenozoospermic males," Niger. Med. J., 2016, doi: 10.4103/0300-1652.193857.

[188] X. Zhang, R. K. Sharma, A. Agarwal, and T. Falcone, "Antioxidant effect of pentoxifylline in reducing oxidative stress induced embryotoxicity," Fertil. Steril., 2004, doi: 10.1016/j.fertnstert.2004.07.878.

[189] M. GAVELLA, V. LIPOVAC, and T. MAROTTI, "Effect of pentoxifylline on superoxide anion production by human sperm," Int. J. Androl., 1991, doi: 10.1111/j.1365-2605.1991.tb01099.x.

[190] M. Gavella and V. Lipovac, "Pentoxifylline-mediated reduction of superoxide anion production by human spermatozoa," Andrologia, 1992, doi: 10.1111/j.1439-0272.1992.tb02606.x.

[191] H. Okada, N. Tatsumi, M. Kanzaki, M. Fujisawa, S. Arakawa, and S. Kamidono, "Formation of reactive oxygen species by spermatozoa from asthenospermic patients: Response to treatment with pentoxifylline," J. Urol., 1997, doi: 10.1016/S0022-5347(01)64697-4.

[192] K. A. McKinney, S. E. M. Lewis, and W. Thompson, "The effects of pentoxifylline on the generation of reactive oxygen species and lipid Peroxidation in human spermatozoa," Andrologia, 1996, doi: 10.1111/j.1439-0272.1996.tb02752.x.

Chapter 4

Antioxidants in Female Reproductive Biology

Banashree Nath and Hirok Roy

Abstract

Human female reproductive biology is a complex system and its pathologies are varied. However, majority of the pathologic processes involves the role of reactive oxygen species (ROS). Imbalance between the ROS and antioxidants results in oxidative stress (OS). OS is the pathognomonic factor in various female reproductive system ailments. OS contributes to the pathophysiology of infertility, pregnancy related complications, endometriosis, ovarian cancers, etc. Evidence of elevated oxidative stress biomarkers can be found in various inflammatory conditions. Numerous strategies have been postulated for management of OS related pathologic conditions. Antioxidants supplementation may play a crucial in prevention and management of these conditions. However, robust evidence is needed to support the role of antioxidants supplementation in various female reproductive disorders.

Keywords: free radicals, oxidative stress, cellular damage, antioxidants, female reproductive tract diseases

1. Introduction

Oxygen is vital for sustaining life. However, its damaging effect on living cells through production of reactive oxygen species is a paradox of cell metabolism [1]. These free radicals with unpaired electrons are toxins that are produced as the body cells uses oxygen to sustain for processing food or reacting to the environment. They have damaging effect through adverse reactions to various components of the cell [2].

Antioxidants also called "free-radical scavengers", are biological and chemical substances that fights the damage to cells caused by free radicals produced in our body. These are metabolites and enzymes that either prevent formation of free radicals or clear them from the body before they exert harmful effects on the integral components of cell such as DNA, proteins and lipids [1, 3]. Ineffective elimination of free radicals leads to oxidative stress. Oxidative stress is the pathognomonic factor in various female reproductive system ailments. Diverse effects of free radicals on female reproductive system are subject to location, concentration and the extent of exposure to these molecules [4]. Oxidative stress can affect manifold physiological mechanisms such as oocyte maturation, fertilization, implantation, embryo development and hence contributes to the pathophysiology of pregnancy related complications, endometriosis, polycystic ovarian disease, unexplained infertility and gynecological cancers [5]. The objective of this chapter is to discuss the influence of antioxidants in

IntechOpen

different physiological processes to maintain healthy female reproductive function and their role in the prevention of various diseases of the female genital tract.

2. Free radicals

Free radicals are products of normal cellular metabolism with an unpaired electron which makes them highly reactive and unstable [6, 7]. They have high tendency to react with other molecules to initiate a chain of reactions resulting in cellular damage and disease [8]. They are mainly of two types: reactive oxygen species (ROS) and reactive nitrogen species (RNS).

2.1 Reactive oxygen species

Reactive oxygen species (ROS) comprise of mainly three types: (a) superoxide anion (O_2^-), (b) hydrogen peroxide (H_2O_2), and (c) hydroxyl radical (HO•) produced due to partial reduction of oxygen [8]. Endogenous sources of free radicals and other ROS in the body originate from the basic reactions of metabolism essential for sustenance of life while exogenous sources are essentially due to hazardous exposure to X-rays, ozone, cigarette smoking, air pollutants, certain drugs and pesticides, and industrial chemicals [9]. Origin of endogenous free radicals may be from: mitochondria, xanthine oxidase, peroxisomes, inflammation, phagocytosis, arachidonate pathways, exercise, ischemia/reperfusion injury [10]. Enzymatic and nonenzymatic reactions both give rise to free radicals in the body. Most of enzymatic reactions occur in respiratory chain, phagocytosis, prostaglandin synthesis and cytochrome P-450 system [11] while nonenzymatic reactions are those of oxygen with organic compounds and ionizing reactions [12].

ROS have been associated with a number of diseases of female reproductive tract as their presence in ovaries, [13–17], fallopian tubes [18] and embryos [19] have been established in various animal and human studies. ROS has been implicated in the regulation of integral functioning of female reproductive organs viz. oocyte maturation, ovarian steroidogenesis, embryo metabolism, corpus luteal function and luteolysis [13, 14, 20].

ROS are formed from normal cellular metabolism and comprises of oxygen ions, free radicals and peroxides. They take part in chemical reactions that remove their unpaired electron. Either an increase in levels of ROS or a decline in the antioxidant defence system of cells causes oxidative stress that induces direct or indirect ROS-mediated macro molecular damage of nucleic acids, proteins, and lipids. This has significant implications in pathogenesis of carcinogenesis [21], neurodegeneration [22, 23], atherosclerosis, diabetes [24], and aging [25]. ROS is assumed to regulate signalling of cellular pathways by which it may contribute to tumour metastasis by gene activation [26]. The knowledge of chemo-interactive processes occurring between the ROS and various molecules involved in the cellular signalling pathways is crucial for understanding the pathogenesis of oxidative stress. Redox reaction between different protein residues and the ROS is the core component of this chemo-interactive process. This redox reaction results in the oxidation of cysteine residues on proteins to form reactive sulfenic acid (–SOH). Further oxidation of sulfenic acid (–SOH) results in the formation of sulfinic ($-SO_2H$) or sulfonic ($-SO_3H$) acid or sulfenamide (in presence of nitrogen). Oxidation of these protein components results in various ultrastructural changes and/or functional alteration. Some of these alterations are reversible with the aid of antioxidant defence mechanism viz. thioredoxin pathways but rest of the alteration especially involving the generation of sulfonic acid results in permanent damage [2].

2.2 Reactive nitrogen species (RNS)

Nitric oxide–derived compounds, which includes nitroxyl anion, nitrosonium cation, higher oxides of nitrogen, *S*-nitrosothiols, and dinitrosyl iron complexes are reactive nitrogen species (RNS). RNS are considered to modulate the physiologic processes of many living cells which may include smooth muscle cells, cardiomyocytes, platelets, and nervous and juxtaglomerular cells. Nitric oxide (NO) is formed when L-arginine is converted to L-citrulline by nitric oxide synthase (NOS) [27–29]. NO plays a vital role in modulating diverse physiological mechanisms such as relaxation of arterial and venous smooth muscles and inhibition of platelet aggregation but excess of NO may not have favourable consequences [28, 30]. NO with an unpaired electron is highly reactive and can induce harmful effects to proteins, carbohydrates, nucleotides and lipids. Along with synergistic effects from other mediators of inflammation, this free radical can cause tissue damage, inflammation and adhesions by inducing nitrosative stress [28].

Nitrosative stress has been linked to inflammatory vascular disease in pregnant women such as preeclampsia where the pathognomonic features include hypertension along with generalized endothelial dysfunction, proteinuria, and foetal growth restriction [31]. There is surge in production of nitric oxide due to vascular inflammation induced by shed membrane particles of leukocytes and platelets along with elevated levels of microparticles from plasma membrane of apoptotic or activated circulating cells or cells of the vascular wall [32, 33] resulting in generation of pro-inflammatory proteins. Platelet microparticles more precisely are pro-inflammatory and hence contribute markedly for nitrosative stress in the vascular wall [34].

3. Antioxidants

To combat the adverse effect of oxidative stress, human body has evolved various defense mechanisms viz. preventive and repair mechanisms, physical defenses, and antioxidant system. Antioxidants can be chemically described as any molecule that can donate electron/s or act as a reducing agent in a redox reaction resulting in conversion of a reactive molecule in to a relatively stable and inert substances. Antioxidants by its virtue as an electron donor can react with ROS, resulting in suppression of oxidative stress [35]. However, this simple way to describe "antioxidants" cannot be justified and it has much wider connotations and complexity. The ability of a molecule to participate in a redox reaction with a ROS is not only the distinguishing feature for an antioxidant. There are numerous molecules which can interact with a ROS resulting from the modulation of inflammatory cascades. Inhibitor molecules for NADPH oxidase and lipoxygenases as well as cofactors for antioxidant enzymes, and metal chelators which can negate the ROS levels, can also be termed as antioxidants. However, it should be remembered that in an appropriate environment, many of these antioxidants may function as a prooxidant due the inherited redox potential of these substances [36, 37]. Hence, proper understanding of these diverse molecules is critically needed prior to formulating rational antioxidant therapies. Antioxidants can broadly be classified as enzymatic and non-enzymatic as depicted in **Table 1**.

Antioxidants, both endogenous and exogenous in origin, counteracts free radicals mediated injury in an interactive and synergistical ways (**Table 2**) [38].

3.1 Enzymatic antioxidants

Enzymatic antioxidants are endogenously synthesized molecules and are more efficacious as free radical scavenging role. These antioxidants have transition

Enzymatic antioxidants	Non-enzymatic antioxidants
Superoxide dismutases (SOD)	a. Endogenous Antioxidants
Peroxidases	• Bilirubin
Catalases	• Uric acid
Thioredoxin (Trx) system	• NADPH and NADH
	• Thiols, e.g., glutathione, N-acetyl cysteine
	• Ubiquinone
	b. Dietary Antioxidants & micronutrients
	• Vitamin A, C, E and the B complex, Zinc, Selenium
	• Beta carotene and other carotenoids
	• Polyphenols, e.g., flavonoids, flavones
	c. Metal Binding Proteins
	• Albumin (copper)
	• Ferritin (iron)
	• Myoglobin (iron)
	• Transferrin (iron)
	• Metallothionein (copper)
	• Ceruloplasmin (copper)

Table 1.
Classification of antioxidants.

ROS	Neutralizing antioxidants
Hydroxyl radical	Vitamin C, Glutathione, Flavonoids, Lipoic acid
Superoxide radical	Vitamin C, Glutathione, Flavonoids, Superoxide dismutase
Hydrogen peroxide	Vitamin C, Glutathione, beta carotene, Vitamin-E, flavonoids, lipoic acid
Lipid peroxides	Beta-carotene, Vitamin-E, Ubiquinone, flavonoids, Glutathione peroxidase

Table 2.
ROS and Neutralizing Antioxidants.

metal core which are capable of transfer of electrons essential for redox reaction with ROS and thereby, effectively neutralizing the adverse effects of ROS. These endogenously produced enzymes include superoxide dismutase enzymes (SODs), glutathione peroxidase, catalases, and glutathione oxidase.

Superoxide dismutase: SOD is an enzyme system that catalyzes the of the superoxide (O2−) radical into ordinary molecular oxygen (O_2) and hydrogen peroxide (H_2O_2). SODs are group of metalloproteins and its enzymatic functions were first discovered by Irwin Fridovich and Joe McCord at Duke University in 1968 [39]. There are various isoforms of this enzyme but in humans, it exists mainly in three isoforms viz. SOD1, SOD2 and SOD3. SOD1 is located in the cytoplasm, SOD2 is predominantly found in the mitochondria, and SOD3 is extracellular. The genes are located on chromosomes 21, 6, and 4, respectively (21q22.1, 6q25.3 and 4p15.3-p15.1). SOD1 is a dimer, whereas SOD2 and SOD3 are tetramers. SOD1 contains a core of two metal cofactors comprising of copper (Cu) and zinc (Zn). Mitochondrial SOD2 contains manganese and is encoded by nuclear DNA. SOD3, the extracellular enzyme, Cu-Zn has in its reactive center.

Glutathione peroxidase: It belongs to a large class of enzyme system called peroxidases. The primary biochemical function of glutathione peroxidase (GPx) is the conversion of lipid hydroperoxides to their corresponding alcohols and to reduce free hydrogen peroxide to water, which is the crucial function as an antioxidant. GPx exists in eight different isoforms in humans and contains selenium as its reactive core. It is a tetrameric enzyme with the exception of GPx4 which is a monomeric enzyme.

Catalases: It is an iron containing enzyme which catalyzes the biotransformation of hydrogen peroxide to non-reactive water and oxygen.

Apart from these endogenous enzymatic antioxidants, thioredoxin plays a central role in humans as a defensive response to ROS. They act as antioxidants by facilitating the reduction of other proteins by cysteine thiol-disulfide exchange. They also play an important role in cell survival [40].

3.2 Nonenzymatic antioxidants

Nonenzymatic antioxidants comprises of various exogenous dietary nutrients as well as endogenous compounds. They may act directly as an antioxidant or as an adjuvant to others molecules which participates in redox reaction.

Vitamin C and vitamin E plays a central role as defense mechanism against ROS. They act synergistically as a redox buffer to reduce the impact of oxidative stress imposed by various ROS. Vitamin C neutralizes superoxide radicals as well as other singlet oxygen species. Vitamin E is a potent scavenger of peroxyl radicals. α-tocopherol has the most potent antioxidant capabilities compared to other tocopherols due to the fact that H+ donating ability of different tocols increases in efficiency with greater ring methyl substitution. Thiols like glutathione is another endogenous antioxidant found in humans and is also can be found in oocytes and embryos in abundant amount. They exert their effect by virtue of its thiol component of cysteine residue which take part in the redox reaction. Moreover, glutathione can act as a cofactor for several antioxidant enzymes viz. glutathione peroxidase (GPx) and glutathione transferase [41]. Various micronutrients like Zn, Se, Cu aids the enzymatic antioxidants to counter the ill-effects of OS. Metal binding proteins like transferrin and ceruloplasmin combines with free iron ions which is a vital component of redox reaction (Fenton). Bilirubin is a tetrapyrrole pigment which possesses potent antioxidant and anti-inflammatory properties. This remarkable antioxidant activity appears likely to stem largely from the inhibitory action of unconjugated bilirubin over common isoforms of NADPH oxidase, which is an active participant of superoxide-generating reactions [42–44]. Another endogenous molecule bearing potent antioxidant property is uric acid. Uric acid is an efficient oxygen radical scavenger. At physiological concentrations, urate reduces the oxoheme oxidant formed by peroxide reaction with hemoglobin, thereby, protecting the erythrocytes from lysis due to lipid peroxidation.

4. Female reproductive diseases

The prooxidants and antioxidants work in synchrony to maintain a balance in the milieu of cellular metabolism. When this mechanism fails, oxidative stress is the sequelae. Prooxidant generation is influenced by cyto- chrome P450, and the corpus luteum is presumed to be one of its key sources [45]. The crucial role of free radicals in regulating the various physiological reproductive processes renders its influence on the oocytes, sperm, and embryos and their microenvironments. These changes in microenvironment has a direct bearing on follicular fluid, hydro salpingeal fluid, and peritoneal fluid which substantially determine the oocytes quality, interaction between sperm and oocyte, implantation of embryo and its early development [46–48]. Hence oxidative stress can affect the prospects of a favourable pregnancy and is also attributed to pathophysiology of endometriosis, hydrosalpinges, polycystic ovary syndrome (PCOS), and unexplained subfertility [49].

4.1 Female subfertility

World Health Organization (WHO) defines Infertility or subfertility as the "failure to achieve a clinical pregnancy after 12 months or more of regular unprotected sexual intercourse" [50]. With 48.5 million couples infertile globally [51], it is a health concern spread worldwide in which female factors are assumed to contribute to 40–50% percent of cases [52, 53]. Ovulatory dysfunction, tubal and pelvic pathology, endometriosis, and poor egg quality are among the most common causes of female subfertility while reproductive age and body mass index (BMI) are vital demographic determinants [54]. Notwithstanding the evidence of obvious pathologies, role of toxic products produced during oxidative stress in the occurrence of female subfertility is well established [55, 56].

ROS however has dual role. It may serve as key modulating agent in numerous physiological processes while in excess may cause cellular damage. The equivalence in the body is maintained by appropriate levels of antioxidants and hence determining the levels of the antioxidants as total antioxidant capacity (TAC) has been investigated in many studies [57–59]. Ovulation is one of key physiologic process in female that is evidenced by high numbers of macrophages and neutrophilic granulocytes in the follicle wall along with fast metabolism of granulosa cells. This gives high probability of ROS generation which may be essential for oocyte development and consequent progression to embryo. ROS are assumed to influence oocyte maturation [60] luteolysis [61, 62] progesterone secretion by the corpus luteum [63, 64] ovulation and follicular atresia [65]. ROS are linked to single follicle generation by stimulating atretic regression of the cohort of newly grown follicles through its action on granulosa cells to exhaust its reactivity to gonadotrophic hormones and steroidogenic function [65]. Pasqualotto et al. [66] found positive correlation of lipid peroxidation (LPO) and total antioxidant capacity (TAC) in pooled FF to pregnancy rate hence concluding high levels of LPO do promote oocyte and embryo development and enhance their quality.

Several studies have documented benefits of supplementary antioxidants in such cases with diverse methods of action. Vitamin E is assumed to improve epithelial growth in blood vessels and in the endometrium [67]. *N*- acetyl-cysteine improves cervical mucus for sperm penetration and also helps in ovulation [68]; L-arginine increases endometrial blood flow for successful implantation [69]; Myo-inositol improves ovarian function by decreasing levels of androgen and increasing sensitivity to insulin [70] while PUFAs promotes prostaglandin and steroid hormone synthesis apart from contributing to formation of cell membranes of the sperm and oocyte essential for fertilisation [71]. Even in Assisted reproductive technology, ROS may arise from cumulus cells, leucocytes, and culture media. Hence IVF cycles will yield better results if patients are screened for oxidative stress levels [72]. Culture medium are supplemented with antioxidants like β-mercaptoethanol, protein, vitamin E, vitamin C, cysteamine, cysteine, taurine and hypotaurine, and thiols to enhance the growth and maturation of embryos by downplaying the effects of ROS. ROS are scavenged by antioxidants and subsequently exert favourable effects by reducing blastocyst degeneration, embryo apoptosis and increasing hatching of blastocysts. Improvement of sperm morphology and preimplantation embryo development as well as reduction of developmental defects are reported with inclusion of antioxidants in the treatment protocol of infertile patients [73].

DOI: http://dx.doi.org/10.5772/intechopen.95937

4.2 Endometriosis

Endometriosis is defined as the presence of endometrial tissue outside of uterine cavity which lead to chronic inflammatory reaction [74]. It affects 6–10% of women in the general female population and is prevalent in 30–45% of patients with infertility or chronic pelvic pain [75, 76]. It is one of the most widespread gynaecological diseases and women present mostly with significant cyclic pelvic pain that escalate just prior to starting of menses and subside with onset of blood flow. In a few atypical cases, patients may not have any complaint and hence poses a dilemma for diagnosis [77]. This oestrogen dependent female pelvic pathology is mainly diagnosed by laparoscopy or laparotomy and confirmed by histopathological examination of retrieved pelvic tissues [78].

There are innumerable theories of the pathophysiology of endometriosis. The origin of OS in endometriosis is assumed to be induced by apoptotic endometrial tissue which get implanted in peritoneal cavity through retrograde menstruation. This tissue along with menstrual effluent are assumed to be antigenic and activate macrophages. Consequently, the number and activity of macrophages in the peritoneal fluid (PF) increase that phagocytose antigens. This results in release of inflammatory cytokines such as interleukin (IL) 2, 4, 10, TNF-a and IFN-g [79, 80] and serum and peritoneal IL-33 in cases of deeply infiltrating endometriosis [81]. Increased inflammatory activity is known to cause OS [82]. Apart from macrophages, there is upregulation of transcription factor NF-kB in endometriosis [83–85] which can activate many genes to further increase inflammation and promote progression of the disease [86]. ROS damage the fragile mesothelium thus facilitating adhesion and implantation of the endometrial cells to further promote progression of the disease [87]. Hence elevated Oxidative stress could be cause or a consequence of one of this debilitating diseases of females of reproductive age group [8].

Despite endometriosis being a disease with benign pathology, there are features in endometriosis identical to cancer such as the invasion of tissues, tendency to evade programmed cell death, distal spread and high propensity of angiogenesis. [88] which renders its close association to ROS reported in numerous studies [89, 90]. The essential feature of angiogenesis and immunity to apoptosis common to both endometriosis and tumorigenesis results in accelerated proliferation rate subsequently producing increased ROS. The pathogenesis of cellular damage by ROS in both endometriosis and cancer cells is same. ROS acts as a second messenger of cell proliferation [91] by activating MAPK signalling pathways to accelerate cell proliferation. Hence this linkage between ROS and cell proliferation in cancer illustrates the definite role of elevated ROS in modulating cell proliferation in endometriosis. To elucidate the fact, Ngô et al. [91] used purified stromal and epithelial cells from ovarian endometrioma and ectopic endometrium of endometriosis to create cell lines. The experiment showed endometriotic cells had high OS levels with increased ROS production and decreased catalase levels. There was increased cellular proliferation and activation of ERK1/2. A group of enzymes called MMPs also contribute to increase ROS in the pathogenesis of endometrial disease. MMPs facilitate implantation of ectopic endometrial cells by degrading the extracellular matrix of the peritoneal mesothelium [92]. Hence the recent strategies to reduce oxidative stress for effective treatment of endometriosis in preference to creating non-oestrogen environment by pharmacological intervention has been gaining evidence. Studies showed there is decrease in symptoms with antioxidant (vitamin E, vitamin C, zinc and selenium) intake [93] as well as improvement in antioxidant markers with antioxidant rich diet [94]. Aminoguanidine through OS reduction prevent adhesion to peritoneal surface.

There are a number of compounds that can act as antioxidants and can manifest its favourable effects in improving the symptoms of endometriosis.

Vitamin C is required for carrying out diverse physiological processes of the body. Humans and other primates acquire it from exogenous sources that acts as co-factor for a number of enzymes, most notably hydroxylases involved in collagen synthesis apart from being an effective antioxidant. Vitamin E is a lipid-soluble antioxidant that scavenges peroxyl radical to eliminate the effect of free radicals and get transformed to tocopheryl radical that is subsequently reduced by a hydrogen donor (as Vitamin C) to return to its reduced state [95].

Resveratrol is a natural polyphenolic flavonoid having antineoplastic, anti-inflammatory and antioxidant properties [96]. It is synthesized by plants following exposure to ultraviolet radiation. Its anti-inflammatory effect is mediated through inhibition of cytokines (tumor necrosis factor-a, IL-6, IL-8), VEGF and monocyte chemotactic protein 1. It inhibits production of ROS by monocytes, macrophages and lymphocytes and regulate cell proliferation and apoptosis by inhibiting NF-kB [97]. It reduces VEGF levels to prevent angiogenesis [98]. Resveratrol is already used in the treatment of several clinical conditions such as cardiovascular diseases, cancer, type-2 diabetes mellitus and neurodegenerative diseases and is being explored for its impact in the treatment of endometriosis.

Melatonin is secreted by pineal gland predominantly during the night and has potent antioxidant effects. It is also shown to stimulate antioxidant enzymes [99]. It can induce down-regulation of MMPs. Hence its mode of action as antioxidant in endometriosis can range from scavenging toxic free radicals [100] to regulating levels of MMPs in ectopic and eutopic endometrial tissue [101, 102]. It can also act as antioxidant enzymes stimulator [99].

N-acetyl-L-cysteine (NAC) is another antioxidant which is precursor of glutathione [103] and is found to inhibit proliferation of endometrial cells [104, 105]. It acts through its ability to limit tissue invasion [106] and suppression of NF-kB activation which acts as a transcriptional factor in the pathophysiology of endometriosis [107]. Its other mode of action is linked to activation of the immune system by increasing IL-2 levels and the expression of CD25 on T cells [107] apart from expression of membrane TNF-a expression [103].

Xanthohumol is extracted from *Humulus lupulus* (species of flowering plant of Cannabaceae) and has antioxidant and anti-inflammatory properties. Rudzitis-Auth et al. suggested Xanthohumol if taken through dietary supplements is effective for selective treatment of endometriotic lesions [108]. It acts by inhibition of NF-kB signaling pathway [109] as well as decreasing production of NO by through suppressing of NO synthase [110].

Epigallocatechin-3-gallate (EGCG) is another antioxidant found in green tea which has also antimitotic and antiangiogenic properties [111]. The effect of EGCG on endometriosis is studied both in vitro and in vivo and is assumed to reduce OS by VEGF reduction and inhibition of angiogenesis. It also inhibits cell proliferation, migration and invasion of endometrial cells [112].

4.3 Pre-ecclampsia

Pre-ecclampsia involves gradual development of hypertension (systolic blood pressure $\geq$ 140 mm Hg and/or diastolic blood pressure $\geq$ 90 mm Hg), or deterioration of pre-existing hypertension, proteinuria (300 mg/L or more in 24 h), generalized oedema, and sometimes blood clotting disorders occurring after 20 weeks of gestation [113]. Severe preeclampsia may progress to eclampsia and the HELLP syndrome, which involves haemolysis, elevated liver enzymes and low platelets. The spectrum of these hypertensive disorders can impose serious foetal morbidity like intrauterine growth restriction and preterm births which has further implications of early neonatal death and infant mortality. The pathophysiology of pre-eclampsia still remains a subject of research. The existing theories suggest incomplete cytotrophoblast invasion into the spiral arteries in the uterus that causes malformed placenta leading to deficient perfusion of placenta. Role of antiplatelet agents and calcium supplements to delay this process are being studied [114, 115]. This inadequate placental perfusion may induce OS with decline in concentrations of antioxidants in plasma and placenta [116, 117]. This complemented with inflammatory response of body cause damage to endothelial cells resulting in signs and symptoms of pre-eclampsia. Antioxidants prevent oxidation of proteins and enzymes, destroy free radicals, and preserve the integrity of cellular membrane [118]. Hence dietary or therapeutic antioxidant supplements in women can possibly eliminate the deleterious effects of OS and uteroplacental endothelial damage evident in preeclampsia. A few recent meta-analysis however failed to show any beneficial role of antioxidant therapy on prevention of PE [119, 120]. More trials are needed to establish the effect of antioxidants on pre-eclampsia and to provide evidence-based information on its adverse effects and long-term consequences on the growth and development of the children.

4.4 Peripheral neuropathy in obstetrics

Pregnant women are prone to a number of neuropathic syndromes due to physical changes resulting from enlargement of the uterus and the gradual growth of the foetus. The subsequential postural changes and nutation of the pelvic girdle and vertebrae due to high concentrations of relaxin released from the tenth week of gestation gives rise to low back pain and entrapment neuropathies. Analgesic drugs and surgery being contraindicated in pregnancy, the best approach to treat such morbidity in pregnancy remains a dilemma. Rehabilitation therapies and neuroprotectors in such cases have proved effective in relieving pain and paraesthesia of peripheral neuropathies [121]. Role of antioxidants as neuroprotective agents are investigated lately. One of such agent is alpha-lipoic acid (ALA) which acts as a powerful antioxidant in the body. It exerts its functions in every cell and tissue in the body due to its solubility in both water and fat. This potent antioxidant can modulate many inflammatory pathways through its inhibitory effect on production of vascular and intracellular adhesion molecules (VCAM-1 and ICAM-1), reducing the expression of CD4 on blood mononuclear cells, secretion of tumour necrosis factor (TNF)-α and inhibition of natural killer (NK) cells [122]. It also has direct inhibitory action on the transcription factor NF-κB which regulates the expression of various genes associated with inflammatory response and cell apoptosis [123]. Hence supplementation with ALA by virtue of its antioxidant and anti-inflammatory action has been shown to relieve pain and paraesthesia in patients with sciatica, carpal tunnel syndrome and diabetic neuropathy [124–127].

ALA supplementation at doses of up to 2400 mg/day and intravenous administration of 600 mg/day seemed to be safe in humans [123]. The safety of this potent antioxidant in pregnant women are yet to be established, however several studies have credited its role in the prevention of premature rupture of membranes, threatened miscarriage and gestational diabetes [128].

4.5 Gynecological (ovarian, endometrial and cervical) cancers

Gynaecological cancers present a diagnostic challenge in early stage since the symptoms appear mostly when the disease has metastasized. Two third cases are diagnosed in advanced stage accounting for high fatality-to-case ratio among all malignancies in women [129]. The process of carcinogenesis occurs in multiple steps starting from normal cell to pre-cancerous stage and finally to an early stage of cancer [130]. A single cell undergoes sequential events in the form of initiation, promotion and progression to finally turn cancerous. ROS can act in all the three stages to stimulate carcinogenesis [131].

Initiation is the first stage of carcinogenesis and is executed as a consequence of an irreversible genetic alteration, that may be either simple mutations, transversions, transitions, and/or small deletions in DNA. DNA damage by oxidation can also occur through hydroxyl radical produced from H_2O_2. Increased oxidative stress may deplete the endogenous antioxidant reserves and activate endonucleases resulting in DNA fragmentation [130]. The second stage of promotion is reversible and it mediates promoter-receptor interactions to influence expression of the genome. Tumour promoters induce production of oxygen radical by modulating metabolic processes of cells. These oxygen radicals through modulation of gene associated with proliferation or cell death can induce the expression of mutated cell clones. However low levels of oxidative stress can promote cell division and tumour growth whereas high levels have cytotoxic effects and can hinder cell proliferation [131, 132]. In the ultimate stage of progression there is karyotypic instability and malignant growth. Progression is characterized by expeditious proliferation of cells, elusion from immune suppression, tissue invasion and metastasis [133]. Genesis of abundant free radicals along with increase in the level of oxidized DNA bases during oxidative stress may incite some tumours to mutate, inhibit anti-proteases and cause damage to local tissues [134]. In fully developed cancer cells, these modified DNA bases may induce genetic instability and metastatic propensity [135].

Diverse natural substances have been recognised to have role in cancer prevention [136] and treatment [137] when supplemented with chemotherapy, radiotherapy, and surgery. The drugs used in radiotherapy and chemotherapy can cause diverse tissue and organ damage through generation of free radicals which can also induce carcinogenesis [138]. Several studies reported that using antioxidants with anticancer drug therapy can significantly decrease these cellular damages and is associated with reduced risk of all-cause mortality and recurrence risk [138, 139].

However, many natural antioxidants may depict conflicting properties in cancer cells. The actions vary according to their concentration. With the possibility of antioxidants causing direct damage to DNA and the cell, speculations are arising on the role of antioxidant in the causation of cancer [140]. Recent studies suggest supplementation of antioxidants in high doses may have ill effects on health. The association of high doses of beta- carotene with lung cancer in smokers and high doses of vitamin E with that of prostate cancer are some examples of health hazards of antioxidants [141].

Hence the biological characteristics of natural antioxidants are assumed being beneficial or harmful depending on their concentration. The natural substances exhibit their antioxidant potential in lower concentration by increasing the expression of ROS scavengers while higher concentration can generate oxidative stress.

4.6 Polycystic ovarian disease

Polycystic ovary syndrome (PCOS) is a major public health disorder affecting 5–21% of women in reproductive age group. This most common endocrine disorder among reproductive-aged women has multitude of manifestations that includes reproductive (hyperandrogenism, hirsutism, anovulation, infertility, and menstrual disturbance), metabolic (obesity, diabetes mellitus and cardiovascular risk), and psychological (mood disorders and decreased quality of life) components [142]. Several studies undertaken still fail to unravel the pathophysiology of PCOS with theories attributing the clinical phenomenon to oxidative stress, inflammation, endothelial injury and genetic mechanisms. Markers of OS are considerably elevated in patients with PCOS and are assumed to play significant role in its pathogenesis [143]. NAC (N-acetyl-cysteine) is an antioxidant which can influence insulin receptor activity and its secretion [144] and also has negative effects on apoptotic activity and can lower homocysteine levels [145]. NAC has shown favourable effects on ovulation induction in PCOS women and can be used as an adjuvant to drugs for ovulation induction [146].

4.7 Diabetes in pregnancy

Gestational diabetes mellitus can pose risk for subsequent development of later-onset DM, metabolic syndrome, and cardiovascular disease [147]. Prevalence of diabetes is nearly 1–14% of pregnancies [148, 149]. Diabetes is a disease condition that could result in production of free radicals through glucose oxidation, alterations in antioxidant defence system, lipid peroxidation, non-enzymatic glycation of proteins and oxidative destruction of glycated proteins [150–151]. Marked deficiency in antioxidant activity have also been reported during the development of gestational diabetes [152]. Levels of antioxidants such as selenium, zinc, and vitamin E are reported to be reduced in GDM [152, 153]. Even adequate intake of antioxidants through diet improves total antioxidant status (TAS) and overall health condition [154].

There are several means by which elevated blood glucose levels induce excess production of ROS [154–156]. High glucose levels during pregnancy can also bring teratogenic changes in foetus through chemical modification and complex rearrangements of DNA. These are brought about by glycation products from elevated glucose levels hence reflecting the significance of genomic injury that can disturb embryonic development. The deficiency states of membrane lipids, changes in biological prostaglandin cascade and the formation of excess free radicals bring about dysmorphogenesis in fetus in diabetic pregnancy [157]. There is decrease in antioxidant defence in women with GDM due to accelerated lipid peroxidation causing membrane damage. Lipid peroxidation generate hydroperoxides that alters prostaglandin cascade of biosynthesis and may contribute to the morbidity by impairing the antioxidant defence system [158, 159]. GDM also induces oxidative stress in the foetus. Hence Increasing antioxidant intake during pregnancy remains an important part of promoting health status during pregnancy. Ahmed M. Maged *et al* reported lowered use of insulin dose for control of blood sugar with antioxidants supplementation in women with GDM. There was markedly improved neonatal outcome with decrease in NICU admission and less cases with RDS [160].

4.8 Abortion

Normal early pregnancy is subject to increase in oxygen concentration with more chances of ROS formation. This occurs from enzymes of respiratory reactions where electrons leak within the mitochondria. The syncytiotrophoblast by virtue of its position on the villous surface is highly vulnerable to OS due to direct exposure to high intervillous PO2. The syncytiotrophoblast consequently suffer loss of function and degeneration. The vulnerability is also high due to lower concentration of antioxidant enzymes in the syncytiotrophoblast when compared to other villous tissues during early pregnancy. Even high levels of antioxidants needed to neutralize and scavenge excessive ROS in women with recurrent abortion contributes to its pathogenesis apart from free radicals formed during the process. Studies reported there is elevated levels of lipoperoxides and significantly decreased vitamin A, E, and beta carotene in women with recurrent pregnancy loss thus indicating that OS may be implicated in the occurrence of recurrent abortion. Studies further reported deficient glutathione peroxidase activity in women with recurrent abortion compared to non-pregnant woman or healthy pregnancies [161–163]. Even concentration of selenium in the hair samples of women with recurrent abortion were found to be significantly lower when compared to healthy viable pregnancies [164].

With many studies affirming OS in the pathogenesis of recurrent abortion, supplementation of antioxidants during pregnancy have gained importance. Optimum dietary intake of antioxidants like vitamins C, E, and A, lycopenes, selenium compounds, lipoic acid, and ubiquinones have a role in the prevention of cellular damage and hence in the occurrence of recurrent pregnancy loss by scavenging ROS. Vitamin C and E are two antioxidants most explored and suggested to have beneficial role in scavenging free radicals and hence reduce the effects of OS in women with pregnancy loss. Both vitamins have been found to increase in normal pregnancy and decrease in conceptions with complications implying their use and consumption while balancing the OS found in such circumstances. However, the determination of appropriate dose and type of antioxidant is essential to prove its favourable effects without causing any harmful effects on the mother or foetus [165, 166].

5. Conclusion

Free radicals and oxidative stress are assumed to influence diverse physiological functions in reproduction, as well as in conditions such as infertility, endometriosis, PCOS, abortion, hydatidiform mole, foetal embryopathies, peripheral neuropathy of pregnancy and other pregnancy complications such as GDM, IUGR and pre-eclampsia. In-vivo evaluation of oxidative stress is still not accurately possible to assess. With many studies reporting role of OS in the physiological processes of reproductive tract, the lowest essential measure of ROS for sustenance of life which is well tolerated need to be specified. Extensive research on the role of different biomarkers in predicting the effects of ROS in averting the complications discussed above shall prove valuable. The effects of antioxidant therapy in preventing complications in deficient and sufficient individuals is indeed subject of research.

Conflict of interest

The authors declare no conflict of interest.

Author details

Banashree Nath[1*] and Hirok Roy[2]

1 Department of Obstetrics and Gynaecology, All India Institute of Medical Sciences, Raebareli, Uttar Pradesh, India

2 Department of Anaesthesiology, All India Institute of Medical Sciences, Raebareli, Uttar Pradesh, India

*Address all correspondence to: nathbanashree@gmail.com

References

[1] Davies KJ (1995). "Oxidative stress: the paradox of aerobic life". Biochemical Society Symposium. 61: 1-31. doi:10.1042/bss0610001. PMID 8660387.

[2] Ray PD, Huang BW, Tsuji Y. Reactive oxygen species (ROS) homeostasis and redox regulation in cellular signaling. Cell Signal. 2012;24(5):981-990. doi:10.1016/j.cellsig.2012.01.008.

[3] Sies H (March 1997). "Oxidative stress: oxidants and antioxidants". Experimental Physiology. 82 (2): 291-295. doi:10.1113/expphysiol.1997.sp004024. PMID 9129943

[4] Aruoma OI, Halliwell B. "Superoxide-dependent and ascorbate-dependent formation of hydroxyl radicals from hy- drogen peroxide in the presence of iron". Biochemistry Journal 241 (1987): 273-278.

[5] Mbah, Chika & Orabueze, Ifeoma & Okorie, Ndiamaka. (2019). Antioxidants Properties of Natural and Synthetic Chemical Compounds: Therapeutic Effects on Biological System. Acta Scientific Pharmaceutical Sciences. 3. 28-42. 10.31080/ASPS.2019.03.0273.

[6] Mbah, Chika & Orabueze, Ifeoma & Okorie, Ndiamaka. (2019). Antioxidants Properties of Natural and Synthetic Chemical Compounds: Therapeutic Effects on Biological System. Acta Scientific Pharmaceutical Sciences. 3. 28-42. 10.31080/ASPS.2019.03.0273.

[7] Cheeseman KH, Slater TF. An introduction to free radicals chemistry. Br Med Bull. 1993;49:481-493. [PubMed: 8221017]

[8] Agarwal A, Gupta S, Sharma RK. Role of oxidative stress in female reproduction. *Reprod Biol Endocrinol*. 2005;3:28. Published 2005 Jul 14. doi:10.1186/1477-7827-3-28

[9] Bagchi K, Puri S. Free radicals and antioxidants in health and disease. East Mediterranean Health Jr. 1998;4:350-360.

[10] Ebadi M. Antioxidants and free radicals in health and disease: An introduction to reactive oxygen species, oxidative injury, neuronal cell death and therapy in neurodegenerative diseases. Arizona: Prominent Press; 2001.

[11] Liu T, Stern A, Roberts LJ. The isoprostanes: Novel prostanglandin-like products of the free radical catalyzed peroxidation of arachidonic acid. J Biomed Sci. 1999;6:226-235. [PubMed: 10420080]

[12] Lobo V, Patil A, Phatak A, Chandra N. Free radicals, antioxidants and functional foods: Impact on human health. Pharmacogn Rev. 2010;4(8):118-126. doi:10.4103/0973-7847.70902

[13] Behrman HR, Kodaman PH, Preston SL, Gao S: Oxidative stress and the ovary. J Soc Gynecol Investig 2001, 8:S40–S42.

[14] Sabatini L, Wilson C, Lower A, Al-Shawaf T, Grudzinskas JG: Superoxide dismutase activity in human follicular fluid after con- trolled ovarian hyperstimulation in women undergoing in vitro fertilization. Fertil Steril 1999, 72:1027-1034.

[15] Shiotani M, Noda Y, Narimoto K, Imai K, Mori T, Fujimoto K, Ogawa K: Immunohistochemical localization of superoxide dis- mutase in the human ovary. Hum Reprod 1991, 6:1349-1353.

[16] Suzuki T, Sugino N, Fukaya T, Sugiyama S, Uda T, Takaya R, Yajima A, Sasano H: Superoxide dismutase in normal cycling human ovaries: immunohistochemical localization and characterization. Fertil Steril 1999, 72:720-726.

[17] Jozwik M, Wolczynski S, Szamatowicz M: Oxidative stress mark- ers in preovulatory follicular fluid in humans. Mol Hum Reprod 1999, 5:409-413.

[18] El Mouatassim S, Guerin P, Menezo Y: Expression of genes encod- ing antioxidant enzymes in human and mouse oocytes dur- ing the final stages of maturation. Mol Hum Reprod 1999, 5:720-725.

[19] Guerin P, El Mouatassim S, Menezo Y: Oxidative stress and pro- tection against reactive oxygen species in the pre-implanta- tion embryo and its surroundings. Hum Reprod Update 2001, 7:175-189.

[20] Ishikawa M: Oxygen radicals-superoxide dismutase system and reproduction medicine. Nippon Sanka Fujinka Gakkai Zasshi 1993, 45:842-848.

[21] Trachootham D, Alexandre J, Huang P. Nat Rev Drug Discov. 2009; 8:579-591. [PubMed: 19478820]

[22] Andersen JK. Nat Med. 2004; 10(Suppl):S18–S25. [PubMed: 15298006]

[23] Shukla V, Mishra SK, Pant HC. Adv Pharmacol Sci. 2011; 2011:572634. [PubMed: 21941533]

[24] Paravicini TM, Touyz RM. Cardiovasc Res. 2006; 71:247-258. [PubMed: 16765337]

[25] Haigis MC, Yankner BA. Mol Cell. 2010; 40:333-344. [PubMed: 20965426]

[26] Ishikawa K, Takenaga K, Akimoto M, Koshikawa N, Yamaguchi A, Imanishi H, Nakada K, Honma Y, Hayashi J. Science. 2008; 320:661-664. [PubMed: 18388260]

[27] Vega M, Johnson MC, Diaz HA, Urrutia LR, Troncoso JL, Devoto L: Regulation of human luteal steroidogenesis in vitro by nitric oxide. Endocrine 1998,8:185-191.

[28] Dong M, Shi Y, Cheng Q, Hao M: Increased nitric oxide in peri- toneal fluid from women with idiopathic infertility and endometriosis. J Reprod Med 2001, 46:887-891.

[29] Rosselli M, Keller PJ, Dubey RK: Role of nitric oxide in the biol- ogy, physiology and pathophysiology of reproduction. Hum Reprod Update 1998, 4:3-24.

[30] Ohl J, Lefebvre-Maunoury C, Wittemer C, Nisand G, Laurent MC, Hoffmann P: Nitric oxide donors for patients undergoing IVF. A prospective, double-blind, randomized, placebo-control- led trial. Hum Reprod 2002, 17:2615-2620.

[31] Harskamp RE and Zeeman GG. Preeclampsia: at risk for remote cardiovascular disease. Am J Med Sci 334: 291-295, 2007.

[32] Martínez MC, Tesse A, Zobairi F, and Andriantsiothaina R. Shed membrane microparticles from circulating and vascular cells in regulating vascular function. Am J Physiol 288: H1004–H1009, 2005.

[33] Meziani F, Tesse A, David E, Martínez MC, Wangesteen R, Schneider F, and Andriantsitohaina R. Shed membrane particles from preeclamptic women generate vascular wall inflammation and blunt vascular contractility. Am J Pathol 169: 1473-1483, 2006.

[34] Martínez MC, Andriantsitohaina R. Reactive nitrogen species: molecular mechanisms and potential significance in health and disease. Antioxid Redox Signal. 2009 Mar;11(3):669-702. doi: 10.1089/ars.2007.1993. PMID: 19014277.

[35] Walczak-Jedrzejowska R, Wolski JK, Slowikowska-Hilczer J. The role of

oxidative stress and antioxidants in male fertility. Central Eur J Urol 2013;66(1):60e7.

[36] Eghbaliferiz S, Iranshahi M. Prooxidant activity of polyphenols, flavonoids, anthocyanins and carotenoids: updated review of mechanisms and catalyzing metals. Phytother Res 2016;30:1379e91.

[37] Gurer-Orhan H, Suzen S. Melatonin, its metabolites and its synthetic analogs as multifaceted compounds: antioxidant, prooxidant and inhibitor of bioactivation reactions. Curr Med Chem 2015;22:490e9.

[38] Mark Percival. 1998 "Antioxidants". Clinical Nutrition Insights, 31: 01-04.

[39] McCord JM, Fridovich I (Nov 1969). "Superoxide dismutase. An enzymic function for erythrocuprein (hein)". The Journal of Biological Chemistry. 244 (22): 6049-6055.

[40] Fujii J, Iuchi Y, Okada F. Fundamental roles of reactive oxygen species and protective mechanisms in the female reproductive system. Reprod Biol Endocrinol. (2005) 3:43. 10.1186/1477-7827-3-43

[41] Valko, M., Leibfritz, D., Moncol, J., Cronin, M.T.D., Mazur, M. & Telser, J. Free radicals and antioxidants in normal physiological functions and human disease. International Journal of Biochemistry and Cell Biology 2007;39(1), 44-84.

[42] Lanone S, Bloc S, Foresti R, et al. Bilirubin decreases nos2 expression via inhibition of NAD(P)H oxidase: implications for protection against endotoxic shock in rats. The FASEB Journal 2005;19:1890-1892. 10.1096/fj.04-2368fje

[43] Matsumoto H, Ishikawa K, Itabe H, et al. Carbon monoxide and bilirubin from heme oxygenase-1 suppresses reactive oxygen species generation and plasminogen activator inhibitor-1 induction. Mol Cell Biochem 2006;291:21-28. 10.1007/s11010-006-9190-y

[44] Jiang F, Roberts SJ, Datla S, et al. NO modulates NADPH oxidase function via heme oxygenase-1 in human endothelial cells. Hypertension 2006;48:950-957. 10.1161/01.HYP.0000242336.58387.1f

[45] Behrman HR, Kodaman PH, Preston SL, Gao S. Oxidative stress and the ovary. J Soc Gynecol Investig 2001;8(Suppl):S40–S42.

[46] Shiotani M, Noda Y, Narimoto K, et al. Immunohistochemical localization of superoxide dismutase in the human ovary. Hum Reprod 1991; 6:1349-1353.

[47] Behrman HR, Kodaman PH, Preston SL, et al. Oxidative stress and the ovary. J Soc Gynecol Investig 2001; 8:S40–S42.

[48] Sugino N, Karube-Harada A, Taketani T, et al. Withdrawal of ovarian steroids stimulates prostaglandin F2alpha production through nuclear factor-kappaB activation via oxygen radicals in human endometrial stromal cells: potential relevance to menstruation. J Reprod Dev 2004; 50:215-225.

[49] Agarwal A, Aponte-Mellado A, Premkumar BJ, Shaman A, Gupta S. The ef- fects of oxidative stress on female reproduction: a review. Reprod Biol Endo- crinol 2012;10:49.

[50] Zegers-Hochschild F, Adamson GD, de Mouzon J, Ishihara O, Mansour R, Nygren K, et al. International Committee for Monitoring Assisted Reproduc- tive Technology (ICMART) and the World Health Oyrganization (WHO) revised glossary of ART terminology, 2009. Fertil Steril 2009;92:1520-1524.

[51] Boivin J, Bunting L, Collins JA, Nygren KG. International estimates of infer- tility prevalence and treatment-seeking: potential need and demand for infertility medical care. Hum Reprod 2007;22:1506-1512.

[52] Inhorn MC, Patrizio P. Infertility around the globe: new thinking on gender, reproductive technologies and global movements in the 21st century. Hum Reprod Update 2015;21:411-426.

[53] Mascarenhas MN, Flaxman SR, Boerma T, Vanderpoel S, Stevens GA. Na- tional, regional, and global trends in infertility prevalence since 1990: a systematic analysis of 277 health surveys. PLoS Med 2012;9:e1001356.

[54] Broekmans FJ, Fauser BCJM. Female infertility: evaluation and management. In: Jameson JL, De Groot LJ, de Krester DM, et al., editors. Endocrinology: adult and pediatric. 7th ed. Philadelphia: Elsevier Saunders; 2016:2260-2274.

[55] Aitken RJ, Clarkson JS. Cellular basis of defective sperm function and its as- sociation with the genesis of reactive oxygen species by human spermatozoa. J Reprod Fertil 1987;81:459-469.

[56] Behrman HR, Kodaman PH, Preston SL, Gao S. Oxidative stress and the ovary. J Soc Gynecol Investig 2001;8(Suppl):S40–S42.

[57] Liu F, He L, Liu Y, Shi Y, Du H. 2013. The expression and role of oxidative stress markers in the serum and follicular fluid of patients with endometriosis. Clin Exp Obstet Gynecol 40:372-376.

[58] Chattopadhayay R, Ganesh A, Samanta J, Jana SK, Chakravarty BN, Chaudhury K. 2010. Effect of follicular fluid oxidative stress on meiotic spindle formation in infertile women with polycystic ovarian syndrome. Gynecologic and Obstetric Investigation 69:197-202

[59] Nasiri N, Moini A, Eftekhari-Yazdi P, Karimian L, Salman-Yazdi R, Zolfaghari Z, Arabipoor A. 2015. Abdominal obesity can induce both systemic and follicular fluid oxidative stress independent from polycystic ovary syndrome. European Journal of Obstetrics & Gynecology and Reproductive Biology 184:112-116.

[60] Riley JC and Behrman HR (1991b) Oxygen radicals and reactive oxygen spe- cies in reproduction. Proc Soc Exp Biol Med 198,781-791.

[61] Riley JC and Behrman HR (1991a) In vivo generation of hydrogen peroxide in the rat corpus luteum during luteolysis. Endocrinology 128,1749-1753.

[62] Sugino N, Takiguchi S, Kashida S, Karube A, Nakamura Y and Kato H (2000) Superoxide dismutase expression in the human corpus luteum during the menstrual cycle and in early pregnancy. Mol Hum Reprod 6,19-25.

[63] Shimamura K, Sugino N, Y oshida Y , Nakamura Y , Ogino K and Kato H (1995) Changes in lipid peroxide and antioxidant enzyme activities in corpora lutea during pseudopregnancy in rats. J Reprod Fertil 105,253-257.

[64] Sawada M and Carlson JC (1996) Intracellular regulation of progesterone secretion by the superoxide radical in the rat corpus luteum. Endocrinol- ogy 137,1580-1584.

[65] Margolin Y, Aten RF and Behrman HR (1990) Antigonadotropic and antister- oidogenic actions of peroxide in rat granulosa cells. Endocrinology 127,245-250.

[66] Pasqualotto EB, Agarwal A, Sharma RK, Izzo VM, Pinotti JA, Joshi NJ and Rose BI (2004) Effect of oxidative stress in follicular fluid on the outcome of assisted reproductive procedures. Fertil Steril 81,973-976.

[67] Ledee-Bataille N, Olivennes F, Lefaix JL, ChaouatG, Frydman R, Delanian S. Combined treatment by pentoxifylline and tocopherol for recipient women with a thin endometrium enrolled in an oocyte donation programme. Human Reproduction 2002;17:1249-1253.

[68] Badawy A, State O, Abdelgawad S. N-acetyl cysteine and clomiphene citrate for induction of ovulation in polycystic ovary syndrome: a cross-over trial. Acta Obstetricia et Gynecologica Scandinavica 2007;86(2):218-222.

[69] Takasaki A, Tamura H, Taniguchi K, Asada H, Taketani T, Matsuoka A, et al. Luteal blood flow and luteal function. Journal of Ovarian Research 2009;2:1.

[70] Nestler JE. Myo-inositolphosphoglycans (IPGs) as mediators of insulin's steroidogenic actions. Journal of BasicClinical Physiological Pharmacology 1998;9(2-4): 197-204.

[71] Wathes DC, Abayasekara DR, Aitken RJ. Polyunsaturated fatty acids in male and female reproduction. Biology of Reproduction 2007;77(2):190-201.

[72] Bedaiwy MA, Falcone T, Mohamed MS, et al. Differential growth of human embryos in vitro: role of reactive oxygen species. Fertil Steril 2004; 82: 593-600.

[73] Agarwal A, Gupta S, Sikka S. The role of free radicals and antioxidants in reproduction. Curr Opin Obstet Gynecol. 2006 Jun;18(3):325-332. doi: 10.1097/01.gco.0000193003.58158.4e. PMID: 16735834.

[74] Kennedy S, Bergqvist A, Chapron C, et al. ESHRE guideline for the diagnosis and treatment of endometriosis. Hum Reprod 2005;20:2698-2704

[75] Houston DE. Evidence for the risk of pelvic endometriosis by age, race and socioeconomic status. Epidemiol Rev 1984;6:167-191

[76] Mehedintu C, Plotogea M, Ionescu S, et al. Endometriosis still a challenge. J Med Life 2014;7:349-357

[77] Abbas S, Ihle P, Koster I, et al. Prevalence and incidence of diagnosed endometriosis and risk of endometriosis in patients with endometriosis-related symptoms: findings from a statutory health insurance-based cohort in Germany. Eur J Obstet Gynecol Reprod Biol 2012;160:79-83

[78] Practice bulletin no. 114: management of endometriosis. Obstet Gynecol 2010;116:223-236

[79] Capobianco A, Rovere-Querini P. Endometriosis, a disease of the macrophage. Front Immunol 2013;4:9

[80] Podgaec S, Abrao MS, Dias JA Jr, et al. Endometriosis: an inflammatory disease with a Th2 immune response component. Hum Reprod 2007;22:1373-1379

[81] Santulli P, Borghese B, Chouzenoux S, et al. Serum and peritoneal interleukin- 33 levels are elevated in deeply infiltrating endometriosis. Hum Reprod 2012;27:2001-2009

[82] Oyinloye BE, Adenowo AF, Kappo AP. Reactive oxygen species, apoptosis, antimicrobial peptides and human inflammatory diseases. Pharmaceuticals (Basel) 2015;8:151-175

[83] Kim SH, Ihm HJ, Oh YS, et al. Increased nuclear expression of nuclear factor kappa-B p65 subunit in the eutopic endometrium and ovarian endometrioma of women with advanced stage endometriosis. Am JReprod Immunol 2013;70:497-508

[84] Tandrasasmita OM, Sutanto AM, Arifin PF, et al. Anti-inflammatory, antiangiogenic, and apoptosis-inducing activity of DLBS1442, a bioactive fraction of Phaleria macrocarpa, in a RL95-2 cell line as a molecular model of endometriosis. Int J Womens Health 2015;7:161-169

[85] Gonzalez-Ramos R, Donnez J, Defrere S, et al. Nuclear factor-kappa B is constitutively activated in peritoneal endometriosis. Mol Hum Reprod 2007;13:503-509

[86] Viatour P, Merville MP, Bours V, et al. Phosphorylation of NF-kappaB and IkappaB proteins: implications in cancer and inflammation. Trends Biochem Sci 2005;30:43-52

[87] Koks CA, Demir Weusten AY, Groothuis PG, et al. Menstruum induces changes in mesothelial cell morphology. Gynecol Obstet Invest 2000;50:13-18

[88] Swiersz LM. Role of endometriosis in cancer and tumor development. Ann N Y Acad Sci 2002;955:281-292

[89] Laurent A, Nicco C, Chereau C, et al. Controlling tumor growth by modulating endogenous production of reactive oxygen species. Cancer Res 2005;65:948-956

[90] Ishikawa K, Takenaga K, Akimoto M, et al. ROS-generating mitochondrial DNA mutations can regulate tumor cell metastasis. Science 2008;320:661-664.

[91] Ngo C, Chereau C, Nicco C, et al. Reactive oxygen species controls endometriosis progression. Am J Pathol 2009;175:225-234

[92] Paul S, Sharma AV, Mahapatra PD, et al. Role of melatonin in regulating matrix metalloproteinase-9 via tissue inhibitors of metalloproteinase-1 during protection against endometriosis. J Pineal Res 2008;44:439-449

[93] Szczepanska M, Kozlik J, Skrzypczak J, et al. Oxidative stress may be a piece in the endometriosis puzzle. Fertil Steril 2003;79:1288-1293

[94] Mier-Cabrera J, Aburto-Soto T, Burrola-Mendez S, et al. Women with endometriosis improved their peripheral antioxidant markers after the application of a high antioxidant diet. Reprod Biol Endocrinol 2009;7:54

[95] Traber MG, Stevens JF. Vitamins C and E: beneficial effects from a mechanistic perspective. Free Radic Biol Med 2011;51:1000-1013

[96] Amaya SC, Savaris RF, Filipovic CJ, et al. Resveratrol and endometrium:a closer look at an active ingredient of red wine using in vivo and in vitro models. Reprod Sci 2014;21:1362-1369

[97] Csaki C, Mobasheri A, Shakibaei M. Synergistic chondroprotective effects of curcumin and resveratrol in human articular chondrocytes: inhibition of IL-1beta-induced NF-kappaB-mediated inflammation and apoptosis. Arthritis Res Ther 2009;11:R165

[98] Rossi T, Gallo C, Bassani B, et al. Drink your prevention: beverages with cancer preventive phytochemicals. Pol Arch Med Wewn 2014;124:713-722

[99] Hardeland R. Antioxidative protection by melatonin: multiplicity of mechanisms from radical detoxification to radical avoidance. Endocrine 2005;27:119-130

[100] Reiter RJ, Tan DX, Manchester LC, et al. Biochemical reactivity of melatonin with reactive oxygen and nitrogen species: a review of the evidence. Cell Biochem Biophys 2001;34:237-256

[101] Collette T, Maheux R, Mailloux J, et al. Increased expression of matrix metalloproteinase-9 in the eutopic endometrial tissue of women

with endometriosis. Hum Reprod 2006;21:3059-3067

[102] Paul S, Bhattacharya P Das Mahapatra P, et al. Melatonin protects against endometriosis via regulation of matrix metalloproteinase-3 and an apoptotic pathway. J Pineal Res 2010;49:156-168

[103] Delneste Y, Jeannin P, Potier L, et al. N- acetyl-L-cysteine exhibits antitumoral activity by increasing tumor necrosis factor alpha-dependent T-cell cytotoxicity. Blood 1997;90:1124-1132

[104] Foyouzi N, Berkkanoglu M, Arici A, et al. Effects of oxidants and antioxidants on proliferation of endometrial stromal cells. Fertil Steril2004;82(Suppl 3):1019-1022

[105] Wu Y, Guo SW. Inhibition of proliferation of endometrial stromal cells by trichostatin A, RU486, CDB-2914, N-acetylcysteine, and ICI 182780. Gynecol Obstet Invest 2006;62:193-205

[106] Albini A, D'Agostini F, Giunciuglio D, et al. Inhibition of invasion, gelatinase activity, tumor take and metastasis of malignant cells by N-acetylcysteine. Int J Cancer 1995;61:121-129

[107] Eylar E, Rivera-Quinones C, Molina C, et al. N-acetylcysteine enhances T cell functions and T cell growth in culture. Int Immunol 1993;5:97-101

[108] Rudzitis-Auth J, Korbel C, Scheuer C, et al. Xanthohumol inhibits growth and vascularization of developing endometriotic lesions. Hum Reprod 2012;27:1735-1744

[109] Dell'Eva R, Ambrosini C, Vannini N, et al. AKT/NF-kappaB inhibitor xanthohumol targets cell growth and angiogenesis in hematologic malignancies. Cancer 2007;110:2007-2011

[110] Zhao F, Nozawa H, Daikonnya A, et al. Inhibitors of nitric oxide production from hops (Humulus lupulus L.).Biol Pharm Bull 2003;26:61-65

[111] Nagle DG, Ferreira D, Zhou YD. Epigallocatechin-3-gallate (EGCG): chemical and biomedical perspectives. Phytochemistry 2006;67:1849-1855

[112] Harlev A, Gupta S, Agarwal A. Targeting oxidative stress to treat endometriosis. Expert Opin Ther Targets. 2015;19(11):1447-1464. doi: 10.1517/14728222.2015.1077226. Epub 2015 Aug 10. PMID: 26256952.

[113] In WHO recommendations for prevention and treatment of pre-eclampsia and eclampsia. 2011. Geneva.

[114] Atallah AN, Hofmeyr GJ, Duley L. Calcium supplementation during pregnancy for preventing hypertensive disorders and related problems. *The Cochrane Database of Systematic Reviews* 2002, Issue 1.Art. No.: CD001059. DOI: 10.1002/14651858.CD001059.pub2.

[115] Knight M, Duley L, Henderson-Smart DJ, King JF. Antiplatelet agents for preventing and treating pre- eclampsia. *The Cochrane Database of Systematic Reviews* 2000, Issue 2.Art. No.: CD000492. DOI: 10.1002/ 14651858.CD000492.pub2.

[116] Hubel CA, Kagan VE, Kisin ER, McLaughlin MK, Roberts JM. Increased ascorbate radical formation and ascorbate depletion in plasma from women with preeclampsia: implications for oxidative stress. Free Radical Biology & Medicine 1997;23:597-609.

[117] Wang Y, Walsh SW. Antioxidant activities and mRNA expression of superoxide dismutase, catalase, and glutathione peroxidase in normal and preeclamptic pregnancies. Journal of the Society for Gynecological Investigation 1996;3:179-184.

[118] Rumbold A, Duley L, Crowther CA, Haslam RR. Antioxidants for preventing pre-eclampsia. Cochrane Database Syst Rev. 2008 Jan 23;2008(1):CD004227. doi: 10.1002/14651858.CD004227.pub3. PMID: 18254042; PMCID: PMC6718237.

[119] Tenório MB, Ferreira RC, Moura FA, Bueno NB, Goulart MOF, Oliveira ACM. Oral antioxidant therapy for prevention and treatment of preeclampsia: Meta-analysis of randomized controlled trials. Nutr Metab Cardiovasc Dis. 2018 Sep;28(9):865-876. doi: 10.1016/j.numecd.2018.06.002. Epub 2018 Jun 9. PMID: 30111493.

[120] Salles AMR, Galvao TF, Silva MT, Motta LCD, Pereira MG. Antioxidants for preventing preeclampsia: a systematic review. Sci World J 2012:1e10. https://doi.org/10.1100/2012/243476.

[121] Lee FH, Raja SN. Complementary and alternative medicine in chronic pain. Pain 2011; 152: 28-30.

[122] Salinthone S, Yadav V, Schillace RV, Bourdette DN, Carr DW. Lipoic acid attenuates inflammation via cAMP and protein kinase A signaling. PloS One 2010; 5: sic.

[123] Goraca A, Huk-kolega H, Piechota A, Kleniewska P, Ciejka E, Skibska B. Lipoic acid--biological activity and therapeutic potential. Pharmacol Rep 2011; 63: 849-858.

[124] Tan EC, Bahrami S, Kozlov AV, Kurvers HA, Ter Laak HJ, Nohl H, Redl H, Goris RJ. The oxidative response in the chronic constriction injury model of neuropathic pain. J Surg Res 2009; 152: 84-88.

[125] Ziegler D, Ametov A, Barinov A, Dyck PJ, Gurieva I, Low PA, Munzel U, Yakhno N, Raz I, Novosadova M, Maus J, Samigullin R. Oral treatment with alpha- lipoic acid improves symptomatic diabetic polyneuropathy: the SYDNEY 2 trial. Diabetes Care 2006; 29:2365-2370.

[126] Di Geronimo G, Caccese Af, Caruso , Oldati A, Passaretti U. Treatment of carpal tunnel syndrome with alpha-lipoic acid. Eur Rev Med Pharmacol Sci 2009; 13: 133-139.

[127] Bertolotto f, Massone a. Combination of alpha lipoic acid and superoxide dismutase leads to physiological and symptomatic improvements in di- abetic neuropathy. Drugs in R&D 2012; 12: 29-34.

[128] Chiara Di Tucci, Mara Di Feliciantonio, Flaminia Vena, Carmela Capone, Michele Carlo Schiavi, Daniela Pietrangeli, Ludovico Muzii & Pierluigi Benedetti Panici (2018): Alpha lipoic acid in obstetrics and gynecology, Gynecological Endocrinology, DOI: 10.1080/09513590.2018.1462320

[129] D'Ambrosio SM, Daniel FB, Hart RW. Cellular repair of DNA damage induced by 7,12-&methylbenz[a]anthracene and its fluoro analogs in vitro. In: Jones PW, Leber P, editors. Polynu- clear aromatic hydrocarbons. Ann Arbor: Ann Arbor Science Publishers, Inc., 1979:793-802.

[130] Schwab M, Amler LC. Amplification of cellular oncogenes: a predictor of clinical outcome in human cancer. Genes Chromo- somes Cancer 1990;1:181-193.

[131] Ratner L, Josephs SF, Wong-Staal F. Oncogenes: their role in neoplastic transformation. Annu Rev Microbiol 1985;39:419-449.

[132] DraganYP,PitotHC.The role of the stages of initiation and promotion in phenotypic diversity during hepatocardnogenesis in the rat. Curcinogenesis 1992;13:739-750.

[133] Pitot HC. Endogenous carcinogenesis: the role of tumor promo- tion. Proc Soc Exp Biol Med 1991;198:661-666.

[134] Farber E,Sarma DSR. Biology of disease: hepatocarcinogenesis. a dynamic cellular perspective. Lab Invest 1987;56:4-22.

[135] Boyd JA,Barrett JC.Genetic and cellular basis of multistep carcinogenesis. Pharmacol Ther 1990;46:469-486.

[136] Asadi-Samani M, Bagheri N, Rafieian-Kopaei M, Shirzad H. Inhibition of Th1 and Th17 Cells by Medicinal Plants and Their Derivatives: A Systematic Review. Phytotherapy Research. 2017;31:1128-1139

[137] Asadi-Samani M, Rafieian-Kopaei M, Lorigooini Z, Shirzad H. A screening of growth inhibitory activity of Iranian medicinal plants on prostate cancer cell lines. BioMedicine. 2018;8:8

[138] Yasueda A, Urushima H, Ito T. Efficacy and interaction of antioxidant supplements as adjuvant therapy in cancer treatment: A systematic review. Integrative Cancer Therapies. 2016;15(1):17-39

[139] Nechuta S, Lu W, Chen Z, Zheng Y, Gu K, Cai H, et al. Vitamin supplement use during breast cancer treatment and survival: A prospective cohort study. Cancer Epidemiology, Biomarkers & Prevention. 2011;20(2):262-271

[140] Watson J. Oxidants, antioxidants and the current incurability of metastatic cancers. Open Biology. 2013;3(1):120144

[141] Antioxidants: MedlinePlus. Available at: https://medlineplus.gov/antioxidants.html.01/03/2018

[142] Amini L, Tehranian N, Movahedin M, Ramezani Tehrani F, Ziaee S. Antioxidants and management of polycystic ovary syndrome in Iran: A systematic review of clinical trials. Iran J Reprod Med. 2015 Jan;13(1):1-8. PMID: 25653669; PMCID: PMC4306978. Mohammadi M.

[143] Oxidative stress and polycystic ovary syndrome: A brief review. Int J Prev Med 2019;10:86.

[144] Bouayed J, Bohn T. Exogenous antioxidants—Double-edged swords in cellular redox state: Health beneficial effects at physiologic doses versus deleterious effects at high doses. Oxid Med Cell Longevity. 2010;3:228-37. [PMCID: PMC2952083] [PubMed: 20972369]

[145] Palacio J, Iborra A, Ulcova-Gallova Z, Badia R, Martinez P. The presence of antibodies to oxidative modified proteins in serum from polycystic ovary syndrome patients. ClinExp Immunol. 2006;144:217-22. [PMCID: PMC1809652] [PubMed: 16634794]

[146] Tuso P, Stoll SR, Li WW. A plant-based diet, atherogenesis, and coronary artery disease prevention. Perm J. 2015;19:62-7. [PMCID: PMC4315380] [PubMed: 25431999]

[147] Hanna FW, Duff CJ, Shelley-Hitchen A, Hodgson E, Fryer AA. Diagnosing gestational diabetes mellitus: implications of recent changes in diagnostic criteria and role of glycated haemoglobin (HbA1c). Clin Med (Lond) 2017;17:108-113.

[148] Ferrara A. Increasing prevalence of gestational diabetes mellitus: a public health perspective. Diabetes Care 2007;30 Suppl 2:S141–S146.

[149] Nilsson C. Gestational diabetes mellitus: future risk for mother and child [doctor's thesis]. Lund: Lund University, Faculty of Medicine; 2013.

[150] Altan N, Dinçel AS, Koca C. Diabetes mellitus ve oksidatif stres. Turk J Biochem 2006;1:51-56.

[151] Maritim AC, Sanders RA, Watkins JB 3rd. Diabetes, oxidative stress, and antioxidants: a review. J Biochem Mol Toxicol 2003;17:24-38.

[152] Suhail M, Patil S, Khan S, Siddiqui S. Antioxidant vitamins and lipoperoxidation in non-pregnant, pregnant, and gestational diabetic women: erythrocytes osmotic fragility profiles. J Clin Med Res 2010;2:266-273.

[153] Huang HY, Appel LJ. Supplementation of diets with α-tocopherol reduces serum concentrations of γ- and δ-tocopherol in humans. J Nutr 2003;133:3137-3140.

[154] Limberaki E, Eleftheriou P, Vagdatli E, Kostoglou V, Petrou C. Serum antioxidant status among young, middle-aged and elderly people before and after antioxidant rich diet. Hippokratia 2012;16:118-123.

[155] Baynes JW. Role of oxidative stress in development of complication in diabetes. Diabetes 1991; 40: 405-412.

[156] Oberley LW. Free radicals and diabetes. Free Radical Biol Med 1988; 5: 113-124.

[157] Reece EA. Maternal Fuels, Diabetic Embryopathy: Pathomechanism and Prevention. Semin Reprod Med 1999; 17(2): 183-194.

[158] Malvy E, Thiébaut R, Marimoutou C, Dabis F. Weight loss and body mass index as predictors of HIV disease progression to AIDS in adults. Aquitaine cohort, France, 1985-1997. J Am Coll Nutr. 2001; 20: 609-615.

[159] Population. C on social security HD criteria and board on the H of select. HIV and Disability: Updating the social security listings. 2010.

[160] Maged AM, Torky H, Fouad MA, GadAllah SH, Waked NM, Gayed AS, Salem AK. Role of antioxidants in gestational diabetes mellitus and relation to fetal outcome: a randomized controlled trial. J Matern Fetal Neonatal Med. 2016 Dec;29(24):4049-4054. doi: 10.3109/14767058.2016.1154526. Epub 2016 Mar 21. PMID: 26999688.

[161] Abdul-Barry J, Al-Rubai SA, Qasim QA. Study of Oxidant-Antioxidant Status in Recurrent Spontaneous Abortion. TQMJ. 2011; 5:35-46.

[162] Mistry HD, Williams PJ. The Importance of Antioxidant Micronutrients in Pregnancy. Oxid Med Cell Longev. 2011; 2011: 841749.

[163] Poston L, Igosheva N, Mistry HD, Seed PT, Shennan AH, Rana S, *et al*. Role of oxidative stress and antioxidant supplementation in pregnancy disorders. Am J Clin Nutr. 2011; 94(6 Suppl): 1980S–1985S.

[164] Al-Kunani AS, Knight R, Haswell SJ, Thompson W, Lindow SW. The selenium status of women with a history of recurrent miscarriage. BJOG. 2001; 108: 1094-1097.

[165] Han M, Pendem S, Teh SL, Sukumaran DK, Wu F, Wilson JX. Ascorbate protects endothelial barrier function during septic insult: Role of protein phosphatase type 2A. Free Radic Biol Med. 2010; 48: 128-135.

[166] Lonn E, Bosch J, Yusuf S, Sheridan P, Pogue J, Arnold JM, *et al.* Effects of Long-term Vitamin E Supplementation on Cardiovascular Events and Cancer: a rondomized clinial trial. JAMA. 2005; 293:1338-1347.

Chapter 5

Thiol Reduction and Cardiolipin Improve Complex I Activity and Free Radical Production in Liver Mitochondria of Streptozotocin-Induced Diabetic Rats

Manjury Jatziry Hernández-Esparza, Claudia Guadalupe Flores-Ledesma, Rocío Montoya-Pérez, Elizabeth Calderón-Cortés, Alfredo Saavedra-Molina, Alain Raimundo Rodríguez-Orozco and Christian Cortés-Rojo

Abstract

Mitochondrial reactive oxygen species (ROS) are involved in diabetic liver disease development. Diabetes impairs complex I activity and increases ROS production in liver mitochondria. The complex I produces ROS in forward electron transfer (FET) or in reverse electron transfer (RET) modes depending on the site of electron transfer blocking and the availability of respiratory substrates. Complex I activity depends on the phospholipid cardiolipin and the redox state of reactive thiols in the enzyme. Neither the underlying factors leading to complex I dysfunction nor the mode of ROS production have been elucidated in liver mitochondria in diabetes. We tested in liver mitochondria from streptozotocin (STZ) -induced diabetic rats if the addition of cardiolipin or β-mercaptoethanol, a thiol reducing agent, recovers complex I activity and decreases ROS production with substrates inducing ROS production in FET or RET modes. Decreased complex I activity and enhanced ROS generation in FET mode was detected in mitochondria from diabetic rats. Complex I activity was fully restored with the combined treatment with cardiolipin plus β-mercaptoethanol, which also abated ROS generation in FET mode. This suggest that therapies restoring cardiolipin and reducing mitochondrial thiols might be useful to counteract impaired complex I activity and excessive ROS production in liver mitochondria in diabetes.

Keywords: diabetes, liver disease, electron transport chain, free radicals, NADH dehydrogenase

1. Introduction

Hyperglycemia causes liver injury in diabetic rats by inducing apoptosis via ERK1/2, p38, and NF-κB pathways [1]. These proteins can be activated by ROS [2].

IntechOpen

The sources of ROS in the diabetic liver includes activated NADPH oxidases [3] and the mitochondrial electron transport chain (ETC) [4]. Mitochondrial ROS are essential for the development diabetic liver injury, as evidenced by the therapeutic effect of mitochondria-targeted antioxidants on non-alcoholic fatty liver disease (NAFLD) [5], which is the manifestation of liver disease in the metabolic syndrome [6].

Diabetes impairs complex I activity in the ETC of liver mitochondria, leading to electron leak and increased ROS production [7–9]. The complex I is a large, L-shaped, multimeric protein that oxidizes NADH via a flavin mononucleotide (FMN) located at the soluble arm of the complex. Electrons are transferred then through a series of Fe-S clusters to a ubiquinone molecule placed in a binding site at the interface of the soluble and membrane arms of the complex I [10]. Complex I activity depends on interactions with the anionic phospholipid cardiolipin, enabling the access of ubiquinone molecules to its binding site and stabilizing the formation of channels for protonation pathways in the ubiquinone-binding site [11]. Lipid peroxidation, a key feature in the diabetic liver [12], modifies the spatial orientation of cardiolipin in the inner mitochondrial membrane, altering specific interactions between protein domains and cardiolipin [13]. Therefore, lipid peroxidation may disrupt electron transfer in the complex I by impairing cardiolipin function. Another factor decreasing complex I activity is the reversible oxidation of reactive thiols, which occurs by a drop in the ratio of reduced-to-oxidized glutathione (GSH/GSSG) in mitochondria. Complex I activity can be recovered by increasing the levels of GSH with a thiol reducing agent [14].

Decreased complex I activity lead to increased mitochondrial ROS production. ROS are produced in FET mode when NADH is oxidized by FMN but electron transfer is blocked at the ubiquinone-binding site in the complex I [15]. ROS may be also produced in RET mode when high succinate concentrations reduces the pool of ubiquinone and forces reverse electron flow from the ubiquinone-binding site to the FMN [16].

Previously, we have observed that diabetes exacerbates lipid peroxidation and decreases GSH/GSSG ratio in liver mitochondria [9]. As these events causes oxidative damage in cardiolipin and the oxidation of thiol groups in the complex I, respectively, the hypothesis of this study is that impaired complex I activity in liver mitochondria of diabetic rats may be restored by the in vitro treatment with cardiolipin and a thiol reducing agent. To address this hypothesis, we have treated isolated liver mitochondria from type 1, STZ-induced diabetic rats with β-mercaptoethanol, a thiol reducing agent [17], or with exogenous cardiolipin, which restitutes normal cardiolipin levels in mitochondria [18]. The results show that β-mercaptoethanol or cardiolipin partially restored complex I activity, while the combination of these agents fully recovers complex I activity. Moreover, diabetes increased ROS production in the complex I only in FET mode, which was inhibited by the combined treatment with β-mercaptoethanol plus cardiolipin. These results are discussed in the context of known structure–activity relationships for complex I and the importance of impaired liver metabolism in the development of insulin resistance.

2. Materials and methods

2.1 Animals and experimental groups

Male Long-Evans rats weighing 300–350 g were housed in a bioterioum with controlled temperature and 12 h/12 h dark/light cycles. The rats were fed ad libitum with a standard rodent chow (Laboratory Rodent Diet 5001, LabDiet, St. Louis, MO, USA) plus free access to water. Before diabetes induction, the animals were fasted overnight. Type 1 diabetes was induced by an intraperitoneal injection of

45 mg/Kg STZ. Five days later, blood glucose was measured and the animals with glucose levels ≥150 mg/dL were selected for the study. Blood glucose levels were assessed with an Accu-Chek glucometer (Roche DC México S.A de C.V.). All the procedures with animals were carried out in accordance with Federal Regulations for the Use and Care of Animals (NOM-062-ZOO-1999) issued by the Mexican Ministry of Agriculture.

2.2 Mitochondria isolation

After 90-days diabetes, rats were fasted by 12 h before the sacrifice. Rats were decapitated, the liver was extracted, weighted, and placed in a medium with 220 mM mannitol, 70 mM sucrose, 2 mM MOPS and 1 mM EGTA (pH 7.4). The liver was cut in small fragments, washed, and homogenized with in a Potter-Elvehjem homogenizer. The liver homogenate was centrifuged at 314 x g for 10 min. The supernatant was recovered and centrifuged at 4410 x g for 10 min. From this centrifugation, the supernatant was discarded, and the pellet was washed and resuspended with a medium containing 220 mM mannitol, 70 mM sucrose and 2 mM MOPS (pH 7.4), and centrifuged at 6350 x g for 10 min. Finally, supernatant from the later centrifugation was discarded and the pellet was resuspended in 500 μL of the latter medium. All the centrifugations were carried out at 4°C. The concentration of mitochondrial protein was assessed by the Biuret method.

2.3 Addition of cardiolipin to isolated mitochondria

Cardiolipin liposomes were fused with liver mitochondria to increase the content of this phospholipid in mitochondrial membranes as reported elsewhere [18]. Briefly, 1.7 mg cardiolipin (Sigma-Aldrich, St. Louis, MO, USA) was added to 1 mL 25 mM KH_2PO_4 (pH 6.7). To obtain liposomes, this mixture was subjected to six cycles of sonication at 40 W for 2.5 min each with a Branson 450 sonifier (Branson Ultrasonics, Danbury, CT USA) under a N_2 stream. Then, 1 mL of freshly prepared liposomes were mixed with 1 mg mitochondrial protein in 25 mM KH_2PO_4 buffer with constant stirring for 40 min. Mitochondria were centrifuged at 13684 x g for 20 min to eliminate cardiolipin excess. Mitochondria were resuspended in 25 mM KH_2PO_4 buffer, and centrifuged again for 10 min at 13684 x g. The pellet was recovered and resuspended in a medium with 250 mM sucrose and 10 mM Tris (pH 7.4).

2.4 Measurement of complex I activity and treatments with β-mercaptoethanol

Mitochondria were solubilized with Triton X-100 as reported previously [9]. Detergent-solubilized mitochondrial protein (0.1 mg/mL) was placed in a quartz cuvette with 1 mL 50 mM KH_2PO_4 buffer (pH 7.6) and incubated with 1 mM KCN and 1 μg antimycin A. After 5 min, 5 mM potassium ferricyanide was added as electron acceptor and the absorbance was registered at 340 nm for 1 min in a Shimadzu UV2550 spectrophotometer (Kyoto, Japan). Next, 1 mM NADH was added and the changes in the absorbance were further registered for 4 min. Complex I activity was calculated from the slopes of the time-traces of NADH oxidation. Mitochondria fused with cardiolipin liposomes were used to determine the effect of exogenously added cardiolipin on complex I activity. For complex I determinations in the presence of a thiol reductant, mitochondria were incubated 15 min before complex I assay in 50 mM KH_2PO_4 buffer (pH 7.6) with 25 or 50 μM β-mercaptoethanol [19]. To evaluate the effect of cardiolipin plus β-mercaptoethanol on complex I activity, mitochondria were first fused with cardiolipin liposomes and then treated with 50 μM β-mercaptoethanol by the procedures described above.

2.5 Determination of ROS production

ROS generation was assessed in isolated mitochondria by measuring the oxidation of the fluorescent probe 2′,7′-dichlorodihydrofluorescein (H_2DCF) as previously described [9], except that some modifications in the experimental conditions were made to identify the mode by which ROS were produced. To assess ROS production in complex I by FET mode, 10 mM glutamate-malate was added as substrate and the fluorescence of H_2DCF was followed for 20 min. To determine ROS production in the complex I by RET mode, 10 mM succinate was added as substrate and the fluorescence was followed for 20 min. ROS production upstream complex I (i.e. in the complex II - complex IV segment of the ETC) was assessed by inhibiting RET with rotenone, a complex I inhibitor, and using succinate as substrate [16], after which the changes in fluorescence were evaluated for 20 min. The rate of ROS generation was expressed like the change in arbitrary units of fluorescence (ΔF) per min^{-1} per mg mitochondrial $protein^{-1}$.

2.6 Statistical analysis

The number of independent experiments using different samples is indicated in the legend to each figure. The results are expressed as the mean ± standard error. Statistical differences between means were analyzed with Student's t-test ($P < 0.05$), using the Sigma Plot (v11.0) software (Systat Software, Inc., San Jose, CA, USA).

3. Results

3.1 Blood glucose and relative liver weight

After 90 days of diabetes induction, blood glucose levels in control and diabetic rats were 98.2 and 347.1 mg/dL, respectively, (**Figure 1A**). Moreover, the liver weight in diabetic rats was 1.3- fold higher than in control rats (**Figure 1B**). This effect was more accentuated when liver-to-body weight ratios were compared, as the value of this parameter was almost two - fold higher in the diabetic rats than in the control animals (**Figure 1C**). These results confirm the presence of hyperglycemia and a pathologic phenotype in the livers of STZ-induced diabetic rats.

3.2 Effects of β-mercaptoethanol and cardiolipin on complex I activity

The effect of diabetes on complex I activity of liver mitochondria is shown in the **Figure 2**. Complex I activity was 1.8 – fold lower in the mitochondria of diabetic rats than in mitochondria from the control group. On the other hand, isolated mitochondria from diabetic rats were incubated with 25 or 50 μM β-mercaptoethanol to evaluate at what extent thiol reduction recovers the activity of the complex I (**Figure 2A**). Both β-mercaptoethanol concentrations partially recovered the enzymatic activity, being this effect statistically significant only with 50 μM of β-mercaptoethanol. Thus, 50 μM of β-mercaptoethanol was chosen for the following experiments. Of note, β-mercaptoethanol concentrations higher than 50 μM impaired complex I activity (data not shown).

Liver mitochondria from diabetic rats were incubated with cardiolipin to determine at what extent this phospholipid recovers complex I activity in diabetic rats (**Figure 2B**). It can be observed that cardiolipin addition restored complex I activity

DOI: http://dx.doi.org/10.5772/intechopen.95112

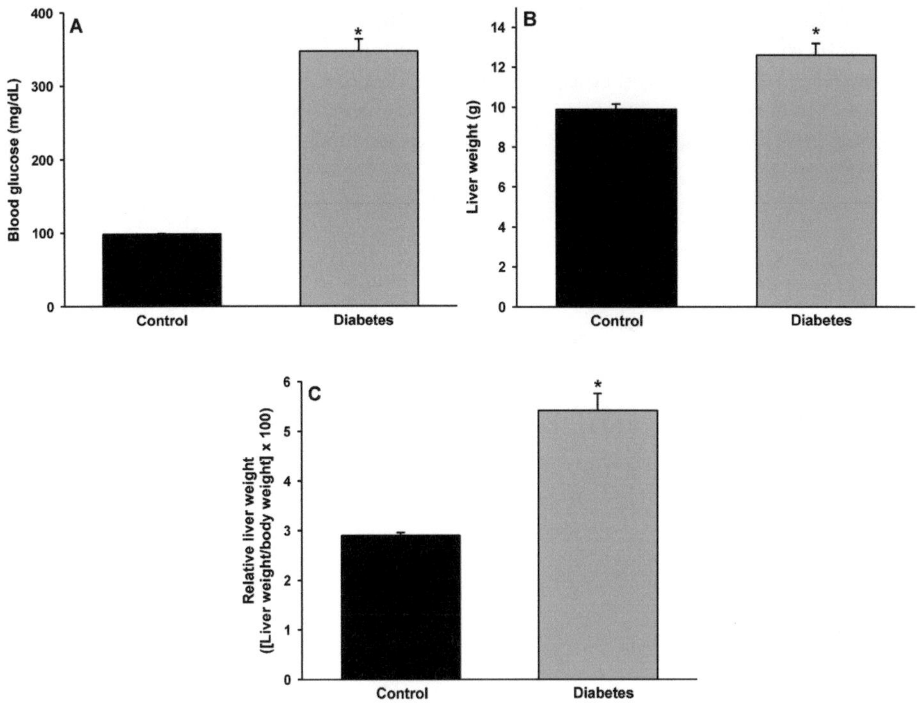

Figure 1.
*Effects of diabetes on blood glucose levels (A), liver weight (B) and relative liver weight (C). Data are presented as the mean ± standard error of n ≥ 4. *P < 0.05 vs. control group (Student's t-test).*

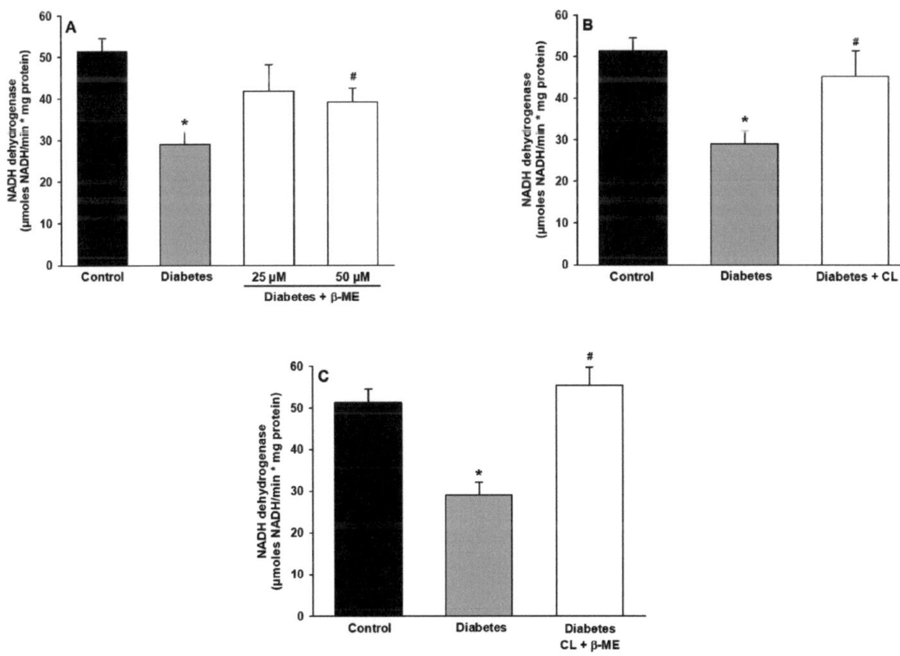

Figure 2.
*Recovery of complex I activity in liver mitochondria from diabetic rats by the incubation with β-mercaptoethanol (β-ME) (A), cardiolipin (CL) (B), or cardiolipin plus 50 µM β-mercaptoethanol (CL+ β-ME) (C). Data are presented as the mean ± standard error of n ≥ 6. *P < 0.05 vs. control; #P < 0.05 vs. Diabetes (Student's t-test).*

without reaching the activity of the control group. In contrast to the individual treatment with β-mercaptoethanol or cardiolipin, the combined treatment with these agents fully recovered complex I activity (**Figure 2C**). These results suggest that impaired complex I activity in mitochondria from diabetic rats may be fully counteracted by supplying cardiolipin and restoring the redox state of mitochondrial thiols.

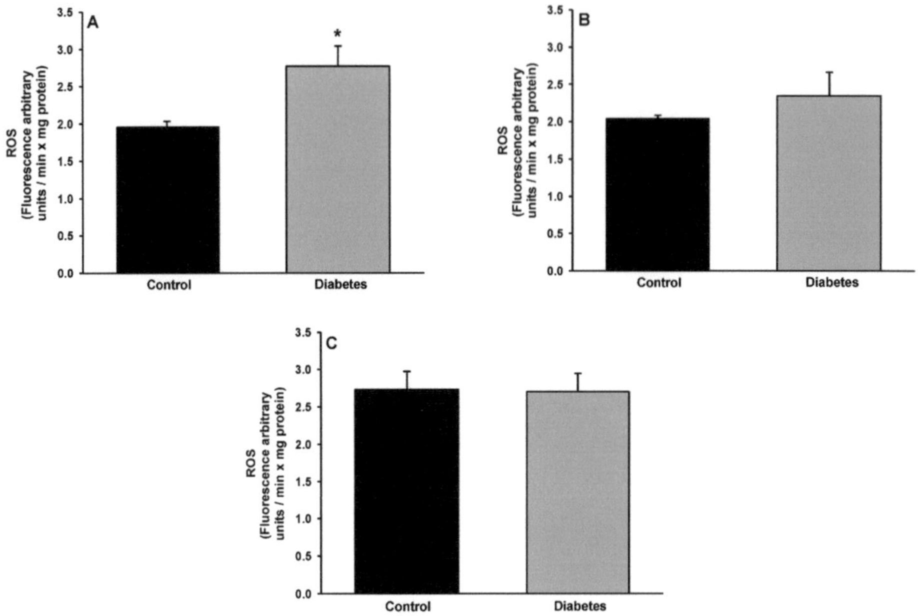

Figure 3.
*ROS production in liver mitochondria in FET mode with glutamate/malate as substrate (A), in RET mode with succinate as substrate (B), and in RET mode blocked with rotenone (C). Data are presented as the mean ± standard error of n = 6. *P < 0.05 vs. control group (Student's t-test).*

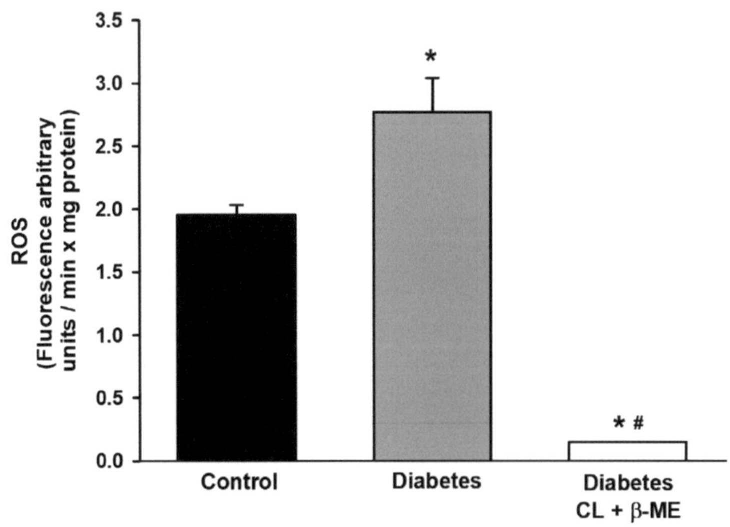

Figure 4.
*Effect of cardiolipin (CL) plus 50 μM β-mercaptoethanol (β-ME) on ROS production in FET mode in liver mitochondria from diabetic rats. Data are presented as the mean ± standard error of n = 6. *P < 0.05 vs. Control; #P < 0.05 vs. Diabetes (Student's t-test).*

3.3 Effect of respiratory substrates on ROS production by complex I

ROS production was determined in isolated liver mitochondria in FET mode using glutamate/malate as substrate for complex I (**Figure 3A**), in RET mode using succinate as complex II substrate (**Figure 3B**), and with succinate plus rotenone (an inhibitor of the ubiquinone-binding site in the complex I) for blocking ROS production in the complex I by RET (**Figure 3C**). In FET mode, ROS production increased 1.4 - fold in mitochondria from diabetic rats in comparison to mitochondria from control rats (**Figure 3A**). No statistically significant changes in ROS production were observed neither in RET mode (**Figure 3B**), nor when RET was blocked with rotenone (**Figure 3C**).

A 19 – fold decrease in ROS production in FET mode was observed in mitochondria from diabetic rats treated with cardiolipin plus β-mercaptoethanol when compared with mitochondria from diabetic rats without any addition (**Figure 4**). These results indicate that diabetes increases ROS production in FET mode, which may be prevented by reducing mitochondrial thiols and supplying mitochondria with cardiolipin.

4. Discussion

The results show that, under our experimental conditions, STZ-induced diabetic rats developed hyperglycemia and abnormal liver weight (**Figure 1**). These events were accompanied by decreased complex I activity (**Figure 2**) and increased ROS generation in FET mode (**Figure 3**), which was reverted by the in vitro treatment with cardiolipin plus β-mercaptoethanol (**Figure 4**). Increased liver weight has been identified as an alteration characterizing liver disease [20]. Moreover, increased blood markers of liver injury have been observed in STZ-induced diabetic rats [1]. All these data indicate that diabetic rats in this study developed liver disease.

There is a close relationship between the development of liver disease and the presence of mitochondrial dysfunction [21]. This agrees with enhanced liver weight (**Figure 1B** and **C**), decreased complex I activity (**Figure 2A**), and higher ROS production (**Figure 3A**) observed in liver mitochondria from diabetic rats. There are two main mechanism modulating complex I activity: the first one is the reversible oxidation of reactive thiols in cysteine residues due to decreased mitochondrial GSH/GSSG ratio. The inhibition of the complex I by thiol oxidation can be reversed in vitro by increasing the concentration of GSH via the addition of thiol reducing agents like dithiothreitol [14]. β-mercaptoethanol is another agent that reduces GSSG to GSH [17], besides, it restores the activity of the ETC complexes after an oxidative insult [19]. Therefore, the partial recovery of complex I activity with 50 μM β-mercaptoethanol (**Figure 2A**) suggests that thiol oxidation in the complex I is part of the mechanism explaining complex I inhibition by diabetes. The second mechanism inhibiting complex I activity is the loss of cardiolipin due to peroxidative damage. An approach to recover impaired complex I activity after cardiolipin loss is the exogenous addition of this phospholipid to isolated mitochondria [18]. This strategy partially recovered complex I activity in liver mitochondria of diabetic rats (**Figure 2B**).

The partial recovery of complex I activity with either β-mercaptoethanol or cardiolipin led us to think that the combined treatment with these two agents may drive to full recovery of complex I activity in liver mitochondria from diabetic rats, which was confirmed in the experiment of the **Figure 2C**. These data suggest that diabetes impaired complex I activity by promoting both the oxidation of reactive thiols in the complex I and the peroxidation of cardiolipin. This suggestion is supported by previous data showing decreased GSH/GSSG ratios and increased lipid peroxidation in liver mitochondria from STZ-induced diabetic rats [9]. As mentioned before, decreased GSH levels lead to the oxidation of reactive thiols in the complex I [14], while lipid peroxidation affects negatively both the structure and function of cardiolipin in the inner mitochondrial membrane [13].

We acknowledge that one of the main limitations of this study is that we did not measure neither cardiolipin levels nor the redox status of thiols in the complex I. Nevertheless, we believe that our results give a clue about the role of cardiolipin and thiol oxidation in the mechanism of complex I inhibition by diabetes, since the experimental approaches used in this study to replenish cardiolipin in mitochondria and to reduce thiols in complex I have been previously validated by direct determinations of both cardiolipin and the redox state of thiols in complex I [14, 18]. On the other hand, there are conflicting studies showing increased complex I activity [22], enhanced content of cardiolipin [23], and decreased superoxide production by complex I [24] in liver mitochondria from STZ-induced diabetic rats. However, it must be pointed out that diabetes was induced in these studies by a shorter, 8 to 9 -weeks period, in comparison with the 12-weeks period used in this study. Thus, it can be hypothesized that the mechanisms responsible for such adaptive responses seen in shorter periods of diabetes might be impaired at longer time periods like in this study.

The complex I produces ROS in FET mode due to electron leak during electron transfer from NADH to ubiquinone. ROS are also produced in the complex I by RET mode when electrons are forced to flow from ubiquinol to NAD^+ [25]. ROS are produced at least in two different sites of the complex I, one situated at the ubiquinone-binding site (I_Q), and the other one located at the flavin mononucleotide (FMN)-binding site (I_F) [16]. The significant increase in ROS levels in mitochondria from diabetic rats only with a substrate for complex I (**Figure 3A**), suggests that diabetes causes an alteration in the complex I that stimulates ROS production in FET mode. This mode of ROS production occurs when electron transfer to ubiquinone is blocked at the I_Q site [16]. In this regard, the access of ubiquinone to the I_Q site is thought to occur via a cardiolipin-dependent mechanism [11]. The recovery of complex I activity (**Figure 2**) and the decrease in ROS production (**Figure 4**) observed with cardiolipin, suggest that diabetes disrupt electron transfer at the I_Q site by a mechanism involving lipid peroxidation, as suggested by the increased levels of lipid peroxidation found in a previous work in liver mitochondria from STZ-induced diabetic rats [9]. Therefore, impaired electron flow in the I_Q site would drive to a more reduced state of the redox centers upstream the I_Q site (i.e. the iron–sulfur clusters and the FMN in the complex I), leading to electron leak and ROS generation, while the replenishment of mitochondria with cardiolipin might improve both the architecture of the I_Q site and electron transfer to ubiquinone, decreasing in this way the electron leak and ROS production.

The inhibition of the complex I during diabetes is not trivial as this enzyme is the main mechanism to maintain high NAD^+/NADH ratios [26]. High NAD^+ levels activates sirtuins proteins, whose deacetylase activity enhances lipid and glucose catabolism and the antioxidant defenses in the liver [27]. On the contrary, low NAD^+ levels impair hepatic catabolism and increases oxidative stress, leading to the development of liver disease and insulin resistance [28]. This reflect the importance of preserving optimal rates of NADH oxidation by the complex I in the diabetic liver, which, according to our results, might be achieved by strategies simultaneously augmenting the levels of cardiolipin and GSH. In this regard, it has been demonstrated that linoleic acid supplementation increases cardiolipin levels in cultured fibroblasts depleted of cardiolipin [29] and increases complex I activity in HeLa cells [30]. On the other hand, phytochemicals like betaine and β-sitosterol have counteracted the negative impact of liver toxicants like ethanol or carbon tetrachloride on the levels of mitochondrial GSH [31, 32]. Therefore, the concomitant targeting of cardiolipin and mitochondrial GSH and its impact on both the complex I function and hepatic lipid metabolism deserves further investigation, given the central role of defective hepatic lipid metabolism in peripheral insulin resistance in diabetes [33].

5. Conclusions

Diabetes induced anormal liver weight in STZ-induced rats, accompanied of mitochondrial alterations in the ETC such as decreased complex I activity and increased ROS production in FET mode. These mitochondrial abnormalities were corrected by the in vitro treatment with cardiolipin plus β-mercaptoethanol, which suggest that alterations in the content of cardiolipin and thiol oxidation may be underlying causes of these mitochondrial alterations. On this basis, is proposed that therapies counteracting mitochondrial alterations in cardiolipin and thiol oxidation might be useful to ameliorate hepatic disturbances elicited by diabetes.

Acknowledgements

This work was supported by a grant from Programa de Investigación 2021, Coordinación de la Investigación Científica - UMSNH, Morelia, Michoacán, México (15798 to C. Cortés-Rojo).

Conflict of interest

The authors declare no conflict of interest.

Author details

Manjury Jatziry Hernández-Esparza[1], Claudia Guadalupe Flores-Ledesma[1], Rocío Montoya-Pérez[1], Elizabeth Calderón-Cortés[2], Alfredo Saavedra-Molina[1], Alain Raimundo Rodríguez-Orozco[3] and Christian Cortés-Rojo[1]*

1 Institute of Chemical and Biological Research, Michoacán University of Saint Nicholas of Hidalgo, Morelia, Mexico

2 Faculty of Nursery, Michoacán University of Saint Nicholas of Hidalgo, Morelia, Mexico

3 Faculty of Medicine, Michoacán University of Saint Nicholas of Hidalgo, Morelia, Mexico

*Address all correspondence to: christian.cortes@umich.mx

References

[1] Manna P, Das J, Ghosh J, Sil PC. Contribution of type 1 diabetes to rat liver dysfunction and cellular damage via activation of NOS, PARP, IkappaBalpha/NF-kappaB, MAPKs, and mitochondria-dependent pathways: Prophylactic role of arjunolic acid. Free Radical Biology & Medicine. 2010;48:1465-1484. DOI: 10.1016/j.freeradbiomed.2010.02.025

[2] Zhang J, Wang X, Vikash V, Ye Q, Wu D, Liu Y, Dong W. ROS and ROS-mediated cellular signaling. Oxidative Medicine and Cellular Longevity. 2016;2016:4350965. DOI: 10.1155/2016/4350965

[3] Dal S, Jeandidier N, Seyfritz E, Bietiger W, Péronet C, Moreau F, Pinget M, Maillard E, Sigrist S. Oxidative stress status and liver tissue defenses in diabetic rats during intensive subcutaneous insulin therapy. Experimental Biology and Medicine. 2016;241:184-192. DOI: 10.1177/1535370215603837

[4] Raza H, John A, Howarth FC. Increased oxidative stress and mitochondrial dysfunction in Zucker diabetic rat liver and brain. Cellular Physiology and Biochemistry. 2015;35:1241-1251. DOI: 10.1159/000373947

[5] Mercer JR, Yu E, Figg N et al. The mitochondria-targeted antioxidant MitoQ decreases features of the metabolic syndrome in ATM+/-/ApoE-/- mice. Free Radical Biology & Medicine. 2012;52:841-849. DOI: 10.1016/j.freeradbiomed.2011.11.026

[6] Yki-Järvinen H. Non-alcoholic fatty liver disease as a cause and a consequence of metabolic syndrome. The Lancet Diabetes Endocrinology. 2014;2:901-910. DOI: 10.1016/S2213-8587(14)70032-4

[7] Lukivskaya O, Patsenker E, Buko VU. Protective effect of ursodeoxycholic acid on liver mitochondrial function in rats with alloxan-induced diabetes: link with oxidative stress. Life Sciences. 2007;80:2397-2402. DOI: 10.1016/j.lfs.2007.02.042

[8] Bouderba S, Sanz MN, Sánchez-Martín C, El-Mir MY, Villanueva GR, Detaille D, Koceïr EA. Hepatic mitochondrial alterations and increased oxidative stress in nutritional diabetes-prone Psammomys obesus model. Experimental Diabetes Research. 2012;2012:430176. DOI: 10.1155/2012/430176

[9] Ortiz-Avila O, Gallegos-Corona MA, Sánchez-Briones LA et al. Protective effects of dietary avocado oil on impaired electron transport chain function and exacerbated oxidative stress in liver mitochondria from diabetic rats. Journal of Bioenergetics and Biomembranes. 2015;47:337-353. DOI: 10.1007/s10863-015-9614-z

[10] Wirth C, Brandt U, Hunte C, Zickermann V. Structure and function of mitochondrial complex I. Biochimica et Biophysica Acta. 2016;1857:902-914. DOI: 10.1016/j.bbabio.2016.02.013.

[11] Jussupow A, Di Luca A, Kaila VRI. How cardiolipin modulates the dynamics of respiratory complex I. Science Advances. 2019;5:eaav1850. DOI: 10.1126/sciadv.aav1850

[12] Dey A, Swaminathan K. Hyperglycemia-induced mitochondrial alterations in liver. Life Sciences. 2010;87:197-214. DOI: 10.1016/j.lfs.2010.06.007.

[13] Vähäheikkilä M, Peltomaa T, Róg T, Vazdar M, Pöyry S, Vattulainen I. How cardiolipin peroxidation alters the properties of the inner mitochondrial

membrane? Chemistry and Physics of Lipids. 2018;214:15-23. DOI: 10.1016/j.chemphyslip.2018.04.005

[14] Mailloux RJ, Xuan JY, McBride S et al. Glutaredoxin-2 is required to control oxidative phosphorylation in cardiac muscle by mediating deglutathionylation reactions. The Journal of Biological Chemistry. 2014;289:14812-14828. DOI: 10.1074/jbc.M114.550574

[15] Lambert AJ, Brand MD. Inhibitors of the quinone-binding site allow rapid superoxide production from mitochondrial NADH:ubiquinone oxidoreductase (complex I). The Journal of Biological Chemistry. 2004;279:39414-39420. DOI: 10.1074/jbc.M406576200.

[16] Wong HS, Monternier PA, Brand MD. S1QELs suppress mitochondrial superoxide/hydrogen peroxide production from site IQ without inhibiting reverse electron flow through Complex I. Free Radical Biology & Medicine. 2019;143:545-559. DOI: 10.1016/j.freeradbiomed.2019.09.006

[17] Janjic D, Wollheim CB. Effect of 2-mercaptoethanol on glutathione levels, cystine uptake and insulin secretion in insulin-secreting cells. European Journal of Biochemistry. 1992;210:297-304. DOI: 10.1111/j.1432-1033.1992.tb17421.x.

[18] Petrosillo G, Portincasa P, Grattagliano I et al. Mitochondrial dysfunction in rat with nonalcoholic fatty liver. Involvement of complex I, reactive oxygen species and cardiolipin. Biochimica et Biophysica Acta. 2007;1767:1260-1267. DOI: 10.1016/j.bbabio.2007.07.011

[19] Cortés-Rojo C, Calderón-Cortés E, Clemente-Guerrero M et al. Electron transport chain of Saccharomyces cerevisiae mitochondria is inhibited by H2O2 at succinate-cytochrome c oxidoreductase level without lipid peroxidation involvement. Free Radical Research. 2007;41:1212-1223. DOI: 10.1080/10715760701635082

[20] Hemmeryckx B, Gaekens M, Gallacher DJ, Lu HR, Lijnen HR. Effect of rosiglitazone on liver structure and function in genetically diabetic Akita mice. Basic & Clinical Pharmacology & Toxicology. 2013;113:353-360. DOI: 10.1111/bcpt.12104

[21] Serviddio G, Bellanti F, Sastre J, Vendemiale G, Altomare E. Targeting mitochondria: a new promising approach for the treatment of liver diseases. Current Medicinal Chemistry. 2010;17:2325-2337. DOI: 10.2174/092986710791698530

[22] Raza H, Prabu SK, John A, Avadhani NG. Impaired mitochondrial respiratory functions and oxidative stress in streptozotocin-induced diabetic rats. International Journal of Molecular Sciences. 2011;12:3133-3147. DOI: 10.3390/ijms12053133.

[23] Ferreira FM, Seiça R, Oliveira PJ, Coxito PM, Moreno AJ, Palmeira CM, Santos MS. Diabetes induces metabolic adaptations in rat liver mitochondria: role of coenzyme Q and cardiolipin contents. Biochimica et Biophysica Acta. 2003;1639:113-120. DOI: 10.1016/j.bbadis.2003.08.001.

[24] Herlein JA, Fink BD, O'Malley Y, Sivitz WI. Superoxide and respiratory coupling in mitochondria of insulin-deficient diabetic rats. Endocrinology. 2009;150:46-55. DOI: 10.1210/en.2008-0404.

[25] Dröse S, Stepanova A, Galkin A. Ischemic A/D transition of mitochondrial complex I and its role in ROS generation. Biochimica et

Biophysica Acta. 2016;1857:946-957. DOI: 10.1016/j.bbabio.2015.12.013

[26] Karamanlidis G, Lee CF, Garcia-Menendez L, Kolwicz SC Jr, Suthammarak W, Gong G, Sedensky MM, Morgan PG, Wang W, Tian R. Mitochondrial complex I deficiency increases protein acetylation and accelerates heart failure. Cell Metabolism. 2013;18:239-250. DOI: 10.1016/j.cmet.2013.07.002.

[27] Li X, Kazgan N. Mammalian sirtuins and energy metabolism. International Journal of Biological Sciences. 2011;7:575-587. DOI: 10.7150/ijbs.7.575.

[28] Akie TE, Liu L, Nam M, Lei S, Cooper MP. OXPHOS-mediated induction of NAD+ promotes complete oxidation of fatty acids and interdicts non-alcoholic fatty liver disease. PLoS One. 2015;10:e0125617. DOI: 10.1371/journal.pone.0125617

[29] Valianpour F, Wanders RJ, Overmars H, Vaz FM, Barth PG, van Gennip AH. Linoleic acid supplementation of Barth syndrome fibroblasts restores cardiolipin levels: implications for treatment. The Journal of Lipid Research. 2003;44:560-566. DOI: 10.1194/jlr.M200217-JLR200.

[30] Oemer G, Edenhofer ML, Lackner K, Leman G, Lindner HH, Dubrac S, Zschocke J, Keller MA. Fatty acyl availability modulates cardiolipin composition and alters mitochondrial function in HeLa cells. BioRxiv. 2020. DOI: 10.1101/2020.02.10.937433

[31] Varatharajalu R, Garige M, Leckey LC, Arellanes-Robledo J, Reyes-Gordillo K, Shah R, Lakshman MR. Adverse signaling of scavenger receptor class B1 and PGC1s in alcoholic hepatosteatosis and steatohepatitis and protection by betaine in rat. The American Journal of Pathology. 2014;184:2035-2044. DOI: 10.1016/j.ajpath.2014.03.005.

[32] Wong HS, Chen JH, Leong PK, Leung HY, Chan WM, Ko KM. β-sitosterol protects against carbon tetrachloride hepatotoxicity but not gentamicin nephrotoxicity in rats via the induction of mitochondrial glutathione redox cycling. Molecules. 2014;19:17649-17662. DOI: 10.3390/molecules191117649.

[33] Fabbrini E, Magkos F, Mohammed BS, Pietka T, Abumrad NA, Patterson BW, Okunade A, Klein S. Intrahepatic fat, not visceral fat, is linked with metabolic complications of obesity. Proceedings of the National Academy of Sciences of the United States of America. 2009;106:15430-15435. DOI: 10.1073/pnas.0904944106.

Chapter 6

Antioxidant and Oxidative Stress

Betül Çalişkan and Ali Cengiz Çalişkan

Abstract

Antioxidants are compounds that eliminate oxidative stress in biological systems. Oxidative stress is caused by various radicals formed in the system as a result of oxygen entering the biological system. Structures with unpaired electron are either free radicals or radical ions. Antioxidants neutralize free radicals or radical ions due to the unpaired electron in their structure. The radical ions formed as a result of oxidation is removed from the system without damaging the biological system with the effect of antioxidants. There are many free radicals and radical ions. Among these radical groups are radical ions formed by oxygen which are important for biological systems. Antioxidants are responsible for the destruction of such radicals.

Keywords: antioxidant, oxidative stress, free radical, radical ions

1. Introduction

1.1 Oxidative stress

Oxidative stress is described as the disturbance of the balance between prooxidants (free radicals) and antioxidants. Oxidative stress occurs with the effect of free radicals and oxidants. Free radicals have unpaired electrons. Therefore, they create the oxidation process in the body. Oxidation causes an oxidative stress to occur. Oxidation processes and free radicals are constantly formed in the body. Oxidation is a process that can be harmful or beneficial. If the increase in free radicals is not balanced with antioxidants, the ground is prepared for the harmful process. It plays an important role in the development of diseases as it causes various damages. It creates DNA, lipid and protein damage.

Aging is an inherent mechanism existing in all living cells. There is a decline in organ functions progressively along with the age-relateddisease development. The twomost important theories related to aging are free radical and mitochondrial theories, and these have passed through the test of time. There is claim by such theories that a vicious cycle is generated within mitochondria wherein reactive oxygen species (ROS) is produced in increased amount thereby augmenting the damage potential [1–6].

The effect of oxidative stress and the interaction of aging and age-related diseases are shown in **Figure 1** [2].

Oxidative stress and disease development are shown in **Figure 2** [3].

Prooxidants are subtances that trigger oxidative stress. Prooxidants are reactive oxygen species (ROS). Prooxidants are studied in two groups. These are exogenous prooxidants and endogenous prooxidants. The exogenous prooxidants are studied in six groups. These are pathogens, drugs, toxicants, dietary ingredients, environmental pollution and climate. The endogenous prooxidants are studied

 IntechOpen

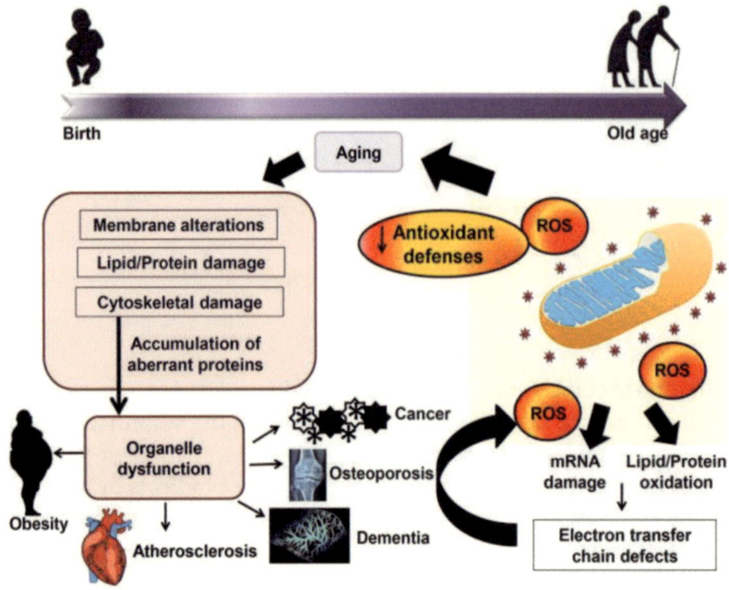

Figure 1.
Effect of oxidative stress and the interaction of aging and age-related diseases.

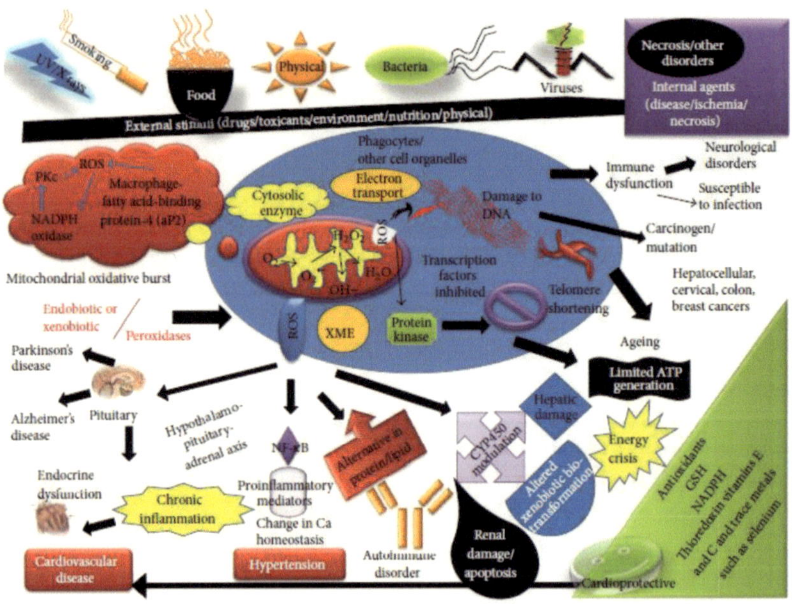

Figure 2.
Oxidative stress and disease development.

in seven groups. These are endogenous metabolites, drug metabolites, cellular metabolism, ion flux, anxiety, pathophysiology and ischemia.

Antioxidants are studied in two groups. These are endogenous antioxidants and exogenous antioxidants. Endogenous antioxdants are studied under two groups. These are enzymatic antioxidants and non-enzymatic antioxidants. Dietary antioxidants derived from fruits, vegetables and grains are exogenous antioxidants.

Contact of living cells with oxygen leads to the formation of reactive oxygen species. Reactive oxygen species are listed in **Table 1** [1–5].

O_2^{-}	Superoxide radical
O_2^{-2}	Peroxide
H_2O_2	Hydrogen peroxide
$HO^{\cdot}$	Hydroxyl radical
OH^{-}	Hydroxyl ion
$^{1}O_2$	Singlet oxygen
$HOO^{\cdot}$	Hydroperoxyl radical
$LOOH$	Alkylhydroperoxide
$LOO^{\cdot}$	Alkylperoxyl radical
$LO^{\cdot}$	Alkoxyl radical
ClO^{-}	Hypochlorite ion
$Fe^{4+}O$	Ferryl ion
$Fe^{5+}O$	Periferryl ion
$NO^{\cdot}$	Nitric oxide
$HOCl$	Hypochlorous acid
$GSOO^{\cdot}$	Glutathione thiylperoxyl radical
$GSO_2^{\cdot}$	Sulfonyl radical
$GSO^{\cdot}$	Sulfinyl radical
$GSO_2OO^{\cdot}$	Sulfonyl-peroxyl radical

Table 1.
Reactive oxygen species.

2. Prooxidants

Reactive oxygen species that cause oxidative stress are called prooxidants. Prooxidants occur for a variety of reasons. These may be internal or external causes. Prooxidants are of two types, exogenous and endogenous.

2.1 Exogenous prooxidants

2.1.1 Pathogens

Pathogens are divided into four groups. These are bacteria, virus, fungus and parasite.

2.1.2 Drugs

Common over-the-counter drug like analgesic (paracetamol) or anticancerous drug (methotrexate) causes oxidative stress.

2.1.3 Toxicants

Toxicants are the man-made harmful substances such as insecticides and many other industrial chemicals which are released to the environment by human activities. Carcinogens, mutagens, allergens, neurotoxin and endocrine disrupters are the different types of toxicants 2 [7]. As an external factor, various toxicants cause oxidative stress.

2.1.4 Dietary ingredients

Dietary ingredients are divided into four groups. These are lipids, carbohydrates, highly processed food and antioxidants.

2.1.5 Environmental pollution

Environmental pollution are divided into three groups. These are transition metals, pesticides and drug residues.

2.1.5.1 Transition metals

These are magnesium, iron, copper, zinc, and so forth.

2.1.5.2 Pesticides

These are BHC, DDT, and so forth.

2.1.5.3 Drug residues

Drug residues cause environmental pollution and trigger oxidative stress.

2.1.6 Climate

Climatic effects such as extreme heat, extreme cold etc. cause oxidative stress.

2.1.7 Cigarette smoke

Cigarette smoke accumulates neutrophils and macrophages in the lungs. Therefore, it is a factor that activates the oxidant mechanism in the body [8].

2.1.8 Ozone exposure

The exposure of the body's airways to ozone causes lipid peroxidation and neutrophil flow in the airway epithelium [9].

2.1.9 Hyperoxia

Hyperoxia is the condition in which the lungs and other tissues have higher oxygen levels. It causes reactive oxygen species (ROS) and reactive nitrogen species (RNS) to form in the body [10, 11].

2.1.10 Ionizing radiation

Ionizing radiation transforms hydroxyl radical, superoxide and organic radicals into hydrogen peroxide and organic hydroperoxides by the effect of O_2 . These hydroperoxide species react with redox active metal ions such as Fe and Cu. Thus, they cause oxidative stress [12, 13].

2.1.11 Heavy metal ions

Heavy metal ions such as cadmium, mercury, nickel, lead and arsenic cause reactive oxygen species in the body.

2.2 Endogenous prooxidants

2.2.1 Endogenous metabolites

Endogenous metabolites are defined as substrates or products of approximately one thousand nine hundred metabolic enzymes encoded in our genome [14–16]. There are several studies showing that most of these metabolites are toxic. These toxic metabolites are classified depending on the method of introducing toxicity to cells. They are expressed as ROS-producing metabolites, reactive metabolites, metabolite analogues, excitotoxins, and not established/unknown biology.

2.2.2 Drug metabolites

Drug metabolism is the term used to describe the biotransformation of pharmaceutical substances in the body so that they can be eliminated more easily. The majority of metabolic processes that involve drugs occur in the liver, as the enzymes that facilitate the reactions are concentrated there. The purpose of metabolism in the body is usually to change the chemical structure of the substance, to increase the ease with which it can be excreted from the body. Drugs are metabolized through various reactions including: Oxidation, reduction, hydrolysis, hydration, conjugation, condensation, isomerization [17].

2.2.3 Cellular metabolism

Cellular metabolism is chemical reactions that occur in living things. They are controlled biochemical reactions in metabolism. Biochemical reactions provide growth, proliferation and preservation of structures.

Thanks to the chemical reactions that occur in metabolism, one chemical is transformed into another chemical under the influence of various enzymes. Enzymes direct chemical processes in living things and are indispensable for living things. Enzymes design down to the finest detail the process of homeostasis called the cell's response to environmental changes.

Cellular metabolism is examined as two processes as anabolism and catabolism. Anabolism is referred to as the constitutive metabolic process. In other words, it is a metabolic process in which a cell uses energy to build various molecules such as enzymes and nucleic acids and to maintain the necessary vital activities. Anabolism consists of three basic stages: The first is the process of making precursors such as amino acids, monosaccharides, isoprenoids, and nucleotides. Second, it includes the process by which precursors such as amino acids, monosaccharides, isoprenoids, and nucleotides are activated to reactive forms. Third, it involves the process by which these precursors combine to form complex molecules.

Catabolism constitutes the second part of the metabolic process. It is the process by which complex molecules are broken down by the cell. Reactions in catabolism provide the energy and substances needed by reactions in anabolism. Catabolic reactions are generally exothermic reactions. Catabolism is divided into several subgroups. These are carbohydrate catabolism, fat catabolism and protein catabolism [18].

2.2.4 Ion flux

Ion channels are pore-forming proteins that warrant controlled and directed flux of ions through membranes. Temporal and spatial coordination of ion movements is essential for a wide range of physiological processes including the generation and propagation of the membrane action potential that is critical for the biomechanical activity of muscle cells. Despite their well-established canonical electrophysiological functions in the heart, recent findings have demonstrated that ion channels also might feature ion flux independent functions during heart development and morphogenesis long before acting as ion-conducting pores [19].

2.2.5 Anxiety

Tension and apprehension cause anxiety. Anxiety disorders can cause low antioxidant defenses and increased oxidative damage to proteins, lipids and nucleic acids pores [20].

2.2.6 Pathophysiology

Pathophysiology means the examination of the causes of the disease, the various effects caused by the disease, and the abnormal changes in body functions that occur with the disease process. Research in the field of pathophysiology has often focused on physical, mental or psychophysiological states that are directly related to disease processes. Topics such as changes in the endocrine system, changes in certain neurotransmitters, or changes in inflammatory parameters related to the activity of the immune system are examples of research in the field of pathophysiology [21].

2.2.7 Ischemia

Ischemia is any reduction in blood flow resulting in decreased oxygen and nutrient supplies to a tissue. Ischemia may be reversible, in which case the affected tissue will recover if blood flow is restored, or it may be irreversible, resulting in tissue death [22].

2.2.8 Physical exercise

Several studies have demonstrated that intense physical exercise causes oxidative stress in animals and humans, being possibly related, for instance, to fatigue and tissue lesions [23].

2.2.9 Antioxidants

There are a number of reasons why high concentrations of antioxidants may be harmful. At high concentrations, antioxidants may act as pro-oxidants, increasing oxidation; protect dangerous cells (such as cancer cells) as well as healthy cells; reduce the health benefits of exercise; have unwanted side effects, such as nausea and headaches, or even reach toxic levels [1–5, 24].

3. Antioxidants

Antioxidants are examined under two headings as natural and synthetic. Natural antioxidants are examined in two groups as enzymatic and non-enzymatic antioxidants.

3.1 Synthetic antioxidants

Synthetic antioxidants make up only one analogue (type) of natural antioxidants and are developed to mimic the most effective analogue of the natural antioxidant. Butylated hydroxyanisole (BHA), butylated hydroxytoluene (BHT), ethoxyquin, propyl gallat and tertiary butylhydroxyquinone (TBHQ) are some of the synthetic antioxidants.

3.2 Natural antioxidants

3.2.1 Exogenous antioxidants

Exogenous antioxidants are prinicipal dietary antioxidants from fruits, vegetables and grains. Exogenous antioxidants are studied in ten groups.

3.2.1.1 Vitamins

Vitamins are examined in two groups as vitamin C and vitamin E.

3.2.1.2 Trace elements

Trace elements are examined in two groups as zinc and selenium.

3.2.1.3 Carotenoids

Carotenoids are examined in four groups as β-carotene, lycopene, lutein and zeaxanthin.

3.2.1.4 Phenolic acids

Chlorogenic acids, gallic acid, cafeic acid, etc. constitute phenolic acids.

3.2.1.5 Flavonols

Quercetin (and their glucosides), kaempferol (and their glucosides) and myricetin (and their glucosides) constitute flavonols.

3.2.1.6 Flavanols

Proanthocyanidins and catechins constitute flavanol.

3.2.1.7 Anthocyanidins

Cyanidin (and their glucosides) and pelagonidin (and their glucosides) constitute anthocyanidins.

3.2.1.8 Isoflavones

Genistein (and their glucosides), daidzein (and their glucosides) and glycitein (and their glucosides) constitute isoflavones.

3.2.1.9 Flavanones

Naringenin (and their glucosides), eriodictyol (and their glucosides) and hesperetin (and their glucosides) constitute flavanones.

3.2.1.10 Flavones

luteolin (and their glucosides) and apigenin (and their glucosides) constituteflavones.

The beneficial and harmful effects of exogenous antioxidants are shown in **Figure 3** [4].

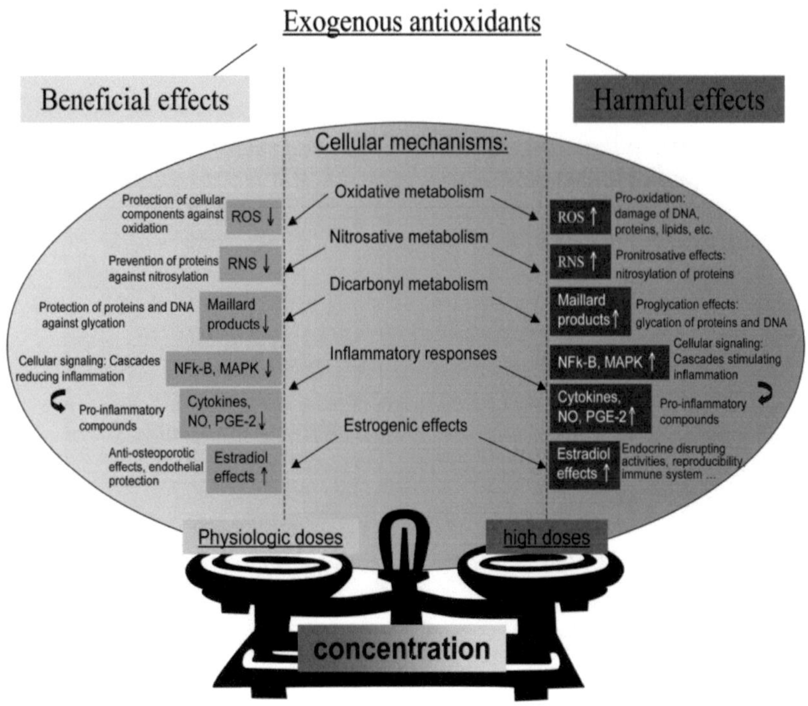

Figure 3.
Beneficial and harmful effects of exogenous antioxidants.

3.2.2 Endogenous antioxidants

Endogenous antioxidants are studied in two groups: enzymatic antioxidants and non-enzymatic antioxidants.

3.2.2.1 Enzymatic antioxidants

Enzymatic antioxidants are studied in five groups.

3.2.2.1.1 Superoxide dismutase (SOD)

Superoxide dismutase (SOD) is enzyme detoxifying superoxide radical (O_2^{-}).

3.2.2.1.2 Catalase (CAT) and glutathione peroxidase (GPx)

Catalase (CAT) and glutathione peroxidase (GPx) are enzymes involved in the detoxification of peroxides (CAT against H_2O_2 and GPx against both H_2O_2 and $ROOH$).

3.2.2.1.3 Glutathione reductase

Glutathione reductase is enzyme involved in the regeneration of glutathione.

3.2.2.1.4 Thioredoxin reductase

Thioredoxin reductase is enzyme involved in the protection against protein oxidation.

3.2.2.1.5 Glucose-6-phosphate dehydrogenase

Glucose-6-phosphate dehydrogenase is enzyme involved in the regeneration of NADPH.

3.2.2.2 Non-enzymatic antioxidants (principal intracellular reducing agents)

Glutathione (GSH), uric acid, lipoic acid, NADPH, coenzyme Q, albumin and bilirubin make up the non-enzymatic antioxidant class [1–5].

4. Conclusion

Oxidative stress is a condition that occurs with the increase of free radicals. Free radicals tend to increase in the body for various reasons. This situation may be caused by exogenous reasons or by various changes in the body (endogenous). As a result of the oxidation process in the body, reactive oxygen species (ROS) are formed. In addition to reactive oxygen species, reactive nitrogen species are also formed in the body. The oxidation process begins with the introduction of food into the body. Oxidation is a process that can be both beneficial and harmful. Oxidation triggers the formation of free radicals, ie reactive oxygen species. If antioxidants do not come into play as a balance element in the body, the increase in free radicals damages the body and causes the formation of the disease process. Depletion of various substances in the body due to age also triggers the formation of reactive oxygen species and the emergence of various diseases. Antioxidants can be various external substances, as well as various enzymes in the body and non-enzymatic substances in the body. With the effect of antioxidants, free radicals are prevented from causing DNA, lipid and protein damage.

Author details

Betül Çalişkan[1]* and Ali Cengiz Çalişkan[2]

1 Department of Physics, Faculty of Arts and Science, Pamukkale University, Denizli, Turkey

2 Department of Chemistry, Faculty of Science, Gazi University, Ankara, Turkey

*Address all correspondence to: bcaliska@gmail.com

References

[1] Yoshikawa T., Naito Y. What is oxidative stress? Journal of the Japan Medical Association (JMAJ) 2012; **45(7):** 271-276. DOI: 10.1093/ndt/21.suppl_4.iv200.

[2] Tan B.L., Norhaizan M.E., Liew W.P.P., Rahman H.S. Antioxidant and oxidative stress: a mutual interplay in age-related diseases. Front. Pharmacol. 2018; **9:**1-28. DOI: 10.3389/fphar.2018.01162.

[3] Rahal A., Kumar A., Singh V., Yadav B., Tiwari R., Chakraborty S., Dhama K. Oxidative stress, prooxidants, and antioxidants: The interplay. BioMed Research International. 2014; Special Issue:1-19. DOI: 10.1155/2014/761264.

[4] Bouayed J., Bohn T. Exogenous antioxidants-Double-edged swords in cellular redox state-Health beneficial effects at physiologic doses versus deleterious effects at high doses. Oxidative Medicine and Cellular Longevity 2010; **3(4):** 228-237. DOI: 10.4161/oxim.3.4.12858.

[5] Birben E, Sahiner Ü.M., Sackesen C., Erzurum S., Kalayci Ö. Oxidative stress and antioxidant defense. World Allergy Organ. J. 2012; **5(1):**9-19. DOI: 10.1097/WOX.0b013e3182439613.

[6] Romano A.D., Serviddio G., Matthaeis A.D, Bellanti F. Vendemiale G. Oxidative stress and aging. J Nephrol. 2010; **23(15):** 29-36.

[7] Toxicants. https://www.imedpub.com/scholarly/toxicants-journals-articles-ppts-list.php, 2021 (accessed 3 Feb 2021).

[8] Church D.F., Pryor W.A. Free-radical chemistry of cigarette smoke and its toxicological implications. Environ Health Perspect. 1985; **64:**111-126. DOI: 10.1289/ehp.8564111.

[9] Hiltermann J.T., Lapperre T.S., van Bree L., Steerenberg P.A., Brahim J.J., Sont J.K., Sterk P.J., Hiemstra P.S., Stolk J. Ozone-induced inflammation assessed in sputum and bronchial lavage fluid from asthmatics: a new noninvasive tool in epidemiologic studies on air pollution and asthma. Free Radic Biol Med. 1999; **27:**1448-1454. DOI: 10.1016/s0891-5849(99)00191-4.

[10] Comhair S.A., Thomassen M.J., Erzurum S.C. Differential induction of extracellular glutathione peroxidase and nitric oxide synthase 2 in airways of healthy individuals exposed to 100% O(2) or cigarette smoke. Am J Respir Cell Mol Biol. 2000;**23(3):**350-354. DOI: 10.1165/ajrcmb.23.3.4076.

[11] Matthay M.A., Geiser T., Matalon S., Ischiropoulos H. Oxidant-mediated lung injury in the acute respiratory distress syndrome. Crit Care Med. 1999;**27(9):**2028-2030. DOI: 10.1097/00003246-199909000-00055.

[12] Biaglow J.E., Mitchell J.B., Held K. The importance of peroxide and superoxide in the X-ray response. Int J Radiat Oncol Biol Phys. 1992;**22(4):**665-669. DOI: 10.1016/0360-3016(92)90499-8.

[13] Chiu SM, Xue LY, Friedman LR, Oleinick NL. Copper ion-mediated sensitization of nuclear matrix attachment sites to ionizing radiation. Biochemistry. 1993;**32(24):**6214-6219. DOI: 10.1021/bi00075a014.

[14] Kanehisa M., Goto S. KEGG: Kyoto Encyclopedia of Genes and Genomes. Nucleic Acids Res. 2000;**28(1):**27-30. DOI: 10.1093/nar/28.1.27.

[15] Possemato R., Marks K.M., Shaul Y.D., Pacold M.E., Kim D., Birsoy K., Sethumadhavan S., Woo H.K., Jang H.G., Jha A.K., Chen W.W., Barrett F.G., Stransky N.,

Tsun Z.Y., Cowley G.S., Barretina J., KalaanyN.Y.,HsuP.P.,OttinaK.,ChanA.M., Yuan B., Garraway L.A., Root D.E., Mino-Kenudson M., Brachtel E.F., Driggers E.M., Sabatini D.M. Functional genomics reveal that the serine synthesis pathway is essential in breast cancer. Nature. 2011;**476(7360)**:346-350. DOI: 10.1038/nature10350.

[16] Lee N., Spears M.E., Carlisle A.E., Kim D. Endogenous toxic metabolites and implications in cancer therapy. Oncogene 2020;**39(35)**:5709-5720. DOI: 10.1038/s41388-020-01395-9.

[17] Smith Y. Drug Metabolism. https://www.news-medical.net/health/Drug-Metabolism.aspx, 2021 (accessed 3 Feb 2021).

[18] Cell Metabolism. https://www.tocris.com/cell-biology/cell-metabolism, 2021 (accessed 3 Feb 2021).

[19] Keßler M., Just S., Rottbauer W. Ion flux dependent and independent functions of ion channels in the vertebrate heart: Lessons Learned from zebrafish. Stem Cells and Ion Channels. 2012; Special Issue: 1-9. DOI: 10.1155/2012/462161.

[20] Fedoce A.D.G, Ferreira F., Bota R.G., Bonet-Costa V., Sun P.Y., Davies K.J.A. The role of oxidative stress in anxiety disorder: Cause or consequence? Free Radic Res. 2018; 52(7): 737-750. DOI: 10.1080/10715762.2018.1475733.

[21] Witthöft M. Pathophysiology. Encyclopedia of Behavioral Medicine. 2013 Edition; Eds. Gellman M.D., Turner J.R. 2013; DOI: 10.1007/978-1-4419-1005-9_43.

[22] Ischemia. https://www.healthgrades.com/right-care/vascular-conditions/ischemia , 2021 (accessed 3 Feb 2021).

[23] de Souza T.P., de Oliveira P.R., Pereira B. Physical exercise and oxidative stress. Effect of intense physical exercise on the urinary chemiluminescence and plasmatic malondialdehyde. Rev Bras Med Esporte 2005; **11(1)**:97-101 http://dx.doi.org/10.1590/S1517-86922005000100010.

[24] Adcock J. What are antioxidants? And are they truly good for us? https://theconversation.com/what-are-antioxidants-and-are-they-truly-good-for-us-86062, 2018 (accessed 3 Feb 2021).

Chapter 7

Natural Antioxidants to the Rescue?

Cenk Aydin and Nilay Seyidoglu

Abstract

Natural antioxidant compounds have different mechanisms of treatment and prevention against various diseases due to their richest ingredients. There are several antioxidants used today, such as phytogenic ingredients, flavonoids, capsaicin, spirulina, beta-glucan, polyphenol etc. Besides the outbreak of diseases, the ability to scavenge oxidative conditions of the natural antioxidants have been notably important. Thereby, therapeutic strategies of diseases have been interested by researchers. Try to seek a kind of effects of natural antioxidants to various diseases, especially viral or pandemic diseases are being important nowadays. This chapter we'll mention about how to viral or pandemic disease's effects on oxidative status in both animals and humans, and what kind of phytochemical ingredients would be a positive effect on. At the same time, the latest advances about these natural antioxidant compounds and pharmaceuticals will be critically highlighted and discussed with newest literatures.

Keywords: natural antioxidants, phytogenic ingredients, essential oils, pandemic, vitamins

1. Introduction

Antioxidants either endogenous or exogenous are essential substances to regulate the oxidative process. The endogenous antioxidants known as glutathione, glutathione peroxidase (GPx), catalase (CAT), and superoxide dismutase (SOD), have an inhibition role on free radicals during oxidation [1]. Nevertheless, either these antioxidant mechanisms are inadequate or for a better healthy life, exogenous antioxidants should be preferred [2]. The exogenous antioxidants which are especially called natural antioxidants such as vitamins, flavonoids, polyphenols, minerals, plants and phytochemicals, are derived from foods and medicinal plants. Over the years, the relationship between natural antioxidants and health has been discussed due to their important efficiencies. Generally, natural antioxidants have a wide range of effects especially antioxidant, antimicrobial, anticancer, immunomodulatory, and antiviral [3–5]. Belong these, natural antioxidants have been drawing great attention for scientific studies.

There are several multidisciplinary studies with natural antioxidants that have focused on human and animal experiments. The researchers have examined to understand the mechanisms of antioxidants on oxidative stress. They have been widely documented the knowledge of free radicals with antioxidants by identifying the oxidative stress pathway, cellular efficiencies and general health impact [6, 7].

Besides, although higher clinical complications have been observed in diseases, the mechanisms for the use of natural antioxidants are still not fully understood.

Since the past century, there have been essential diseases needed to determine how diseases progress and how the world could control them. Environmental factors, insufficient water, climate changes or new viruses influence the spread of contagious disease, and thereby cause epidemics. Nevertheless, The World Health Organization (WHO) has been still working on epidemiological studies to identify the possible sources of outbreaks, and to observe the pathogens spread from one region to different regions of the world [8]. Throughout history, there have been many significant pandemics recorded in human history. Some examples of the most up to date are Influenza virus (H1N1), Severe Acute Respiratory Syndrome (SARS), the Middle East Respiratory Syndrome (MERS), Ebola, Zika, Yellow Fever, Cholera, Malaria, and Tuberculosis [9].

Today, in response to pandemics, people have been transformed into plants and phytochemicals to protect their health. Also, researchers have advocated that these natural foods could meet antioxidant protection. However, studies are still ongoing. This chapter aims to summarize the essential natural antioxidants, their mechanism, and their effects on pandemic diseases.

2. The reality of diseases in the 21st century

In recent years, climate change, lack of safe drinking water, poor living conditions and food insecurity have been the main causes of illness, epidemics and pandemics. Besides, there are also many chemicals or toxins, which can contaminate food, drink, and medicines that cause death, injury or harm to organs. The WHO reported that besides environmental changes, many diseases can occur in animals and can be transmitted if animals and people come into close contact, for example, animal husbandry, wildlife trade, etc. Also, urbanization and air travel are essential factors for outbreaks nowadays. First and foremost, flights across the world can cause illness in other countries. This means that the pathogen has a new home, and a pandemic is realized within hours [8].

The WHO indexed the 21st century's serious diseases, which threaten public health and have no therapeutic strategies, especially vaccines or new medicines, in 2018. Some important as follows: Influenza virus (H1N1), Severe Acute Respiratory Syndrome (SARS), Middle East Respiratory Syndrome (MERS), Ebola, Zika, Yellow Fever, Cholera, Malaria, Tuberculosis. It was also reported that in the 21st century, epidemics can spread faster and farther than ever. Besides that, the last announced one, coronavirus-disease 2019 (COVID-19), was accepted as a pandemic disease by the WHO.

The global strategy is to eliminate and eradicate these illnesses through vaccines or medical investments. The WHO also recommends fresh foods and healthy nutrition during pandemics, which positively affect immunity [10]. The key vision of the relationship between nutrition, their role in immunity, and stress management was highlighted. Recent advances are also being critically demonstrated in antioxidant compounds, herbal ingredients, and pharmaceutical products with literature. The coronavirus diseases such as MERS, SARS, and COVID-19, it was reviewed that vitamin C, D and E, have an important role in the regulation of T cell differentiation in immunity [11]. Also, Leite Diniz et al. [12] reviewed that several natural antioxidants can have antiviral properties on metabolic modulation, and can treat the clinical symptoms in SARS, MERS, and COVID-19.

Nevertheless, it was reviewed that some herbal remedies such as geranium, green tea, pomegranate or Echinacea may be safer than drugs against influenza infections due to the anti-inflammatory, antibacterial and antioxidant activities of herbs and their extracts [13]. Also, it was showed that all these herbs and extracts have potential effects on respiratory complications and pro-inflammatory cytokines. Kaihatsu et al. [14] reported that natural phenolic compounds and coffee ingredients can inhibit the influenza virus by possessing radical scavenging activity. Moreover, flavonoids in citrus fruits have anti-inflammatory and antioxidant activities on the pulmonary system which showed by a bronchial epithelium model study [15].

The effect of thyme and its volatile oils may affect the penetration of the virus into the host cell or block viral proteins that are necessary for the virus to enter the host cells. Thyme may also act as an antiviral against intracellular viruses. In the meantime, evidence shows that natural compounds have plays a key role in alternative treatments to fight SARS-CoV-2. Recently determined that SARS-CoV-2 has spike glycoprotein consisted of two units. The first unit initiating virus attachment to the host cell surface and the second unit responsible for the virus-host membrane. Subunits are of great clinical importance as inhibition of the receptor binding domain which is the first step to hinder viral infections. Studies have shown that carvacrol, anethole, cinnamaldehyde, thymol, camphene, pulegone, ocimene and menthol showed good binding affinities and those natural compounds may contribute to the stability of the complex protein ligand [16, 17].

Furthermore, the potential effects of marine algal antioxidants on viral diseases has been reported [18]. Besides, some researchers reported that natural foods and natural compounds can have antibacterial and antiviral effects on cellular and molecular pathways, and thereby immunity is improved in several outbreaks such as Ebola, Cholera, Malaria and Tuberculosis [19–21].

Pandemics are old as humanity as well as natural antioxidants. Several natural foods and antioxidants have been used for healthy nutrition. However, the impact of several pandemics in the last century, there has been a growing interest between healthy food, nutrition, natural antioxidants and disease. Researchers studied the new therapeutic possibilities of the natural antioxidant for this purpose.

3. Life related to free radicals, oxidative stress and antioxidants

A healthy life is associated with the oxidative status of the organism. In a cellular mechanism, the oxidative process starts with oxygen generation to energy. Thereby, free radicals occur as a consequence of energy in mitochondria. The rest products are reactive oxygen species (ROS) and reactive nitrogen species (RNS) which have a role in toxicological and pathological conditions. On the contrary, both ROS and RNS positively affect the cellular mechanism and immune system when they are at low levels, which means a normal metabolic process. Free radicals produce against stress conditions and antioxidants during the normal healthy condition, which is also called homeostasis. So, the body tries to maintain the oxidant and antioxidant balance.

Oxidative stress markers, ROS and RNS, produce homeostasis through enzymatic and non-enzymatic reactions. Enzymatic reactions include cellular oxidase system like peroxidase, NADPH oxidase, hydrogen peroxidase. On the other side, the non-enzymatic process is based on organic compounds of the organism; for example, oxidative phosphorylation in mitochondria [22, 23]. ROS and RNS are formed from endogenous and exogenous sources that belong to several physiological and psychological mechanisms. Endogenous sources are generally occurring by immune cell activation, infection, excessive exercise, aging, or mental stress. However, environmental pollutants, drugs, heavy metals or radiation are exogenous sources, and are metabolized in free radical processes [22, 24].

The oxidative mechanism interacts with the antioxidant, endogenous, or exogenous mechanism. Both antioxidant mechanisms are capable of neutralizing free radicals and protecting the body. Endogenous antioxidant activity is the organism's first defensive system against free radicals. SOD, GPx, glutathione reductase, and CAT are the most important endogenous antioxidant in a healthy organism. Exogenous antioxidants are nutrients produced from foods and supplements, particularly vitamins E and C, flavonoids, phytochemicals, and certain essential plant-based antioxidants. These compounds can inactivate oxidizing agents and also inhibit inflammatory activation. They can modulate the enzymatic process and inflammatory mediators, including cytokines and peptides [25].

4. Oxidative stress in diseases

Oxidative stress, which includes significant bodily activities, is an imbalance between the oxidizing and antioxidant processes. If the oxidative stress cannot be regulated, several damages occur in an organism. While free radicals and oxidants are in excess production, antioxidant reactions are limited, thereby oxidative stress is generated. Several membranes or cellular structures and systems are also adversely affected by this status. Cellular proteins, lipids, lipoproteins, DNA or RNA, and oxidizing compounds, and also critical systems such as cardiovascular, neurological, or immunity, are damaged. For instance, the chains of free radicals react, and the peroxidation of lipids exists. Besides, protein damage affects the structure of the cell membrane as well as the lower antibody output. Also, enzyme activity is reduced due to proteins and occurs in several molecular and cellular mutations. These changes reflect body systems, and diseases can be occur [25].

There are several significant diseases reviewed for oxidative stress in both humans and animals (**Figure 1**). Cancer is one of the most important one, creates complex changes in an organism such as chromosomal defects or induced free radicals activation. Another critical disease is cardiovascular disease related to stress, hypertension, hypercholesterolemia, diabetes, etc. Studies showed that cardiac structure changes, especially heart failure, hypertrophy, ischemia, or atherosclerosis, generate oxidative stress [26, 27]. Nevertheless, oxidative status and its generation have been described for neurological, pulmonary, and other diseases. It was reported that loss of neuron production and progression stimulates the oxidative process, thereby neurological diseases are presented [28]. The pulmonary diseases

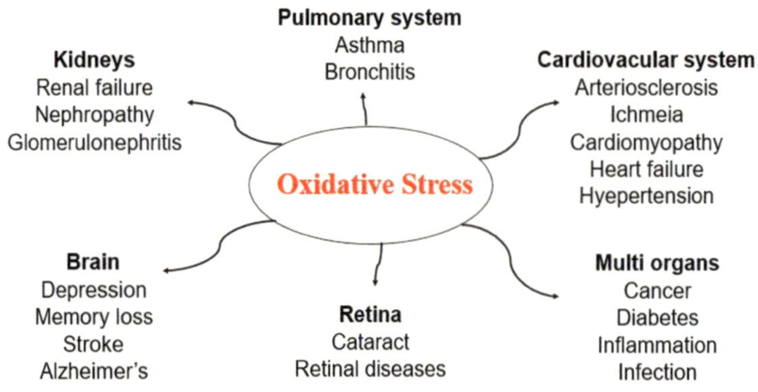

Figure 1.
Oxidative stress related diseases.

are qualified by inflammation and activation of redox transcript factors [29]. Also, researchers have been studied the generation of ROS and RNS in autoimmune and renal diseases, or several other diseases [30–32]. The importance of the immune system is interested in low antibody production and low protein which concluded in increasing the risks of diseases. Besides that, macrophages' infiltration of activated immune cells causes inflammation and oxidative damage [30]. Nevertheless, some drugs, heavy metals, or lipid peroxidation molecules are accepted as strong free radicals inducers [33]. The fact that oxidative stress has a large place during inflammation and diseases is inevitable.

Oxidative stress has a crucial role in disease onset and development. During viral infections, there may be an increase in the production of oxidizing species not neutralized by the antioxidant system, causing oxidative stress that promotes cell damage [34–36]. However, it was reviewed that in viral diseases, viruses can control oxidative stress on their benefits in cellular replication [37]. Viruses especially can change the activation of the immune system signaling pathway in oxidative status [38, 39]. ROS and RNS production are triggered by cytokines, and thereby, cell death occurs due to the imbalance between the production of reactive species and the host's anti-oxidative status. Also, RNA viruses bring about changes in the body's antioxidant defense system. Viruses are responsible for this by affecting enzymes like SOD and CAT, as well as lowering ascorbic acid, carotenoids and reduced glutathione [40–42]. Recently, in a pandemic disease COVID-19, lung damage occurs due to the release of pro-inflammatory cytokines, which alter the oxidative stress [43]. Zhao [44] also determined that another immune response of pro-inflammatory cytokines against oxidative stress is activated phagocytes cells in COVID-19. Nevertheless, generated oxidative stress is also associated with nucleic acid damage in viral mutations. It was reported that human coronavirus disease (HCoVs) and SARS are identified by genetic mutations, and also mutations in spike protein [45]. Nevertheless, influenza viruses have been demonstrated with induced oxidative stress with the activation of the Nrf2 pathway in nuclear translocation, and expression in alveolar epithelial cells [46]. Similarly, the hepatitis C virus (HCV) has been linked with genes and phosphorylation of Nrf2 [47]. It was reviewed that the Nrf2 pathway has a critical inhibition role of viral genes [37].

Management of pathogenic effects of viral diseases can be described by the mutual interaction between oxidant and antioxidant status control. Therefore this interaction is also associated with a healthy environment, balanced nutrition, and exogenous antioxidants.

5. The truth regarding antioxidants

The antioxidant process begins with oxidation when it damages a free radical compound, and then it follows by attempting to restore the body. An antioxidant may act as a pro-oxidant, which has generated ROS and RNS into two ways; breaking the chain and preventing it [48]. A chain breaking antioxidant may stabilize the formation of free radicals in the oxidative state, e.g., lipid peroxidation. Vitamins C and E, or carrots may be accepted in these anti-oxidants that break the chain. On the other hand, endogenous antioxidant enzymes such as glutathione, GPx, CAT, and SOD, may inhibit the initiation and propagation steps, consequently delaying the oxidant process.

Along with current literature, there have been several natural antioxidants reviewed for diseases or pandemic diseases [12, 49]. Each of these antioxidant properties is the neutralization capability of oxidative stress (**Table 1**).

Natural Antioxidants			
Vitamins	**Minerals**	**Plants**	**Phtyochemicals**
Vitamin E	Selenium	Garclic	Polyphenols
Vitamin C	Zinc	Ginger	Flavonoids
Beta carotene	Copper	Thyme	Carotenoids
Lycopene	Iron	Echinacea	
		Spirulina	
		Liquorice	

Table 1.
Natural antioxidants.

5.1 Vitamins

Vitamins, C, E and beta-carotene, which also called as primary antioxidants, have the beneficial effect either in health or diseases. Nevertheless, excessive doses of vitamins can be harmful rather than safe. So there has been ongoing research on nutritional antioxidants. WHO recommends antioxidants for malnutrition, disease, and pandemic-related needs [10]. Besides, nutritionists have endorsed antioxidant foods for humans first, while they have also pointed out that supplements may help.

Vitamins E and C have a higher antioxidative capacity among vitamins. Vitamin E (also known as tocopherol or alpha-tocopherol) has been reported to protect cellular membranes from lipid peroxide. Studies have suggested that vitamin E may be used in breast cancer, arthritis, some cardiovascular and neurological diseases. Besides, it was determined that the long-term use of vitamin E is acceptable as being available. Sources of vitamin E include vegetable oils, walnuts, cereals, eggs, poultry, and meat [50].

Nonetheless, vitamin C, called ascorbic acid, is essential for carnitine, neurotransmitter biosynthesis, and collagen. This vitamin has antioxidant, anti-carcinogenic, and immunomodulatory effects, which has also reduced the incidence of cancers. Also, vitamin C acts alongside vitamin E to quench free radicals. Vitamin C is found throughout natural sources such as fruits, vegetables, and tomatoes [51].

Beta-carotene, which is an active ingredient of pro-vitamin A, is a powerful antioxidant. Beta-carotene has the potential to quench oxygen during oxidative stress. This pro-vitamin has an antioxidant effect on cardiovascular diseases and cancer in particular. Beta-carotene comprises many foods, mainly green plants, spinach, carrots, oils, mangoes, apricots, and a watermelon [52, 53]. Another essential carotenoid, lycopene, is a vegetable nutrient that has protective effects on pulmonary cells and cancer. Lycopene was shown to be capable of balancing free radicals. The best source of lycopene is cooked tomato, juice, and sauce [54]. What are more, more red and pink fruits have this vitamin, like watermelon, grapefruit.

High doses of vitamins are recommended for using safely during pandemics. It was reported that especially Vitamin C has used for the treatment of cardiovascular, pulmonary disease as well as sepsis or nephropathy. It was evaluated that vitamin C can improve the mechanical ventilation of patients [55].

5.2 Minerals

There are several antioxidant minerals, in particular, selenium, zinc, copper, and iron. Selenium is an essential mineral in several vegetables, mushrooms, meat, and seafood, with anticarcinogenic and immunomodulatory effects. Selenium also plays a crucial role in thyroid function, gastrointestinal, cardiovascular, and pulmonary diseases [48]. Selenium contains about 35 antioxidant proteins, which reduce free radicals and allow cytoprotective antioxidant genes [56]. The mineral targets hydrogen peroxide and transforms it into water.

The other minerals Mn, Cu, Zn, and Fe, can maintain the endogenous antioxidants. Fe and Cu can suppress free radicals' formation by keeping bound to transport proteins. A high dose of Fe may negatively affect Zn's absorption to damage the immune system. It was reported that the increase of Zn in the cell has an antiviral effect in COVID-19 [57]. Also, Te Velthuis et al. [58] determined that a low dose of Zn inhibits replicating the virus in SARS.

Nevertheless, Cu is an essential mineral for cellular respiration, iron metabolism, and reducing oxidative stress. It was observed that Cu has an antiviral effect in some diseases such as COVID-19, human immunodeficiency virus (HIV), or bronchitis [59, 60]. On the other hand, according to some kinds of literature, Fe and Cu may be toxic due to an increase of viral replication and mortality in diseases, for example, HIV or COVID-19 [60]. Therefore, it was accepted that Cu and Fe must be taken in sufficient doses for the biological mechanism [61].

As the pandemic diseases continuing, humans should boost their immune system by taking sufficient minerals. Optimal nutrition can exist with dietary nutrient intake including especially vitamins and minerals.

5.3 Plants and phytochemicals

Earlier scientific studies have shown that commonly used wild edible plants, spices and herbal teas have high antiviral activity against a variety of viruses. There is also evidence that some of these drugs are used for various types of coronavirus diseases as potential phyto antiviral agents [62].

Natural antioxidants can alternate the multiple pathological processes in oxidative stress, primarily oxidative damage, inflammation, genetic changes, growth factors, etc. It was reviewed that natural antioxidants, mostly plants, and phytochemicals, can improve either oxidant status or antioxidant capacity [12]. Several plants are alternative medicines, such as ginger, garlic, curcumin, thyme, licorice, *Echinacea purpurea* or Spirulina, etc. These plants are recommended to strengthen immunity and reduce oxidative status. It was reported that these medicinal plants have essential roles in pandemic diseases, especially HIV, SARS and, COVID-19 [62–64].

Garlic, which is the most crucial spice worldwide, has a remarkably enhanced immune system booster. It may boost the activity of natural killer cells during immune deficiency. This medicinal herb has been approved as a therapeutic agent for homeostasis [65]. Furthermore, garlic has been used against cancer and cardiovascular disease [66]. This interesting spice, which has been used as a seasoning herb and traditional medicine in immunity and viral diseases, has several compounds such as saponin, cardio glycoside, and flavonoids [67–69]. Antiviral effects in garlic depend on inhibition of viral replication effects, viral protein synthesis, and viral DNA polymerization [70]. Also, garlic and its extracts have been shown to improve CAT and GPx enzymes and act as a collector of hydroxyl radicals [71]. It was reviewed that garlic and its extracts may be an alternative medicinal herbs against COVID-19 [72].

Ginger is a well-known herb with several effects such as treating sickness, colic, and appetite, controlling gastrointestinal problems, and respiratory infections. It is also accepted as a neuroprotectant, antidiabetic, anti-inflammatory, antioxidant, antiviral, and anticancer [73, 74]. This herb can maintain homeostasis by cooling the body, and reduce high fever. It was also reported that ginger shows its effect by inhibiting productions of nitric oxide and superoxide [75, 76]. Chang et al. [77] reported that ginger can block the viral attachment in respiratory epithelium, and is effective in human respiratory syncytial virus.

A blue-green microalga named Spirulina is a popular superfood with several beneficial effects such as antioxidant, antiviral, immunomodulatory, etc. [5]. It was reported that Spirulina could inhibit viral replication by blocking replication [78]. Hernández-Corona et al. [79] found that Spirulina inhibited the viral cell penetration and replication in a virus disease named herpes simplex virus type-1 (HSV-1). It was reviewed that the antiviral features of Spirulina are belonged to acidic polysaccharides extract such as calcium spirulina. Moreover, studies suggested that Spirulina may be safe for managing influenza outbreaks, however, additional investigations are needed [80–82].

Essential oils are aromatic oily liquids derived from plant material. These natural products have been widely used, in particular fragrances, cosmetics, aromatherapy, and herbal medicine, spices, nutrition, and agriculture. Essential oils have a known biological activity, including antibacterial, antiviral, anti-fungal, and anti-inflammatory effects [83].

Echinacea purpurea, a popular natural food worldwide, includes essential oils, flavonoids, tannin, saponin, betain, etc. According to studies, this herbal medicine can reduce the symptoms of respiratory diseases. Antiviral and immunomodulatory effects in SARS and COVID-19 have been reported [84, 85].

Thyme, curcumin, and licorice have been used for decades safely for both therapeutic and treatments. The ingredients of the essential oils of the origanum species were linalol, γ terpinene, p-cymenon, thymol and myrcene. Thymus's essential oil consists primarily of thymol. Other components found other than thymol are carvacrol, linalyl acetate, linalool, γ-terpinene, p-cymene and geraniol. Numerous studies have been carried out over the application of detected phenolic compounds as an antioxidant and antiviral activities have been tested, and it shows the antiviral effects against respiratory syncytial virus, Coxsackie virus, and herpes simplex virus type 1 [86]. Zhang et al. [86] reported that a significant ingredient of thyme has antiviral and antioxidant features. Curcumin is an active supplement to inhibit the activation of cytokines and neutrophils in the lungs. Many clinical studies have evaluated its effect on inflammation, immunity, microbial, and viral conditions [87]. It was also reported that curcumin could induce the glutathione level as a scavenger of free radicals [37]. On the other hand, an exciting herb named licorice can grow in many geographical structures worldwide. It was reported that licorice could reduce hepatocellular damage in hepatitis B and C. Nevertheless, it has an antiviral effect on HIV and SARS virus [88]. Also, licorice has an immunomodulatory effect, and it can induce respiratory activity [89]. It was determined that licorice shows these activities by its extracts named triterpene, saponins, and flavonoids [90].

Scientific studies on different species of cistus have shown that different species of the plant contain useful phytochemical products. Plant-derived polyphenols have been shown to be strong antioxidant, antibacterial, antifungal, anti-inflammatory, anti-viral, cytotoxic and anti-cancer properties with potential health benefits [91]. *Cistus creticus* is a naturally occurring plant native to Turkey with phenolic substances and flavonoids. Plant-derived polyphenols are strong antioxidants, and have protective effects on DNA. Various reports have appeared on the antiviral and antibacterial potential, including several reports describing the antiviral activity of polyphenols against the parainfluenza 3 virus [92].

Begun to be remembered with the existence of human beings, the olive was the symbol of peace and healthy life in every period of life from antiquity. Olive leaf traditionally used against hypertension, diuretic, antipyretic, appetizing and against constipation [93]. The olive leaf contains much more oleuropein than other parts. It has demonstrated that it is a phytochemical active against numerous diseases. Principal active constituents of the olive leaf are oleanolic acid and calcium elenolate compounds. These compounds have been shown to have anti-viral activity against many viruses such as parainfluenza, herpes simplex, pseudorabies, polioviruses (type-1, −2, and − 3), rhinoviruses, mycoviruses, coxsackievirus [94].

Phytochemicals are produced in plants, which are also referred to as naturally occurring plant chemicals. Several studies have demonstrated that flavonoids or phytochemicals may block these diseases' enzymatic activities [12, 95]. The most significant phytochemical compounds, polyphenols, flavonoids, and carotenoids, have been identified as antioxidants [96]. Polyphenols referred to as resveratrol and ellagic acid, are natural compounds in green tea, red wine, whole grains, grapes, and berries. They have potent antioxidants, metabolic, and cardiovascular effects. They can inhibit the proliferation of lung cancer cells by increasing autophagy [97, 98]. Resveratrol and ellagic acid may also help protect DNA and balance cell cycles. Also, it was reported that there is insufficient information on side effects and efficacy. Hence, traditional treatments need to be discussed before treatment.

Nevertheless, it was reported that flavonoids have an inhibition role in macrophages against inflammatory cytokines production in viral diseases [99]. There are some crucial plants included flavonoids, such as green tea, grapes, apples, and *Ginkgo biloba*. Also, the richest flavonoids, catechin and quercetin, are found in green tea. Catechin in green tea has anti-inflammatory features, which increases the glucocorticoids in pulmonary diseases, especially in the lung [100]. Quercetin is extracted from some plants such as *Rubus fruticosus*, *Passiflora subpeltata*, *Hypericum perforatum*, or Lagerstroemia. It was reported that quercetin could inhibit oxidative stress by increased endogenous antioxidants SOD, CAT, and GPx, and decreased lipid peroxidation. This flavonoid can also improve the function of non-enzymatic antioxidants such as vitamin C and E, and glutathione [101–103]. It was reported that another green tea metabolite named gallocatechin could reduce nitric oxide synthesis and oxidative status, and increase antioxidant capacity, especially catalase level [104, 105]. *Ginkgo biloba*, another popular herb, is a bioflavonoid compound, and also its extract named amentoflavone has a high antioxidant capacity, especially for lung diseases due to its improvement effect on SOD and glutathione [106]. Besides, some foods such as carrots, cabbage, and apple, which has luteolin, causes an increase in glutathione, SOD, and CAT. Luteolin also can improve lipid peroxidation during oxidative status in cancer and lung diseases [107].

Plant carotenoids were considered in terms of their role as mediators of free radicals through oxidation or oxygenation [108]. Furthermore, carotenoids act as chemical quench, which is necessary for the antioxidant function. They may reduce the risk of disease, in particular cancer and cardiovascular disease. The most important carotenoids are lycopene, lutein, zeaxanthine, beta-carotene found in tomatoes, carrots and watermelon.

Traditional medicinal herbs are rich compounds used in the development of medicines. They have centuries of experience with the use of herbal remedies for prevention and treatment. There are many medicinal herbs scattered geographically throughout the world. As such, further investigations are necessary to identify differences.

6. Future perspectives

Several clinical approaches have been agreed upon to deal with oxidative stress. Lately, for healthy living, the use of antioxidant supplements has been targeted to provide adequate homeostasis for humans and animals in many diseases or pandemics. Besides the prevention strategies such as isolation, hygiene, and control, nutrition, mostly natural antioxidants, is essential for improving antiviral activity against viral and pandemic diseases such as SARS, COVID-19 and, HIV etc.

Natural antioxidants have been used in many therapeutic practices because of their enzyme inhibition and their inhibitory effect on viral protein receptors. In addition, natural antioxidants may enhance immunity during diseases. As well, they have been the subject of multidisciplinary studies [109]. The WHO also acknowledged that there was insufficient evidence of herbal medicines for the treatment or treatment of viral diseases in humans, especially COVID-19 [110].

7. Conclusion

Throughout history, there have been significant pandemic diseases such as the 1918 influenza pandemic (H1N1 virus), HIV and COVID-19. During pandemics, nutrition is as important as health, hygiene, or self-isolation standards. To that end, predominantly natural antioxidants have been used in therapeutic practices. Many herbal medicines, plants, and their extracts have inhibitory effects on pandemic diseases or their symptoms. These nutrients have been investigating their immune-modulating, antiviral, and antioxidant effects for decades. However, all these effects of natural antioxidants are not equal. Research into the health performance of these nutrients is therefore necessary.

Conflict of interest

The authors declare no conflict of interest.

Acronyms and abbreviations

WHO	The World Health Organization
H1N1	Influenza virus
SARS	Severe Acute Respiratory Syndrome
Mers-Cov	Middle East Respiratory Syndrome Coronavirus
COVID-2019	Coronavirus-disease 2019
hCoVs	Human coronavirus disease
SARS-CoV-2	Severe acute respiratory syndrome coronavirus
HIV	Human immunodeficiency virus
ROS	Reactive oxygen species
RNS	Reactive nitrogen species
GPx	Glutathione peroxidase
CAT	Catalase
SOD	Superoxide dismutase
HCV	Hepatitis C Virus
Cu	Copper
Fe	Ferrous
Zn	Zinc

Appendices and nomenclature

Ascorbic acid	Vitamin C
Tocopherol	Vitamin E

Beta carotene	provitamin A
Blue-green algae	Spirulina
Thymus	Thymol
Olive leaf	Oleanolic acid and calcium elenolate compounds
Green tea	Gallocatechin
Ginkgo biloba	Bioflavonoid compound
Phytochemical compounds	Polyphenols, flavonoids, carotenoids
Essential oils	Linalol, γ terpinene, p-cymenon, thymol, myrcene
Endogenous antioxidant	Superoxide dismutase, glutathione peroxidase, glutathione reductase, catalase
Cistus creticus	Polyphenols
Flavonoids	Catechin, quercetin

Author details

Cenk Aydin[1]* and Nilay Seyidoglu[2]

1 Department of Physiology, Faculty of Veterinary Medicine, Bursa Uludag University, Bursa, Turkey

2 Department of Physiology, Faculty of Veterinary Medicine, Tekirdag Namik Kemal University, Tekirdag, Turkey

*Address all correspondence to: caydin@uludag.edu.tr

References

[1] Birben E, Sahiner UM, Sackesen C, Erzurum S, Kalayci O. Oxidative stress and antioxidant defense. World Allergy Organ J. 2012;5(1):9-19. doi: 10.1097/WOX.0b013e3182439613.

[2] WHO/ FAO Report 2002. Dietary antioxidants: a consideration of factors influencing requirements. In: Human Vitamin and Mineral Requirements. Rome, 2002 Report of a joint FAO/WHO expert consultation Bangkok, Thailand. Avaliable from: http://www.fao.org/3/Y2809E/y2809e0n.htm

[3] Chehue Romero A, Olvera Hernández EG, Flores Cerón T, Álvarez-Chávez A. The exogenous antioxidants. In: Morales-González JA, editor. Oxidative Stress and Chronic Degenerative Diseases—A Role for Antioxidants. Croatia: InTechOpen; 2013. p. 33.

[4] Zheng J, Zhou Y, Li, Y, Xu DP, Li S, Li HB. Spices for prevention and treatment of cancers. Nutrients. 2016;8:495. DOI: 10.3390/nu8080495

[5] Seyidoglu N, Aydin C. 2020. Stress, Natural Antioxidants and Future Perspectives. In: Salanta CL, editor. The Health Benefits of Foods - Current Knowledge and Further Development. London: Intechopen; 2020. p. 149-165.

[6] Lobo V, Patil A, Phatak A, Chandra N. Free radicals, antioxidants and functional foods: Impact on human health. Pharmacogn Rev. 2010;4(8):118-126. DOI: 10.4103/0973-7847.70902.

[7] Huang D. Dietary Antioxidants and Health Promotion. Antioxidants (Basel). 2018;7(1):9. DOI: 10.3390/antiox7010009.

[8] WHO (World Health Organization, Food and Agricultural Organization of the United Nations). Managing epidemics [Internet]. 2018. Available from: https://www.who.int/emergencies/diseases/managing-epidemics-interactive.pdf [Accessed: 2020-12-12]

[9] WHO (World Health Organization, Food and Agricultural Organization of the United Nations). [Internet]. 2020a. Available from: https:// https://www.who.int/emergencies/diseases/en/ [Accessed: 2020-12-30]

[10] WHO (World Health Organization, Food and Agricultural Organization of the United Nations). [Internet]. 2004. Available from: https://www.who.int/nutrition/publications/micronutrients/9241546123/en/ [Accessed: 2020-12-30]

[11] Fernandes IG, de Brito CA, Silva dos Reis VM, Sato MN, Pereira NZ. SARS-CoV-2 and Other Respiratory Viruses: What Does Oxidative Stress Have to Do with It?. Oxidative Medicine and Cellular Longevity. 2020;ID 8844280:13. DOI: 10.1155/2020/8844280

[12] Leite Diniz LR, Bezerra Filho CSM, Fielding BC, de Sousa DP. Natural Antioxidants: A Review of Studies on Human and Animal Coronavirus. Oxid Med & Cellular Longevity. 2020;Id3173281:14pages. DOI: 10.1155/2020/3173281

[13] Hudson JB. The use of herbal extracts in the control of influenza. Review. Journal of Medicinal Plants Research. 2009;3(13):1189-1195

[14] Kaihatsu K, Kawakami C, Kato N. Potential Anti-Influenza Virus Agents Based on Coffee Ingredients and Natural Flavonols. Nat Prod Chem Res. 2014;2:2. DOI: 10.4172/2329-6836.1000129

[15] Liu X, Wang N, Fan S, Zheng X, Yang Y, Zhu Y, Lu Y, Chen Q, Zhou H, Zheng J. The citrus flavonoid naringenin confers protection in a murine

endotoxaemia model through AMPK-ATF3-dependent negative regulation of the TLR4 signaling pathway. Scientific Reports. 2016;6:39735. DOI: 10.1038/srep39735.

[16] Zhang Y, Kutateladze TG. Molecular structure analyses suggest strategies to therapeutically target SARS-CoV-2. Nat. Commun. 2020;11(1):2920. doi: 10.1038/s41467-020-16779-4.

[17] Kulkarni SA, Nagarajan SK, Ramesh V, Palaniyandi V, Selvam SP, Madhavan T. Computational evaluation of major components from plant essential oils as potent inhibitors of SARS-CoV-2 spike protein. J. Mol. Struct. 2020:1221:128823. DOI: 10.1016/j.molstruc.2020.128823

[18] Sansone C, Brunet C, Noonan DM, Albini A. Marine Algal Antioxidants as Potential Vectors for Controlling Viral Diseases. Antioxidants (Basel). 2020;9(5):392. DOI: 10.3390/antiox9050392.

[19] Qui X, Kroeker A, He S, Kozak R. Prophylactic Efficacy of Quercetin 3-β-O-d-Glucoside against Ebola Virus Infection. Antimicrobial Agents and Chemotherapy. 2016;60(9):AAC.00307-16. DOI: 10.1128/AAC.00307-16

[20] Khalil A, Tazeddinova D. The upshot of Polyphenolic compounds on immunity amid COVID-19 pandemic and other emerging communicable diseases: An appraisal. Natural Products and Bioprospecting. 2020;10:411-429. DOI: 10.1007/s13659-020-00271-z

[21] Garcia S. Pandemics and Traditional Plant-Based Remedies. A Historical-Botanical Review in the Era of COVID19. Front. Plant Sci. 2020;11:571042. DOI: 10.3389/fpls.2020.571042

[22] Valko M, Leibfritz D, Moncola J, Cronin MD, Mazur M, Telser J. Free radicals andantioxidants in normal physiological functions and human disease. Review. Int J Biochem Cell Biol. 2007;39:44-84. DOI: 10.1016/j.biocel.2006.07.001

[23] Dröge W. Free radicals in the physiological control of cell function. Review. Physiol Rev. 2002;82:47-95. DOI: 10.1152/physrev.00018.2001

[24] Halliwell B. Biochemistry of oxidative stress. Biochem Soc Trans. 2007;35:1147-1150. DOI: 10.1042/BST0351147

[25] Pham-Huy LA, He H, Pham-Huy C. Free Radicals, Antioxidants in Disease and Health. Int J Biomed Sci. 2008;4(2):89-96. PMCID: PMC3614697

[26] Bahorun T, Soobrattee MA, Luximon-Ramma V, Aruoma OI. Free radicals and antioxidants in cardiovascular health and disease. Internet J Med. 2006;1(2):1-17. DOI: 10.4314/ijmu.v1i2.39839

[27] Ceriello A. Possible role of oxidative stress in the pathogenesis of hypertension. Review. Diabetes Care. 2008;31 (Suppl 2):S181–S184. DOI: 10.2337/dc08-s245

[28] Butterfield DA. Amyloid beta-peptide (1-42)-induced oxidative stress and neurotoxicity: implications for neurodegeneration in Alzheimer's disease brain. A review. Free Radic Res. 2002;36:1307-1313. DOI: 10.1080/1071576021000049890

[29] MacNee W. Oxidative stress and lung inflammation in airways disease. Eur J Pharmacol. 2001;429:195-207. DOI: 10.1016/s0014-2999(01)01320-6

[30] Walston J, Xue Q, Semba RD, Ferrucci L, Cappola AR, Ricks M, Guralnik J, Fried LP. Serum antioxidants, inflammation, and total mortality in older women. Am J Epidemiol. 2006;163:18-26. DOI: 10.1093/aje/kwj007

[31] Meyer CH, Sekundo W. Nutritional supplementation to prevent cataract formation. Dev Ophthalmol. 2005;38:103-119. DOI: 10.1159/000082771

[32] Braekke K, Harsem NK, Staff AC. Oxidative stress and antioxidant status in fetal circulation in preeclampsia. Pediatr Res. 2006;60:560-564. DOI: 10.1203/01.pdr.0000242299.01219.6a

[33] Galle J. Oxidative stress in chronic renal failure. Nephrol Dial Transplant. 2001;16:2135-2142. DOI: 10.1093/ndt/16.11.2135

[34] Sies H. Oxidative stress: a concept in redox biology and medicine. Redox Biology. 2015;4:180-183. DOI: 10.1016/j.redox.2015.01.002.

[35] Gravier-Hernández R, Gil-del Valle L, Valdes-Alonso L, Hernández-AyalaN,Bermúdez-AlfonsoY, Hernández-Requejo D, Rosell-Guerra T, Hernández-González-Abreu MC. Oxidative stress in hepatitis C virus–human immunodeficiency virus co-infected patients. Annals of Hepatology. 2020;19(1):92-98. DOI: 10.1016/j.aohep.2019.05.009

[36] Zhang Z, Rong L, Li YP. Flaviviridae Viruses and Oxidative Stress: Implications for Viral Pathogenesis. Oxid Med Cell Longev. 2019:1409582. DOI: 10.1155/2019/1409582.

[37] Lee W, Loo C, Bebawy M, Luk F, Mason R, Rohanizadeh R. Curcumin and its derivatives: Their application in neuropharmacology and neuroscience in the 21st century. Curr Neuropharmacol. 2013;11:338-378. DOI: 10.2174/1570159X11311040002

[38] Rehermann B, Nascimbeni M. Immunology of hepatitis B virus and hepatitis C virus infection. Nature Reviews Immunology. 2005;5(3):215-229. DOI: 10.1038/nri1573

[39] Imai Y, Kuba K, Greg Neely G, Yaghubian Malhami R, Perkmann T, van Loo G, Ermolaeva M, Veldhuizen R, Leuing YHC, Wang H, Liu H, Sun Y, Pasparakis M, Kopf M, Mech C, Bavari S, Perisi JSM, Slutsky AS, Akira S, Hultqvist M, Holmdahl R, NichollsJ,JiangC,BinderCJ,PenningerJM. Identification of oxidative stress and Toll-like receptor 4 signaling as a key pathway of acute lung injury. Cell. 2008;133(2):235-249.

[40] Bogden JD, Baker H, Frank O, Perez G, Kemp F, Bruening K, Louria D. Micronutrient status and human immunodeficiency virus (HIV) infection. Ann N Y Acad Sci. 1990;587:189-195. DOI: 10.1111/j.1749-6632.1990.tb00146.x

[41] Chrobot AM, Szaflarska-Szczepanik A, Drewa G. Antioxidant defense in children with chronic viral hepatitis B and C. Med Sci Monit. 2000;6(4):713-718.

[42] Reshi ML, Su YC, Hong JR. RNA Viruses: ROS-Mediated Cell Death. Int J Cell Biol. 2014;2014:467452. DOI: 10.1155/2014/467452

[43] Xiaowei Li, Manman G, Yizhao P, Liesu M, Shemin L. Molecular immune pathogenesis and diagnosis of COVID-19. J Pharm Anal. 2020;10(2):102-108. DOI: 10.1016/j.jpha.2020.03.001

[44] Zhao M. Cytokine storm and immunomodulatory therapy in COVID-19: role of chloroquine and anti-IL-6 monoclonal antibodies, Int. J. Antimicrob. Agents. 2020;55(6):105982. DOI: 10.1016/j.ijantimicag.2020.105982.

[45] Xu D, Zhang Z, Chu F, Li Y, Jin L, Zhang L, Gao GF, Wang FS. Genetic variation of SARS coronavirus in Beijing hospital, Emerg. Infect. Dis. 2004;10:789-794. DOI: 10.3201/eid1005.030875

[46] Kosmider B, Messier EM, Janssen WJ, Nahreini P, Wang J, Hartshorn KL, Mason RJ. Nrf 2 protects human alveolar epithelial cells against injury induced by influenza A virus. Respiratory Research. 2012;13(1):43. DOI: 10.1186/1465-9921-13-43

[47] Burdette D, Olivarez M, Waris G. Activation of transcription factor Nrf2 by hepatitis C virus induces the cell-survival pathway. J Gen Virol. 2010;91(Pt 3):681-690. DOI: 10.1099/vir.0.014340-0

[48] Young I, Woodside J. Antioxidants in health and disease. J. Clin.Pathol. 2001;54:176-186. DOI: 10.1136/jcp.54.3.176

[49] Derouiche S. Oxidative Stress Associated with SARS-Cov-2 (COVID-19) Increases the Severity of the Lung Disease - A Systematic Review. Infect Dis Epidemiol. 2020;6(3):1-6. DOI: 10.23937/2474-3658/1510121

[50] Zhou Z, Xi W, Hu Y, Nie C, Zhou Z. Antioxidant activity of citrus fruits, review. Food Chemistry. 2016;196:885-896. DOI: 10.1016/j.foodchem.2015.09.072

[51] Coulter ID, Hardy ML, Morton SC, Hilton LG, Tu W, Valentine D, Shekelle PG. Antioxidants vitamin C and vitamin E for the prevention and treatment of cancer. Journal of General Internal Medicine. 2006;21(7):735-744. DOI: 10.1111/j.1525-1497.2006.00483.x

[52] Gaziano JM, Hennekens CH. The role of beta-carotene in the prevention of cardiovascular disease. Annals of the New York Academy of Sciences. 1993;691:148-155. DOI: 10.1111/j.1749-6632.1993.tb26166.x

[53] Ozsoy N, Candoken E, Akev N.Implications for degenerative disorders: Anti oxidative activity, total phenols, flavonoids, ascorbic acid, beta-carotene and beta-tocopherol in Aloe vera. Oxidative Medicine and Cellular Longevity. 2009;2:99-106. DOI: 10.4161/oxim.2.2.8493

[54] Donaldson MS. Nutrition and cancer: A review of the evidence for an anti-cancer diet. Nutr. J. 2004;3:19-25. DOI: 10.1186/1475-2891-3-19

[55] Hemilä H, Chalker E. Vitamin C can shorten the length of stay in the ICU: a meta-analysis. Nutrients. 2019;11(4):708. DOI: 10.3390/nu11040708

[56] Nakamura H. Thioredoxin and its related molecules: Updated 2005. Antioxidants and Redox Singaling. 2005;7(5-6):823. DOI: 10.1089/ars.2005.7.823

[57] Skalny AV, Rink L, Ajsuvakova OP, Aschner M, Gritsenko VA, Alekseenko SI, Svistunov AA, Petrakis D, Spandidos DA, Aaseth J, Tsatsakis A, Tinkov AA. Zinc and respiratory tract infections: Perspectives for COVID-19 (Review). International Journal of Molecular Medicine. 2020;46:17-26. DOI: 10.3892/ijmm.2020.4575

[58] te Velthuis AJW, van den Worm SHE, Sims AC, Baric RS, Snijder EJ, van Hemert MJ. Zn2+ inhibits coronavirus and arterivirus RNA polymerase activity in vitro and zinc ionophores block the replication of these viruses in cell culture. PLOS Pathogens. 2010;4;6(11):e1001176. DOI: 10.1371/journal.ppat.1001176

[59] Raha S, Mallick R, Basak S, Duttaroy AK. Is copper beneficial for COVID-19 patients? Medical Hypotheses. 2020;142:109814. DOI: 10.1016/j.mehy.2020.109814

[60] Dalamaga M, Karampela I, Mantzoros CS. Commentary: Could iron chelators prove to be useful as

an adjunct to COVID-19 treatment regimens? Metabolism Clinical and Experimental. 2020;108:154260. DOI: 10.1016/j.metabol.2020.154260

[61] Li C, Li Y, Ding C. The role of copper homeostasis at the host-pathogen axis: From bacteria to fungi. International Journal of Molecular Sciences. 2019;20(1):175. DOI: 10.3390/ijms20010175

[62] Sekeroglu N, Gezici S. Coronavirus Pandemic and Some Turkish Medicinal Plants. Anadolu Kliniği Tıp Bilimleri Dergisi. 2020;25(1):163-182. DOI: 10.21673/anadoluklin.724210 (Turkish)

[63] Vellingiri B, Jayaramayy K, Iyer M, Narayanasamy A, Govindasamy V, Giridharane B, Ganesan S, Venugopal A, Venkatesan D, Ganesan H, Rajagopalan K, Rahman PKSM, Cho SG, Kumar NS, Subramaniam MD. COVID-19: A promising cure for the global panic. Sci. Total Environ. 2020;725:138277. DOI: 10.1016/j.scitotenv.2020.138277

[64] Babich O, Sukhikh S, Prosekov A, Asyakina L, Ivanova S. Medicinal Plants to Strengthen Immunity during a Pandemic. Pharmaceuticals. 2020;13:313. DOI: 10.3390/ph13100313

[65] Kyo E, Uda N, Kasuga S, Itakura Y. Immunmodulator effects of agedgarlic extract. J. Nutr. 2001;131(3s):1075S–1079S. DOI: 10.1093/jn/131.3.1075S

[66] Amagese H. Clarifying the real bioactive cconstituents of garlic. J. Nutr. 2006;136:716S–725S. DOI: 10.1093/jn/136.3.716S

[67] Kun S. Seetaha S, Pongsanarakul S, Hannongbua Si Shoowongkomon K. Anti HIV-1 reverse tanscriptase activities of hexane etracts from some Asian medicinal plants. Journal of Medicinal Plants Research. 2011;5(19):4899-4960. DOI: 10.5897/JMPR.9000098

[68] Rehman R, Saif S, Hanif MA, Riaz M. Garlic. In: Hanif M, Nawaz H, Khan M, Byrne H, editors. Medicinal plants of South Asia. Amsterdam: Elsevier BV; 2019. p. 301-315. DOI: 10.1016/B978-0-08-102659-5.00023-9

[69] Rouf R, Uddin SJ, Sarker DK, Islam MT, Ali ES, Shilpi JA, Nahar L, Tiralongo E, Sarker SD. Antiviral potential of garlic (Allium sativum) and its organosulfur compounds: A systematic update of pre-clinical and clinical data. Trends in Food Science & Technology. 2020;104 (2020):219-234. DOI: 10.1016/j.tifs.2020.08.006

[70] Mehrbood P, Ideris A, Amini E, Eslami T, Bande F, Kheiri M. Assessment of direct immınofluoresence assay in detection of antiviral effect of grlic extract on influenca virus. Africa Journal of microbiology research. 2013;7:2608-2612. DOI: 10.5897/AJMR12.2329

[71] Prasad K, Haxdal A, Yu M, Raney BL. Antioxidant activity of allicin, an active principle in garlic. Mol Cell Biochem. 1995;148:183-189. DOI: 10.1007/BF00928155

[72] Oladele JO, Ajayi EI, Oyeleke OM, Oladele OT, Olowookere BD, Adeniyi BM, Oyewole OI, Oladiji AT. A systematic review on COVID-19 pandemic with special emphasis on curative potentials of Nigeria based medicinal plants. Heliyon. 2020;6(9):e04897. DOI: 10.1016/j.heliyon.2020.e04897

[73] Sornpet B, Potha T, Tragoolpua Y, Pringproa K. Antiviral activity of five Asian medicinal pant crude extracts against highly pathogenic H5N1 avian influenza virus. Asian Pac J Trop Med. 2017;10:871-876. DOI: 10.1016/j.apjtm.2017.08.010

[74] Abiyana S, Gayatri Devi R, Lakshmanan G. Knowledge and awareness about ginger and turmeric as a herbal cure for COVID-19. Int. J.

Pharm. Res. 2020;(12): 768-777. DOI: 10.31838/ijpr/2020.SP2.093

[75] Ippoushi K, Azuma K, Ito H, Horie H, Higashio H. [6]-Gingerol inhibits nitric oxide synthesis in activated J774.1 mouse macrophages and prevents peroxynitrite-induced oxidation and nitration reactions. Life Sci. 2003;14;73(26):3427-37. doi: 10.1016/j.lfs.2003.06.022

[76] Rahmani AH, Al Sharbrmi FM, Aly SM. Active ingredients of ginger as potential candidates in the prevention and treatment of diseases via modulation of biological activities. Int J Physiol Pathophysiol Pharmacol. 2014;6(2):125-136. PMCID: PMC4106649

[77] Chang JS, Wang KC, Yeh CF, Shieh DE, Chiang LC. Fresh ginger (Zingiber officinale) has anti-viral activity against human respiratory syncytial virus in human respiratory tract cell lines. J Ethnopharmacol. 2013;145(1):146-151. DOI: 10.1016/j.jep.2012.10.043

[78] Hayashi K., Hayashi T., Kojima I. A natural sulfated polysaccharide, calcium spirulan, isolated from Spirulina platensis: in vitro and ex vivo evaluation of anti-Herpes simplex virus and anti-human immunodeficiency virus activities. AIDS Research and Human Retroviruses. 1996;12:1463-1471. DOI: 10.1089/aid.1996.12.1463

[79] Hernández-Corona A, Nieves I, Meckes M, Chamorro G, Barron BL. Antiviral activity of Spirulina maxima against herpes simplex virus type 2. Antiviral Res. 2002;56(3):279-285. DOI: 10.1016/S0166-3542(02)00132-8

[80] Singh S, Dwivedi V, Sanyal D, Dasgupta S. Therapeutic and Nutritional Potential of Spirulina in Combating COVID-19 Infection. AIJR prints. 2020;49(1). DOI: 10.13140/RG.2.2.16527.41127

[81] Deng F, Lu JJ, Liu HY, Lin LP, Ding J. Zhang JS. Synthesis and antitumor activity of novel salvicine analogues. Chin Chem Lett. 2011;22:25-28. DOI: 10.1016/j.cclet.2010.07.009

[82] Chen YH, Chang GK, Kuo SM, Huang SY, Yu IC, Lo YL, Shih SR. Well-tolerated Spirulina extract inhibits influenza virus replication and reduces virus-induced mortality. Scientific Reports. 2016;6:24253. DOI: 10.1038/srep24253

[83] Sengezer E, Gungor T. Essential oils and their effects on animals. Lalahan Hay. Araşt. Enst. Derg. 2008;48(2):101-110 (Turkish). Avaliable from: Retrieved from https://dergipark.org.tr/tr/pub/lahaed/issue/39442/465209

[84] David S. Cunningham, R. Echinacea for the prevention and treatment of upper respiratory tract infections: A systematic review and meta-analysis. Complement. Ther. Med. 2019:44:18-26. DOI: 10.1016/j.ctim.2019.03.011

[85] Li SJ, Wang YL, Xue J, Zhao N, Zhu TS. The impact of COVID-19 epidemic declaration on psychological consequences: A study on active Weibo users. Int. J. Environ. Res. Public Health. 2020;17(6):2032. DOI: 10.3390/ijerph17062032

[86] Zhang XL, Guo YS, Wang CH, Li GQ, Xu JJ, Chung HY, Ye WC, Li YL, Wang GC. Phenolic compounds from Origanum vulgare and their antioxidant and antiviral activities. Food Chem. 2014; 152:300-306. DOI: 10.1016/j.foodchem.2013.11.153

[87] Boskabady MH, Shakeri F, Naghdi F. The effects of Curcuma Longa L. and its constituents in respiratory disorders andmolecular mechanisms of their action. In: Rahman A, editor. Studies in Natural Products Chemistry. Oxford, UK: Elsevier; 2020;65:239-269. DOI: 10.1016/B978-0-12-817905-5.00007-X

[88] Fiore C, Eisenhut M, Krausse R, Ragazzi E, Pellati D, Armanini D, Bielenberg J. Antiviral effects of Glycyrrhiza species. Phytother Res. 2008;22(2):141-148. DOI: 10.1002/ptr.2295

[89] Fiore C, Eisenhut M, Ragazzi E, Zanchin G, Armanini D. A history of the therapeutic use of liquorice in Europe. J Ethnopharm. 2005;99(3):317-324. DOI: 10.1016/j.jep.2005.04.015

[90] Wang C, Chen L, Xu C, Shi J, Chen S, Tan M, Chen J, Zou L, Chen C, Liu Z, A Comprehensive Review for Phytochemical, Pharmacological, and Biosynthesis Studies on Glycyrrhiza spp. (Review). Am. J. Chin. Med. 2020;48:17-45. DOI: 10.1142/S0192415X20500020

[91] Stępień A, Aebisher D, Bartusik-Aebisher D. Biological properties of "Cistus species". Eur J Clin Exp Med. 2018; 16(2):127-132. DOI: 10.15584/ejcem.2018.2.8

[92] Kilic DD, Siriken B, Erturk O, Tanrikulu G, Gül M, Başkan C. Antibacterial, Antioxidant and DNA Interaction Properties of Cistus creticus L. Extracts. J Int Environ Appl Sci. 2019; 14(3):110-115.

[93] Wyk BE, Wink M. Medicinal Plants of the World: An Illustrated Scientific Guide to Important Medicinal Plants and Their Uses. 1st ed. Portland, Oregon. USA: Timber Press; 2004. 480 p.

[94] AMR. Alternative Medicine Review. Olive Leaf Monograph-Foundational Med Rev. 2009;14(1):62-66. Available from: https://www.foundationalmedicinereview.com/wp-content/uploads/2019/02/v14-1-62.pdf [Accessed:2020-12-10]

[95] Jo S, Kim S, Shin DH, Kim MS. Inhibition of SARSCoV 3CL protease by flavonoids. Journal of Enzyme Inhibition and Medicinal Chemistry. 2020;35(1):145-151. DOI: 10.1080/14756366.2019.1690480

[96] Miller AL. Antioxidant Flavonoids: Structure, Function and Clinical Usage. Alt. Med. Rev. 1996;1:103-111.

[97] Han DH, Lee MJ, Kim JH. Antioxidant and Apoptosis-inducing Activities of Ellagic Acid. Anticancer Research. 2006;26:3601-3606. DOI: 10.1007/s11356-019-07352-8

[98] Duan J, Zhan JC, Wang GZ, Zhao XC, Huang WD, Zhou GB. The red wine component ellagic acid induces autophagy and exhibits anti-lung cancer activity in vitro and in vivo. Journal of Cellular and Molecular Medicine. 2018;23(1):143-154. DOI: 10.1111/jcmm.13899

[99] Yahfoufi N, Alsadi N, Jambi M, Matar C. The immunomodulatory and anti-inflammatory role of polyphenols. Nutrients. 2018;10:1618. DOI: 10.3390/nu10111618

[100] Lugt T, Weseler AR, Vrolijk MF, Opperhuizen A, Aalt B. Dietary advanced glycation endproducts decrease glucocorticoid sensitivity in vitro. Nutrients. 2020;12:441. DOI: 10.3390/nu12020441

[101] Kucharíková A, Kusari S, Sezgin S, Spiteller M, Čellárová E. Occurrence and distribution of phytochemicals in the leaves of 17 in vitro cultured Hypericum spp. adapted to outdoor Conditions. Frontiers in Plant Science. 2016;27;7:1616. DOI: 10.3389/fpls.2016.01616

[102] Meng LQ, Yang FY, Wang MS. Shi BK, Chen DX, Chen D, Zhou Q, He QB, Ma LX, Cheng WL, Xing NZ. Quercetin protects against chronic prostatitis in rat model through NF-κB and MAPK signaling pathways. Prostate. 2018;78(11):790-800. DOI: 10.1002/pros.23536

[103] Zahoor M, Shah AB, Naz S, Ullah R, Bari A, Mahmood HM. Isolation of quercetin from rubus fruticosus, their concentration through nf/ro membranes, and recovery through carbon nanocomposite. a pilot plant study. BioMed Research International. 2020;2020(11):1-7. DOI: 10.1155/2020/8216435

[104] Pan Y, Long X, Yi R, Zhao X. Polyphenols in Liubao tea can prevent CCl4-induced hepatic damage in mice through its antioxidant capacities. Nutrients. 2018;10;10(9):1280. DOI: 10.3390/nu10091280

[105] Bulboaca AE, Boarescu PM, Porfire AS, Dogaru G, Barbalata C, Valeanu M, Munteanu C, Râjnoveanu RM, Nicula CA, Stanescu IC. The effect of nano-epigallocatechin-gallate on oxidative stress and matrix metalloproteinases in experimental diabetes mellitus. Antioxidants. 2020;9(2):172. DOI: 10.3390/antiox9020172

[106] Bajpai VK, Park IW, Lee JI, Shukla S, Nile SH, Chun HS, Khan I, Oh SY, Lee H, Huh YS, Na MK, Han YK. Antioxidant and antimicrobial efficacy of a biflavonoid, amentoflavone from Nandina domestica in vitro and in minced chicken meat and apple juice food models. Food Chemistry. 2019;271:239-247. DOI: 10.1016/j.foodchem.2018.07.159

[107] Kang KA, Piao MJ, Ryu YS, Hyun YJ, Park JE, Shilnikova K, Zhen AX, Kang HK, Koh YS, Jeong YJ, Hyun JW. Luteolin induces apoptotic cell death via antioxidant activity in human colon cancer cells. International Journal of Oncology. 2017;51(4):1169-1178. DOI: 10.3892/ijo.2017.4091

[108] Fiedor J, Burda K. Potential Role of Carotenoids as Antioxidants in Human Health and Disease. Nutrients. 2014;6:466-488. DOI: 10.3390/nu6020466

[109] Thomford NE, Dzobo K, Chimusa E, Andrae-Marobela K, Chirikure S, Wonkam A, Dandara C. Personalized herbal medicine? a roadmap for convergence of herbal and precision medicine biomarker innovations. OMICS: A J Integrative Biology. 2018;22(6):375-391. DOI: 10.1089/omi.2018.0074.

[110] WHO (World Health Organization, Food and Agricultural Organization of the United Nations). Myth busters. [Internet]. 2020b. Available from: https://www.who.int/westernpacific/emergencies/covid-19/information/mythbusters [Accessed: 2020-12-25]

Chapter 8

An Antioxidant Defense System in Radiation-Resistant Bacterium *Deinococcus geothermalis* against Oxidative Stress

Chanjae Lee, Min K. Bae and Sung-Jae Lee

Abstract

A radiation-resistant bacterium, *Deinococcus geothermalis* has various stress response mechanisms, including antioxidation. Features that maintain vitality at high radiation doses include the following: enzymatic scavengers of ROS such as catalase, SOD, and peroxidase; strain-specific DNA repair systems such as Deinococcal unique proteins; non-enzymatic responses such as manganese complexes, carotenoids, and DNA-binding proteins. This chapter summarizes the primary response mechanism by redox balance centered on the cystine transporter. It also reviews action characteristics of DNA-binding protein Dps and a putative LysR family protein, and effects on loss of function of the carotenoid biosynthesis genes by transposition of insertion sequences. Environmental adaptation and molecular evolution of radiation-resistant bacterium are also considered to explain the potentials of molecular behavior induced by oxidative stress.

Keywords: cystine ABC transporter, Dps, LysR regulator, oxidative stress, redox-potential, transposition

1. Introduction

The radiation-resistant bacterium of genus *Deinococcus* is an essential resource for research to understand responses to oxidative stress and mechanisms for recovering direct double-strand break damage to DNA caused by gamma-radiation [1–3]. High gamma-ray resistance is caused by the unique DNA-damage repair proteins and various protective mechanisms in these radiation-resistant *Deinococcus* bacteria [4–6]. Many researchers have studied the properties of their unique proteins. These studies have expanded our scientific understanding [7–9]. Technological advances have recently been made to understand life phenomena through genomics, metabolomics, and proteomics studies [10–12]. Despite the remarkable progress in recent omics studies, it is still difficult to fully understand these cell recovery characteristics from various cellular stress damages. The accumulation of various creative research results will eventually lead to a complete understanding of such characteristics.

Only 20% of DNA damage is directly caused by radiation. In comparison, the remaining 80% is indirectly caused by reactive oxygen species (ROS) such as

IntechOpen

superoxide and hydroxyl radicals which are chemically reactive molecules that can damage cell structures such as cell membrane, proteins, and nucleic acids (DNA and RNA) [1, 10]. Bacteria have a natural ROS scavenging system composed of enzymatic antioxidants (e.g. catalase, peroxidase, superoxide reductase, and superoxide dismutase (SOD)), and non-enzymatic antioxidants (e.g. intracellular manganese, pyrroloquinoline quinone, carotenoids), small antioxidant thiols (e.g. cystine, bacillithiol, or mycothiol), and DNA-protecting proteins [2, 13–15].

Specific regulators tightly control many stress response defense systems. Enzymatic ROS scavengers are regulated by the global transcriptional regulator OxyR, a LysR family regulator [16–20]. OxyR of *Deinococcus radiodurans* is a 1-Cys-type that can activate the transcription of genes encoding catalase (*katE*), ferrous iron transporter (*feoB*), and iron(III) dicitrate transporter (drb0125). It is also a repressor of *dps* and *mntH* transcription to control antioxidant functions and Mn/Fe ion homeostasis [21].

These gene regulation systems are also susceptible to intracellular redox balance through specific ABC transporters and chemical modification of low-molecular-weight (LMW) thiol compounds using unique enzyme reactions. The cystine importer is one of the redox controlling ABC transporters [22–25]. It could sense the redox balance and affect gene regulation for enzymatic defense through the OxyR activation [15, 20]. There are also some exceptional OxyR regulons in bacteria [26–28].

This redox balance affects various enzymatic and chemical modification processes through a progressive transformation. For example, acetylation is a conserved modification used to regulate various cellular pathways such as gene expression, protein synthesis, detoxification, and virulence. Acetyltransferase enzymes can transfer an acetyl moiety, usually from acetyl coenzyme A (AcCoA), onto a target substrate, thereby modulating the activity or stability [29]. Gcn5-related N-acetyltransferase (GNAT) members can acetylate the amino group of an extensive range of substrates. They are classified into three groups: (1) small molecule acetyltransferases such as aminoglycosides and mycothiol; (2) peptide acetyltrandferases such as the peptidoglycan that is part of the cell wall; and (3) protein acetyltransferases such as the histone family [30]. In Gram-positive *Actinomycetes* and *Firmicutes*, alternative LMW thiols such as mycothiol (MSH) and bacillithiol (BSH) play related as glutathione surrogates of Gram-negative bacteria, respectively [31].

As antioxidant substances, carotenoid compounds also act as scavengers of ROS. *Deinococcales* species generally have a reddish color phenotype due to carotenoid biosynthesis. The metabolic pathway in *Deinococcus* is well conserved and industrially applicable [32].

As one of bacterial nucleoid proteins in gene expression specificity of growth phase-dependent manner, Dps (DNA-binding protein from starved cells) is initially suppressed at the exponential cell growth phase. It is then expressed in large quantities in the stationary growth phase to become the major protein [33, 34]. These sequential nucleoid protein transitions and overexpression of a particular protein demonstrate the function of a defense mechanism that can protect against cell damage during stress due to increased ROS and reduced nutrients that cells can consume. Dps proteins are found almost ubiquitously in bacterial genomes. Each bacterial genome contains species-specific Dps genes. Dps has multifaceted roles such as DNA binding, iron sequestration, and ferroxidase activity in various stress responses [35–37]. Dps was described initially in *Escherichia coli* as a protein that could protect the bacteria in a malnourished environment by DNA-binding [38]. Dps has a shell-like structure with a spherical hollow cavity in the center. This hollow cavity of Dps acts as an iron storage compartment and iron sequestration that is important in iron detoxification and homeostasis. Dps is a small DNA-binding protein having approximately 150 to 300 amino acid residues with a positive charge along the entire chain. While Dps is a significant protein when it is over-expressed, Dps plays another essential role in condensing and protecting the stationary-phase nucleoid from severe environmental stress such as oxidative and radioactive damages [34, 39, 40]. Therefore, many bacteria express more than one Dps depending on environmental factors around them. How the condensed DNA is untangled when proteins are expressed remains unclear. It merits further studies.

Bacterial insertion sequence (IS) elements consist of a gene encoding transposase (one or two), terminal inverted repeats (TIR), and direct repeats (DR). Their lengths are less than 3 kb [41, 42]. According to the database of IS finding platform such as ISfinder, IS types vary [43]. IS densities are significantly less in chromosomes than in plasmids in bacteria. Perhaps plasmids are the primary IS carrier [44]. These IS elements can be transferred by high temperature, γ-irradiation, oxidative stress, and substances that could damage DNA and result in gene breakdown [45–47]. Regulation of IS transposition is also affected by various factors such as transcriptional repressors and inhibitors, ribosome frameshifting, methylation, mRNA stability, and target sequences [48–51]. Gene breakdown by transposition of IS elements does not just have deleterious aspects. IS-mediated gene inhibition offers various advantages such as virulence, antibiotic/xenobiotic resistance, metabolism, and small promoter obtained by IS migration in the genome of a strain [52].

A comprehensive paper on *D. radiodurans*'s antioxidant mechanism and control systems of specific regulator proteins in response to oxidation stress has been published during the preparation of this chapter [53]. Here, we will focus on antioxidation mechanisms in *Deinococcus geothermalis*, a radiation-resistant bacterium used within the research destination's scope [54]. We characterized the cystine importer and used transcriptomics analysis to detect the critical players in intracellular antioxidant responses. The putative Dps protein and LysR family regulator's functional role was then determined and IS transposition events were selected on carotenoid biosynthesis path defect (**Figure 1**). Understanding the

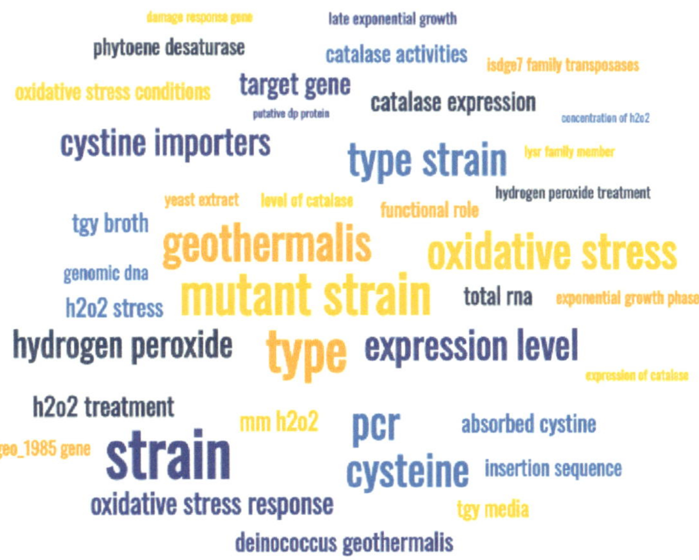

Figure 1.
WordCloud analysis of our owns four published papers [25, 55, 61, 62] by the WordCloud generator 40 quantity of MonkeyLearn.

sophisticated antioxidant system of living organisms is a problematic and challenging study like a puzzle game.

2. An antioxidant defense system in a radiation-resistant bacterium

2.1 A cystine importer, redox balance and control of gene expression

D. geothermalis contains a cystine importer as a substrate-binding protein and a membrane permease Dgeo_1986-87 which is highly expressed at the late exponential growth phase [25, 55]. Its intracellular total thiol level is affected by the expression level of this cystine importer. *Deinococcus* has specific genes that can repair when DNA is damaged. Using *dgeo*_1986-87 a cystine importer disrupted mutant strain, we have detected the expression levels of unique DNA repair proteins, *ppr*A, *ddr*A, and *ddr*B. These DNA repair proteins were highly up-regulated under oxidative stress conditions induced by 50 mM H_2O_2 [55]. However, when cystine importer expression is enhanced in a mutant Dgeo_1985R strain, DNA repair proteins are entirely down-regulated [25]. The increased intracellular thiol concentration strongly repressed the expression level of these DNA repair-related unique genes, excluding *rec*A gene in *Deinococcus* through overexpressed cystine transporter. Therefore, unique DNA repair proteins in *Deinococcus* are controlled by redox potential levels. If there is a direct controlling system for unique DNA repair genes, maybe it is repressed by the reduced redox potential through the cystine transporter's overexpression.

In general, the primary antioxidant enzyme, e.g. catalase, is highly induced by an oxidative stress condition. It is positively controlled by a global transcriptional regulator OxyR [16]. In *D. radiodurans*, the redox sensor OxyR has a single cysteine residue in the active site. It controls the expression of catalase and iron/manganese uptake proteins positively [21]. However, in *D. geothermalis* wild-type and Δ*dgeo*_1986-87 cystine importer disrupted strain, expression level of *oxyR* is strongly induced. OxyR is not proportionally affected on catalase expression level. Thus, OxyR is not a positive regulator of catalase.

The strain's cystine transport has been found to be dependent on the growth phase. In other words, some features are often expressed in the latter half of the exponential phase. In a mutant with the importer gene removed, it reacts relatively sensitive to oxidative stress. However, if the importer is overexpressed, its resistance to hydrogen peroxide is increased. A mutant that artificially overexpression the importer shows increased resistance to hydrogen peroxide without being affected by catalase expression, which results from an increase in the content of total thiol entering the cell through the cystine importer [15]. Therefore, the intracellular reduction state through enhancing thiol contents is a primary defense system of *D. geothermalis* against oxidative stress without induction of enzymatic ROS defense factors.

2.2 Hints from transcriptomic analysis

We performed transcriptomic analysis using RNA-Seq technology to define functional roles of bacterial TrmB (Dgeo_1985), Dps (Dgeo_0257), a cystine importer (Dgeo_1986-87), and LysR family regulator (Dgeo_2840). We constructed target gene disrupted mutants. Expression levels of all genes at OD_{600} 4.0 as a late exponential growth phase in mutants were then compared to those in wild-type *D. geothermalis* [55]. Data have been deposited in NCBI's Gene Expression Omnibus. They are accessible through GEO series accession number GSE151903.

First, a transcriptomic study was done to compare gene expression levels between wild-type and cystine importer deleted mutant of *D. geothermalis*. Genes up-regulated more than 3.0-fold of log value are listed in **Table 1**. Both CRISPR-Cas system gene clusters, Dgeo_0233-38 gene cluster and Dgeo_0956-65 gene cluster, were up-regulated 35.1-105.5-fold and 10.3-65.2-fold, respectively. Iron transporter Dgeo_2443 and 2444 genes were up-regulated 4.69 and 12.42-fold, respectively. Three gene clusters for GCN5, Dgeo_0369-70, 2125, and 2313, were up-regulated 12.53, 3.73, and 11.2-fold, respectively. Four MFS transporters, Dgeo_0249, 0530, 1968, and 2330, were up-regulated 3.75, 6.41, 5.57, and 3.22-fold, respectively. Four ABC transporters, Dgeo_0543, 0647, 1805, and 2581, were up-regulated 3.34, 6.96, 8.03, and 3.6-fold, respectively.

Δ*dgeo*_0257 and Δ*dgeo*_2840 mutant strains were revealed many no effect and several fluctuated patterns. The CRISPR-Cas system's slightly upregulated expression was also found in the LysR family regulator Dgeo_2840 disrupted mutant, but not in a putative Dps gene Dgeo_0257 disrupted mutant. In the case of Δ*dgeo*_2840 mutant, a different iron transporter *dgeo*_1370 was up-regulated 3.35-fold. However, gene expression levels of GCN5 and MFS transporter gene clusters were not affected in Δ*dgeo*_0257 or Δ*dgeo*_2840 mutant strain. When the intracellular redox potential was reduced through disruption of a cystine importer, why these gene clusters with several distinct physiological functions showed dramatic overexpression? Do they somehow have a relationship with antioxidant responses? These questions are interesting. Future studies in this field of antioxidation research are needed. We focused on two antioxidant biosynthesis pathways for bacillithiol and mycothiol because these pathways are related to up-regulated GCN5 gene clusters.

Gene clusters	Genes	Δ*dgeo*_1986-87	Δ*dgeo*_0257	Δ*dgeo*_2840
CRISPR-Cas	Dgeo_0233-38	35.1–105.6	—	3.36
	Dgeo_0956-65	10.3–65.2	—	4.59–5.46
Iron transporter	Dgeo_1370	—	—	3.35
	Dgeo_2443-44	4.69–12.42	—	—
GCN5	Dgeo_0369-70	12.53	—	—
	Dgeo_2125	3.73	—	—
	Dgeo_2313	11.2	—	—
MFS transporter	Dgeo_0249	3.75	—	—
	Dgeo_0530	6.41	—	—
	Dgeo_1968	5.57	—	—
	Dgeo_2330	3.22	—	—
ABC transporter	Dgeo_0543	3.34	0.35	1.62
	Dgeo_0647	6.96	1.54	—
	Dgeo_1805	8.03	—	—
	Dgeo_2581	3.60	0.69	—
RpiR family	Dgeo_2822	—	—	3.20
	Dgeo_2619	0.20	0.29	0.28

Table 1.
Transcriptomics analysis for some target genes among wild-type and mutants.

2.3 Mycothiol as a major under oxidation state

D. geothermalis genome contains 28 GNAT proteins [56]. Four GNAT genes, *dgeo*_0369-0370, 2125, and 2313, contribute to its redox-balancing regulation. In Δ*dgeo*_1986-87 mutant, these four GNAT genes were up-regulated over 3.0-fold (**Table 1**). Dgeo_2125 is an acetyltrans_3 family member. However, its function has not been characterized yet. Dgeo_0370 is a putative phosphinothricin acetyltransferase, a broad-spectrum herbicide that acts as a competitive inhibitor of glutamine synthetase. Dgeo_0369 is a putative RimI which is a S18 ribosomal protein acetylation enzyme. Dgeo_2313 is a putative mycothiol synthase MshD (**Table 2**). Thus, Dgeo_2313 is a gene direct-related to redox potential because mycothiol acts as a total thiol balance. Mycothiol is the main LMW thiol in most *Actinomycetes*, including *Mycobacterium tuberculosis* [31]. MshD and MshC were strongly induced in Δ*dgeo*_1986-87 mutant with the absence of hydrogen peroxide. However, when hydrogen peroxide was present, MshD expression was strongly down-regulated to be under 0.3-fold.

Somehow, intracellular redox potential affects these GNAT regulations. If two artificial conditions such as oxidation and reduction are provided, the expression levels of redox potential-dependent GNAT genes would be detected. These variable expression levels of GNAT genes will provide stress response control. At the moment, the physiological roles of these four GNAT proteins remain unclear. In general, proteins in the GNAT superfamily have broad-spectrum physiological functions. Their amino acid sequence identities are very low. Thus, predicting their functional roles through protein sequence similarities is difficult.

How about expression levels of bacillithiol (BSH) biosynthesis-related genes in the transcriptome of *D. geothermalis*? The genome of *D. geothermalis* contains BSH biosynthesis enzymes BshA (Dgeo_1099; BSH biosynthesis glycosyltransferase), BshB1 (Dgeo_2305; BSH biosynthesis deacetylase), BshC (Dgeo_1276; BSH biosynthesis cysteine-adding enzyme), and BstA (Dgeo_1829; BSH transferase) as Drad BSH-related genes. It also contains BSH reductase (Dgeo_2331; YpdA) and bacilliredoxin (Dgeo_1464; YtxJ). Despite all genes involved in BSH biosynthesis and degradation pathway, expression levels of these genes were not affected in the intracellular oxidation state of Δ*dgeo*_1986-87 strain. However, they might be affected by other stressors such as heat shock and hydrogen peroxide treatment.

2.4 Dps and its mysterious roles

D. radiodurans have two paralogous Dps proteins, each known to play a different role. DrDps1 (DR2263) binds to both linear and coiled DNA. However, DrDps2 (DRB0092) preferentially binds to coiled DNA, forming different conformation of protein-DNA complexes to protect DNA against ROS, although its protection occurs at different iron to protein ratios. The difference between two DrDps could result from the fact that DrDps1 has higher iron oxidation rate in the presence of hydrogen

Genes	Δ*dgeo*_1986-87	Δ*dgeo*_0257	Δ*dgeo*_2840
MshA (Dgeo_2307)	0.79	0.98	0.69
MshB (Dgeo_1021)	1.14	1.00	1.10
MshC (Dgeo_1714)	10.78	0.88	1.36
MshD (Dgeo_2313)	11.2	1.21	0.99

Table 2.
Expression levels of MSH biosynthesis-related genes.

peroxide and higher affinity to bind DNA than DrDps2 [37]. In summary, DrDps1 may function in DNA metabolism, while DrDps2 may protect against exogenously derived ROS [57].

D. geothermalis has two Dps proteins homologous to Dps proteins of *D. radiodurans*. Dgeo_0281 is homologous to DrDps1 (DR_2263). The novel Dgeo_0257 has been proposed to be one of Dps DNA-binding proteins in *D. geothermalis*. It probably has different roles from DrDps1 homologous protein, Dgeo_0281. Dgeo_0257 shares 72% amino acid sequence identity to DR_0528 of *D. radiodurans*, suggesting the need for research as another candidate protein of DrDps. The DrDps2 (DR_B0092) did not share any significant sequence identities with proteins of *D. geothermalis*. Dgeo_0281 and Dgeo_0257 share only 11.5% amino acid sequence identity, lower than 16% amino acid sequence identity shared between DrDps1 and DrDps2.

We prepared both *dps* genes disrupted mutant strains, Δ*dgeo*_0257 and Δ*dgeo*_0281, and they were more susceptible to H_2O_2 than the wild-type strain. The novel putative Dps Dgeo_0257 might play a role in DNA protection and antioxidant reactions such as Dgeo_0281. DNA-binding capacities of purified Dgeo_0257 and Dgeo_0281 proteins were then determined by electrophoretic mobility shift assay (EMSA). Gel filtration assay was also performed for conformational determination [58]. Dgeo_0257 protein has a 5-fold higher DNA-binding affinity than Dgeo_0281. Interestingly, both Dps proteins were found to have similar metal-sensing behavior (**Figure 2**). When ferrous ion was present, Dps proteins could not bind to DNA. Their DNA-binding activity was found to be non-specific for DNA sequence. To determine the physiological functions of these two Dps proteins, we performed quantitative real-time (qRT)-PCR analysis for both *dgeo*_0257 and *dgeo*_0281 genes in wild-type, Δ*dgeo*_0257, and Δ*dgeo*_0281 mutant strains at different growth phase in a time-course study. Surprisingly, the *dgeo*_0281 gene was early expressed at OD_{600} 2.0. Its expression then gradually reduced at OD_{600} 4.0 and 8.0. However, *dgeo*_0257 was dramatically induced in a stationary phase at OD_{600} 8.0. Thus, we predicted that both Dps proteins of *D. geothermalis* had growth phase-dependent specificity.

2.5 Active transposition of insertion sequences under oxidative stress condition

Various selectable approaches have detected transposition events of ISs. For example, IS*Dra2* was induced by irradiation, causing the *thyA* (thymidylate synthase) gene to be destroyed in *D. radiodurans*. As a result, *thyA* mutant became

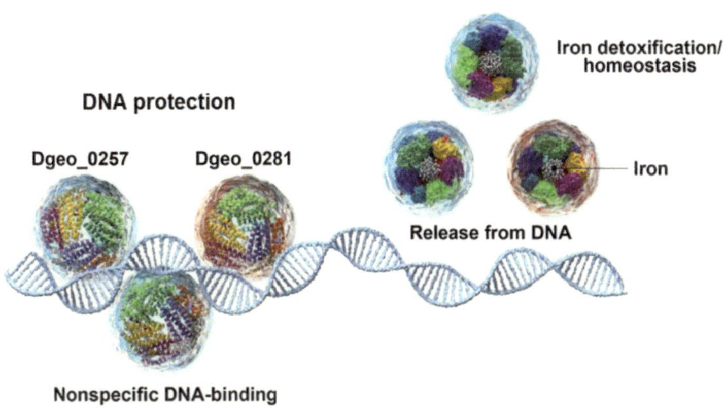

Figure 2.
Illustration of DNA protection and iron detoxification roles of two Dps proteins in D. geothermalis.

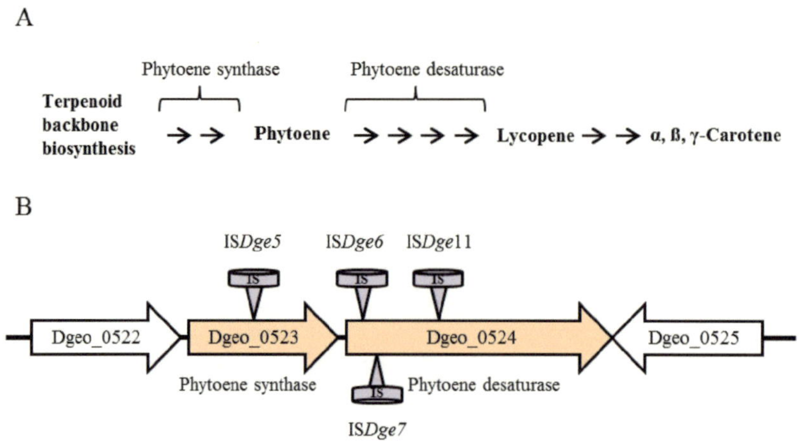

Figure 3.
Brief scheme of metabolic pathway (A) and the ISs integrated loci in the gene cluster for carotenoid biosynthesis (B).

resistant to trimethoprim [47, 59]. In the case of antibiotic-resistant phenotype, a certain IS element was integrated into *rsmG* gene disrupted by IS*Tth7* of IS5 family in *Thermus thermophilus*, resulting in streptomycin-resistance [60].

The genome of *D. geothermalis* contains a total of 73 ISs. *Deinococcus* species were found to have pink or reddish colored colonies. However, *D. geothermalis* wild-type, Dps-like gene disrupted mutant (Δ*dgeo*_0257 mutant), and LysR gene disrupted mutant (Δ*dgeo*_2840 mutant) were found to have white-colored colonies under an oxidative stress condition. The reason was that phytoene desaturase function of Dgeo_0524 as a carotenoid pathway-related gene was interrupted by the transposition of each IS element: IS*Dge6* for Δ*dgeo*_2840 mutant, IS*Dge7* for Δ*dgeo*_0257 mutant, and IS*Dge11* for wild-type (**Figure 3**) [32, 61, 62]. Among down-regulated genes in RNA-seq, two genes (*dgeo*_0928 and *dgeo*_1785) were disturbed by IS*Dge5* in the Δ*dgeo*_0257 mutant strain. A new biomarker for finding transposition loci with antibiotic streptomycin-resistance was also used easily to selecting colonies on streptomycin contained media. When the IS*Dge6* element was inserted into the *rsmG* gene (*dgeo*_2335) encoding ribosomal RNA small subunit methyltransferase and a point mutation or frameshift mutation on *rsmG* gene occurred, mutant strains were resistant to 50 μg/ml streptomycin (prepared manuscript). In the current discovery, IS*Dge5*, IS*Dge6*, IS*Dge7*, and IS*Dge11* were all replicating transposition modes through PCR detection of target genes. We found that each IS element was transposed, explicitly depending on DNA-binding proteins from these active transposition events. There is an open question. Although the genome of *D. geothermalis* contains a high copy number of IS elements such as IS*Dge2*, IS*Dge3*, IS*Dge4*, and IS*Dge13*, transposition events have not been found yet. Nevertheless, in the case of IS*Dge2*, its transposase gene expression was strongly induced by oxidative stress. Thus, it is a big challenge to detect DNA-binding protein-dependent IS transposition occurrence. We can imagine that when the environmental factor is changed from oxidative stress to others such as other source radiations, gravity, pressure, and certain chemicals, specialized IS elements might be transposed into other loci in the genome.

3. Conclusion

As a model for oxidative stress response, *Deinococcus* species is a beneficial model organism to understand its survival strategies in the presence of harsh environmental stressors such as ionizing radiation, desiccation, and ultraviolet light. It is also a useful model organism to understand DNA damage repair mechanisms and industrial application such as bioremediation of toxic substances. For these reasons, many researchers are interested in applying extreme conditions, including microgravity and universe exposure outside the international space station, to a type strain of *D. radiodurans* recently. Here, we focused on several aspects of oxidative stress defense systems dependent on our research destination, for example, intracellular redox balance through a cystine importer, antioxidant substance carotenoid biosynthesis, DNA protecting and iron detoxification protein Dps, and transposition of IS elements under oxidative stress. We hope this chapter will provide an opportunity to open up a new horizon in traditional research as we learn about the phenomena linked differently to known antioxidant response mechanisms in radiation-resistant strains.

Acknowledgements

This study was supported by the National Research Foundation of Korea Grant funded by the Korean government (MSIT) (2020R1F1A1070779) and SJL thanks Kyung Hee University's support.

Conflict of interest

The authors declare no conflict of interest.

Author details

Chanjae Lee, Min K. Bae and Sung-Jae Lee*
Department of Biology, Kyung Hee University, Seoul, Korea-South

*Address all correspondence to: sungjaelee@khu.ac.kr

References

[1] Battista JR, Earl AM, Park MJ. Why is *Deinococcus radiodurans* so resistant to ionizing radiation? Trends in Microbiology. 1999;7:362-365. DOI:10.1016/s0966-842x(99)01566-8.

[2] Blasius M, Hubscher U, Sommer S. *Deinococcus radiodurans*: what belongs to the survival kit? Crit Rev Biochem Mol Biol. 2008;43:221-238. DOI: 10.1080/10409230802122274.

[3] Agapov AA, Kulbachinskiy AV. Mechanisms of stress resistance and gene regulation in the radioresistant bacterium *Deinococcus radiodurans*. Biochem. (Mosc.) 2015;80:1201-1216. DOI: 10.1134/S0006297915100016.

[4] Cox MM, Battista JR. *Deinococcus radiodurans* - the consummate survivor. Nat Rev Microbiol. 2005; 3:882-892. DOI: 10.1038/nrmicro1264.

[5] Daly MJ. A new perspective on radiation resistance based on *Deinococcus radiodurans*. Nat Rev Microbiol. 2009;7:237-245. DOI: 10.1038/nrmicro2073.

[6] Slade D, Radman M. Oxidative stress resistance in *Deinococcus radiodurans*. Microbiol. Mol Biol Rev. 2011;75:133-191. DOI: 10.1128/MMBR.00015-10.

[7] Hua Y, Narumi I, Gao G, Tian B, Satoh K, Kitayama S, Shen S. PprI: a general switch responsible for extreme radioresistance of *Deinococcus radiodurans*. Biochem Biophys Res Comm. 2003;306:354-360. DOI: 10.1016/s0006-291x(03)00965-3.

[8] Tanaka M, Earl AM, Howell HA, Park MJ, Eisen JA, Peterson SN, Battista JR. Analysis of *Deinococcus radiodurans*'s transcriptional response to ionizing radiation and desiccation reveals novel proteins that contribute to extreme radioresistance. Genetics. 2004;168:21-33. DOI: 10.1534/genetics.104.029249.

[9] Selvam K, Duncan JR, Tanaka M, Battista JR. DdrA, DdrD, and PprA: components of UV and mitomycin C resistance in *Deinococcus radiodurans* R1. PLoS One. 2013;8:e69007. DOI: 10.1371/journal.pone.0069007.

[10] Luan H, Meng N, Fu J, Chen X, Xu X, Feng Q, other authors. Genome-wide transcriptome and antioxidant analysis on gamma-irradiated phases of *Deinococcus radiodurans* R1. PLoS One. 2014;9:e85649. DOI: 10.1371/journal.pone.0085649.

[11] Lim S, Jung J-H, Blanchard L, de Groot A. Conservation and diversity of radiation and oxidative stress resistance mechanisms in *Deinococcus* species. FEMS Microbiol Rev. 2019;43:19-52. DOI:10.1093.femsre/fuy037.

[12] Ott E, Kawaguchi Y, Ozgen N, Yamagishi A, Rabbow E, Rettberg P, Weckwerth W, Milojevic T. Proteomic and metabolomics profiling of *Deinococcus radiodurans* recovering after exposure to stimulated low earth orbit vaccum conditions. Front Microbiol. 2019;10:909. DOI: 10.3389/fmicb.2019.00909.

[13] Chiancone E, Ceci P. The multifaceted capacity of Dps proteins to combat bacterial stress conditions: detoxification of iron and hydrogen peroxide and DNA binding. Biochim Biophys Acta. 2010;1800:798-805. DOI: 10.1016/j.bbagen.2010.01.013.

[14] Helmann JD. Bacillithiol, a new player in bacterial redox homeostasis. Antioxid Redox Signal. 2011;15:123-133. DOI: 10.1089/ars.2010.3562.

[15] Hillion M, Antelmann H. Thiol-based redox switches in prokaryotes.

Biol Chem. 2015;396:415-444. DOI: 10.1515/hsz-2015-0102.

[16] Christman MF, Storz G, Ames BN. OxyR, a positive regulator of hydrogen peroxide-inducible genes in *Escherichia coli* and Salmonella typhimurium, is homologous to a family of bacterial regulatory proteins. Proc Nat Acad Sci. USA. 1989;86:3484-3488. DOI: 10.1073/pnas.86.10.3484.

[17] Storz G, Tartaglia LA, Ames BN. The OxyR regulon. Antonie van Leeuwenhoek. 1990;58:157-161. doi: 10.1007/bf00548927. DOI: 10.1007/BF00548927.

[18] Schell MA. Molecular biology of the LysR family of transcriptional regulators. Annu Rev Microbiol. 1993;47:597-626. DOI: 10.1146/annurev.mi.47.100193.003121.

[19] Åslund F, Zheng M, Beckwith J, Storz G. Regulation of the OxyR transcription factor by hydrogen peroxide and the cellular thiol disulfide status. Proc Natl Acad Sci USA. 1999;96:6161-6165. DOI: 10.1073/pnas.96.11.6161.

[20] Kim SO, Merchant K, Nudekman R, Beyer Jr WF, Keng T, DeAngelo J, Hausladen A, Stamler JS. OxyR: a molecular code for redox-related signaling. Cell. 2002;109:383-396. DOI: 10.1016/s0092-8674(02)00723-7.

[21] Chen H, Xu G, Zhao Y, Tian B, Lu H, Yu X, Xu Z, Ying N, Hu S, Hua Y. A novel OxyR sensor and regulator of hydrogen peroxide stress with one cysteine residue in *Deinococcus radiodurans*. PLoS One. 2008;3:e1602. DOI: 10.1371/journal.pone.0001602.

[22] Burguière P, Auger S, Hullo MF, Danchin A, Martin-Verstraete I. Three different systems participate in L-cystine uptake in *Bacillus subtilis*. J Bacteriol. 2004;186:4875-4884. DOI: 10.1128/JB.186.15.4875-4884.

[23] Ohtsu I, Kawano Y, Suzuki M, Morigasaki S, Saiki K, Yamazaki S, Nonaka G, Takagi H. Uptake of L-cystine via an ABC transporter contributes defense of oxidative stress in the L-cystine export-dependent manner in *Escherichia coli*. PLoS One. 2015;10:e0120619. DOI: 10.1371/journal.pone.0120619.

[24] Chonoles Imlay KR, Korshunov S, Imlay JA. Physiological roles and adverse effects of the two cystine importers of *Escherichia coli*. J Bacteriol. 2015;197:3629-3644. DOI: 10.1128/JB.00277-15.

[25] Kim M, Jeong S, Lim S, Sim J, Rhie HG, Lee S-J. Oxidative stress response of *Deinococcus geothermalis* via a cystine importer. J Microbiol. 2017;55:137-146. DOI: 10.1007/s12275-017-6382-y.

[26] Loprasert S, Vattanaviboon P, PratuanW,ChamnongpolS,MongkolsukS. Regulation of the oxidative stress protective enzymes, catalase and superoxide dismutase in *Xanthomonas*-a review. Gene. 1996;179:33-37. DOI: 10.1016/s0378-1119(96)00427-1.

[27] Milse J, Petri K, Rückert C, Kalinowski J. Transcriptional response of *Corynebacterium glutamicum* ATCC 13032 to hydrogen peroxide stress and characterization of the OxyR regulon. J Biotechnol. 2014;190:40-54. DOI: 10.1016/j.jbiotec.2014.07.452.

[28] Liu X, Sun M, Cheng Y, Yang R, Wen Y, Chen Z, Li J. OxyR is a key regulator in response to oxidative stress in *Streptomyces avermitilis*. Microbiol. 2016;162:707-716. DOI: 10.1099/mic.0.000251.

[29] Burckhardt RM, Escalante-Semerena JC. Small-molecule

acetylation by GCN5-related N-acetyltransferases in bacteria. Microbiol Mol Biol Rev. 2020;84:e00090–e00019. DOI: 10.1128/MMBR.00090-19.

[30] Favrot L, Blanchard JS, Vergnolle O. Bacterial GCN5-related N-acetyltransferases: from resistance to regulation. Biochem. 2016;55:989-1002. DOI: 10.1021/acs.biochem.5b01269.

[31] Imber M, Pietrzyk-Brzezinska AJ, Antelmann H. Redox regulation by reversible protein S-thiolation in Gram-positive bacteria. Redox Biol. 2019;20:130-145. DOI: 10.1016/j.redox.2018.08.017.

[32] Tian B, Hua Y. Carotenoid biosynthesis in extremeophilic *Deinococcus-Thermus* bacteria. Trends in Microbiol. 2010;18:512-520. DOI: 10.1016/j.tim.2010.07.007.

[33] Azam TA, Ishihama A. Twelve species of the nucleoid associated protein from *Escherichia coli*: sequence recognition specificity and DNA binding affinity. J Biol Chem. 1999;274:33105-33113. DOI: 10.1074/jbc.274.46.33105.

[34] Ishihama A. The nucleoid: an overview. EcoSal Plus. 2009;3. DOI:10.1128/ecosalplus.2.6.

[35] Zhao G, Ceci P, Ilari A, Giangiacomo L, Laue TM, Chiancone E, Chasteen ND. Iron and hydrogen peroxide detoxification properties of DNA-binding protein from starved cells. A ferritin-like DNA-binding protein of *Escherichia coli*. J Biol Chem. 2002;277:27689-27696. DOI: 10.1074/jbc.M202094200.

[36] Chiancone E, Ceci P. The multifaceted capacity of Dps proteins to combat bacterial stress conditions: detoxification of iron and hydrogen peroxide and DNA binding. Biochim Biophys Acta. 2010;1800:798-805. DOI: 10.1016/j.bbagen.2010.01.013.

[37] Santos SP, Mitchell EP, Franquelim HG, Castanho MARB, Abreu IA, Romao CV. Dps from *Deinococcus radiodurans*: oligomeric forms of Dps1 with distinct cellular functions and Dps2 involved in metal storage. FEBS J. 2015;282:4307-4327. DOI: 10.1111/febs.13420.

[38] Almirón M, Link AJ, Furlong D, Kolter R. A novel DNA binding protein with regulatory and protective roles in starved *Escherichia coli*. Genes Dev. 1992;6:2646-2654. DOI:10.1101/gad.6.12b.2646.

[39] Wolf SG, Frenkiel D, Arad T, Finkel SE, Kolter R, Minsky A. DNA protection by stress-induced biocrystallization. Nature. 1999;400:83-85. DOI: 10.1038/21918.

[40] Ceci P, Cellai S, Falvo E, Rivetti C, Rossi GL, Chiancone E. DNA condensation and self-aggregation of *Escherichia coli* Dps are coupled phenomena related to the properties of the N-terminus. Nucleic Acids Res. 2004;32:5935-5944. DOI: 10.1093/nar/gkh915.

[41] Mahillon J, Chandler M. Insertion sequences. Microbiol Mol Biol Rev. 1998;62:725-774.

[42] Siguier P, Gourbeyre E, Varani A, Ton-Hoang B, Chandler M. Everyman's guide to bacterial insertion sequences. Microbiol Spectrum. 2015;3:MDNA3-0030-2014. DOI: 10.1128/microbiolspec.MDNA3-0030-2014.

[43] Siguier P, Perochon J, Lestrade L, Mahillon J, Chandler M. ISfinder: the reference centre for bacterial insertion sequences. Nucleic Acids Res. 2006;34:D32–D36. DOI: 10.1093/nar/gkj014.

[44] Siguier P, Gourbeyre E, Chandler M. Bacterial insertion sequences: their genomic impact and diversity. FEMS Microbiol Rev. 2014;38:865-891. DOI: 10.1111/1574-6976.12067.

[45] Narumi I, Cherdchu K, Kitayama S, Watanabe H. The *Deinococcus radiodurans* uvrA gene: identification of mutation sites in two mitomycin-sensitive strains and the first discovery of insertion sequence element from deinobacteria. Gene. 1997;198:115-126. DOI: 10.1016/s0378-1119(97)00301-6.

[46] Ohtsubo Y, Genka H, Komatsu H, Nagata Y, Tsuda M. High-temperature-induced transposition of insertion elements in *Burkholderia multivorans* ATCC17616. Appl Environ Microbiol. 2005;71:1822-1828. DOI: 10.1128/AEM.71.4.1822-1828.2005.

[47] Pasternak C, Ton-Hoang B, Coste G, Bailone A, Chandler M, Sommer S. Irradiation-induced *Deinococcus radiodurans* genome fragmentation triggers transposition of a single resident insertion sequence. PLoS Genetics. 2010;6:e1000799. DOI: 10.1371/journal.pgen.1000799.

[48] Roberts D, Hoopes BC, McClure WR, Kleckner N. IS10 transposition is regulated by DNA adenine methylation. Cell. 1985;43:117-130. DOI: 10.1016/0092-8674(85)90017-0.

[49] Escoubas JM, Prere MF, Fayet O, Salvignol I, Galas D, Zerbib D, Chandler M. Translational control of transposition activity of the bacterial insertion sequence IS1. EMBO J. 1991;10:705-712.

[50] Kleckner N, Chalmers RM, Kwon D, Sakai J, Bolland S. Tn10 and IS10 transposition and chromosome rearrangements: Mechanism and regulation *in vivo* and *in vitro*. In: Transposable Elements. Curr Top Microbiol Immunol. 1996;204:49-82. DOI: 10.1007/978-3-642-79795-8_3.

[51] Kiss J, Nagy Z, Toth G, Kiss GB, Jakab J, Chandler M, Olasz F. Transposition and target specificity of the typical IS30 family element IS1655 from *Neisseria meningitidis*. Mol Microbiol. 2007;63:1731-1747. DOI: 10.1111/j.1365-2958.2007.05621.x.

[52] Vandecraen J, Chandler M, Aertsen A, Van Houdt R. The impact of insertion sequences on bacterial genome plasticity and adaptability. Crit Rev Microbiol. 2017;43:709-730. DOI: 10.1080/1040841X.2017.1303661.

[53] Qi H, Wang W, He J, Ma Y, Xiao F, He S. Antioxidative system of *Deinococcus radiodurans*. Res Microbiol. 2020;171:45-54. DOI: 10.1016/j.resmic.2019.11.002.

[54] Makarova KS, Omelchenko MV, Gaidamakova EK, Matrosova VY, Vasilenko A, other authors. *Deinococcus geothermalis*: the pool of extreme radiation resistance genes shrinks. PLoS One. 2007;2:e955. DOI: 10.1371/journal.pone.0000955.

[55] Choo K, Kim M, Abdi Nansa S, Bae MK, Lee C, Lee S-J. Redox potential change by the cystine importer affected on enzymatic antioxidant protection in *Deinococcus geothermalis*. Antonie van Leeuwenhoek. 2020;113:779-790. DOI: 10.1007/s10482-020-01388-4.

[56] Ud-Din AIMS, Tikhomirova A, Roujeinikova A. Structure and functional diversity of GCN5-related N-acetyltransferases (GNAT). Int J Mol Sci. 2016;17:1018. DOI: 10.3390/ijms17071018.

[57] Reon BJ, Nguyen KH, Bhattacharyya G, Grove A. Functional comparison of *Deinococcus radiodurans* Dps proteins suggests distinct in vivo roles. Biochem J. 2012;447:381-391. DOI: 10.1042/BJ20120902.

[58] Bae MK. Purification and characterization of DNA binding proteins from starved cell (Dps) of *Deinococcus geothermalis* [thesis]. Seoul: Kyung Hee University; 2020.

[59] Mennecier S, Servant P, Coste G, Bailone A, Sommer S. Mutagenesis via IS transposition in *Deinococcus radiodurans*. Mol Microbiol. 2006;59:317-325. DOI: 10.1111/j.1365-2958.2005.04936.x.

[60] Gregory ST, Dahlberg AE. Transposition of an insertion sequence, ISTth7, in the genome of the extreme thermophile *Thermus thermophiles* HB8. FEMS Microbiol Lett. 2008;289:187-192. DOI: 10.1111/j.1574-6968.2008.01389.x.

[61] Lee C, Choi N, Bae MK, Choo K, Lee S-J. Transposition of insertion sequences was triggered by oxidative stress in radiation-resistant bacterium *Deinococcus geothermalis*. Microorganisms. 2019;7:446. DOI: 10.3390/microorganisms7100446.

[62] Lee C, Choo K, Lee S-J. Active transposition of insertion sequences by oxidative stress in *Deinococcus geothermalis*. Front Microbiol. 2020;11:558747. DOI:10.3389/fmicb.2020.558747.

Chapter 9

The Two Sides of Dietary Antioxidants in Cancer Therapy

Musbau Adewumi Akanji, Heritage Demilade Fatinukun, Damilare Emmanuel Rotimi, Boluwatife Lawrence Afolabi and Oluyomi Stephen Adeyemi

Abstract

Cancer is a major cause of mortality around the world, representing about 13% of deaths on the planet. Among the available cancer treatments, chemotherapy is most frequently utilized compared to other treatments such as surgery and radiotherapy. Many dietary antioxidants have proven to effectively prevent oxidative stress, which has been noted in many disease pathogeneses, including cancer. However, during chemotherapy or radiotherapy treatment of cancer patients, antioxidants are used as an adjuvant treatment. The use of a proof-based technique is advised in determining the supplements most suited to cancer patients. Though there are numerous opinions about the dangers and advantages of antioxidants, it is reasonable to conclude that side effects caused by antioxidants, for now, remain unclear for patients during cancer treatment, aside from smokers during radiotherapy. In this report, details of the effectiveness of antioxidants on cancer treatment aiding in the reduction of cancer therapy side effects are discussed.

Keywords: antioxidants, chemotherapy, dietary supplements, polyphenolics, radiotherapy

1. Introduction

Cancer is a wide collection of diseases that can begin in practically any organ or tissue of the body when abnormal cells develop and move beyond their space to attack surrounding areas and also spread to different organs [1]. There are numerous types of cancer such as breast cancer, skin cancer, bone cancer, lung cancer, colon cancer, prostate cancer and if left untreated, it results in serious harm and could eventually lead to death [2]. Different causes of cancer include hereditary variables, way of life, diet, exposure to various kinds of synthetic compounds, and radiation. The American Cancer Society has estimated the number of new cancer cases for the year 2020 in the United States is 1,806,590 cases and 606,520 deaths. Previously, the cancer death rate increased up until the year 1991, at which point, the numbers dropped ceaselessly from 2017, bringing about a general decrease of about 29% which is equivalent to 2.9 million fewer cancer deaths than as projected. This was attributed to the long-term decrease in death rates for the 4 main cancer types (colorectal, prostate, breast, and lung cancer) [3]. Among the reasons that can be mentioned for the reduction in the mortality rate of cancer patients are the various techniques being used for treatment such as chemotherapy, surgery, and radiotherapy. Various kinds of cancer can proceed in abnormal ways, develop at different rates, and react to treatment differently, hence, each cancer treatment is focused on the specific cancer type. Cancer therapy used in the treatment of cancer patient includes surgery, chemotherapy, radiotherapy and more recently antioxidant have been proposed to benefit cancer patients during cancer therapy [2].

Antioxidants are substances that can neutralize the production of free radicals and counteract the oxidation process. Antioxidants can be classified based on their source; endogenous source (enzymes) and exogenous diets (carotenoids, flavonoids, phenolics, minerals, and vitamins) [4]. Antioxidants are naturally found abundant in dietary sources, and their consumption possesses great health benefits [5]. The use of dietary antioxidants mitigates oxidative stress which contributes majorly to several diseases. Plant nutrients including organic products, vegetables, tea, grains, red wine, nuts, spices, and flavors give a huge sum and variety of antioxidants by preventing diseases. Dietary antioxidants are also a complex mixture of minerals (selenium, zinc, or copper) and micronutrients (vitamins A, C, and E) [6]. There are recommended antioxidants intake either as a diet with antioxidant activities or combined with antioxidant enzymes. Metals such as iron, zinc, manganese, copper, and selenium are considered cofactors of various enzyme antioxidants, and some nutrients (β-carotene, α-tocopherol, ascorbic acid, and folic acid) as sequestrate of reactive oxygen species (ROS) [7]. In light of this, this review discusses dietary antioxidants in cancer therapy in light of merits and demerits.

2. Oxidative stress

A free radical is a particle capable of existing independently and has at least one unpaired electron in its outer shell. Most free radicals are profoundly reactive and unsteady as a result of the number of electrons. Therefore, they rapidly react with different substances to attain stability. Free radical attacks the nearest steady particle and acquire its electron, meanwhile, the attacked particle can turn into a free radical by loosing its electron and start a chain reaction course harming the living cells. Examples of free radicals are superoxide anion, lipid alkoxyl, lipid peroxide, lipid peroxyl, and hydroxyl radical. Reactive oxygen species (ROS) are radical subordinates, for example, hydrogen peroxide and singlet oxygen [8]. Free radicals are fundamentally reactive oxygen species (ROS) or reactive nitrogen species (RNS) comprising of singlet oxygen, hydrogen peroxide, superoxide radicals, intermediary nitrite, and nitric oxide (NO) [9]. The primary reactive oxygen species (ROS) are the superoxide (O2-), singlet oxygen (O2), hydrogen peroxide (H2O2), hydroxyl radicals (HO-), peroxyl and alkoxyl radicals (ROS- and RO-), and natural peroxides (ROOH). In the event of cellular damage caused by free radicals, for example, involving cellular amino acids, lipids, and DNA, reactive oxygen species (ROS) can activate enzymatic and non-enzymatic cell reactions, with the possibility of tampering with different metabolic processes and interfering with gene expression among other things.

Oxidative stress is an aftereffect of a variation in reactive oxygen species (ROS) and antioxidant resistances. Oxidative stress takes control of the development and function of the cell which can contribute to the pathogenesis of various conditions like neurodegenerative sickness, Parkinson's dementia, diabetes, cancer, immune system ailments, Alzheimer's ailment, cardiovascular diseases, carcinogenesis, asthma [10]. Oxidative stress predisposes cellular harm through oxidation of proteins, nucleic acids, and lipid, structural adjustment of the membranes, the harm induced may extend to the organs and become systemic [11]. Countering the effect of free radicals can be through a large intake of dietary antioxidants and specific antioxidant supplements as part of the diet. Though, some reports have suggested that combining several antioxidants is more viable in the long-term than single antioxidant substances. Therefore, antioxidants provide a great advantage in improving personal health by hindering several diseases conditions [12].

2.1 Antioxidants

Antioxidants act as scavengers of free radical or reactive oxygen species (ROS) and avert oxidation leading to several disease conditions. An antioxidant hinders the oxidation of lipids, DNA, sugar, and proteins at low concentrations. Antioxidants are found in plants, numerous foods, and some are synthesized in the body [13, 14]. In recent times, there has been increased utilization of natural products and reports have indicated that consumption of vegetables and fruits that contains antioxidants might be related to the decreased frequency of diseases activated by reactive oxygen species (ROS), such as cardiovascular diseases, cancer, etc. Oxidative stress and its damaging effects can be averted through the consumption of naturally occurring antioxidants [15]. Polyphenols and carotenoids (natural antioxidants) reveal natural activities as anti-atherosclerosis, anti-aging, anti-inflammatory, and anticancer [16]. Antioxidants function in the body to promote health and strength, particularly during old age. They ensure protection from damage to the tissues, and skin caused by the production of free radicals. In industries, they help to expand the food shelf-life and are added in the skin-care products for anti-aging purposes [13].

The antioxidant system comprises of enzymatic and non-enzymatic antioxidants. Among the enzymatic antioxidants, are superoxide dismutase (SOD), glutathione peroxidase (GPx), and catalase (CAT). The non-enzymatic antioxidant also contributes to the cellular redox balance, examples include hormones such as estradiol, melatonin, as well as certain nutrients, for example, vitamins E and C [17].

The antioxidants are grouped into three fundamental classes:

1. The principal line guard antioxidants which involve superoxide dismutase (SOD), glutathione reductase (GR), catalase (CAT), and minerals like Zn, Se, and Cu, etc.

2. The second line safeguard antioxidants which involve glutathione (GSH), flavonoids, carotenoids, vitamin C, vitamin E, etc.

3. The third line safeguards antioxidants which involve a complex combination of chemicals responsible for fixing the damaged DNA, proteins, oxidized lipids, and peroxides. Examples are DNA repair enzymes, methionine sulphoxide reductase, protease, lipase, transferases, and so on [10].

2.2 Dietary antioxidants

Dietary antioxidants are substances found in food and it ensures the protection of cells, tissues, and DNA against oxidative harm of free radicals. Dietary antioxidant supplements involve protein, starch, sodium, fiber, fat as well as minerals and vitamins. Dietary antioxidants having both antioxidant and pro-oxidant impacts involve nutrients (tocopherol, carotenoids, pro-vitamin A, ascorbic acid, basic micronutrients with physiological roles) and also involve phytochemicals and polyphenols. In a review, dietary consumption of anthocyanins (an antioxidant found in berries) was revealed about 8% decrease in hypertensive condition [18]. Dietary nutrients have also shown significant improvement in bodily functions such as brain health, improved nervous system metabolism, and so on [19].

Since scientific evidence established the role of free radicals in the pathogenesis of diseases such as cardiovascular diseases, cancer among others, there have been considerable studies towards natural antioxidant properties to ameliorate such effects. The dietary antioxidant can have useful impacts on the body by scavenging free radicals and also the redox potential if they are available in tissues at adequate concentrations. For some dietary phytochemicals, direct antioxidants intake for some disease condition might be less significant to health than others as well as its consequences on cell signaling and gene expression [20]. There is a concern that the global consumption of fruits and vegetables is insufficient, leading to a decreased intake of antioxidants and predisposes to degenerative diseases [21].

2.3 Examples of dietary antioxidants and their sources

2.3.1 Vitamin C

Vitamin C (ascorbic acid) is vital to the health of the body by acting as an intense scavenger of radical. Ascorbic acid is a water-soluble vitamin and a huge supplement for quick intestinal absorption. It is needed for the collagen synthesis in the body, essential in regulating norepinephrine from dopamine and function in tyrosine digestion. Insufficient intake of vegetables and fruits, the main sources of vitamin C, can prompt the inadequacy of this crucial nutrient in the body. Ascorbic acid is quickly exhausted and oxidized during oxidative stress. Examples of natural sources rich in vitamin C are grapefruits, pineapple, cherries, citrus fruits, potatoes, pepper, strawberries, gooseberry, broccoli, kiwi fruit, and paprika, etc. [22].

2.3.2 Vitamin D

Vitamin D is a fat-soluble vitamin known to assume an important role in bone and calcium homeostasis and function as an anti-inflammatory agent since it represses invulnerable the expression of cell cytokine and prompts monocyte/macrophage to emit molecules which have a firm antibiotic impact. Its insufficiency can expand the danger of infectious diseases. Almost 95% of vitamin D is gathered in the epidermis of the skin on exposure to the sun, the rest is gotten from different dietary sources. In food, oily fish contains the largest amount of vitamin D, other sources include milk, orange, etc. [22].

2.3.3 Vitamin E

Vitamin E also called tocopherol is a fat-soluble vitamin. Vitamin E has an extremely wide capacity of preserving biological membrane and nucleic acids in the body from the attacks of free radicals. Vitamin E is rich in vegetables, vegetable oil, almonds, walnuts, etc. Vitamin E has been discovered to have repressive capacity on tumors [23].

2.3.4 Flavonoids

Plants have numerous flavonoids essential to mitigate the development of diseases. Basic flavonoids compounds involve anthocyanins, isoflavones, flavones, etc. Flavonoids destroy the free radicals by transforming them into phenolic radicals (inactive) after providing hydrogen to lipid compound radicals. Foods containing a large number of flavonoids involve herb, onions, blueberries, banana, and all citrus fruits, etc. [23].

2.3.5 Carotenoids

These are dietary antioxidants that have exhibited action of photoprotection. In plants, these compounds are found in the photosynthetic parts where they are classified as extra light-collecting shades and shield from harm caused by sunlight. The photoprotective impacts of carotenoid-rich eating routine have been researched for its capacity to diminish the erythema (skin redness) size upon UV radiation exposure, though an extended period is necessary for a successful mediation. Among carotenoids, beta-carotene, lycopene, and lutein are gotten from various plant sources, for example, tomato, carrots, etc. [24].

2.3.6 Polyphenols

There has been developing interest upheld by various epidemiological tests, on the possible gainful impacts of polyphenols on brain health. Polyphenol is micronutrients abundant in plant-determined nourishment which is also strong antioxidants. Fruits and beverages, for example, coffee, cocoa, and tea, and so on are significant dietary sources of polyphenols. Polyphenols are noted for their neuroprotective activities; protecting neurons against damage induced by neurotoxins, can suppress neuroinflammation, and the possibility to advance memory, learning, and psychological capacity. Recent evidence suggests that their beneficial impact includes a reduction in oxidative stress, an increase in defensive signaling, prompting the expression of genes that encode antioxidant enzymes, neurotrophic factors, and protective protein [7].

3. Cancer

Cancer is a major medical issue globally and is the second leading cause of death in the United States. A century ago, cancer was not all that normal, however, since the last few decades, its frequency has been rising alarmingly, presumably because of our evolving way of life and habits. Cancer is among the most dreaded illnesses of the 20th century and grows forward with the increasing rate in the 21st century. Cancer is the abnormal development of cells. Cancers are made of small cells that have lost the capacity to stop developing and can emerge from any body structure or organ. Caner is not easily detected in its early stages but might be recognized by chance via a laboratory test or radiological routine test [25].

Cancer is a general term used in describing a group of diseases portrayed through independent development and the spread of a somatic clone. In this light, cancer must approach different cell pathways that empower it to disregard the typical requirements on cell development, change the local microenvironment to support its growth, attack through tissue boundaries, spread to different organs, and avoid immune system observation. No single cell program coordinates these behaviors, rather, there is a wide mass of pathogenic abnormalities from which singular cancers draw their combination, the shared traits of macroscopic features across tumors give a false representation of a huge heterogeneous scene of cell abnormalities [1].

Any time a cell divides, errors during the DNA replication process suggest that new mutations are present in the genomes of the daughter cells. Epigenetic marks (e.g. DNA methylation) are also replicated with limited precision. Larger-scope chromosol or part-chromosome losses or modifications [somatic copy number alternation (SCNAs)] and other structural modifications also occur at a standard frequency in many cancers. It is naturally occurring in the genetic modification that records the history of the cells in the tumor and since tumors are clonally derived; the entire cells in the tumor will carry the mutations in the main cancer cell, thus later-emerging subclones are recognizable by their sharing of a specific arrangement of variants, therefore, the order of clone advancement can be constructed by comparing the arrangement of mutation present in various cell tumor [26]. Cancer cells to meet their energy requirements, they depend on aerobic metabolism and also combined fatty acids, proteins, and nucleotides. Therefore, there is a constant need to expand the glucose supply needed to uphold diseases like diabetic-related hyperglycemia [27].

3.1 Cancer types

3.1.1 Lung cancer

Lung cancer is the most dangerous tumor, and the principal reason for cancer death worldwide in both genders combined. Globally, lung cancer occurrence and mortality on the general populace are essentially dictated by tobacco usage, the fundamental etiological factor in lung carcinogenesis [28]. The hazard factors for lung cancer involve ecological and hereditary hazard factors, all of which have an impact on tumor advancement and additionally influence patients' treatment [29]. Ladies have some unique hazard factors for lung cancer compared to men, and lung tumors in ladies have different pathologic conduct, results, and visualization in comparison to lung cancer growth in men [30]. The viability of lung cancer growth screening, utilizing computed tomography (CT) or chest X-ray (CXR), involving extra aides or not, such as sputum cytology, has been explored in various studies as asymptomatic at-risk populations [31].

3.1.2 Breast cancer

Breast cancer is the commonest cancer analyzed in the female population (excluding skin cancer) and reported the second highest cause of death among ladies after lung cancer [32]. There have been numerous analytic techniques for diagnosing early-stage breast cancer such as biopsy, breast MI, MRI, PET, ultrasonography, and mammography [33]. There are various hazardous factors, for example, sex, maturing, estrogen, family history, gene mutation, and an unhealthy lifestyle, which can contribute to the risk of breast cancer. Most breast cancers occur in ladies and the quantity of cases is multiple times more in ladies than that of men [34]. Various treatments can be utilized, for example, targeted therapy, hormonal therapy, radiation treatment, surgery, and chemotherapy [35].

3.1.3 Prostate cancer

Prostate cancer is another deadly cancer diagnosed in men and the fifth-highest cause of death around the world. Prostate cancer might show no symptoms in the beginning phase, regularly has slow movement, and may require little or even no treatment. Problems with urination have been the most common issue, however, records indicate that it may emerge from prostatic hypertrophy [36]. Screening for prostate cancer is initiated by measuring prostate-specific antigen (PSA) protein levels in the blood. A raised prostate-specific antigen (PSA) level indicates prostate cancer and other conditions, such as inflammation of the prostate and amplified prostate [37]. Prostate cancer has more victims of older men. Numerous patients with prostate cancer in the beginning stages obtain good results after various treatments involving prostatectomy, radiation therapy, hormonal therapy, etc. [38].

3.1.4 Colon cancer

Colon cancer is the third most commonly diagnosed and second deadliest cancer for all genders joined. Natural affiliations and hereditary are the main risk factors. In patients, screening colonoscopy is required for tissue biopsy neurotic affirmation of colon carcinoma, such as baseline computed tomography (CT) of the chest, mid-region, and pelvis, and carcinoembryonic antigen (CEA) are favored cost-effective [39]. Chemotherapy and Surgery are the fundamental treatment choices for colon cancer, depending on the cancer stages and tumor area, as well as the health qualities of the patients [40].

3.1.5 Pancreatic cancer

Pancreatic cancer is one of the highest causes of cancer deaths in developed nations and one of the deadliest cancers worldwide. The two-fundamental tumors; pancreatic endocrine tumors (less than 5% of cases) and pancreatic cancer are adenocarcinoma (about 85% of cases) [41]. Finding the tumor at a treatable stage is extremely difficult, patients do not usually show symptoms and tumors do not show sensitivity or signals to help in early discovery [42].

Other types of cancer including skin cancer, kidney cancer, lymphoma, bone cancer, leukemia, liver cancer, etc.

3.2 Causes

Cancer is caused by changes to the DNA within cells which are influenced by factors such as unhealthy diet, alcohol intake, tobacco use, infections, genetic tendency, ionizing radiation, toxins, obesity, inactive lifestyle, and other environmental factors [43] (**Figures 1** and **2**).

3.3 Cancer therapy

Cancer is among the primary causes of deaths globally, and in the previous years, numerous researches have concentrated on discovering new treatments other than the customary treatments which carry side effects. There are still numerous issues that must be addressed to improve cancer treatment, though much advancement has been accomplished in medication [44]. The number of cancer survivors continues to grow in the United States, notwithstanding the general declining age-normalized rates in men and stable rates in women. This shows an expanding number of new cancer analysis methods coming from the developing population as well as an increase in cancer survival due to advances in early detection and treatment. Many cancer survivors must adapt to the physical impacts of cancer and its treatment, possibly prompting functional and intellectual exhaustion [45]. There are numerous types of cancer treatment techniques based on the type of cancer and stage it has progressed to. There is no specific treatment or procedure rivaling cancer, in some cases, the treatment plan may utilize a mix of the treatment techniques to have a more effective treatment. Every one of the techniques has its side effect on the patient [46].

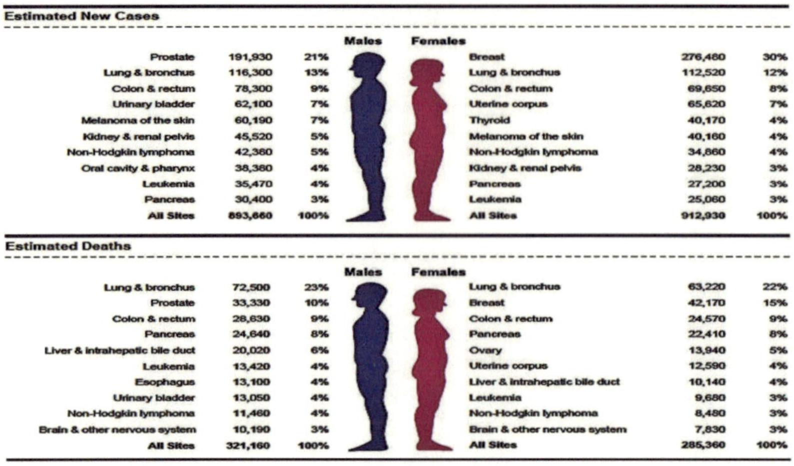

Figure 1.

Estimation of new cancer cases and deaths by sex, specifically the ten Main types of cancer in the United States, 2020. Estimates are regulated to the closest 10 and avoid basal cell, squamous cell skin tumors, and cancer which have not undergone metastasis except for urinary bladder [43].

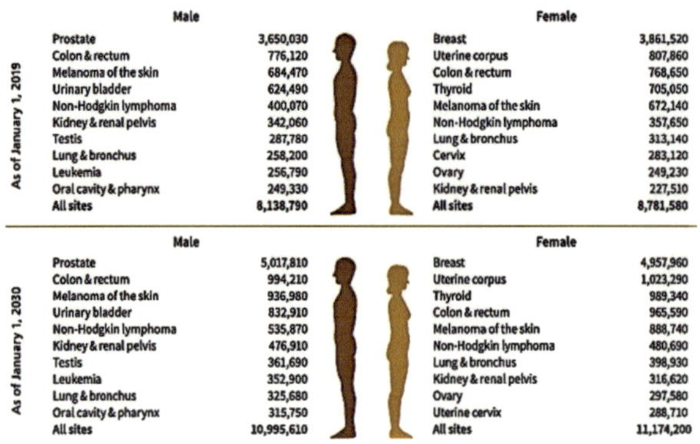

Figure 2.

Estimated amount of US cancer survivors. Evaluations exclude cancer which has not undergone metastasis, except for urinary bladder and exclude basal cells or squamous cell skin cancer [45].

3.3.1 Available cancer treatments

3.3.1.1 Surgery

Treatment of cancer by surgery is usually operated on non-hematological cancers. By surgical technique, the specialist expels the cancer tissues from the body. The surgical methodology can give a total or fractional fix for cancer. There might be side effects of the surgery based on the kind of cancer and the patients' health status. If cancer is metastasized to different areas of the body, at that point expelling cancer by the surgical process is impossible. The development of the cancer cells follows the Halstedian model of cancer progression where the tumors begin developing locally and spreading to the lymph nodes and the rest of the body. The treatment of cancer by surgery should be possible to cancers that are limited to an area and the tumor is small in size [47].

3.3.1.2 Chemotherapy

The technique of chemotherapy is done using drugs, generally known as anticancer medications, to destroy or pulverize the cancer cells. These medications interfere with the development of tumors and even damage the cancer cells. Chemotherapy is commonly considered a powerful technique for the treatment of cancer, though it can cause extreme side effects as it can also damage healthy cells or tissues. The side effects caused by chemotherapy depend on the type of cancer, its areas, and the patients' reaction to the specific kinds of chemotherapy treatment. The side effects on the cancer patient do not represent the viability of the treatment and disappear once the treatment process is finished. For the most part, chemotherapy medicines are recommended to a subject in an estimated amount over a time frame. In some cases, chemotherapy is administered at least two different medications at a time, this method is known as combination chemotherapy [48].

3.3.1.3 Immunotherapy

Immunotherapy is a technique for cancer treatment that causes the immune system to fight cancer. This is otherwise called biologic therapy, which excites the immune system of the patient to fight cancer. Several studies have been conducted on immunotherapy for treating cancer, for example, monoclonal antibodies that block specific protein work by constraining to cancer cells, which train the immune system to perceive and fight the cancer cells. This technique for treatment does not have any significant side effects. Immunotherapy is divided into two principle immunotherapeutic; passive and active. The grouping depends on the component of the therapeutic agent utilized, as well as the status of the patients' immune system. The passive immunotherapeutic is utilized in cancer patients with feeble, unresponsive, or low responsive immune systems. To apply active immunotherapeutic, the patients' immune system should be able to react strongly when opposed, be adequately stimulated, and resolve effector capacities [49].

3.3.1.4 Radiation therapy

Radiation therapy utilizes high portions of ionizing radiation to kill cancer cells and destroy the tumor tissues. This treatment is regularly utilized as a medical procedure to evacuate or lessen the size of the tumors. The radiation treatment is usually administered externally and internally to the target area and can be harmful to ordinary cells and prompt a reaction from ordinary cells because of these ionizing radiations. The radiation treatment utilizes unique equipment to carry estimated portions of radiation to the cancer cells. The radiation treatment destroys tumor cells by damaging their DNA either directly or by harming free radicals inside the cells which can hence damage the DNA. This treatment utilizes high energy ionizing radiation, for example, x-rays. This treatment has significant side effects that have different approaches in both grown-ups and children [50].

3.3.1.5 Hormone therapy

The hormone treatment fights cancer by evolving the number of hormones in the body to treat particular types of cancer that depend on the chemicals to develop and spread. This treatment technique is utilized for treating cancers of the breast, reproductive system, and prostate. The side effects depend on the type of cancer, age, sex, and the sort of medication utilized in the treatment [51].

3.3.1.6 Targeted therapy

The targeted treatment of cancer focuses on the cells that re-empower the cancer cells to develop, separation, and spread. The targeted treatment utilizes specific agents for the deregulated proteins of cancer cells. The small atoms of targeted therapy medication are inhibitors of enzymatic areas on the change, overexpressed, or critical proteins inside the cancer cells [52].

Other treatments include bone marrow transplant, cryoablation, and radiofrequency ablation.

4. Roles of dietary antioxidants in cancer therapy

Numerous types of cancer have been associated with the relation between free radicals and DNA which can cause harmful impacts on the cell cycle and also prompt dire threats. Antioxidants in suitable portions indicate that they have a generally good effect in making the tumors progressively responsive towards chemotherapy and radiation therapy. They can repress the development of tumors specifically without interfering with typical cells. Antioxidants can ensure protection against the toxicity caused by chemotherapy by hindering cell expansion. Additionally, antioxidants have demonstrated to hold an advantageous ability to decrease harm by oxidative stress, lessening the issues joined with the production of ROS and neurodegenerative issues [53].

ROS are chemically reactive particles containing oxygen, created by cellular metabolism. A moderate amount of ROS assumes a fundamental role in managing cell multiplication and cell survival. Nonetheless, an increase in ROS levels can harm cell components, for example, lipids, proteins, and DNA causing an imbalance between cell reduction–oxidation (redox) conditions and cause disturbance of homeostasis. Constantly, increased reactive oxygen species (ROS) prompt extreme cell harm and lead to carcinogenesis by regulating cell signaling such as cell expansion, angiogenesis, and metastasis [54].

There are two kinds of antioxidant dosages utilized in cancer treatment; a preventive low portion, which restrains typical cells as well as tumor cells from developing, and a remedial high portion, which restrains the development of cancer cells without impacting typical cells. Ongoing tests demonstrated that certain conditions should be met before involving antioxidants in chemotherapy. Moreover, they do not hinder but improve the cytotoxic effect of chemotherapy while protecting the typical tissue which subsequently increases the patients' survival and therapeutic response [55].

Research has indicated that 35% of cancer can be prevented by dietary adjustments. Fruits and vegetables, which are wealthy in antioxidants, act defensively against some types of cancer. Plant nutrients that contain polyphenols have demonstrated to be viable antioxidant agents for the body, they appear to oppose cancer growth in prostate, lung, breast, tongue, gastric, larynx, and colon cancers [56]. Besides, supplements such as nutrients and minerals can lessen the risk of cancer by stimulating antioxidant activity, restraining the multiplication of cancerous cells, tending to DNA methylation, and advancing cell-cycle capture. In patients recently treated for cancer, a healthy eating routine rich in fruits and vegetables can alter biomarkers of cancer growth [57]. Notably, the redox status of the cancer cell which is under stress is not the same as the ordinary cell. Ordinary cells keep up cell homeostasis by the endogenous antioxidant mechanism which perfectly makes redox balance between the beginning and end of an overabundance of reactive oxygen species (ROS). Unfortunately, the remedial technique utilized in cancer treatment could cause an increased ROS level and also increases the endogenous ROS threshold level in cancer cells and may render ordinary cells of certain organs such as the kidney, liver, and heart ineffective against oxidative toxicity caused by oxidative stress. However, current research aims to distinguish the properties which may improve oxidative stress in cancer cells and protect ordinary cells from

DOI: http://dx.doi.org/10.5772/intechopen.94988

oxidative harm. Extensive research conducted in recent years has indicated that plant-based nutrients have a high substance of phytochemicals such as flavonoids and polyphenols with chemopreventive properties that focus on some key factors associated with the improvement of cancer [58].

Some chemo-preventive compounds having antioxidant properties have been noted to have the potential to mitigate the cytotoxic effect of radiation treatment in cancerous cells while reducing its harm to ordinary cells and tissues. In such a manner, different research has demonstrated that phytochemicals soy isoflavones such as glycitein, show anti-carcinogenic properties to an extent using their antioxidant activities, and can be utilized as powerful radio-sensitizers to improve the viability of radiotherapy-mediated suppression of the development and metastatic capacity of tumors. As cancer patients experience treatment some unfavorable side effects may develop such as weight reduction, or loss of appetite, and so on [59].

4.1 The equivocal of dietary antioxidants in cancer therapy

The ability of antioxidants to shield the cells from ROS created the premise of its production in food supplement enterprise, with the increase in the scientific literature on its helpful impacts and wide acknowledgment among the general public. Nonetheless, present research in cancer shows two different aspects of antioxidants. Antioxidants are both helpful as a treatment system for the cancer patient and also involve harmful impacts of expanding the cancer cell growth [60].

DNA protection utilizing antioxidant therapy has been a productive choice for clinical trials. Flavonoids and phenolic acid are being noted as effective agents against the side effects of chemotherapy. A strong antioxidant such as coenzyme Q is mainly applied as a treatment in cancer, inflammation, and maturing. Application of coenzyme Q, for example on human epidermal cells, ensures protection against cell death initiated by reactive oxygen species (ROS) [61]. Supplements of vitamin C, one of the most abundant dietary antioxidants, have been found to ensure protection against oxidative harm caused by tobacco smoking reducing the risk factor of cancer. The relation between reactive oxygen species and cancer initiation is long-established. Other than the significant levels of ROS in environmental carcinogens such as tobacco smoking, reactive oxygen species (ROS) have been demonstrated to be basic for the transformation of cells caused by a gene that can transform a cell into a tumor cell or a loss of tumor suppressors. For instance, the downregulation of the p53 gene (a tumor suppressor) prompts increased reactive oxygen species (ROS) levels and antioxidant-related medications hinder tumor formation in mice lacking this gene. Though every tumor is unique and the role of reactive oxygen species (ROS) and antioxidants can differ depending on hereditary, epigenetic, and environmental variation [62].

Discovery is being made implying that the impact which antioxidants have on cancer patients is truly harmful. It is important to note that a few antioxidants do behave as pro-oxidants under certain conditions. Another study showed that the b-carotene, a likely antioxidant, should be utilized cautiously, clear from its extremely reactive carotenoid radical development during the searching system of free radicals. The investigation indicated that the carotenoid radical structure which is scavenged through vitamin C can have harmful impacts on the initiation of cancer by UV-radiation with altering levels of vitamin C. The research implies that when antioxidants are taken by healthy persons, they present gainful impacts, however, when there is a beginning of tumor development, high portions of antioxidants should be avoided to stop the increase in expansion of tumor cells. It is also important to note that the antioxidants utilized as the cream can turn unstable through the responses related to UV-radiation which can prompt harmful impacts. These facts raise issues concerning antioxidant treatment, a potential solution could be the intake of selected antioxidants according to the cancer cells movement and utilizing standard eating routine involving such antioxidants instead of the intake of direct supplements [14].

Adequate verification is required to determine the efficacy of different anticancer agents combined with antioxidant supplements. In a recent study, no reports have shown that they cause cancer growth or an increase in mortality rate. However, if antioxidant supplements are to be utilized as aids for cancer patients, more research is required for the combination of cancer therapy and dietary supplement. The use of unauthorized supplements should be avoided [60].

5. Conclusion

There is uncertainty in determining whether antioxidants may have positively affected cancer treatment outcomes or prevent the harmful impacts of chemotherapy and radiotherapy. At first, it is important to consider all options of treatment and some patients are usually in good condition to endure the side effects of antioxidants. On second thought, some patients are not ready to endure the side effects of antioxidants, and to use treatment certain to work to some degree is more advisable. However, to be able to manage the side effects, these conditions should be revised; the dosage and types of antioxidants, the background and condition of the patient, and type of cancer and anticancer therapy. It is advisable to utilize a proof-based technique to choose the most appropriate supplement for cancer patients. Even though there are many opinions on the good and bad of antioxidants, it is difficult to clinically conclude that dietary antioxidants enhance therapeutic toxicities and also, there is no evidence of dietary antioxidant causing harm with cancer treatment, aside from smokers experiencing radiotherapy.

Conflict of interest

The authors declare no conflict of interest.

Author details

Musbau Adewumi Akanji[1], Heritage Demilade Fatinukun[2], Damilare Emmanuel Rotimi[2], Boluwatife Lawrence Afolabi[2] and Oluyomi Stephen Adeyemi[2*]

1 Department of Biochemistry, University of Ilorin, Ilorin, Nigeria

2 Department of Biochemistry, Medicinal Biochemistry and Toxicology Laboratory, Landmark University, Omu-Aran, Nigeria

*Address all correspondence to: yomibowa@yahoo.com

References

[1] The, I. C. G. C, of Whole, T. P. C. A, Genomes Consortium, Pan-cancer analysis of whole genomes. Nature. 2020;578:(7793), 82. DOI: 10.1038/s41586-020-1969-6.

[2] Subrahmanyam V, Ramachandran, R. P, Significance of Dietary Antioxidants in Averting Cancer. J Carcinogen Mutagen. 2011;2:127. DOI: 10.4172/2157-2518.1000127.

[3] Siegel R. L, Miller K. D, Jemal A, Cancer statistics, CA: a cancer journal for clinicians. 2020;70:1:7-30. DOI: 10.3322/caac.21590.

[4] He L, He T, Farrar S, Ji L, Liu T, Ma X, Antioxidants maintain cellular redox homeostasis by elimination of reactive oxygen species. Cellular Physiology and Biochemistry. 2017;44:2:32-553. DOI: 10.1159/000485089.

[5] Yeung A. W. K, Tzvetkov N. T, El-Tawil O. S, Bungău S. G, Abdel-Daim M. M, Atanasov, A. G, Antioxidants: scientific literature landscape analysis. Oxidative medicine and cellular longevity, 2019;2-13. DOI: 10.1155/2019/8278454.

[6] Goni I, Hernandez-Galiot A, Intake of Nutrient and Non-Nutrient Dietary Antioxidants. Contribution of Macromolecular Antioxidant Polyphenols in an Elderly Mediterranean Population. Nutrients. 2019;11:9:2165. DOI: 10.3390/nu11092165.

[7] Lalkovicova M, Danielisova V, Neuroprotection and antioxidants. Neural regeneration research, 2016;11:6:865. DOI: 10.4103/1673-5374.184447.

[8] Arulselvan P, Fard M. T, Tan W. S, Gothai, S, Fakurazi S, Norhaizan M. E, Kumar S. S, Role of antioxidants and natural products in inflammation. Oxidative medicine and cellular longevity. 2016;4-16. DOI: 10.1155/2016/5276130.

[9] Rahimi-Madiseh M, Malekpour-Tehrani A, Bahmani M, Rafieian-Kopaei M, The research and development on the antioxidants in prevention of diabetic complications. Asian Pacific journal of tropical medicine. 2016;9:9:825-831. DOI; 10.1016/j.apjtm.2016.07.001.

[10] Sindhi V, Gupta V, Sharma K, Bhatnagar S, Kumari R, Dhaka N, Potential applications of antioxidants–A review. Journal of Pharmacy Research. 2013;7:9:828-835. DOI: 10.1016/j.jopr.2013.10.001.

[11] Domazetovic V, Marcucci G, Iantomasi T, Brandi M. L, Vincenzini M. T, Oxidative stress in bone remodeling: role of antioxidants. Clinical Cases in Mineral and Bone Metabolism. 2017;14:2:209. DOI: 10.11138/ccmbm/2017.14.1.209.

[12] Alam M. N, Bristi N. J, Rafiquzzaman M, Review on in vivo and in vitro methods evaluation of antioxidant activity. Saudi pharmaceutical journal. 2013;21:2:43-152. DOI: 10.1016/j.jsps.2012.05.002.

[13] Aversa R, Petrescu R. V, Apicella A, Petrescu F. I, One can slow down the aging through antioxidants. American Journal of Engineering and Applied Sciences. 2016;9:4. DOI: 10.3844/ajeassp.2016.1112.1126.

[14] Sarangarajan R, Meera S, Rukkumani R, Sankar P, Anuradha G, Antioxidants: Friend or foe? Asian Pacific Journal of Tropical Medicine. 2017;10:12:1111-1116. DOI: 10.1016/j.apjtm.2017.10.017.

[15] Olas B, Berry phenolic antioxidants–implications for human health?

Frontiers in pharmacology. 2018;9:78. DOI: 10.3389/fphar.2018.00078.

[16] Xu D. P, Li Y, Meng X, Zhou T, Zhou Y, Zheng J, Li H. B, Natural antioxidants in foods and medicinal plants: Extraction, assessment and resources. International journal of molecular sciences. 2017;18:1:96. DOI: 10.3390/ijms18010096.

[17] Addor F. A. S. A, Antioxidants in dermatology. Anais brasileiros de dermatologia. 2017;92:3:356-362. DOI: 10.1590/abd1806-4841.20175697.

[18] Peluso I, Dietary Antioxidants: Micronutrients and Antinutrients in Physiology and Pathology. 2019;4:6. DOI: 10.3390/antiox8120642.

[19] Huang Q, Liu H, Suzuki K, Ma S, Liu C, Linking what we eat to our mood: A review of diet, dietary antioxidants, and depression. Antioxidants. 2019;8:9:376. DOI: 10.3390/antiox8090376.

[20] Gordon M. H, Significance of dietary antioxidants for health. International Journal of Molecular Sciences. 2012;13:1:173-179. DOI: 10.3390/ijms13010173.

[21] Varadharaj S, Kelly O. J, Khayat R. N, Kumar P. S, Ahmed N, Zweier J. L, Role of dietary antioxidants in the preservation of vascular function and the modulation of health and disease. Frontiers in cardiovascular medicine. 2017;4:64. DOI: 10.3389/fcvm.2017.00064.

[22] Kaur G, Kathariya R, Bansal S, Singh A, Shahakar D, Dietary antioxidants and their indispensable role in periodontal health. Journal of food and drug analysis. 2016;24:2:239-246. DOI: 10.1016/j.jfda.2015.11.003.

[23] Li S, Chen G, Zhang C, Wu M, Wu S, Liu Q, Research progress of natural antioxidants in foods for the treatment of diseases. Food Science and Human Wellness. 2014;3:3-4:110-116. DOI: 10.1016/j.fshw.2014.11.002.

[24] Petruk G, Del-Giudice R, Rigano, M. M, Monti D. M, Antioxidants from plants protect against skin photo aging. Oxidative medicine and cellular longevity. 2018;2;6. DOI: 10.1155/2018/1454936.

[25] Roy P. S, Saikia B. J, Cancer and cure: A critical analysis. Indian journal of cancer. 2016;53:3:441. DOI: 10.4103/0019-509X.200658.

[26] Graham T. A, Sottoriva A, Measuring cancer evolution from the genome. The Journal of pathology. 2017;241:2:183-191. DOI: 10.1002/path.4821.

[27] Avgerinos K. I, Spyrou N, Mantzoros C. S, Dalamaga M, Obesity and cancer risk: Emerging biological mechanisms and perspectives. Metabolism. 2019;92:121-135. DOI: 10.1016/j.metabol.2018.11.001.

[28] Malhotra J, Malvezzi M, Negri E, La-Vecchia C, Boffetta P, Risk factors for lung cancer worldwide. European Respiratory Journal. 2016;48:3:889-902. DOI: 10.1183/13993003.00359-2016.

[29] Tsao A. S, Scagliotti G. V, Bunn J. P. A, Carbone D. P, Warren G. W, Bai C, Adusumilli P. S, Scientific advances in lung cancer 2015. Journal of Thoracic Oncology. 2016;11:5:613-638. DOI: 10.1016/j.jtho.2016.03.012.

[30] De Groot P. M, Wu C. C, Carter B. W, Munden R. F, The epidemiology of lung cancer. Translational lung cancer research. 2018;7:3:220. DOI: 10.21037/tlcr.2018.05.06.

[31] Blandin-Knight S, Crosbie P. A, Balata H, Chudziak J, Hussell T, Dive C, Progress and prospects of early detection in lung cancer. Open biology. 2017;7:9:170070. DOI: 10.1098/rsob.170070.

[32] DeSantis C, Siegel R, Bandi P, Jemal, A, Breast cancer statistics, 2011. CA: a cancer journal for clinicians. 2011;61:6:408-418. DOI: 10.3322/caac.20107.

[33] Wang L, Early diagnosis of breast cancer. Sensors. 2017;17:7:1572. DOI: 10.3390/s17071572.

[34] Sun Y.S, Zhao Z, Yang Z.N, Xu F, Lu H.J, Zhu Z.Y, Shi W, Jiang J, Yao P.P, Zhu H.P, Risk factors and preventions of breast cancer. International journal of biological sciences. 2017;13:11:1387. DOI: 10.7150/ijbs.21635.

[35] Akram M, Iqbal M, Daniyal M, Khan A. U, Awareness and current knowledge of breast cancer. Biological research. 2017;50:1:33. DOI: 10.1186/s40659-017-0140-9.

[36] Rawla P, Epidemiology of prostate cancer. World journal of oncology. 2019;10:2:63. DOI: 10.14740/wjon1166.

[37] Grossman D. C, Curry S. J, Owens D. K, Bibbins-Domingo K, Caughey A. B, Davidson K. W, Krist A. H, Screening for prostate cancer: US Preventive Services Task Force recommendation statement. Jama. 2018;319:18:1901-1913. DOI: 10.1001/jama.2018.3710.

[38] Fujita K, Hayashi T, Matsushita M, Uemura M, Nonomura N, Obesity, inflammation, and prostate cancer. Journal of Clinical Medicine. 2019; 8:2:201. DOI: 10.1001/jama.2016.5989.

[39] Recio-Boiles A, Waheed A, Cagir B, Cancer, colon. In StatPearls [Internet]. StatPearls Publishing. Treasure Island (FL): StatPearls Publishing. 2020. https://www.ncbi.nlm.nih.gov/books/NBK470380/.

[40] Hu T, Li Z, Gao C. Y, Cho C. H, Mechanisms of drug resistance in colon cancer and its therapeutic strategies. World journal of gastroenterology. 2016;22:30:6876. DOI: 10.3390/jcm8020201.

[41] Ilic M, Ilic I, Epidemiology of pancreatic cancer. World journal of gastroenterology. 2016;22:44:9694. DOI: 10.3748/wjg.v22.i30.6876.

[42] Kleeff J, Korc M, Apte M, La-Vecchia C, Johnson C. D, Biankin A. V, Neoptolemos J. P, Pancreatic cancer. Nature reviews Disease primers. 2016;2:1:1-22. DOI: 10.1038/nrdp.2016.22.

[43] Siegel R. L, Miller K. D, Jemal A, Cancer statistics, 2020. CA: a cancer journal for clinicians. 2020;70:1:7-30. DOI: 10.6004/jnccn.2020.0032.

[44] Pucci C, Martinelli C, Ciofani G, Innovative approaches for cancer treatment: current perspectives and new challenges. Ecancermedicalscience. 2019;13:5-13. DOI: 10.3332/ecancer.2019.961.

[45] Miller, K. D, Nogueira L, Mariotto A. B, Rowland J. H, Yabroff K. R, Alfano C. M, Siegel R. L, Cancer treatment and survivorship statistics, 2019. CA: a cancer journal for clinicians. 2019;69:5:363-385. DOI: 10.3322/caac.21551.

[46] Roma-Rodrigues C, Mendes R, Baptista P. V, Fernandes A. R, Targeting tumor microenvironment for cancer therapy. International journal of molecular sciences. 2019;20:4:840. DOI: 10.3390/ijms20040840.

[47] Tringale K. R, Pang J, Nguyen Q. T, Image-guided surgery in cancer: A strategy to reduce incidence of positive surgical margins. Wiley Interdisciplinary Reviews: Systems Biology and Medicine. 2018;10:3:e1412. DOI: 10.1002/wsbm.1412.

[48] Wang J. J, Lei K. F, Han F, Tumor microenvironment: recent advances in various cancer treatments. Eur. Rev.

Med. Pharmacol. Sci. 2018;22:3855-3864. DOI: 10.3390/ijms20040840.

[49] Papaioannou N. E, Beniata O. V, Vitsos P, Tsitsilonis O, Samara P, Harnessing the immune system to improve cancer therapy. Annals of translational medicine. 2016;4:14:4-14. DOI: 10.21037/atm.2016.04.01.

[50] Baskar R, Itahana K, Radiation therapy and cancer control in developing countries: Can we save more lives? International journal of medical sciences. 2017;14:1:13. DOI: 10.7150/ijms.17288.

[51] Deli T, Orosz M, Jakab A, Hormone replacement therapy in cancer survivors–review of the literature. Pathology & Oncology Research. 2019;1-16. DOI: 10.1007/s12253-018-00569-x.

[52] Ke X, Shen L, Molecular targeted therapy of cancer: The progress and future prospect. Frontiers in Laboratory Medicine. 2017;1:2:69-75. DOI: 10.1016/j.flm.2017.06.001.

[53] Gummadi P, Role of Antioxidants on Cancer and Neurodegenerative Disorders. Journal of Medical & Health Science. 2016;5:3:1-6. DOI: 10.2174/1570159097876O2823.

[54] Kim S. J, Kim H. S, Seo Y. R, Understanding of ROS-inducing strategy in anticancer therapy. Oxidative Medicine and Cellular Longevity. 2019. DOI: 10.1155/2019/5381692.

[55] Ammar H. O, Shamma R. N, Elbatanony R. S, Khater B, Antioxidants in Cancer Therapy: Recent Trends in Application of Nanotechnology for Enhanced Delivery. Scientia Pharmaceutica. 2020;88:1:5. DOI: 10.3390/scipharm88010005.

[56] Singh K, Bhori M, Kasu Y. A, Bhat G, Marar T, Antioxidants as precision weapons in war against cancer chemotherapy induced toxicity–Exploring the armoury of obscurity. Saudi Pharmaceutical Journal. 2018;26:2:177-190. DOI: 10.1016/j.jsps.2017.12.013.

[57] Liu Z, Ren Z, Zhang J, Chuang C. C, Kandaswamy E, Zhou, T, Zuo L, Role of ROS and nutritional antioxidants in human diseases. Frontiers in physiology. 2018;9:477. DOI: 10.3389/fphys.2018.00477.

[58] Fatima S, Cancer Treatment with Pro and Antioxidant Agents. CPQ Cancer. 2018;1:4:01-06.

[59] Thyagarajan A, Sahu R. P, Potential contributions of antioxidants to cancer therapy: immunomodulation and radio sensitization. Integrative cancer therapies. 2018;17:2:210-216. DOI: 10.1177/1534735416681639.

[60] Yasueda A, Urushima H, Ito T, Efficacy and interaction of antioxidant supplements as adjuvant therapy in cancer treatment: a systematic review. Integrative cancer therapies. 2016;15:1:17-39. DOI: 10.1177/1534735415610427.

[61] Chowdhury W, Arbee S, Debnath S, Bin Zahur S, Akter S, Potent Role of Antioxidant Molecules in Prevention and Management of Skin Cancer. J Clin Exp Dermatol Res. 2017;8:3. DOI: 10.4172/2155-9554.1000393.

[62] Walton E. L, The dual role of ROS, antioxidants and autophagy in cancer. Biomedical Journal. 2016;39:2:89-92. DOI: 10.1016/j.bj.2016.05.001.

Chapter 10

Antioxidant and Infertility

Huda Mahmood Shakir

Abstract

Unexplained sub-fertility is commonly identified if couples fail to conceive after 1 yr. of everyday unprotected sexual intercourse even though investigations for ovulation, tubal patency and semen evaluation are ordinary. Many previous studies had shown that oxidative stress plays an important role in human fertility. Free radicals are neutralized by an elaborate antioxidant defense system. In a healthy body, pro-oxidants and antioxidants maintain a ratio and a shift in this ratio towards pro-oxidants gives rise to oxidative stress. There are two types of antioxidants in the human body: enzymatic and non-enzymatic antioxidants. Under normal conditions, antioxidants convert ROS to H_2O to prevent overproduction of ROS. All cells in the human body are capable of synthesizing glutathione specially the liver. Free radicals appear to have a physiological role in female reproductive system in many different processes such as: oocyte maturation, fertilization, luteal regression, endometrial shedding and progesterone production by the corpus luteum. Protection from ROS is afforded by scavengers present in both male and female reproductive tract fluids, as well as in seminal plasma elevated concentrations of ROS in these environments may have detrimental effects on the spermatozoa, oocytes, sperm oocyte interaction and embryos both in the Fallopian tube and the peritoneal cavity; therefore oxidative stress modulates a host of reproductive pathologies affecting natural fertility in a woman's life.

Keywords: ROS, reactive oxygen species, OS, oxidative stress, NO, nitric oxide, NO_2, nitrogen dioxide, MDA, malondiadehyde

1. Introduction

Reproductive failure is a significant public health concern. Infertility, carries significant personal, societal and financial consequences. One of the most important and underappreciated reproductive health problems in developing countries is the high rate of infertility and childlessness.

Causes of infertility can be found in about 90% of cases, about 10% of patients do not know why they can not conceive this is called unexplained infertility [1].

Unexplained infertility is a diagnosis of exclusion, when the standard investigation of both the female and male partner has ruled out other infertility diagnosis.

A couple is considered to have unexplained infertility if the woman ovulated and had a normal and hysterosalpingogram, and the man a normal semen analysis. Critical factors to be considered in evaluating and managing unexplained infertility are the duration of infertility and female age [2].

In case of unexplained infertility, any form of treatment is speculated.

A period of three years of unexplained infertility is generally accepted as minimum duration before active intervention is considered.

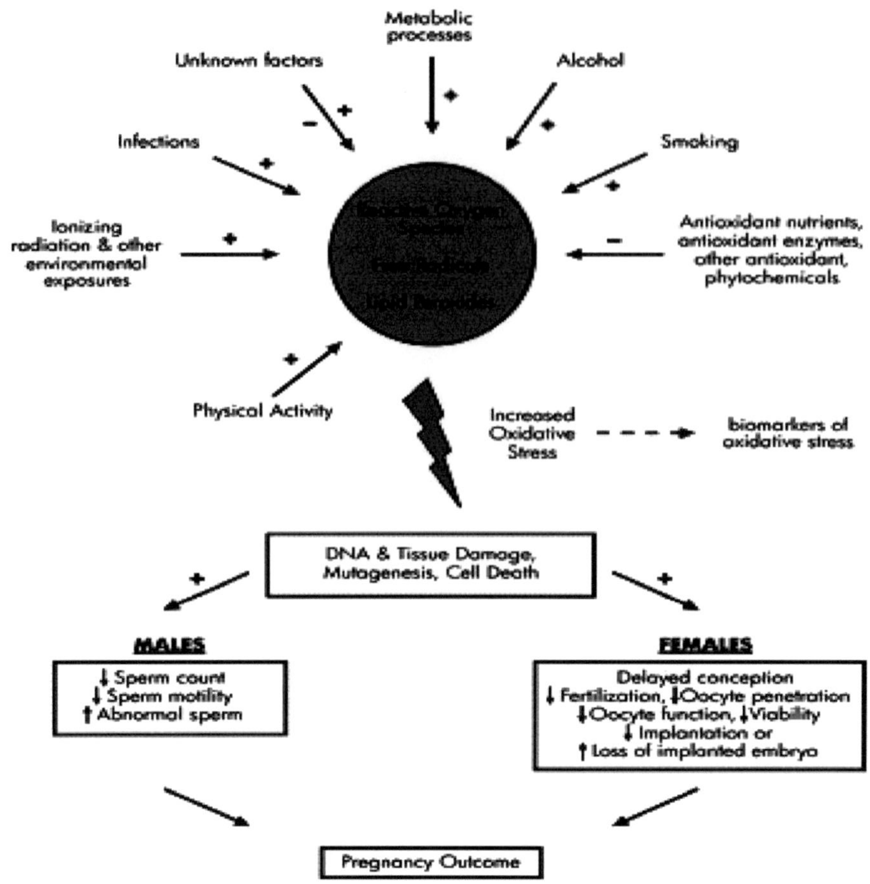

Figure 1.
Role of oxidative stress in fertility.

Empirical treatment with clomiphene,intrauterine insemination are used in treatment of unexplained infertility, if failed, invitro fertilization is considered.

Because female ovary is the source of oocytes and regulating hormones, free radicals in the gynecologic environment is likely to be an important mediator of conception. Recently there is a growing evidence of possible role of highly reactive products of oxygen, termed free radicals, in infertility [3].

A free radical is any atom (e.g. oxygen, nitrogen) with at least one unpaired electron in the outermost [4]. Free radicals are neutralized by an elaborate antioxidant defense system. In a healthy body, pro-oxidants and antioxidants maintain a ratio and a shift in this ratio towards pro-oxidants gives rise to oxidative stress [3].

In this case free radical species which are unstable and highly reactive, will become stable by acquiring electrons from nucleic acids, lipids, proteins, carbohydrates or any nearby molecule causing a cascade of chain reactions resulting in cellular damage and diseas [5]. Because free radicals are unstable, and difficult to measure, traditional indices of oxidative stress include downstream markers of oxidative damage to macromolecules such as lipids, proteins and DNA. Oxidative stress is also indirectly assessed by estimating capacity for antioxidant defense in serum, or other body fluids. Such measures include assessment of enzymatic antioxidant activity and individual assessment of circulating non-enzymatic antioxidant levels [6].

Successful initiation of pregnancy requires the ovulation of a mature oocyte, production of competent sperm, proximity of sperm and oocyte in the reproductive tract, fertilization of the oocyte, transport of the conceptus into the uterus, and implantation of the embryo into a properly prepared, healthy endometrium. A dysfunction in any one of these complex biological steps can cause infertility [7].

Free radicals can affect the female fertility potential in number of ways which can contribute negatively to a number of reproductive processes including folliculogenesis, oocyte maturation, sperm DNA damage, necrozoospermia, asthenospermia, endometriosis [8]. High levels of ROS play an important role in the etiology of male and female infertility. It has been proposed that the imbalance between antioxidants and ROS, favoring the latter, is responsible for increased OS levels that induce infertility [9]. Fissore *et al* [10] have found that OS is associated with maternal aging and postovulatory aging of the ova. The Role of oxidative stress in fertility is shown in **Figure 1**.

The role of Oxidative Stress in female reproductive diseases and infertility is under intense investigations [8]. Whenever there is imbalance in the levels of ROS and antioxidants, damage can occur to oocytes and embryos through various pathological mechanisms [11].

2. Role of free radicals in unexplained infertility

2.1 Free radicals

A free radical is any atom (e.g. oxygen, nitrogen) with at least one unpaired electron in the outermost shell [4].

Free radical atoms are unstable and highly reactive. They become stable by acquiring electrons from nucleic acids, lipids, proteins, carbohydrates or any nearby molecule causing a cascade of chain reactions resulting in cellular damage and disease [5]. The terms free radical and ROS are commonly used in an interchangeable manner, despite the fact that not all ROS are free radicals [12]. For example, hydrogen peroxide (H_2O_2) is considered a ROS but it is not a free radical since it does not contain unpaired electrons. In addition, there is a sub-class of free radicals derived from nitrogen [13].

There must be a balance between oxidants and antioxidants, generation of an excess of free radical results in oxidative stress [14].

2.2 Types of free radical species

There are two major types of free radical species: reactive oxygen species (ROS) and reactive nitrogen species (NOS).

2.3 Reactive oxygen species (ROS)

The Oxygen centered free radicals are class of powerful oxidants in the human body. The most common ROS include: the superoxide anion (O_2^-), the hydroxyl radical ($OH^\cdot$), singlet oxygen ($1O_2$), and a number of related species, such as hydrogen peroxide (H_2O_2), that do not themselves contain unpaired electrons but are often involved in the generation of free radicals [15].

2.4 Reactive nitrogen species

The two common examples of reactive nitrogen species are nitric oxide (NO) and nitrogen dioxide (NO_2). Nitric oxide is a highly reactive free radical results in cells and tissues damage [16].

2.5 Sources of free radicals in human body

The main four endogenous normal sources appear to account for most of the oxidants produced by cells; are aerobic respiration in mitochondria, Phagocyte, Peroxisomes and Cytochrome P450 enzymes. Exogenous sources may significantly increase the large endogenous oxidant load which include: Iron and copper salts [17]; smoking and alcohol; normal diets (fried food, caffien) [18]; radiation, sunlight; pollution and xenobiotics (Drugs,pesticides, anesthetics,andindustrial solvents) [19].

2.6 Pathological damage of free radicals

Interaction of free radicals with other compounds results in a chain reactions of oxidation and reduction which ultimately can lead to cellulardamage [6].

Oxidation of DNA molecules, for example, can result in mutation where as oxidation of protein can result in protein cross-linking and loss function [20].

Reactive oxygen species can attack polyunsaturated fatty acids of the cell membrane leading to a chain of chemical reactions called lipid peroxidation and this will lead to decrease structural fluidity of these compounds, thus resulting in loss of integrity of cellular membranes [6]. It is possible to measure the extent of peroxidative damage by estimatingthe stable end products of lipid peroxidation such as MDA (malondiadehyde) [3].

2.7 Types of antioxidants

There are two types of antioxidants in the human body: enzymatic and non-enzymatic antioxidants [11]:

2.7.1 Enzymatic antioxidants

Enzymatic antioxidants are also known as natural antioxidants. They are mainly composed of:

- Superoxide dismutase.
- Catalase.
- Glutathione peroxidase.

Antioxidant enzymes may act in a coordinate manner to defend living tissue from oxidant [21].

Superoxide dismutase is a protein dimer,destroys the free radical superoxide by converting it to peroxide [22].

Catalase is a hemoprotein enzyme of the oxidoreductase class that catalyzes the convertion of hydrogen peroxide to water and oxygen, active H_2O_2 [23].

Glutathione peroxidase, is a tetramer protein containing selenium, and uses glutathione as a co-substrate. Glutathione peroxidase is a cytosolic enzyme and also eliminates H_2O_2; but, in comparison to catalase, has a wider range of substrates including lipid peroxides. Glutathione peroxidase primarily functions to detoxify low levels of H_2O_2 in the cell [24].

2.7.2 **Non-enzymatic antioxidants**

Non-enzymatic antioxidants are also known as synthetic antioxidants or dietary supplements. The body's complex antioxidant system is influenced by dietary intake of antioxidant vitamins and minerals such as vitamin C, vitamin E, selenium, zinc, glutathione and beta carotene [11].

2.7.2.1 Vitamin C (Ascorbic acid)

Vitamin C is a water soluble vitamin found in many fruit and vegetable.

Vitamin C is required for optimal functions of number of enzymes;deficiency cause scurvy and poor wound repair. It is also considered a chain breaking antioxidant that stops the propagation of the peroxidative process. Vitamin C also helps recycle oxidized vitamin E and glutathione, It is an unstable,easily oxidized acid and can be destroyed by oxygen, alkaline and high temperature. Humans cannot synthesize vitamin C, so they take it from exogenous supplement or diet found in many fruit and vegetable [25].

Tocopherol and Glutathione (GSH),also rely on vitamin C for regeneration back to their active isoforms. The relationship between vitamin C and Glutathione is unique. Vitamin C reduces GSH back to the active form. Once reduced, Glutathione will regenerate vitamin C from its oxidized state. Vitamin C protects the DNA of the cells from the damage caused by free radicals and mutagens. It prevents harmful genetic alterations within cells [26, 27].

2.7.2.2 Vitamin E

Vitamin E is the collective name for a set of at least eight related tocopherols and tocotrienols compounds with similar biological antioxidants activity. Vitamin E is the first line of defense against lipid peroxidation. Moreover, it plays a very important function in lending red blood cells flexibility as they make their way through the arterial network and helps prolong the life of erythrocytes, immune function, and has positive effects in the fertility [28].

Vitamin C regenerates Vitamin E and Vitamin C is,in turn by regenerated glutathione [29].

2.8 Antioxidant defense system

Organisms have developed efficient protective mechanisms against excessive accumulation of free radicals called antioxidants [30].

Free radicals are neutralized by an elaborate antioxidant defense system. In a healthy body, pro-oxidants and antioxidants maintain a ratio and a shift in this ratio towards pro-oxidants gives rise to oxidative stress. Whenever ROS levels become pathologically elevated, antioxidants begin to work and help minimize the oxidative damage, repair it or prevent it [31]. An antioxidant can be defined as any substance that, when present at low concentration compared to those of an oxidizable substance, significantly delays or prevents the oxidation of that substrate [32].

Under normal conditions, antioxidants convert ROS to H_2O to prevent overproduction of ROS.

The different possible mechanisms by which antioxidants may offer protection against free radical damage include:

- Prevention of formation of free radicals.

- Interception of free radicals by scavenging the reactive metabolites and converting them to less reactive molecules.

- Facilitating the repair of damage caused by free radicals.
- Providing a favorable environment for effective functioning of other antioxidants [33].

2.9 Oxidative stress in female reproduction

- The presence of oxidant and antioxidant systems in various reproductive tissues has evoked great interest in the role of OS in human reproduction. The role of ROS and antioxidants in relation to female reproductive function has, in contrast, received relatively little attention [8].
- Oxidative stress influences the entire reproductive span of women's life and even thereafter (i.e. menopause).
- Free radicals appear to have a physiological role in female reproductive system in many different processes such as: oocyte maturation, fertilization, luteal regression, endometrial shedding and progesterone production by the corpus luteum [34]. Protection from ROS is afforded by scavengers present in both male and female reproductive tract fluids, as well as in seminal plasma [35].

2.9.1 Free radicals, antioxidants, and reproductive processes in women

The production of a viable oocyte is modulated by a complex interaction of endocrine, paracrine and autocrine factors, leading to follicular maturation, granulosa cell maturation, ovulation and luteinization [36]. Elevated concentrations of ROS in these environments may have detrimental effects on the spermatozoa, oocytes, sperm oocyte interaction and embryos both in the Fallopian tube and the peritoneal cavity;therefore oxidative stress modulates a host of reproductive pathologies affecting natural fertility in a woman's life [37]. Free radicals plays a role in the physiology of ovarian function [36]. They may have a regulatory role in oocyte maturation, folliculogenesis, ovarian steroidogenesis and luteolysis. There is a delicate balance between ROS and antioxidant enzymes in the ovarian tissues [11]. Vitamin C deficiency characteristically produces ovarian atrophy and extensive follicular atresia [36]. Glutathione has been identified as critical for oocyte maturation and formation of the male sperm pronucleus (PN) [4]

- Glutathione in mature oocytes is thought to be a highly relevant biochemical marker for the viability of mammalian oocytes [38]. Hence, Follicular ROS initiate apoptosis; whereas follicular Glutathione, in addition to FSH, protect against apoptosis in cultured pre-ovulatory rat follicles [39]. The secreted Glutathione would protect oocytes against excessively produced ROS that occurs during the ovulation, thus maintaining fertilization potency [40].
- [41] observe that integrity of the antioxidant defenses within the different stages of oocyte development may contribute significantly to the overall quality of the oocytes. One consequence of an excess of ROS in the ovary may be plasma membrane damage of the oocytes. The significance of such damage for female fertility, however, is unknown.

DOI: http://dx.doi.org/10.5772/intechopen.95791

- Glutathione peroxidase may also maintain low levels of free radicals inside the follicle and thus play an important role in gametogenesis and fertilization [11]. Glutathione is considered the major source of redox potential in the oocyte [14].

- Oocytes are also rich in glutathione reductase [24].

- Reactive oxygen species are produced during luteal regression [28]. Because the corpus luteum produces much of the progesterone; ROS are produced as a byproduct [28]. The detoxification of the produced ROS by GSH in conjunction with antioxidative enzymes would be particularly important for the corpus luteum and surrounding cells (**Figure 2**) [42].

Reactive oxygen species may act as important mediators in hormone signaling, ovarian steroidogenesis and germ cell function [43].

Oxidative stress may affect theca-interstitial cells by inducing their proliferation and growth. Higher doses of Oxidative stress inhibited the proliferation of the theca-interstitial cells while antioxidants stimulate the release of gonadotrophins from the adenohypophysis [44].

Cells involved in steroidogenesis such as theca cells, granulosa lutein cells, and hilus cells show stronger oxidative enzyme activity [45]. Over-exposure of the ovary to H_2O_2 causes the LH receptor to uncouple from adenyle cyclase, thereby impairing protein synthesis and cholesterol utilization by mitochondria [28].

Data suggest that vitamin C has defined functions in hormone secretion, gamete protection, and gonadal tissue remodeling [26]. Steroidogenesis appears to be ascorbate-dependent [27] and the reduced concentrations of antioxidants often coincide with poor fertilization success rates [46].

Reactive oxygen species therefore play a role in the formation of the corpus luteum and steroidogenesis. Imbalance in redox leading to luteal regression that results in lack of luteal support to pregnancy [37].

Endogenous NO system exists in the fallopian tubes [36]. NO has a relaxing effect on smooth muscles and it has similar effects on tubular contractility. Deficiency of NO may lead to tubal motility dysfunction, resulting in retention of the ovum,

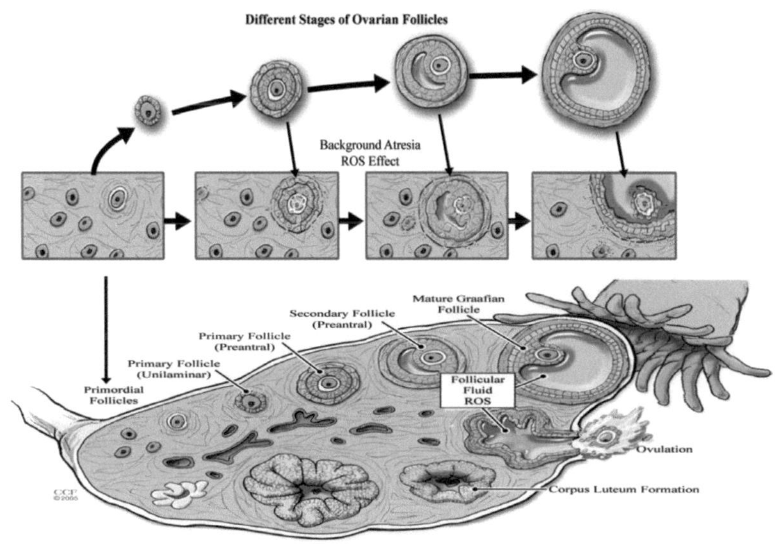

Figure 2.
Reactive oxygen species in folliculogenesis in women ovary [43].

delayed sperm transport and infertility. Increased NO levels in the fallopian tubes are cytotoxic to the invading microbes and also may be toxic to spermatozoa [11].

In male, ROS cause infertility by two principal mechanisms:

- Reactive oxygen species damage the sperm membrane which, in turn, reduces the sperm's motility and ability to fuse with the oocyte.

- Damage sperm DNA, compromising the paternal genomic contribution to the embryo [13].

The percentage of sperm with DNA damage is negatively correlated with the fertilization rate [47]. Oocytes can repair DNA damage to some extent, but when the damage is severe, embryo death and miscarriages can occur.

The inability of sperm to fuse with an oocyte appears to be due to the effects of ROS on the sperm membrane. As a result of lipid peroxidation process, spermatozoa are unable to initiate the necessary biochemical reactions associated with acrosome reaction, zona pellucida binding and oocyte penetration [29].

In addition, ROS brings about changes in the endometrium that prepare it for implantation [36]. Nitric oxide functions as an important vasodilator, neurotransmitter, regulator of implantation [8] and may also contribute as an anti-platelet agent during implantation [48].

3. The effect of some factors on free radicals levels

3.1 Body weight

The effects of body weight and weight change on OS have only recently been investigated. More studies on this topic are needed, since both inadequate and excessive energy intakes have been associated with reduced fertility among women [49].

Research has focused on the effects of energy intake on hormonal patterns and menstrual cycles, ovulatory dysfunction and later age at menarche have been associated with both low and high body mass index (BMI, calculated as kg/m^2), energy intake and high levels of physical activity [50].

3.2 Age

It has been suggested that the age-related decline in fertility is modulated by OS. Moreover, there is an age related decline in the number and quality of follicles in females [51].

Several studies have investigated if there is an age-associated increase in the generation of oxidants by mitochondria [11]. Free radical activity of human follicular fluid increases with age [10] as does apoptosis (programmed cell death) of human granulosa and cumulus cells [9]. Carbone,*et al.* [52] find that a reduction in the expression of glutathione and CAT activity is demonstrated in older women compared with young controls. Yeh et al. [53] show alterations in antioxidant defense with age. It is hypothesized that diminished antioxidant status may induce apoptosis during luteal regression and lead to decreased progesterone synthesis.

3.3 Smoking

Smoking is known to decrease fertility in women [51], likely through an increase in OS. A history of smoking is associated with high levels of oxidative stress [36].

The oxides of nitrogen (NO) in cigarette smoke damage macromolecules and deplete antioxidant. This is likely to contribute significantly to the pathology of smoking [11].

Dietary intakes of smokers; however, are different from non-smokers, confounding this relationship [11]. It is found that intrafollicular exposure to cigarette smoking metabolites was associated with a significant increase in follicular lipid peroxidation and decrease in the local antioxidative potential [3]. Smoking significantly reduced glutathione peroxidase concentration in the follicular fluid [24]. Consequently, OS imbalance may be responsible for impaired folliculogenesis in female smokers [43].

4. Overcoming OS in female infertility

Oxidative stress can be overcome by reducing generation of ROS or increasing the amounts of antioxidants available [11]. So prior to the treatment of female infertility, ROS levels should be assessed. By estimating ROS levels, it may be possible to identify the causes of infertility, especially in cases of idiopathic infertility [43]. It is important to identify the source of increased ROS generation [3]. Patients with history of smoking should be advised to stop smoking. In addition, Any exposure to drugs, toxic substances and radiation should be checked and patients should be advised to stop exposure to them.

Infections of the reproductive tract should be treated with appropriate antibiotics [11]. Initially, specific therapeutic options directed against the etiological cause of raised ROS should be tried [3]. After treating the primary cause, patients can be advised to take antioxidant supplementation. Antioxidants can be started directly when a specific etiology cannot be identified (unexplained infertility) [43]. Considerable interest has been generated in the use of antioxidants to overcome the adverse and pathological results of OS. Some studies that used nutritional supplements and antioxidants, like vitamin C supplementation to protect against ROS and OS. However, there is a lack of consensus on the type and dosage of antioxidants to be used [3]. In vivo antioxidants may be helpful in smoker infertile women [24]. A study, impact of a nutritional supplement, containing vitamin E, iron, zinc and selenium, is examined. The patients receiving the supplement experienced a significant increase in ovulation rates and pregnancy rates compared with the placebo group [28]. Indirect evidence of the importance of OS and its control with antioxidant intake is provided by studies that have shown that preconceptional multivitamin supplementation may enhance fertility, perhaps by increasing menstrual cycle regularity [44] or via prevention of ovulatory disorders [46]. In general, when supplemental vitamins C and E are given to older mice, the age-associated reduction in ovulation is partially prevented [51]. There is sufficient evidence to hypothesize that diet, particularly its constituent antioxidants, and OS may influence the timing and maintenance of a viable pregnancy [4].

5. Conclusion

- Assessment of OS as a cause of unexplained female infertility must be carried out to discriminate OS infertility from other causes of infertility.

- There is inverse significant relationship between GSH level with age and duration of infertility increment in patients with unexplained infertility.

- There is an inverse significant relationship between Vitamine C and age increment in patients with unexplained infertility.

Author details

Huda Mahmood Shakir
Department of Obstetrics and Gynaecology, Ibn Sina University for Medical and Pharmaceuticals Sciences, Iraq

*Address all correspondence to: hudaalfatal2010@gmail.com

References

[1] Siristatidis ,C. and Bhattacharya,S. (2007). Unexplained infertility: does it really exist? Does it matter?. Human Reproduction J., 22(8)2084-2087.

[2] Smith,S.; Pfiefer, S.M. and Collins, J. (2003). Diagnosis and management of female infertility. J.A.M.A. ,290:17.

[3] Agarwal, A. and Allamaneni, S.S.(2004).Role of free radicals in female reproductive diseases and assisted reproduction.Reproductive BioMedicine Online, 9:338-347.

[4] Ruder,E.; Hartman' J.; Blumberg ,J. and Goldman ,M.(2008). Oxidative stress and antioxidants: exposure and impact on female fertility. Human Reproduction and Embryology J.

[5] Van Langendonckt, A.; Casanas-Roux, F.; Donnez, J.(2002). Oxidative stress and peritoneal endometriosis. Fertil. Steril. J.,77:861-870.

[6] Janiki,Dj.(2008).oxidative stress. pittsburgh mind body center.

[7] Goldman, M.B.; Missmer, S.A. and Barberi ,R.L. (2000). Infertility. In:Women and Helath . San Diego: Academic Press., 196-214.

[8] Guerin, P.; El Mouatassim, S. and Menezo, Y. (2001). Oxidative stress and protection against reactive oxygen species in the pre-implantation embryo and its surroundings. Hum. Reprod. Update, 7:175-189.

[9] Savita, S. M.; Anitha, S. K.; Chaya ,S. D. and Bharati,A . (2009). Oxidative stress-mediated essential polyunsaturated fatty acid alterations in female infertility .Human Fertility,12 (1)28-33.

[10] Fissore, R. A.; Kurokawa, M.;Knott, J.; Zhang, M. and Smyth, J.(2002). Mechanisms underlying oocyte activation and postovulatory ageing. Reproduction J., 124:745-754.

[11] Agarwal, A., Gupta, S. and Sharma, R.(2005). Oxidative stress and its implications in female infertility - a clinician's perspective. Reprod. Biomed. Online,11(5): 641-650

[12] Cheeseman ,K.H. and Slater, T.F. (1993). An introduction to free radical biochemistry. Med Bull , 49:481-493.

[13] Tremellen, J. (2008). Oxidative stress and male infertility—a clinical perspective .Hum. Reprod. J. , 14(3):243-258.

[14] Fujii, J.; Iuchi, Y. and Okada, F.(2005). Fundamental roles of reactive oxygen species and protective mechanisms in the female reproductive system. Reprod. Biol. Endocrinol., 3:43-53.

[15] Christophersen, A. G.; Jun, H.; Jŕgensen, K., and Skibsted, L. H. (1991). Photobleaching of astaxanthin and canthaxanthin: quantum-yields dependence of solvent, temperature, and wavelength of irradiation in relation to packageing and storage of carotenoid pigmented salmonoids. Z. Lebensm. Unters. Forsch., 192:433-439

[16] Dong, M.; Shi, Y. and Cheng, Q. (2001). Increased nitric oxide in peritoneal fluid from women with idiopathic infertility and endometriosis. J Reprod Med, 46:887-891.

[17] Lauffer, R. B. (1992). Iron and Human Disease. CRC, Boca Raton, FL.

[18] Ames, B. N.; Profet, M. and Gold, L. S. (1990). Proc. Natl. Acad. Sci. USA ,87: 7777-7781.

[19] Bruce, N. Mark, K. and Tory, M. (1993). Oxidants, antioxidants, and the degenerative diseases of aging(cancer/mutation/endogenous DNA adducts/

oxygen radicals). Proc. Natl. Acad. Sci. USA, 90: 7915-7922.

[20] Bergamini, C.M.; Gambetti, S.; Dondi, A. and Cervellati, C.(2004). Oxygen, reactive oxygen species and tissue damage. Curr. Pharm. Des.,10: 1611-1626.

[21] Quinlan, T.; Spivack, S. and Mossman, B.T (1994). Regulation of Antioxidant Enzymes in Lung after Oxidant Injury. Environmental Health Perspectives, 102(2):77-81.

[22] Benov, L. and Fridovich, I. (1998). Growth in iron-enriched medium partially compensates Escherichia coli for the lack of manganese and iron superoxide dismutase. Bio.l Chem. J., 273: 10313-10316.

[23] Brioukhanov, A.; Netrusov, A. and Eggen, R. (2006). The catalase and superoxide dismutase genes are transcriptionally up-regulated upon oxidative stress in the strictly anaerobic archaeon Methanosarcina barkeri. Microbiology, 152: 1671-1677.

[24] Paszkowski, T.; Traub, A.I.; Robinson, S.Y. and McMaster, D. (1995). Selenium dependent glutathione peroxidase activity in human follicular fluid. Clin. Chim. Acta., 236: 173-180

[25] Eidan, B.; almukhtar, N.; Altemimmi, H. (2009), relashionship betwwen cervical and blood free radicals concentration in unexplained infertility.

[26] Franceschi, R.T. (1992). The role of ascorbic acid in mesenchymal differentiation. Nutr. Rev. , 50:65-70

[27] Tsuji, M.; Ito, Y.; Terada, N. and Mori H.(1989). Ovarian aromatase activity in scorbutic mutantrats unable to synthesize ascorbic acid. Acta. Endocrinol. (Copenh) , 121:595-602.

[28] Behrman, H.R.; Kodaman, P.H.; Preston, S.L. and Gao, S.(2001). Oxidative stress and the ovary. J. of the Society for Gynecol. Investigation, 8: S40-42.

[29] Griveau, J.F and Le Lannou, D. (1997). Reactive oxygen species and human spermatozoa: physiology and pathology. Int. J. Androl., 20:61-69.

[30] Ebisch, I.M.; Thomas, C.M.; Peters, W.H.; Braat, D.D. and Steegers-Theunissen, R.P. (2007). The importance of folate, zinc and antioxidants in the pathogenesis and prevention of subfertility. Hum. Reprod. Update, 13:163-174.

[31] Zini, A.; Garrels, K. and Phang, D. (2000). Antioxidant activity in the semen of fertile and infertile men. Urology J.,55:922-6.

[32] Lunec, J. (1990). Review Article, Ann Clin. Biochem., 27:173.

[33] Battino, M.; Ferreiro, M.S.; Galalrdo, I. ; Newman, H.N. and Bullon, P.(2002).The antioxidant capacity of saliva. J. Clin. Periodontol., 29:189-194.

[34] Sugino, N.; Nakata, M. and Kashida, A.(2000). Decreased superoxide dismutase expression and increased concentration of lipid peroxide and prostaglandin F2" in the deciduas of failed pregnancy. Mol. Hum. Reprod., 6(7): 642-647

[35] Urner, F.; and Sakkas, D. (2005). Involvement of the pentose phosphate pathway and redox regulation in fertilization in the mouse. Mol. Reprod. Dev., 70,494-503.

[36] Agarwal, A.; Saleh, R.A. and Bedaiwy, M.A.(2003).Role of reactive oxygen species in the pathophysiology of human reproduction. Fertil. Steril. J., 79: 829-843.

[37] Agarwal, A; Gupta, S.; Malhotra, N.; Sharma, D. and Chandra, A. (2009). Oxidative Stress and its Role in Female

Infertility and Assisted Reproduction: Clinical Implications. International Journal of Fertil. and Steril., 2(4): 147-164.

[38] Zuelke, K.A.; Jeffay, S.C.; Zucker, R.M. and Perreault, S.D.(2003). Glutathione (GSH) concentrations vary with the cell cycle in maturing hamster oocytes, zygotes, and pre-implantation stage embryos. Mol. Reprod. Dev., 64:106-112.

[39] Turton. M. and Luderer. U. (2006). Opposing Effects of Glutathione Depletion and FSH on Reactive Oxygen Species and Apoptosis in Cultured Preovulatory Rat Follicles. Endocrinology, 147:1224-1236.

[40] Ikeda, S.; Kitagawa, M.; Imai, H. and Yamada, M.(2005). The roles of vitamin A for cytoplasmic maturation of bovine oocytes. J. Reprod. Dev., 51:23-35.

[41] Goto, T.; Jones, G.M.; Lolatgis, N.; Pera, M.F.; Trounson ,A.O. and Monk M.(2002).Identification and characterisation of known and novel transcripts expressed during the final stages of human oocyte maturation. Mol. Reprod .Dev., 62:13-28.

[42] Tatemoto, H.; Sakuraim N. and Muto, N.(2000). Protection of porcine oocytes against apoptotic cell death caused by oxidative stress during In vitro maturation: role of cumulus cells. Biology of Reproduction ,63 805-810.

[43] Agarwal, A.; Gupta, S.; Sekhon, L. and Shaha,R.(2008).Redox Considerations in Female Reproductive Function and Assisted Reproduction: From Molecular Mechanisms to Health Implications. Antioxidants and redox signaling J., 10(8):1376-1396

[44] Duleba, A.J.; Foyouzi, N. and Karaca, M.(2004). Proliferation of ovarian theca-interstitial cells is modulated by antioxidants and oxidative stress. Human Reproduction, 19:1519-1524.

[45] Cohen, G.; Dembiec, D. and Marcus, J. (1970). Measurement of catalase activity. Analyt.Biochem., 34 : 30-38.

[46] Paszkowski, T.; Clarke, R. and Hornstein, M. (2002). Smoking induces oxidative stress inside the Graafianfollicle. J. Obstet. Gynecol. Reprod. Biol.,17(4):921-925

[47] Sun, J.G.; Jurisicova, A. and Casper, R.F.(1997). Detection of deoxyribonucleic acid fragmentation in human sperm: correlation with fertilization in vitro.Biol. Reprod., 56:602-607

[48] Cameron, I.T. and Campbell, S. (1998). Nitric oxide in the endometrium. European Society of Hum. Reprod. and Embryology, 4(5):565.

[49] Allaire, C.(2006). Endometriosis and infertility. Reprod. Med. J., 51:164-168.

[50] De Souza, M.J. and Williams, .I. (2004). Physiological Aspects and Clinical Sequelae of Energy Deficiency and Hypoestrogenism in Exercising Women. Human Reproduction Update, 10(5):433-448.

[51] Tarin, J.; Ten, J.; Vendrell, F.J.; de Oliveira, M.N. and Cano, A. (1998). Effects of maternal ageing and dietary antioxidant supplementation on ovulation, fertilisation and embryo development in vitro in the mouse. Reprod. Nutr. Dev. , 38:499-508.

[52] Carbone, M.C.; Tatone, C. and Monache, S.(2003). Antioxidant enzymatic defences in human follicular fluid: characterization and age-dependent changes. Hum. Reprod., 9:639-643.

[53] Yeh, J.; Bowman, M.J.; Browne, R.W. and Chen, N. 2005. Reproductive aging results in a reconfigured ovarian antioxidant defense profile in rats. Fertil. Steril. J.; 84(2):1109-1113.

Section 2

Antioxidant Compounds

Chapter 11

The Role of Lycopene in Chronic Lung Diseases

Emilio Balbuena, Junrui Cheng and Abdulkerim Eroglu

Abstract

Lycopene, a naturally occurring non-provitamin A carotenoid pigment, is responsible for the red to pink colors in tomato, watermelon, red bell peppers, and pink guava. There are many health benefits attributed to lycopene including but not limited to its antioxidant activity. According to the American Lung Association's State of Lung Cancer, lung cancer is still the leading cause of cancer death in the United States. Other chronic lung diseases such as asthma, emphysema, and chronic obstructive pulmonary disease are high prevalence. This chapter summarizes lycopene's protective role against lung diseases in both *in vitro* and *in vivo* studies. While it has been demonstrated that circulating lycopene can be used as a biomarker for several lung diseases, further studies are warranted to establish that. We aim to provide insights into how lycopene can remedy for lung diseases, including lung cancer.

Keywords: lycopene, lung diseases, oxidative stress, lung cancer, antioxidants, carotenoids

1. Introduction

1.1 Lycopene: chemical definition and metabolism

Lycopene, a major dietary carotenoid pigment responsible for the red color, is synthesized by plants and microorganisms [1]. It is mostly found in tomatoes and tomato products, albeit there is a small amount of lycopene in few other fruits, including watermelon, papaya, guava, and pink grapefruit [2]. Lycopene is one of the six most abundant carotenoids (others being α-carotene, β-carotene, β-cryptoxanthin, lutein, and zeaxanthin) in circulation in humans [3]. It has been shown that lycopene exerts cancer-preventive or chemopreventive properties against several cancer types, including prostate, lung, and colon cancers [4].

Lycopene has a chemical formula of $C_{40}H_{56}$, tetraterpene comprised of eight isoprene units that are purely containing carbon and hydrogen [5]. Lycopene can undergo isomerization from *trans* to *cis* by heat, light, and chemical reactions, although the all-*trans* isomeric form is the main isomer in nature [6].

Lycopene can be cleaved via two pathways (**Figure 1**). It can be metabolized by central cleavage, catalyzed by beta-carotene-15,15′-oxygenase (BCO1), yielding apo-15′-lycopenal [7]. It also can be metabolized by eccentric cleavage, catalyzed by beta-carotene-9′,10′-oxygenase (BCO2) yielding apo-10′-lycopenal, which can be either further oxidized into apo-10′-lycopenoic acid or reduced to apo-10′-lycopenol [8]. It has also been shown apo-lycopenals at various chain lengths can also be derived from the absorption of apo-lycopenals directly from food [9].

IntechOpen

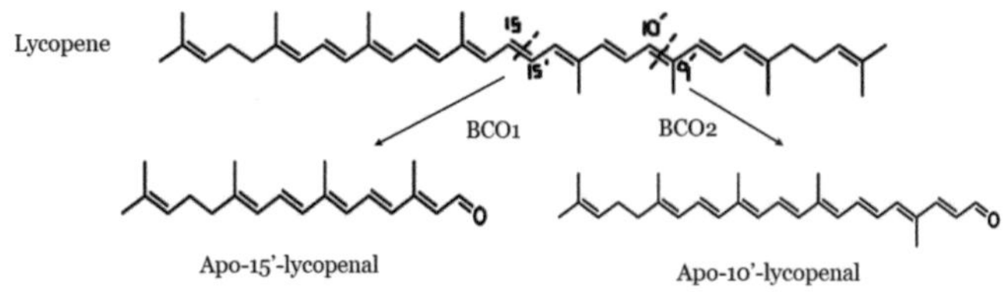

Figure 1.
Central and eccentric cleavage of lycopene. Oxidative cleavage of lycopene at the central 15, 15′ double bond is catalyzed by beta-carotene-15,15′-oxygenase 1 (BCO1) leading to the generation of two molecules of apo-15′-lycopenal [7]. Eccentric cleavage takes place at the 9′-10′ double bond and is catalyzed by beta-carotene-9, 10′-oxygenase 2 (BCO2) yielding apo-10′-lycopenal [8].

1.2 Lycopene: its antioxidant function

Lycopene is a linear, unsaturated hydrocarbon carotenoid with eleven and two unconjugated double bonds, making it highly reactive against oxygen and free radicals [10]. Lycopene displays the highest physical quenching rate constant of singlet oxygen ($k_q = 31 \times 10^9$ M^{-1} s^{-1}) *in vitro*, while rate constants for α-carotene, β-carotene, and lutein were 19, 14, and 8, respectively [10]. Also, lycopene's antioxidant activity in liposomes was found to be greater than α-tocopherol [11]. It is worth highlighting its high quenching rate constant of singlet oxygen because lycopene's concentration in the circulation is 0.7 μM in humans. Lycopene can also scavenge hypochlorous acid, a precursor of free radicals in respiratory stress pathology [12]. It has been documented that tomato products with olive oil increased human plasma antioxidant activity [13]. The authors used the Ferric Reducing Antioxidant Power (FRAP) assay, a quantitative assay for measuring the antioxidant potential, to demonstrate the antioxidant activity of tomato products with olive oil, and it was increased from 930 to 1118 mmol/L [13]. Finally, lycopene could enhance the production of endogenous antioxidant enzymes, e.g., glutathione peroxidase (Gpx), glutathione reductase (GR), and superoxide dismutase (SOD) [14].

1.3 Lycopene: its dietary intake and bioavailability

Although lycopene can be consumed through various sources, processed tomato products (e.g., ketchup, tomato source, tomato juices, tomato extract) are the major dietary lycopene source in the United States [15]. Indeed, the mean lycopene content in these products is more than 90% [16]. The average lycopene intake in the U.S. is 6.6–10.5 mg/day in males and 5.7–10.4 mg/day in females [17].

Dietary lycopene intake amount is not always correlated with circulating lycopene levels because multiple factors can affect its bioavailability. Processed tomato products, for example, contain more lycopene than fresh fruits and vegetable [18]. While the lycopene content in ketchup is 9.9–13.44 mg lycopene/100 g [19], lycopene content in fresh tomatoes ranges from 1.82–11.9 mg/100 g wet weight [20]. Also, lycopene is more bioavailable in processed foods than in raw materials since the transformation of the all-*trans* isomer into the *cis*-isomer renders lycopene elevated solubility in bile acids [21, 22]. Since lycopene is a lipid-soluble compound, a diet with high levels of lipids may increase lycopene bioavailability. It has been shown that the addition of avocado to salad significantly increased lycopene absorption in humans, although the increase of lycopene bioavailability was not correlated with avocado co-consumption in a dose–response manner [23].

There has been growing research interest in genetic variant studies in recent years and the association between genetic variation and lycopene bioavailability.

In a study with 33 subjects, researchers revealed that 72% of the variance in the postprandial plasma lycopene response was explained by 28 single nucleotide polymorphisms (SNPs) in 16 genes [24]. Among these genes, ATP binding cassette subfamily a member 1 (ABCA1), lipoprotein lipase (LPL), insulin-induced gene 2 (INSIG2), solute carrier family 27 member 6 (SLC27A6), lipase C (LIPC), cluster of differentiation 36 molecule (CD36), and apolipoprotein B (APOB) play critical roles in cellular lipid intake and transportation, indicating that the bioavailability of lycopene is likely to depend on lipid metabolism. Another study found that although SNP genotypes were unrelated to usual dietary lycopene intake, two BCO1 SNPs predicted the plasma lycopene changes after subjects were given the same amount of tomato juice [25]. Such finding is intriguing because the activity of BCO1 is lower than BCO2 toward non-provitamin A carotenoids such as lycopene [26], so further studies are warranted to explore the underlying mechanism by which BCO1 SNPs led to different postprandial lycopene response.

Lycopene is widely distributed in various tissues in humans. However, the distribution is uneven, with liver, adipose tissue, testes, adrenal glands, and circulating blood being the major storage pools [27, 28] while lung and kidney have relatively low lycopene concentration [19]. It has been shown that familial resemblances were found in plasma lycopene, indicating that lycopene distribution variance is due to genetic and environmental factors [29]. Cigarette smoke, for example, decreased plasma carotenoid concentrations in humans [30, 31]. A lower serum lycopene concentration was reported in ever-smokers than in never-smokers [32], and lycopene concentration was even substantially lower in smokers who take more than three cigarettes per day [33]. Other factors, including aging, air pollution, and the initiation of diseases such as cardiovascular disease and diabetes, may also deplete lycopene levels due to increased oxidative stress and elevated reactive oxygen species (ROS) [34, 35]. While numerous studies reported the lycopene levels in patients with lung diseases, there is a gap in providing the overall picture. Therefore, our current work aims to shed light on the association between lung diseases and lycopene concentration and how lycopene supplementation affects lung disease initiation/development, offering further research directions.

2. Lycopene and lung diseases

2.1 *In vitro* and *in vivo* evidence

2.1.1 Asthma

Asthma is characterized as the narrowing or blockage of the airways, leading to breathing difficulties like shortness of breath, coughing, or wheezing. The onset of asthma is associated with elevated pulmonary inflammation, which characteristically involves airway infiltration of related inflammatory cells through the activation of Th2-type lymphocytes, eosinophils, and mast cells [36]. A combination of these immunological activities with genetic and environmental factors can lead to the progression of asthma.

To investigate strategies to potentially mitigate the effects of asthma, two *in vivo* studies utilized dietary lycopene supplementation within a murine model induced with this lung condition. These studies involved intraperitoneal (i.p.) injection of ovalbumin (OVA) to induce airway inflammation in BALB/c mice and demonstrated that subsequent lycopene supplementation of 8 and 16 mg/kg body weight (BW)/day alleviated such inflammatory cell infiltration into the bronchoalveolar lavage fluid (BALF) [37] as well as into the lung tissue and blood supply [38].

Lycopene treatment at both of these dosages decreased the expression of eosinophil peroxidase (EPO) and the gelatinolytic activity of matrix metalloproteinase-9 (MMP-9) caused by the i.p. injection of OVA [37]. Lycopene administration at both dosages also inhibited the OVA-specific release of Th2-associated cytokines interleukin-4 (IL-4) and interleukin-5 (IL-5) [37, 38]. The data presented in these studies revealed that dietary lycopene intervention could inhibit the infiltration of inflammatory immunocytes and alleviate asthma's pathogenesis and progression.

2.1.2 COPD and emphysema

Chronic obstructive pulmonary disease (COPD) is a coined term that governs a group of inflammatory lung conditions such as bronchiolitis and emphysema [39]. Bronchiolitis involves fibrosis-related obstruction of small air passages, while emphysema is characteristic of alveolar enlargement and alveolar wall damage. COPD symptoms commonly consist of a chronic cough, shortness of breath, excess phlegm or sputum, and chest tightness [40].

One of COPD's most prevalent risk factors is cigarette smoking, which can be usefully incorporated into *in vivo* studies to investigate potential remedies to alleviate proinflammatory symptoms and this chronic condition's progression. Due to its documented antioxidant capabilities, lycopene treatment can be utilized to reduce the oxidative stress induced by cigarette smoke. A study utilizing a ferret model investigated the efficacy of dietary lycopene stimulation upon both bronchiolitis and emphysema-related aspects of COPD [41]. Through i.p. injection of tobacco carcinogen nicotine-derived nitrosamine ketone (NNK) at 200 mg/kg BW/day and cigarette smoke exposure five days a week for four months, the COPD model was established in ferrets. Lycopene was administered via 10% w/w beadlets at a low dosage of 2.2 mg/kg BW/day and a high dosage of 6.6 mg/kg BW/day over 22 weeks. Following this exposure and treatment period, the findings illustrated that the high dose of lycopene decreased the incidence of NNK/cigarette smoke-induced bronchiolitis and emphysema in ferrets [41].

Tackling the issue of emphysema in particular, two *in vivo* studies investigated the antioxidant/anti-inflammatory efficacy of dietary lycopene supplementation on chronic cigarette smoke exposure alone in murine models. Lycopene administration at 25 and 50 mg/kg BW/day in C57BL/6 mice appeared to alleviate the detrimental effects of chronic cigarette smoke exposure (12 cigarettes/day) over 60 days [42]. Lycopene treatment at both dosages appeared to have improved redox balance and decreased lipid peroxidation and DNA damage; activities of SOD, catalase (CAT), and glutathione (GSH) were increased via lycopene treatment. Lycopene also decreased interleukin-10 (IL-10), tumor necrosis factor-alpha (TNF-α), and interferon-gamma (IFNγ) levels at both dosages. On the other hand, the weight loss that occurred due to the smoke exposure was not recovered by lycopene treatment at either dosage. The same research team had previously conducted a short-term smoke exposure study [43] for just five days, not long enough to establish emphysema, that employed the same dosages of lycopene treatment (25 and 50 mg/kg BW/day). This earlier study described that lycopene administration decreased neutrophil initiation and macrophage influx into the BALF as well as similarly decreased levels of IL-10, TNF-α, and IFNγ at both dosages.

Another *in vivo* study investigated the association of age-related progression with emphysema development within a senescence-accelerated mouse (SAM) model [44]. Utilizing the SAM model that mimics the senile mouse lung, the study aimed to determine if the dietary lycopene supplementation could prevent the onset of emphysema through chronic cigarette smoke exposure (30 min/day, five days/week, for eight weeks). Tomato juice (containing 5 mg of lycopene) administration in place of tap water was shown to have an inhibitory effect on the onset of cigarette smoke-induced emphysema.

Collectively, dietary lycopene supplementation appears to have alleviating effects upon chronic obstructive pulmonary disease, cigarette smoke-induced bronchiolitis, and emphysema due to its potent antioxidant and anti-inflammatory activities.

2.1.3 Acute lung injury

Acute lung injury (ALI) is an acute inflammatory pulmonary disorder that causes endothelial and epithelial barrier disruption, leading to compromised alveolar-capillary membrane integrity [45]. Factors such as lung infection, aspiration, sepsis, trauma, and shock can contribute to ALI's onset. Due to the loss of the alveolar-capillary membrane integrity, further complications characteristic of ALI can involve increased pulmonary edema permeability, increased infiltration of neutrophils, and increased release of pro-inflammatory cytotoxic mediators.

Several *in vivo* studies have been conducted utilizing dietary lycopene supplementation to determine potential treatment in alleviating the damage associated with acute lung injury. One method of generating ALI in these animals was through the administration of lipopolysaccharide (LPS). One study investigated the synergistic protective efficacy of lycopene and matrine, an alkaloid found in kinds of Sophora plants, against LPS-induced ALI compared to the corticosteroid dexamethasone (DEX) in BALB/c mice [46]. Mice were intraperitoneally injected with DEX (5 mg/kg BW), matrine (25 mg/kg BW), lycopene (100 mg/kg BW), or a combination of the matrine + lycopene treatments for seven days before a final dosage of LPS (5 mg/kg BW). Following 6 hours after LPS administration, the combined treatment of matrine and lycopene appeared to have similar beneficial effects. Furthermore, the combined treatment inhibited NF-κB p65 activity and reduced the expression of malondialdehyde (MDA), myeloperoxidase (MPO), interleukin-6 (IL-6), and TNF-α while simultaneously upregulating GSH.

Sarcandra glabra (SG), an herb native to Southeast Asia which is used for treating various oxidative stress diseases, was incorporated within another study in conjunction with lycopene to combat LPS-induced ALI in a rat model [47]. The rats were treated similarly as the other study with supplementation of SG (2.5 mg/kg BW) and lycopene (5 mg/kg BW) individually or in combination for two weeks before LPS (6 mg/kg BW) administration. Like the study involving matrine, the combination of SG and lycopene led to a significant decrease in LPS-induced histopathological injuries, as well as reduced levels of IL-6, TNF-α, NF-κB, and mitogen-activated protein kinase (MAPK). Furthermore, the combination treatment increased anti-oxidative activity and helped reverse the abnormal metabolism back towards normal status. Courtesy of the findings from these studies, lycopene treatment has the potential to alleviate LPS-induced acute lung injury. As lipopolysaccharide is not the only way to induce acute lung injury, other studies have incorporated alternative methods to study lycopene's effect. A study investigated the effects of Redivio® capsules (lycopene in 10% fluid suspension) against oleic acid (OA)-induced ALI in Wistar rats [48]. Over five weeks, the rats were treated with 100 mg/kg BW/day OA and 20 mg/kg BW/day lycopene. Lycopene supplementation decreased neutrophilic infiltration and decreased perivascular and alveolar edema. Lycopene treatment also decreased serum and tissue MDA, serum and tissue SOD, and increased tissue CAT levels; however, there was no effect on serum and tissue Gpx. ALI can additionally be brought on by hyperoxia, which was investigated in a study involving newborn rats that were housed in conditions of normoxia (ambient air) or hyperoxia and supplemented with 50 mg lycopene in olive oil/kg BW/day for 11 days [49]. Despite the expected antioxidant effects of lycopene in these conditions, this treatment did not improve hyperoxia-induced injury as MDA, SOD, and IL-6 levels were not changed; interleukin-1β (IL-1β) and Gpx levels were not affected by hyperoxia or lycopene.

2.1.4 Pulmonary fibrosis

Lung fibrosis, or idiopathic pulmonary fibrosis (IPF), is considered an interstitial lung disease. It involves alveolar epithelial damage and scarring of the lungs due to excess deposition of extracellular matrix by myofibroblasts [50]. The alveolar epithelial degradation is considered an indicative initiating factor of IPF, and the associated damage can lead to interstitial pneumonia. Patients with IPF have a 20% higher risk of developing lung cancer, which can take approximately 2–4 years to reach end-stage respiratory insufficiency [51]. In this case, a treatment regime is quite crucial to shunt this detrimental progression.

Bleomycin (BLM), a polypeptide antitumor agent, can mimic lung fibrosis's pathological effects and can be incorporated within studies to study treatment efficacy. One *in vivo* study utilized this model via intratracheal instillation of BLM (4 mg/mL) in Sprague–Dawley rats to induce IPF [52]. Lycopene extracted from tomatoes was administered over 28 days at a dosage of 5 mg/kg BW/day appeared to alleviate the damage attributed to BLM-induced oxidative stress partially. Such lycopene treatment inhibited the extent of free radical injury, fibrosis, and alveolitis. Furthermore, supplemental lycopene decreased plasma and tissue levels of TNF-α and decreased plasma levels of MDA and nitric oxide (NO). Since lung fibroblasts can contribute to the onset of pulmonary fibrosis, this cell type can be studied within an *in vitro* context to identify methods of regulating their abnormal activity. Two *in vitro* studies capitalized on this cell line type by inducing DNA damage in Chinese lung fibroblasts, V79 cells, through peroxynitrite administration [53] and catechol estrogen [54]. The cells were pre-treated with β-carotene and lycopene at concentrations of 0–5 μM and 0–10 μM 24 hours before the damage. The treatment of these carotenoids decreased the DNA damage in these fibroblast cells by inhibiting single-strand breaks [53, 54] and decreasing the inflammation oxidative stress [53].

2.1.5 Lung cancer

Lung cancer is the leading cause of cancer mortality in the United States, constituting nearly one fourth of all cancer deaths [55]; thus bringing about the need to finding remedies in any way possible. In terms of carotenoid treatment, supplementation of lycopene and its metabolites may demonstrate some anti-cancer efficacy within both *in vitro* and *in vivo* settings by inhibiting carcinoma severity and progression; such a trend has been seen in multiple cell types including prostate, breast, hepatoma, stomach, colon and oral cancer cells [56–58]. In the studies regarding lung cancer, the models typically involve lung cancer cell lines, cigarette smoke exposure, and the administration of carcinogenic agents. As non-small cell lung cancer (NSCLC) accounts for the most lung cancer-related deaths, various *in vitro* studies have utilized cell lines that characterize this cell type. In these cases, lycopene and its metabolites appeared to be a potent inhibitor of cancer cell growth and proliferation [59–62], even more so than either α- carotene or β-carotene [59], by arresting the cell cycle at the G1 checkpoint [62]. In cigarette smoke-induced oxidative stress, the formation of reactive oxygen species (ROS) could lead to damage of cellular macromolecules, notably to genomic DNA that can cause mutations. Like in the case of the Chinese hamster fibroblasts [50], lycopene's antioxidant potential was shown as its capability to quench ROS and upregulate enzymes related to base excision repair, such as DNA glycosylases [63].

Through the classic model of cancer-induction via cigarette smoke exposure *in vivo*, treatment of lycopene at both a low dose (1.1 mg/kg BW/day) and a high dose (4.3 mg/kg BW/day) for nine weeks reduced the extent of lung squamous metaplasia via apoptosis in a ferret model [64]. The apoptosis was attributed to the upregulation of plasma insulin-like growth factor binding protein-3 (IGFBP-3) levels and reduction of the IGF-1/IGFBP-3 ratio.

An alternate method of inducing tumorigenesis in animal models can be achieved through the administration of carcinogenic agents like benzo[a]pyrene (BaP), NNK, and dimethylhydrazine (DMH) [62–64]. An *in vivo* study utilized the DMH method of tumor-induction via subcutaneously injecting 20 mg/kg BW DMH into B6C3F1 mice, the F1 generation of a cross between C57BL/6 J females and C3H/HeJ males [65]. For 32 weeks, the mice were administered with DMH twice a week for five weeks and then lycopene (25 or 50 ppm in drinking water) starting at week 21. After this treatment period, anticancer effects were primarily seen in males as the high lycopene dose (50 ppm) decreased DMH-related tumor development and decreased multiplicities for lung adenomas and carcinomas [65]. Another two *in vivo* studies utilized the treatment of lycopene-enriched tomato oleserin (LTO) in models involving tumorigenesis induction via BaP only [66] or BaP and NNK [67]. In one of those particular studies, a proprietary MutaMouse model consisting of the F1 generation of a cross between BALB/c and DBA/2 mice was injected with 125 mg/kg BaP and treated with LTO (3.7% lycopene) at different doses in their diets (7 and 14 g LTO/kg diet, 0.5 and 1.0 mmol lycopene/kg diet). However, the BaP-induced lung mutagenesis was found to have increased with LTO supplementation, especially at the high dosage [66]. On the other hand, a study incorporating BaP and NNK-induced carcinogenesis into A/J mice investigated the effect of LTO (5.9% lycopene) at different doses in their diets (185 ppm, 1850 ppm, 9260 ppm). In this case, there was no overall effect on the weight gain or survivability of the mice; furthermore, none of the LTO-enriched treatments given before, during, or after BaP and NNK administration had any effect on tumor incidence or multiplicity [67]. The minimal or lack of effect that lycopene has on these carcinogenic agents may indicate that this carotenoid's anticancer efficacy is better suited against cigarette smoke exposure, possibly due to its antioxidant properties.

While lycopene is typically utilized within these carotenoid treatment studies, its metabolites have shown some anticancer efficacy, especially apo-10′-lycopenoic acid. In a joint *in vitro* and *in vivo* study, apo-10′-lycopenoic acid was shown to inhibit cell cycle progression in non-small cell lung cancer (NSCLC) and lung tumor multiplicity in A/J mice [62]. Approaching the *in vitro* aspect, normal human bronchial epithelial cells (NHBE), BEAS-2B-immortalized normal bronchial epithelial cells, and non-small cell lung cancer, A549 cells, were treated with 0–10 μM apo-10′-lycopenoic acid for five days; this treatment regime appeared to have decreased cyclin E and inhibited cell cycle progression from G1 to S phases as seen with lycopene previously [59]. Furthermore, cell cycle mediators (p21 and p27) were increased, indicating promoted mediation of checkpoint regulation.

Lycopene also appears to be involved in tumorigenesis suppression through several pathways, such as inhibiting NF-κB, activating sirtuin-1, or modulating reverse cholesterol transport mechanism by inhibiting 3-hydroxy-3-methylglutaryl–coenzyme A (HMG-CoA) reductase expression [1, 68, 69]. Furthermore, lycopene and its metabolites have been shown to upregulate retinoic acid receptor β (RARβ) activation [63], leading to reduced cell proliferation, increased apoptosis [70], and enhanced gap junction communication (GJC) by upregulating connexin-43 (Cx43) [63, 71].

3. Lycopene and lung diseases in human

To conclude the association between circulating lycopene and lung diseases, we performed a systematic review and meta-analysis by following the PRISMA guideline [72]. We conducted a comprehensive search of the following electronic databases: MEDLINE, Web of Science, EMBASE, and Google Scholar from inception up to November 8, 2020. We employed an integration of Medical Subject Heading (MeSH) terms and/or keywords to article-searching in these databases. The search terms are listed as follows:

("lung diseases"[MeSH Terms (MeSH), title or abstract (ti/ab)] OR (("lung"[MeSH] OR "lung"[All Fields]) AND "cancer*"[MeSH Terms]) OR "pulmonary disease, chronic obstructive"[MeSH, ti/ab] OR "pulmonary disease, chronic obstructive"[MeSH, ti/ab] OR "pulmonary disease, chronic obstructive"[MeSH, ti/ab] OR ("pulmonary emphysema"[MeSH, ti/ab] OR "emphysema"[MeSH, ti/ab]) OR "asthma"[MeSH, ti/ab] OR "acute lung injur*"[MeSH] OR "cystic fibrosis"[MeSH, ti/ab] OR "pulmonary fibrosis"[MeSH, ti/ab]) AND "lycopene"[MeSH, ti/ab].

3.1 Methods

3.1.1 Eligibility

We used these inclusion criteria while carrying out a meta-analysis and systematic review:

- patients with confirmed lung diseases including asthma, acute lung injuries, emphysema, COPD, lung fibrosis, and lung cancer;
- used one of the following study designs: randomized controlled trial (RCT), cohort study, case–control study, nested case–control study, and cross-sectional study;
- reported circulating lycopene level, dietary lycopene intake, dietary consumption of lycopene-enriched foods (e.g., tomato products);
- outcomes related to the incidence or development of lung diseases;
- provided statistical reports

When multiple studies included subjects from the same cohort, only the publication reported the most updated results were selected. *In vitro* studies and animal studies were excluded. Review articles were also excluded.

3.1.2 Data extraction

Data extraction was performed by two independent researchers (J. Cheng, A. Eroglu) by utilizing a structured form. A third investigator (E. Balbuena) would be involved if discrepancies occurred. The following information was collected from eligible studies: study characteristics (author, year of the study, study design, name of the cohort), subject characteristics (a type of lung disease, subject age), treatment information, and primary results, which included means, comparison of the groups, relative ratio (RR)/odds ratio (OR)/hazard ratio (HR), and the measure of variability (95% confidence interval and p-value). For studies that used both univariate analysis and multivariate analysis, only the multivariate analysis results were extracted. A table was constructed (**Table 1**) to summarize the data.

3.1.3 Statistical analysis

We only included the studies that reported OR/RR/HR and 95% confidence interval to perform statistical analysis. Studies that failed to provide such information were excluded from meta-analysis but were still included in our systematic review with detailed information listed in **Table 1**. According to the rare disease assumption, the prevalence of lung diseases is low, and the relative risk approaches the odds ratio [73]. Therefore, we reported all risk estimates in our current meta-analysis as OR for simplicity. With the possibility that the variance between the studies was caused by heterogeneity, the pooled ORs of the risk of lung diseases were estimated using a random-effects model. Two-tailed p-values <0.05 were considered statistically significant. We performed statistical analyses by employing RevMan 5.4.1.

3.2 Results

The process of study selection was displayed in the flow chart (**Figure 2**). The search for the four databases yielded 105 articles, of which 101 were eventually screened (**Figure 2**). Forty-eight articles were included for final screening after we excluded 53 in vitro or animal studies. Among them, 11 articles were excluded with various rationales: the exposure is not lycopene-related (N = 1), outcomes are not related to lung diseases (N = 3), review articles (N = 3), full text unavailable (N = 1), or studies that used the same cohort (N = 4) which led to 37 papers included in this systematic review (**Figure 2**).

3.2.1 Asthma

A total of 13 articles reported the relation between asthma and lycopene concentration, or dietary lycopene intake [74–86]. Among them, 9 studies are observational studies: cross-sectional (N = 1), nested case–control (N = 1), or case–control studies (N = 7) [74–82], whereas other studies are randomized clinical trials (RCTs) [83–86].

In total, eight case–control (including nested case–control) studies included 1,280 current asthma patients and explored circulating lycopene levels in cases versus matched controls. Additionally, one cross-sectional study with 218 subjects reported the association between serum lycopene concentration and asthma severity [77]. In four studies, a significantly lower circulating lycopene concentration was observed in cases than in healthy controls [76–79]. Nevertheless, other case–control studies reported similar circulating lycopene levels in asthma patients than the matched control group, indicating that the risk of asthma was unrelated to circulating lycopene levels [74, 75, 81, 82]. Such discrepancy might be due to the heterogeneity of disease characteristics. Wood et al. showed a trend of higher plasma lycopene concentration in asthma patients with airway hyper-responsiveness [80]. It was also reported that plasma lycopene concentration was higher in atopic asthma subjects than in non-atopic asthma subjects [76]. Therefore, a high proportion of hyper-responsive asthma patients or atopic asthma patients may decrease the probability of observing a significant difference.

Two studies reported the correlation between circulating lycopene concentration and the severity of asthma. Forced expiratory volume in one second (FEV1) is defined as the volume of breath exhaled during a forced breath within one second.

Author, Year	Lung disease	Study Design	Subject (N*)	Age (mean,yr)*	Treatment	Duration	Results
Rohan, 2002	Lung cancer	Nested case–control	196	40–59	NA	8	Lycopene intake was unrelated to lung cancer risk (RR = 1.04, 95% CI: 0.61–1.76, P trend = 0.233)
Sackesen, 2008	Asthma	Case–control	164	9.65 ± 1.55	NA	NA	• Plasma lycopene concentration was higher in children with atopic asthma vs. non-atopic asthma (0.46 ± 0.2 μmoL/L vs. 0.45 ± 0.2 μmoL/L, P = 0.027) • Plasma lycopene concentration was lower in cases vs. controls (P < 0.001)
Voorrips, 2000	Lung cancer	Nested case–control	939	55–69	NA	6.3 years	• Lycopene intake was lower in cases than in controls (983 ± 1517 μg/d vs. 1050 ± 1560 μg/d, P = NR) • A lower lycopene intake was correlated with higher lung cancer risk (RR = 1.12, 95% CI: 0.77–1.71, P trend = 0.04). However, after adjusted for folate intake, the correlation was not statistically significant (RR = 1.05, 95% CI: 0.75–1.46, P trend = 0.14)
Wood, 2005	Asthma	Case–control	15	48.4 ± 4.3	NA	NA	• Cases had a lower lycopene level vs. controls in whole blood (29 ug/L vs. 247 ug/L P 0.05) or whole sputum (31 ug/L vs. 9 ug/L, P > 0.05) • Daily lycopene intake was similar in cases vs. controls (3.90 mg/d vs. 2.51 mg/d, P > 0.05)
Kodama, 2015	Asthma-COPD overlap syndrome Bronchial asthma	Case–control	• 39 COPD patients • 21 patients with ACOS (asthma-COPD overlap syndrome) • 15 patients with BA (bronchial asthma)	• 72.7 ± 6.9 (COPD) • 66.8 ± 8.4 (ACOS) • 56.4 ± 13.7 (BA)	NA	NA	• Plasma lycopene concentration was lower in COPD subjects vs. controls (P 0.05) • Plasma was lycopene concentration similar in ACOS subjects vs. healthy controls (P > 0.05) • Plasma lycopene concentration was similar in BA subjects vs. healthy controls (P > 0.05)
Schock, 2003	Asthma	Case–control	78	7.2 ± 3.3	NA	NA	Lycopene concentration in the BAL was similar between cases vs. controls (0.146 μmoL/L vs. 0.156 μmoL/L, P = 0.33)

Author, Year	Lung disease	Study Design	Subject (N*)	Age (mean,yr)*	Treatment	Duration	Results
Ochs-Balcom, 2006	Asthma COPD	Cross-sectional	• 68 asthma patients • 121 COPD patients • 29 asthma and COPD patients	61.7 ± 10.3	NA	NA	• Serum lycopene was positively associated with %FVC (P 0.05) • Dietary lycopene intake was positively associated with %FEV1 and %FEV1/FVC (P 0.05)
Jun, 2020	Pulmonary function	Cross-sectional	15,792	54.1 ± NR	NA	NA	• Lycopene dietary intake was not correlated with FEV1/FVC ratio (P = 0.283) • The consumption of lycopene & lutein/zeaxanthin foods were not correlated with FEV1/FVC ratio (P = 0.518)
Ford, 2014	COPD	Prospective study	1,492	55.7 ± 0.7	NA	14 years	• Serum lycopene concentration was similar in cases vs. controls (0.41 ± 0.03 μmoL/L vs. 0.46 ± 0.01 μmoL/L, P = 0.120) • A higher serum lycopene concentration was correlated with a lower all-cause mortality among adults with obstructive lung function (HR = 0.80, 95% CI: 0.67–0.95, P = 0.013)
Ito, 2005	Lung cancer	Prospective study	3,182	39–79	NA	10.5 years	• Serum lycopene concentration was lower in lung cancer deaths vs. the survivors (0.229 ± NR μmoL/L vs. 0.328 ± NR μmoL/L, P = 0.007) • Serum lycopene concentration was unrelated to lung cancer mortality (HR = 0.93, 95% CI: 0.39–2.24, P trend = 0.76)
Stefani, 1993	Lung cancer	Case–control	541	30–89	NA	NA	• Lycopene intake was similar in cases vs. controls (1603.4 ± 1416 μg/d vs. 1666.6 ± 1439 μg/d, P = 0.47) • Dietary lycopene intake was unrelated to lung cancer risk (OR = 0.83, 95% CI: 0.56–1.21, P trend = 0.18) • A higher dietary tomato intake frequency was correlated with lower lung cancer risk (OR = 0.76, 95% CI: 0.55–1.07, P trend = 0.09)

Author, Year	Lung disease	Study Design	Subject (N*)	Age (mean,yr)*	Treatment	Duration	Results
Holick, 2002	Lung cancer	Prospective study	27,084	57.2	NA	14 years	• A higher dietary lycopene intake was correlated with lower lung cancer risk (Age-adjusted: RR = 0.63, CI 0.54–0.75, P trend <0.0001; Multivariate: RR = 0.72, 95% CI: 0.61–0.84, P trend <0.0001) • In subgroup analysis, a higher lycopene intake was correlated with lower lung cancer risk in subjects who took 5–19 cigarettes (RR = 0.65, 95% CI: 0.49–0.87, P for trend = 0.01), 20–29 cigarettes (RR = 0.81, 95% CI: 0.64–1.02, P for trend = 0.009), ≥30 cigarettes (RR = 0.63, 95% CI: 0.45–0.88, P for trend = 0.008)
Yuan, 2003	Lung cancer	Prospective study	63,257	63 ± NR	NA	8 years	Lycopene dietary intake was unrelated to lung cancer risk (RR = 0.89, 95% CI: NR, P trend: NR)
Asbaghi, 2015	Lung cancer	Case–control	55	NR	NA	NA	• Daily lycopene intake was lower in cases than in controls (P = 0.001) • Serum lycopene concentration was lower in cases than in controls (P = 0.004)
Talwar, 1997	Lung cancer	Case–control	22	66	NA	NA	Plasma lycopene concentration was lower in cases than in controls (<0.02 ± NR μmoL/L vs. 0.37 ± NR μmoL/L, P < 0.001)
Falk, 2005	Asthma	RCT	19	13.0 ± 2.15	Placebo Lycopene (30 mg/d)	1 week	Lycopene supplementation did not change FVC, predicted %FVC, FEV1, predicted %FEV1, PEF1, predicted %PEF1, FEF25–75, or predicted %FEF25–75 (P values were NR) among subjects who had exercise-induced asthma
Garcia-Closas, 1998	Lung cancer	Case–control	103	63	NA	NA	Dietary lycopene intake was unrelated to lung cancer risk (OR = 0.56, 95% CI: 0.26–1.24, P trend = 0.15)
Michaud, 2000	Lung cancer	Prospective study	46,924 men 77,283 women	NR	NA	10 years (men) 12 years (women)	• Lycopene intake was unrelated to lung cancer in males (RR = 0.86, 95% CI: 0.59–1.25, P = 0.51) or females (RR = 0.80, 95% CI: 0.64–0.99, P = 0.10) • In lag analysis, lycopene intake was not correlated with lung cancer risk (0–4-y lag: RR = 0.93, 95% CI: 0.76–1.15; 8–12-y lag: RR = 0.87, 95% CI: 0.61–1.24), except for in 4–8-y lag (RR = 0.68, 95% CI: 0.53–0.88)

Author, Year	Lung disease	Study Design	Subject (N*)	Age (mean,yr)*	Treatment	Duration	Results
Shareck, 2017	Lung cancer	Case–control	1,105	64.3 ± 7.8	NA	NA	Dietary lycopene intake was lower in cases vs. control (male: 15,888 ± 10,878 vs. 16,969 ± 9,285, P: NR; female: 11,911 ± 11,902 vs. 16,175 ± 10,985, P: NR) A higher lycopene intake was correlated with a lower lung cancer risk (OR = 0.75, 95% CI: 0.59–0.95, P = 0.03)
Satia, 2009	Lung cancer	Prospective study	521	67.0 ± 6.8	NA	3 years	• Lycopene supplementation frequency was similar between total lung cancer cases vs. controls (multivitamin use: HR = 1.06, CI 0.86–1.30; individual supplement use: HR = 0.98, 95% CI: 0.25–3.96, P trend = 0.61) • Lycopene supplementation frequency was similar between NSCLC cases vs. controls (multivitamin use: HR = 1.14, 95% CI: 0.90–1.44; individual supplement use: HR = 1.32, CI 0.33–5.30, P trend = 0.25) • Lycopene supplementation frequency was similar between SCLC cases vs. controls (multivitamin use: HR = 0.97, 95% CI: 0.55–1.71; individual supplement use data NR, P trend = 0.81) • Lycopene supplementation frequency was similar between other lung cancer cases vs. controls (multivitamin use: HR = 0.67, 95% CI: 0.33–1.37; individual supplement use data NR, P trend = 0.24)
Ito, 2005	Lung cancer	Nested case–control	211	40–79	NA	10 years	• In male, serum lycopene concentration was lower in cases vs. controls (0.06 μmoL/L vs. 0.07 μmoL/L, Univariate model: P = 0.025; Multivariate model: P = 0.032) • In female, serum lycopene concentration was similar in cases vs. controls (0.10 μmoL/L vs. 0.412 μmoL/L, Univariate model: P = 0.20; Multivariate model: P = 0.33) • In male, a higher serum lycopene concentration was correlated with a lower lung cancer risk (OR = 0.44, CI 0.19–1.05, P trend = 0.03) • In female, serum lycopene concentration was unrelated to lung cancer risk (OR = 0.82, CI 0.12–3.25, P trend = 0.5)

Author, Year	Lung disease	Study Design	Subject (N*)	Age (mean,yr)*	Treatment	Duration	Results
Wood, 2008	Asthma	Randomized, cross-over trial	32	52.1 ± 2.4	Low antioxidant diet then placebo, or tomato extract (45 mg lycopene/day), or tomato juice (45 mg lycopene/day)	• 10 days of low antioxidant diet • 7 days for each treatment • 10 days for each washout	• Low antioxidant diet: ↓ predicted %FEV1 (P = 0.004), %FVC (P = 0.0032), asthma control score (P = 0.0035), sputum %neutrophils (P = 0.038), %macrophages (P = 0.06); unchanged biomarkers including FEV1/FVC (P = 0.407), sputum PD15 (P = 0.838), total cell count (P = 0.401), %eosinophils (P = 0.894), exhaled nitric oxide (P = 0.975), and neutrophil elastase (P = 0.961) • Tomato juice supplementation ↓ sputum %neutrophils (P 0.05) • Tomato extract supplementation ↓ sputum %neutrophils (P < 0.05) and neutrophil elastase activity (P < 0.05)
Wood, 2012	Asthma	RCT	137	High-antioxidant diet (54 ± 14) Low-antioxidant diet (58 ± 14)	Low-antioxidant diet (<=2 servings of vegetables and 1 serving of fruit/day), then placebo or lycopene (45 mg/d)	14 weeks or until an exacerbation occurred	• Tomato extract supplementation ↓ plasma CRP (P = 0.010), IL-6 (P = 0.093), TNF-a (P = 0.070) • Tomato extract supplementation did not change %FEV1 (P = 0.948), %FVC (P = 0.534), %FEV1/%FVC (P = 0.918), DRS (P = 0.954), ACQ (P = 0.597), exhaled NO (P = 0.296), sputum %eosinophils (P = 0.299), eosinophil count (P = 0.384), IL-8 (P = 0.874), NE (P = 0.968), or 8-isoprostane (P = 0.720)
Larkin, 2015	Asthma	Nested case–control	150	52.5 ± 8.7	NA	8 years	• Plasma lycopene concentration was similar in cases vs. controls (6.8 mg/dl vs. 6.7 mg/dl, P = 0.79) • Plasma lycopene concentration was not correlated with asthma risk (OR = 0.9w6; 95% CI, 0.84–1.11)
Kentson, 2018	COPD	Case–control	66	70 ± NR	NA	NA	• Plasma lycopene concentration was similar between cases vs. controls (0.41 ± 0.20 µmoL/L vs. 0.48 ± 0.21 µmoL/L, P > 0.05) • Plasma lycopene concentration was positively correlated with blood oxygenation saturation in the COPD patients (P < 0.05)

DOI: http://dx.doi.org/10.5772/intechopen.95468

Author, Year	Lung disease	Study Design	Subject (N*)	Age (mean,yr)*	Treatment	Duration	Results
Riccioni, 2007	Asthma	Case–control	40	37.1 ± 12.5	NA	NA	• Tomato intake was similar in the cases vs. controls (raw tomatoes: 18.1 g vs. 16.8 g, $P > 0.05$) • Serum lycopene was lower in cases vs. controls (0.10 ± 0.7 μmoL/L vs. 0.16 ± 0.8 μmoL/L, $P < 0.001$)
Riccioni, 2006	Asthma	Case–control	22	35.1 ± 11.7	NA	NA	Plasma lycopene concentration was lower in asthma patients vs. controls (8.12 ± 2.63 lg/dl vs. 18.13 ± 3.67 lg/dl, $P < 0.001$)
Yuan, 2001	Lung cancer	Nested case–control	209	64.8 ± NR	NA	12 years	• Serum lycopene concentration was lower in ever-smokers than in never-smokers ($P = 0.0002$) • A higher serum lycopene concentration was correlated with lower lung cancer risk in all subjects (OR = 0.46, 95% CI: 0.27–0.79, P trend = 0.003), but the adjusted OR was not statistically significant (OR = 0.15, 95% CI: 0.31–1.14, $P = 0.15$)
Wood, 2010	Asthma	Case–control	41	49 ± 3.4	NA	NA	• There was a trend of higher plasma lycopene concentration in hyper-responsive asthma patients vs. non-hyper-responsive asthma patients (0.115 ± 0.45 mg/L vs. 0.084 ± NR mg/L, $P = 0.098$) • Plasma lycopene concentration was similar in patients with asthma controlled or partly controlled vs. uncontrolled (0.10 mg/L vs. 0.08 mg/L, $P = 0.581$) • Plasma lycopene concentration was similar in patients with mild–moderate asthma vs. severe asthma (0.10 mg/L vs. 0.09 mg/L, $P = 0.862$)
Neuman, 2000	Asthma	RCT	20	23 ± 9	Placebo Lycopene (30 mg/d)	1 week	Lycopene supplementation increased forced expiratory volume in 1 s among patients who had exercise-induced asthma ($P < 0.05$)

Author, Year	Lung disease	Study Design	Subject (N*)	Age (mean,yr)*	Treatment	Duration	Results
Ford, 2004	Asthma	Case–control	• 771 current asthma • 352 former asthma	• 44.8 ± 0.7 (current asthma) • 44.2 ± 1.0 (former asthma)	NA	NA	• Plasma lycopene concentration was similar between current asthma patients vs. controls (0.44 ± 0.01 μmoL/L vs. 0.44 ± 0.00 μmoL/L) • Plasma lycopene concentration was similar between former asthma patients vs. controls (0.47 ± 0.04 μmoL/L vs. 0.44 ± 0.00 μmoL/L)
Klarod, 2011	Lung cancer	Case–control	49	58.8 ± NR	NA	NA	• Serum lycopene concentration was lower in total cases than in controls ($P < 0.001$) • Serum lycopene concentration was lower in both early stage patients ($P = 0.09$) and advanced stage patients ($P = 0.001$) than in controls. • Serum lycopene concentration was similar in early stage patients vs. advanced stage patients ($P = 0.749$)
Comstock, 2008	Lung cancer	Nested case–control	258	25–65	NA	15 years (CLUE I) 3 years (CLUE II)	• Serum lycopene concentration was similar in cases vs. controls ($P = 0.76$) • Serum lycopene concentration was unrelated to lung cancer risk (OR = 1.01, 95% CI: NR, P trend = 0.99) • In subgroup analysis, serum lycopene concentration was unrelated to lung cancer risk (Male: OR = 0.32, 95% CI: NR, P trend = 0.25; Female: OR = 0.83, CI NR, P trend = 0.83)
Marchand, 1989	Lung cancer	Case–control	332	NR	NA	NA	• A lower tomato (including tomato juice) intake was correlated with higher lung cancer risk in males (OR = 2.3, 95% CI: NR, P trend = 0.002) and females (OR = 3.7, 95% CI: NR, P trend <0.001)
Steinmetz, 1993	Lung cancer	Nested case–control	138	55–69	NA	4 years	• The consumption of the 'high-lycopene' foods was unrelated to lung cancer risk (OR = 1.21, 95% CI: 0.69–2.10, P trend = 0.53) • Tomato consumption was unrelated to lung cancer risk (OR = 1.00, 95% CI: 0.61–1.64. P trend = 0.99)

Author, Year	Lung disease	Study Design	Subject (N*)	Age (mean,yr)*	Treatment	Duration	Results
Schut, 1997	Lung cancer	Case–control	19	NR	NA	NA	Serum lycopene concentration was lower in lung cancer patients vs. controls (0.13 ± 0.10 μmoL/L vs. 0.42 ± 0.41 μmoL/L, $P < 0.01$)
Kawchak, 1999	Cystic fibrosis	Nested case–control	24	NR	Standard nutrition care and vitamin supplements that included 5,000 IU retinol	3 years	At the baseline, serum lycopene concentration was lower in cases vs. controls (0.05 ± 0.05 μmoL/L vs. NR, range 0.15–0.39 μmoL/L, P 0.05).

**Significance values presented individually in each study's result column.*

Table 1.
A table was constructed to summarize the data of clinical trials including study characteristics (author, year of the study, study design, name of the cohort), subject characteristics (a type of lung disease, subject age), treatment information, and primary results.

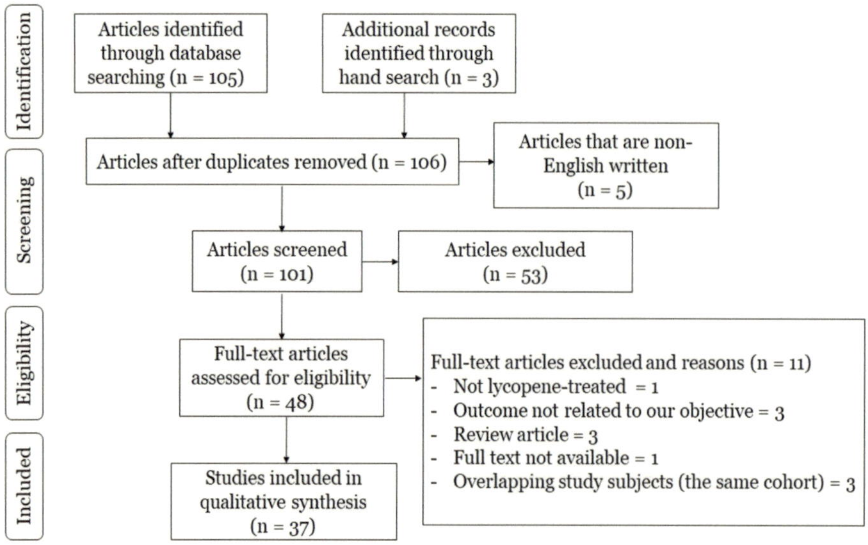

Figure 2.
Flow diagram of study selection according to the PRISMA guideline.

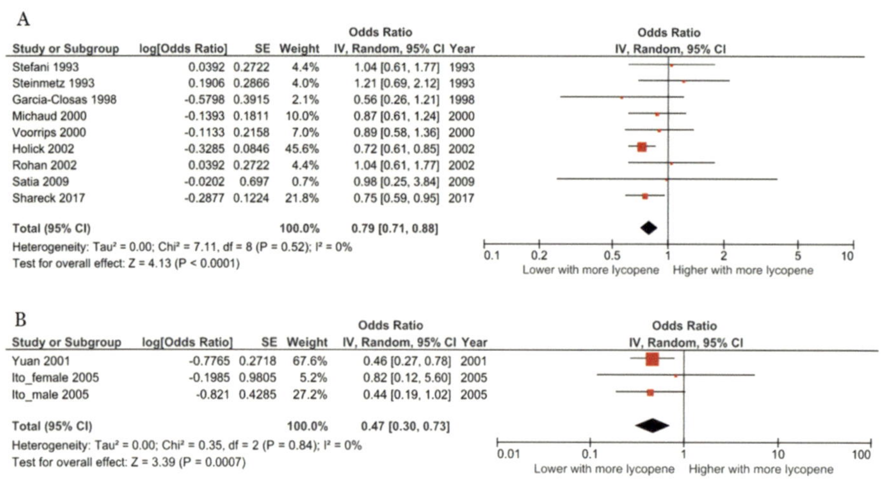

Figure 3.
Forest plots for lung cancer risk in (A) subjects with lower lycopene intake vs. subjects with higher lycopene intake, and (B) subjects with lower circulating lycopene levels vs. subjects with higher circulating lycopene levels.

Forced vital capacity (FVC) is the full air exhaled in the entire timeframe [87]. A low percentage predicted FEV1/FVC ratio is an indicator of reduced pulmonary function. Ochs-Balcom et al. reported a lack of association between serum lycopene concentration and %FEV1/FVC ratio in 22 asthma cases, indicating that circulating lycopene concentration is not correlated with pulmonary function [77]. Similarly, Wood et al. depicted that plasma lycopene concentration was similar in moderate asthma patients than patients with severe asthma [80]. Also, no difference was found in plasma lycopene levels between asthma controlled or partly controlled patients vs. uncontrolled patients [80], indicating that circulating lycopene levels are unrelated to asthma development.

Four RCTs supplemented asthma patients with lycopene or lycopene-enriched foods to investigate the effect of dietary lycopene on asthma [83–86]. They examined their pulmonary function at the end of the study [83–86]. Two studies addressed exercise-induced asthma, where researchers gave asthma patients lycopene at a dosage of 30 mg/d for one week [80, 81]. Although one study found that lycopene supplementation increased %FEV1 [83], Falk et al. failed to observe any significant differences in pulmonary function indicators between patients with lycopene supplementation and the placebo group [84]. Such inconsistency may have resulted from the inadequate intensity of the exercise challenge in the study. In the study by Falk et al., the participants performed an eight-minute treadmill exercise at a load of 85% of the predicted maximal heart rate [84]. Such intensity may not be strenuous enough to induce exercise-induced bronchoconstriction, especially in physically active people [88]. Also, only 19 subjects were included in the trial, leading to a loss of power. Therefore, additional studies with larger samples size and higher exercise challenges are warranted to examine the effect of lycopene supplementation on exercise-induced asthma.

With a growing interest in investigating the synergistic effect of various antioxidants on lung diseases, Wood et al. provided the subjects with a 10-day low antioxidant diet, followed by either placebo or tomato extract (or tomato juice) supplementation that contains 45-mg lycopene for another ten days [85]. As a result, the low antioxidant diet significantly increased sputum neutrophils, decreased with tomato juice or tomato extract supplementation [85]. Furthermore, a reduced level of sputum neutrophil elastase activity was found in patients supplemented with tomato extract [85]. The neutrophil elastase released by neutrophils is a serine proteinase that may act as a biomarker of inflammation and pathogen invasion [89]. Since this enzyme is involved in lung tissue destruction, by inhibiting neutrophil elastase activity, tomato extract supplementation may hinder pulmonary inflammation, subsequently mitigate the swell of the airways and decrease mucus production [90], leading to alleviated asthma manifestations. Indeed, in a follow-up study with 137 subjects, Wood et al. portrayed decreased levels of plasma C-reactive protein (CRP), IL-6, and IL-1β in the asthma patients who consumed tomato extract that contains 45 mg/d lycopene [86]. Intriguingly, the repeated-measures analysis by time point showed a reduced risk of disease exacerbation in the patients with tomato extract supplementation compared to the placebo group. Additionally, the decrease of %FEV1 and %FVC from baseline was only observed in the placebo group, but not in the tomato extract-supplemented group [86].

Collectively, the results generated from these clinical trials did not show a consistent association between circulating lycopene and the initiation or development of asthma. Besides, there is a lack of evidence that dietary lycopene supplementation alleviating asthma progression. Whole foods that contain a high concentration of lycopene, such as tomato extract, showed beneficial efficacies against asthma. However, both RCTs subjects had a low-antioxidant diet at baseline to deplete their antioxidant levels, meaning that a similar alleviating effect may not be observed in people with normal circulating antioxidant concentrations. It is also important to note that tomato extract and tomato juice are high in lycopene and other antioxidants, such as ascorbic acid or β-carotene. Thus, lycopene itself may lack the capability of mitigating asthma. It should be noted that the combination of lycopene with other antioxidants produces a synergistic effect that can further inhibit pulmonary inflammation and lessen asthma manifestations.

3.2.2 COPD

Both asthma and COPD cause swelling in the airways and difficulties to breathe [91]. Several studies focused on tackling COPD and asthma-COPD overlap syndrome (ACOS) due to the similarities between the two diseases.

At the end of article screening, two case–control studies, one cross-sectional study, and one prospective study depicted the association between circulating lycopene concentration and COPD [75, 77, 81, 92]. Overall, 105 COPD patients and 21 ACOS patients were included in the case–control studies [77, 81], whereas the cross-sectional study included 218 subjects (68 asthma patients, 121 COPD patients, and 29 ACOS patients). The prospective study used the data from the Third National Health and Nutrition Examination Survey (NHANES III), recruiting 1,492 COPD patients [75].

In one case–control study, Kodama et al. reported a significantly lower plasma lycopene concentration in the COPD subjects than the healthy controls [81]. However, such an association was not observed in the ACOS subjects [81]. Interestingly, another case–control study did not find any differences in plasma lycopene levels between the COPD patients and the controls [92]. However, they demonstrated a positive correlation between plasma lycopene concentration and blood oxygenation saturation in COPD patients [92], indicating that circulating lycopene concentration may be related to COPD severity. Similarly, the cross-sectional study conducted by Ochs-Balcom et al. also reported that serum lycopene concentration was positively associated with %FVC, but not %FEV1 or %FEV1/FVC ratio [77]. In 2014, Ford et al. reported that although the COPD patients and the healthy controls appeared to have similar serum lycopene levels, they observed an inverse correlation between serum lycopene concentration and all-cause mortality among people with obstructive lung function [75]. With a large sample size and prospective study design, these findings highlighted the possibility that serum lycopene concentration could be a potential biomarker predicting COPD's development and prognosis.

3.2.3 Lung cancer

In total, 19 studies met our inclusion criteria and provided information on lycopene and lung cancer [32, 93–110]. Among them, there are 8 case–control studies that included 2,226 lung cancer patients [93, 95, 99, 100, 104, 105, 107, 110], 6 nested case–control studies that included 1,951 lung cancer cases [32, 94, 98, 102, 106, 108], and 5 prospective studies that included 218,251 subjects [96, 97, 101, 103, 109].

Among the studies that reported the association between lycopene intake and lung cancer risk, nine studies provided detailed study estimates [95, 96, 101–106, 108] (**Figure 3A**). Our meta-analysis results showed that the meta-OR of lung cancer with a higher dietary lycopene intake was 0.79 (95% CI: 0.71–0.88, overall $P < 0.0001$). The p-value of the Chi-squared (Chi^2) test is 0.52, and the between-study variance (I2) for lung cancer incidence is 0%, meaning that there was a minimum of heterogeneity in the studies. Two case–control studies found that lycopene or lycopene-enriched tomato juice's daily consumption was lower in lung cancer cases than in healthy controls [93]. In contrast, the Singapore Chinese Health Study failed to observe a significant correlation between lycopene dietary intake and lung cancer risk [109]. Multiple factors may contribute to the non-significant findings. In the case–control studies, studies that used the Food Frequency Questionnaire (FFQ) to collect lycopene intake frequencies may undergo recall bias, which led to a loss of power. It is also likely to observe a significant difference in lycopene consumption between cases and controls by including subjects who had a low baseline circulating lycopene level or dietary lycopene intake. Rohan et al. observed significantly different lycopene intake between the cases and the controls when the subjects' daily lycopene intake was between 983 μg to 1,050 μg [102]. However, by including the subjects who reported a baseline daily dietary lycopene intake at 15.8 mg to 16.9 mg, which is about twice the amount of average daily lycopene intake in the U.S. [17], Shareck et al. found the dietary lycopene intake was comparable between the cases and the controls [104].

Three case–control studies [93, 99, 107] and three nested case–control studies [32, 94, 97] reported the association between circulating lycopene concentration and lung cancer risk. Two studies provided estimates [32, 98], thus were included in the meta-analysis. Since Ito et al. only reported the estimates in the male and female subgroups [98], we pooled the two subgroups and another study [32] to explore the relationship between circulating lycopene concentration and lung cancer risk by performing the meta-analysis. Our results showed that the meta-odds ratio of lung cancer with a higher circulating lycopene level was 0.47 (95% CI: 0.30–0.73, overall $P = 0.0007$), with the Chi^2 p-value at 0.84, and the I2 at 0% (**Figure 3B**). Such data indicates that a higher circulating level of lycopene is correlated with a lower risk of lung cancer. Intriguingly, the other three studies that were not included in the meta-analysis consistently showed that lung cancer cases had a significantly lower circulating lycopene concentration than the healthy controls [93, 99, 110]. Only one study reported a similar lycopene concentration in lung cancer subjects and the controls [94]. One possible explanation for this negative result is that Comstock et al. did not stratify the subjects according to the stage of lung cancer. Although serum lycopene concentration was comparable in the early stage patients and the advanced stage patients, serum lycopene concentration was more significant between the advanced lung cancer patients and the healthy controls [99]. If the majority of the patients included by Klarod et al. were cancer patients at an early stage, the difference of circulating lycopene level between the cases and the controls would be unapparent. One prospective study showed that serum lycopene concentration was lower in the lung cancer deaths than in the cancer survivors; however, such difference disappeared after the researchers adjusted the model for sex, age, smoking habit, and serum levels of total cholesterol and alanine aminotransferase (ALT) activity [97] suggesting that the association between lycopene and lung cancer mortality might be influenced by multiple factors, which warrants further investigation.

In conclusion, we found consistent reports showing that dietary lycopene intake, or the consumption of lycopene-enriched foods, was inversely related to lung cancer risk. Our systematic review and meta-analysis showed that the circulating lycopene level might be a potential biomarker predicting lung cancer risk.

4. Concluding remarks

We summarized the association between circulating lycopene and chronic lung diseases in a comprehensive manner. To accomplish this task, we first have screened both *in vitro* reports and *in vivo* animal models to delineate lycopene's role in chronic lung diseases including asthma, COPD, emphysema, acute lung injury, pulmonary fibrosis, and lung cancer. Dietary lycopene intervention could potentially decrease the infiltration of pro-inflammatory cytokines in ovalbumin-induced airway inflammation in a murine model of asthma [37, 38]. Lycopene was also found to inhibit smoke-induced bronchitis and emphysema through reverse cholesterol transport in the COPD model in ferrets [41]. In a murine model (C57BL/6 mice) for emphysema, lycopene administration lessened the detrimental effects of chronic cigarette smoke exposure [42]. Lycopene treatment was found to ease LPS-induced acute lung injury (ALI) in murine animal models [46], BALB/c mice, and LPS-induced ALI in a rat model [47]. Lycopene extracted from tomatoes could reduce the burden of lung fibrosis's pathological effects in a rodent study [52]. In terms of lung cancer, lycopene could decrease the extent of squamous metaplasia in a ferret model using the conventional method of induction of lung cancer by cigarette smoke [64]. Alternative models using carcinogenic agents were not definitive in showing its chemoprevention capabilities [62–67].

Next, we conducted a systematic review and meta-analysis to reveal the link between lycopene concentration and lung diseases in clinical trials using multiple electronic databases. While several case–control studies reported markedly lower lycopene concentration in asthma patients [76–79], others found that asthma progression was not related to lycopene in the circulation [74, 75, 77, 80–82], suggesting that the association between asthma and lycopene concentrations in humans was not conclusive. We came across several epidemiological studies, including case–control, cross-sectional, and prospective studies, to demonstrate the association between lycopene concentration in the circulation and COPD in our meta-analysis. These trials reported similar lycopene concentrations in healthy subjects vs. COPD patients [75, 77, 81, 92]. Finally, we found that dietary lycopene is inversely associated with lung cancer risk, particularly in subjects with low lycopene in their circulation [93, 102, 104]. Furthermore, circulating lycopene displayed a significant association between advanced lung cancer patients and early-stage patients [99].

5. Future perspective

Overall, our comprehensive review in this chapter provides convincing evidence on the role of lycopene in chronic lung diseases including lung cancer. This chapter also contributes confirmatory data to the as yet unsettled proof on the hypothesized associations between lycopene in circulation and lung diseases. The health benefits of lycopene can be attributed to its antioxidant function as highlighted in this chapter. Lycopene can be used as a preventive and therapeutic compound by itself or in combination with other compounds to improve lung diseases. Further investigations and well-designed clinical trials are needed to confirm whether there is a casual relation between the disease and the circulating lycopene in humans.

Acknowledgements

The authors gratefully *acknowledge* the financial support of North Carolina State University. We also thank Baxter Miller for searching the research literature.

Abbreviations

FRAP	Ferric Reducing Antioxidant Power
Gpx	glutathione peroxidase
GR	glutathione reductase
SOD	superoxide dismutase
SNPs	single nucleotide polymorphisms
ABCA1	ATP binding cassette subfamily a member 1
LPL	lipoprotein lipase
INSIG2	insulin-induced gene 2
SLC27A6	solute carrier family 27 member 6
LIPC	lipase C
CD36	cluster of differentiation 36 molecule
APOB	apolipoprotein B

ROS	reactive oxygen species
i.p.	intraperitoneal
OVA	ovalbumin
BW	body weight
BALF	bronchoalveolar lavage fluid
EPO	eosinophil peroxidase
MMP-9	matrix metalloproteinase-9
IL-4	interleukin-4
IL-5	interleukin-5
COPD	Chronic obstructive pulmonary disease
NNK	nicotine-derived nitrosamine ketone
CAT	catalase
GSH	glutathione
IL-10	interleukin-10
TNF-α	tumor necrosis factor-alpha
IFNγ	interferon-gamma
SAM	senescence-accelerated mouse
ALI	Acute lung injury
LPS	lipopolysaccharide
MDA	malondialdehyde
MPO	myeloperoxidase
IL-6	interleukin-6
SG	Sarcandra glabra
MAPK	mitogen-activated protein kinase
OA	oleic acid
IL-1β	interleukin-1β
IPF	idiopathic pulmonary fibrosis
BLM	Bleomycin
NO	nitric oxide
NSCLC	non-small cell lung cancer
ROS	reactive oxygen species
BaP	insulin-like growth factor binding protein-3, benzo[a]pyrene
DMH	dimethylhydrazine
LTO	lycopene-enriched tomato oleserin
NHBE	normal human bronchial epithelial cells
HMG-CoA	3-hydroxy-3-methylglutaryl–coenzyme A
RARβ	retinoic acid receptor β
GJC	gap junction communication
Cx43	connexin-43
RCT	randomized controlled trial
RR	relative ratio
OR	odds ratio
HR	hazard ratio
FEV1	Forced expiratory volume in one second
FVC	Forced vital capacity
ACOS	asthma-COPD overlap syndrome
NHANES III	National Health and Nutrition Examination Survey
ALT	alanine aminotransferase

Author details

Emilio Balbuena[1,2,†], Junrui Cheng[1,†] and Abdulkerim Eroglu[1,2*]

1 Plants for Human Health Institute, North Carolina State University, Kannapolis, NC, USA

2 Department of Molecular and Structural Biochemistry, College of Agriculture and Life Sciences, North Carolina State University, Raleigh, NC, USA

*Address all correspondence to: aeroglu@ncsu.edu

† Balbuena and Cheng contributed equally to this work.

References

[1] Palozza, P., et al., *Tomato Lycopene and Inflammatory Cascade: Basic Interactions and Clinical Implications.* Curr Med Chem, 2010. **17**(23): p. 2547-2563.

[2] Rao, A.V. and A. Ali, *Biologically Active Phytochemicals in Human Health: Lycopene.* International Journal of Food Properties, 2007. **10**(2): p. 279-288.

[3] Eroglu, A. and E.H. Harrison, *Carotenoid metabolism in mammals, including man: formation, occurrence, and function of apocarotenoids.* J Lipid Res, 2013. **54**(7): p. 1719-1730.

[4] Rowles, J.L., 3rd and J.W. Erdman, Jr., *Carotenoids and their role in cancer prevention.* Biochim Biophys Acta Mol Cell Biol Lipids, 2020. **1865**(11): p. 158613.

[5] Olson, J.A. and N.I. Krinsky, *Introduction: the colorful, fascinating world of the carotenoids: important physiologic modulators.* Faseb j, 1995. **9**(15): p. 1547-1550.

[6] Palozza, P., et al., *Lycopene modulation of molecular targets affected by smoking exposure.* Curr Cancer Drug Targets, 2012. **12**(6): p. 640-657.

[7] Narayanasamy, S., et al., *Synthesis of apo-13- and apo-15-lycopenoids, cleavage products of lycopene that are retinoic acid antagonists.* J Lipid Res, 2017. **58**(5): p. 1021-1029.

[8] Hu, K.Q., et al., *The biochemical characterization of ferret carotene-9',10'-monooxygenase catalyzing cleavage of carotenoids in vitro and in vivo.* J Biol Chem, 2006. **281**(28): p. 19327-19338.

[9] Kopec, R.E., et al., *Identification and quantification of apo-lycopenals in fruits, vegetables, and human plasma.* J Agric Food Chem, 2010. **58**(6): p. 3290-6.

[10] Di Mascio, P., S. Kaiser, and H. Sies, *Lycopene as the most efficient biological carotenoid singlet oxygen quencher.* Arch Biochem Biophys, 1989. **274**(2): p. 532-538.

[11] Stahl, W., et al., *Carotenoid mixtures protect multilamellar liposomes against oxidative damage: synergistic effects of lycopene and lutein.* FEBS Lett, 1998. **427**(2): p. 305-308.

[12] Pennathur, S., et al., *Potent antioxidative activity of lycopene: A potential role in scavenging hypochlorous acid.* Free Radic Biol Med, 2010. **49**(2): p. 205-213.

[13] Lee, A., D.I. Thurnham, and M. Chopra, *Consumption of tomato products with olive oil but not sunflower oil increases the antioxidant activity of plasma.* Free Radic Biol Med, 2000. **29**(10): p. 1051-1055.

[14] Subhash, K., C. Bose, and B.K. Agrawal, *Effect of short term supplementation of tomatoes on antioxidant enzymes and lipid peroxidation in type-II diabetes.* Indian J Clin Biochem, 2007. **22**(1): p. 95-98.

[15] Clinton, S.K., *Lycopene: chemistry, biology, and implications for human health and disease.* Nutr Rev, 1998. **56**(2 Pt 1): p. 35-51.

[16] Soares, N.d.C.P., et al., *Comparative Analysis of Lycopene Content from Different Tomato-Based Food Products on the Cellular Activity of Prostate Cancer Cell Lines.* Foods (Basel, Switzerland), 2019. **8**(6): p. 201.

[17] Porrini, M. and P. Riso, *What are typical lycopene intakes?* J Nutr, 2005. **135**(8): p. 2042s–5s.

[18] Kamiloglu, S., D. Boyacioglu, and E. Capanoglu, *The effect of food processing on bioavailability of tomato antioxidants.* Journal of Berry Research, 2013. **3**: p. 65-77.

[19] Başaran, N., M. Bacanlı, and A. Ahmet Başaran, *Chapter 28 - Lycopenes as Antioxidants in Gastrointestinal Diseases*, in *Gastrointestinal Tissue*, J. Gracia-Sancho and J. Salvadó, Editors. 2017, Academic Press. p. 355-362.

[20] Marković, K., M. Hruškar, and N. Vahčić, *Lycopene content of tomato products and their contribution to the lycopene intake of Croatians.* Nutrition Research, 2006. **26**(11): p. 556-560.

[21] Gärtner, C., W. Stahl, and H. Sies, *Lycopene is more bioavailable from tomato paste than from fresh tomatoes.* Am J Clin Nutr, 1997. **66**(1): p. 116-122.

[22] Danuta, G., et al., *Lycopene in tomatoes and tomato products.* Open Chemistry, 2020. **18**(1): p. 752-756.

[23] Unlu, N.Z., et al., *Carotenoid absorption from salad and salsa by humans is enhanced by the addition of avocado or avocado oil.* J Nutr, 2005. **135**(3): p. 431-436.

[24] Borel, P., et al., *Lycopene bioavailability is associated with a combination of genetic variants.* Free Radical Biology and Medicine, 2015. **83**: p. 238-244.

[25] Moran, N.E., et al., *Single Nucleotide Polymorphisms in β-Carotene Oxygenase 1 are Associated with Plasma Lycopene Responses to a Tomato-Soy Juice Intervention in Men with Prostate Cancer.* The Journal of Nutrition, 2019. **149**(3): p. 381-397.

[26] Wang, X.-D., *Lycopene metabolism and its biological significance.* The American journal of clinical nutrition, 2012. **96**(5): p. 1214S–1222S.

[27] Moran, N.E., J.W. Erdman, Jr., and S.K. Clinton, *Complex interactions between dietary and genetic factors impact lycopene metabolism and distribution.* Archives of biochemistry and biophysics, 2013. **539**(2): p. 171-180.

[28] Story, E.N., et al., *An update on the health effects of tomato lycopene.* Annual review of food science and technology, 2010. **1**: p. 189-210.

[29] Tremblay, B.L., et al., *Genetic and Common Environmental Contributions to Familial Resemblances in Plasma Carotenoid Concentrations in Healthy Families.* Nutrients, 2018. **10**(8): p. 1002.

[30] Rust, P., P. Lehner, and I. Elmadfa, *Relationship between dietary intake, antioxidant status and smoking habits in female Austrian smokers.* Eur J Nutr, 2001. **40**(2): p. 78-83.

[31] Lagiou, P., et al., *Plasma carotenoid levels in relation to tobacco smoking and demographic factors.* Int J Vitam Nutr Res, 2003. **73**(3): p. 226-231.

[32] Yuan, J.M., et al., *Prediagnostic levels of serum beta-cryptoxanthin and retinol predict smoking-related lung cancer risk in Shanghai, China.* Cancer Epidemiol Biomarkers Prev, 2001. **10**(7): p. 767-773.

[33] Rao, A.V. and S. Agarwal, *Effect of diet and smoking on serum lycopene and lipid peroxidation.* Nutrition Research, 1998. **18**(4): p. 713-721.

[34] Petyaev, I.M., *Lycopene Deficiency in Ageing and Cardiovascular Disease.* Oxidative medicine and cellular longevity, 2016. **2016**: p. 3218605-3218605.

[35] Steck-Scott, S., et al., *Plasma and lung macrophage responsiveness to carotenoid supplementation and ozone exposure in humans.* Eur J Clin Nutr, 2004. **58**(12): p. 1571-1579.

[36] Holgate, S.T., *The airway epithelium is central to the pathogenesis of asthma.* Allergol Int, 2008. **57**(1): p. 1-10.

[37] Lee, C.M., et al., *Lycopene suppresses ovalbumin-induced airway inflammation in a murine model of asthma.* Biochem

Biophys Res Commun, 2008. **374**(2): p. 248-252.

[38] Hazlewood, L.C., et al., *Dietary lycopene supplementation suppresses Th2 responses and lung eosinophilia in a mouse model of allergic asthma.* J Nutr Biochem, 2011. **22**(1): p. 95-100.

[39] Barnes, P.J., et al., *Chronic obstructive pulmonary disease.* Nat Rev Dis Primers, 2015. **1**: p. 15076.

[40] Vestbo, J., et al., *Global strategy for the diagnosis, management, and prevention of chronic obstructive pulmonary disease: GOLD executive summary.* Am J Respir Crit Care Med, 2013. **187**(4): p. 347-365.

[41] Mustra Rakic, J., et al., *Lycopene Inhibits Smoke-Induced Chronic Obstructive Pulmonary Disease and Lung Carcinogenesis by Modulating Reverse Cholesterol Transport in Ferrets.* Cancer Prev Res (Phila), 2019. **12**(7): p. 421-432.

[42] Campos, K.K.D., et al., *Lycopene mitigates pulmonary emphysema induced by cigarette smoke in a murine model.* J Nutr Biochem, 2019. **65**: p. 93-100.

[43] Campos, K.K.D., et al., *The antioxidant and anti-inflammatory properties of lycopene in mice lungs exposed to cigarette smoke.* J Nutr Biochem, 2017. **48**: p. 9-20.

[44] Kasagi, S., et al., *Tomato juice prevents senescence-accelerated mouse P1 strain from developing emphysema induced by chronic exposure to tobacco smoke.* Am J Physiol Lung Cell Mol Physiol, 2006. **290**(2): p. L396–L404.

[45] Johnson, E.R. and M.A. Matthay, *Acute lung injury: epidemiology, pathogenesis, and treatment.* J Aerosol Med Pulm Drug Deliv, 2010. **23**(4): p. 243-252.

[46] Li, W.W., et al., *Synergistic protection of matrine and lycopene against lipopolysaccharide-induced acute lung injury in mice.* Mol Med Rep, 2019. **20**(1): p. 455-462.

[47] Liu, T.Y. and S.B. Chen, *Sarcandra glabra combined with lycopene protect rats from lipopolysaccharide induced acute lung injury via reducing inflammatory response.* Biomed Pharmacother, 2016. **84**: p. 34-41.

[48] Türkoğlu, S., et al., *Effects of lycopene on the model of oleic acid-induced acute lung injury.* Tuberk Toraks, 2012. **60**(2): p. 101-107.

[49] Bastug, O., et al., *Effects of Lycopene in Hyperoxia-Induced Lung Injury in Newborn Rats.* Int J Vitam Nutr Res, 2018. **88**(5-6): p. 270-280.

[50] Ballester, B., J. Milara, and J. Cortijo, *Idiopathic Pulmonary Fibrosis and Lung Cancer: Mechanisms and Molecular Targets.* Int J Mol Sci, 2019. **20**(3).

[51] Ley, B., H.R. Collard, and T.E. King, Jr., *Clinical course and prediction of survival in idiopathic pulmonary fibrosis.* Am J Respir Crit Care Med, 2011. **183**(4): p. 431-440.

[52] Zhou, C., et al., *Lycopene from tomatoes partially alleviates the bleomycin-induced experimental pulmonary fibrosis in rats.* Nutr Res, 2008. **28**(2): p. 122-130.

[53] Muzandu, K., et al., *Effect of lycopene and beta-carotene on peroxynitrite-mediated cellular modifications.* Toxicol Appl Pharmacol, 2006. **215**(3): p. 330-340.

[54] Muzandu, K., et al., *Lycopene and beta-carotene ameliorate catechol estrogen-mediated DNA damage.* Jpn J Vet Res, 2005. **52**(4): p. 173-184.

[55] Jemal, A., et al., *Global cancer statistics.* CA Cancer J Clin, 2011. **61**(2): p. 69-90.

[56] Kim, L., A.V. Rao, and L.G. Rao, *Effect of lycopene on prostate LNCaP cancer cells in culture.* J Med Food, 2002. **5**(4): p. 181-187.

[57] Park, Y.O., E.S. Hwang, and T.W. Moon, *The effect of lycopene on cell growth and oxidative DNA damage of Hep3B human hepatoma cells.* Biofactors, 2005. **23**(3): p. 129-139.

[58] Fornelli, F., et al., *The influence of lycopene on the proliferation of human breast cell line (MCF-7).* Toxicol In Vitro, 2007. **21**(2): p. 217-223.

[59] Levy, J., et al., *Lycopene is a more potent inhibitor of human cancer cell proliferation than either alpha-carotene or beta-carotene.* Nutr Cancer, 1995. **24**(3): p. 257-266.

[60] Choi, S.H., et al., *Changes in free amino acid, phenolic, chlorophyll, carotenoid, and glycoalkaloid contents in tomatoes during 11 stages of growth and inhibition of cervical and lung human cancer cells by green tomato extracts.* J Agric Food Chem, 2010. **58**(13): p. 7547-7556.

[61] Reddy, M.K., R.L. Alexander-Lindo, and M.G. Nair, *Relative inhibition of lipid peroxidation, cyclooxygenase enzymes, and human tumor cell proliferation by natural food colors.* J Agric Food Chem, 2005. **53**(23): p. 9268-9273.

[62] Lian, F., et al., *Apo-10'-lycopenoic acid inhibits lung cancer cell growth in vitro, and suppresses lung tumorigenesis in the A/J mouse model in vivo.* Carcinogenesis, 2007. **28**(7): p. 1567-1574.

[63] Cheng, J., et al., *Lycopene Protects against Smoking-Induced Lung Cancer by Inducing Base Excision Repair.* Antioxidants (Basel), 2020. **9**(7).

[64] Liu, C., et al., *Lycopene supplementation inhibits lung squamous metaplasia and induces apoptosis via up-regulating insulin-like growth factor-binding protein 3 in cigarette smoke-exposed ferrets.* Cancer Res, 2003. **63**(12): p. 3138-3144.

[65] Kim, D.J., et al., *Chemoprevention by lycopene of mouse lung neoplasia after combined initiation treatment with DEN, MNU and DMH.* Cancer Lett, 1997. **120**(1): p. 15-22.

[66] Hecht, S.S., et al., *Evaluation of butylated hydroxyanisole, myo-inositol, curcumin, esculetin, resveratrol and lycopene as inhibitors of benzo[a] pyrene plus 4-(methylnitrosamino)-1-(3-pyridyl)-1-butanone-induced lung tumorigenesis in A/J mice.* Cancer Lett, 1999. **137**(2): p. 123-130.

[67] Guttenplan, J.B., et al., *Effects of a lycopene-rich diet on spontaneous and benzo[a]pyrene-induced mutagenesis in prostate, colon and lungs of the lacZ mouse.* Cancer Lett, 2001. **164**(1): p. 1-6.

[68] Li, C.C., et al., *Tomato Powder Inhibits Hepatic Steatosis and Inflammation Potentially Through Restoring SIRT1 Activity and Adiponectin Function Independent of Carotenoid Cleavage Enzymes in Mice.* Mol Nutr Food Res, 2018. **62**(8): p. e1700738.

[69] Lim, J.Y. and X.D. Wang, *Mechanistic understanding of β-cryptoxanthin and lycopene in cancer prevention in animal models.* Biochim Biophys Acta Mol Cell Biol Lipids, 2020. **1865**(11): p. 158652.

[70] Palozza, P., et al., *Modulation of apoptotic signalling by carotenoids in cancer cells.* Arch Biochem Biophys, 2004. **430**(1): p. 104-109.

[71] Stahl, W., et al., *Stimulation of gap junctional communication: comparison of acyclo-retinoic acid and lycopene.* Arch Biochem Biophys, 2000. **373**(1): p. 271-274.

[72] Moher, D., et al., *Preferred reporting items for systematic reviews and*

meta-analyses: the PRISMA statement. BMJ, 2009. **339**: p. b2535.

[73] Greenland, S. and D.C. Thomas, *On the need for the rare disease assumption in case-control studies.* Am J Epidemiol, 1982. **116**(3): p. 547-553.

[74] Schock, B.C., et al., *Antioxidants and oxidative stress in BAL fluid of atopic asthmatic children.* Pediatr Res, 2003. **53**(3): p. 375-381.

[75] Ford, E.S., D.M. Mannino, and S.C. Redd, *Serum antioxidant concentrations among U.S. adults with self-reported asthma.* J Asthma, 2004. **41**(2): p. 179-187.

[76] Wood, L.G., et al., *Airway and circulating levels of carotenoids in asthma and healthy controls.* J Am Coll Nutr, 2005. **24**(6): p. 448-455.

[77] Ochs-Balcom, H.M., et al., *Antioxidants, oxidative stress, and pulmonary function in individuals diagnosed with asthma or COPD.* Eur J Clin Nutr, 2006. **60**(8): p. 991-999.

[78] Riccioni, G., et al., *Plasma lycopene and antioxidant vitamins in asthma: the PLAVA study.* J Asthma, 2007. **44**(6): p. 429-432.

[79] Sackesen, C., et al., *A comprehensive evaluation of the enzymatic and nonenzymatic antioxidant systems in childhood asthma.* J Allergy Clin Immunol, 2008. **122**(1): p. 78-85.

[80] Wood, L.G. and P.G. Gibson, *Reduced circulating antioxidant defences are associated with airway hyper-responsiveness, poor control and severe disease pattern in asthma.* Br J Nutr, 2010. **103**(5): p. 735-741.

[81] Kodama, Y., et al., *Antioxidant nutrients in plasma of Japanese patients with chronic obstructive pulmonary disease, asthma-COPD overlap syndrome and bronchial asthma.* Clin Respir J, 2017. **11**(6): p. 915-924.

[82] Larkin, E.K., et al., *New risk factors for adult-onset incident asthma. A nested case-control study of host antioxidant defense.* Am J Respir Crit Care Med, 2015. **191**(1): p. 45-53.

[83] Neuman, I., H. Nahum, and A. Ben-Amotz, *Reduction of exercise-induced asthma oxidative stress by lycopene, a natural antioxidant.* Allergy, 2000. **55**(12): p. 1184-1189.

[84] Falk, B., et al., *Effect of lycopene supplementation on lung function after exercise in young athletes who complain of exercise-induced bronchoconstriction symptoms.* Ann Allergy Asthma Immunol, 2005. **94**(4): p. 480-485.

[85] Wood, L.G., et al., *Lycopene-rich treatments modify noneosinophilic airway inflammation in asthma: proof of concept.* Free Radic Res, 2008. **42**(1): p. 94-102.

[86] Wood, L.G., et al., *Manipulating antioxidant intake in asthma: a randomized controlled trial.* Am J Clin Nutr, 2012. **96**(3): p. 534-543.

[87] Vaz Fragoso, C.A., et al., *The ratio of FEV1 to FVC as a basis for establishing chronic obstructive pulmonary disease.* American journal of respiratory and critical care medicine, 2010. **181**(5): p. 446-451.

[88] Beck, K.C., M.J. Joyner, and P.D. Scanlon, *Exercise-Induced asthma: diagnosis, treatment, and regulatory issues.* Exerc Sport Sci Rev, 2002. **30**(1): p. 1-3.

[89] Thulborn, S.J., et al., *Neutrophil elastase as a biomarker for bacterial infection in COPD.* Respir Res, 2019. **20**(1): p. 170.

[90] Murdoch, J.R. and C.M. Lloyd, *Chronic inflammation and asthma.* Mutation research, 2010. **690**(1-2): p. 24-39.

[91] Cukic, V., et al., *Asthma and Chronic Obstructive Pulmonary Disease (COPD) - Differences and Similarities.* Materia socio-medica, 2012. **24**(2): p. 100-105.

[92] Kentson, M., et al., *Oxidant status, iron homeostasis, and carotenoid levels of COPD patients with advanced disease and LTOT.* Eur Clin Respir J, 2018. **5**(1): p. 1447221.

[93] Asbaghi, S., et al., *Dietary Intake and Serum Level of Carotenoids in Lung Cancer Patients: A Case-Control Study.* Nutr Cancer, 2015. **67**(6): p. 893-898.

[94] Comstock, G.W., et al., *The risk of developing lung cancer associated with antioxidants in the blood: ascorbic acids, carotenoids, alpha-tocopherol, selenium, and total peroxyl radical absorbing capacity.* Am J Epidemiol, 2008. **168**(7): p. 831-840.

[95] Garcia-Closas, R., et al., *Intake of specific carotenoids and flavonoids and the risk of lung cancer in women in Barcelona, Spain.* Nutr Cancer, 1998. **32**(3): p. 154-158.

[96] Holick, C.N., et al., *Dietary carotenoids, serum beta-carotene, and retinol and risk of lung cancer in the alpha-tocopherol, beta-carotene cohort study.* Am J Epidemiol, 2002. **156**(6): p. 536-547.

[97] Ito, Y., et al., *Cancer mortality and serum levels of carotenoids, retinol, and tocopherol: a population-based follow-up study of inhabitants of a rural area of Japan.* Asian Pac J Cancer Prev, 2005. **6**(1): p. 10-15.

[98] Ito, Y., et al., *Lung cancer mortality and serum levels of carotenoids, retinol, tocopherols, and folic acid in men and women: a case-control study nested in the JACC Study.* J Epidemiol, 2005. **15 Suppl 2**: p. S140–S149.

[99] Klarod, K., et al., *Serum antioxidant levels and nutritional status in early and advanced stage lung cancer patients.* Nutrition, 2011. **27**(11-12): p. 1156-1160.

[100] Le Marchand, L., et al., *Vegetable consumption and lung cancer risk: a population-based case-control study in Hawaii.* J Natl Cancer Inst, 1989. **81**(15): p. 1158-1164.

[101] Michaud, D.S., et al., *Intake of specific carotenoids and risk of lung cancer in 2 prospective US cohorts.* Am J Clin Nutr, 2000. **72**(4): p. 990-997.

[102] Rohan, T.E., et al., *A cohort study of dietary carotenoids and lung cancer risk in women (Canada).* Cancer Causes Control, 2002. **13**(3): p. 231-237.

[103] Satia, J.A., et al., *Long-term use of beta-carotene, retinol, lycopene, and lutein supplements and lung cancer risk: results from the VITamins And Lifestyle (VITAL) study.* Am J Epidemiol, 2009. **169**(7): p. 815-828.

[104] Shareck, M., et al., *Inverse Association between Dietary Intake of Selected Carotenoids and Vitamin C and Risk of Lung Cancer.* Front Oncol, 2017. 7: p. 23.

[105] Stefani, E.D., et al., *Dietary antioxidants and lung cancer risk: a case-control study in Uruguay.* Nutr Cancer, 1999. **34**(1): p. 100-110.

[106] Steinmetz, K.A., J.D. Potter, and A.R. Folsom, *Vegetables, fruit, and lung cancer in the Iowa Women's Health Study.* Cancer Res, 1993. **53**(3): p. 536-543.

[107] Talwar, D., et al., *Effect of inflammation on measures of antioxidant status in patients with non-small cell lung cancer.* Am J Clin Nutr, 1997. **66**(5): p. 1283-5.

[108] Voorrips, L.E., et al., *A prospective cohort study on antioxidant and folate intake and male lung cancer risk.* Cancer Epidemiol Biomarkers Prev, 2000. **9**(4): p. 357-365.

[109] Yuan, J.M., et al., *Dietary cryptoxanthin and reduced risk of lung cancer: the Singapore Chinese Health Study.* Cancer Epidemiol Biomarkers Prev, 2003. **12**(9): p. 890-898.

[110] Bakker Schut, T.C., et al., *Intracellular carotenoid levels measured by Raman microspectroscopy: comparison of lymphocytes from lung cancer patients and healthy individuals.* Int J Cancer, 1997. **74**(1): p. 20-25.

Chapter 12

Management of Diabetic Eye Disease Using Carotenoids and Nutrients

Drake W. Lem, Dennis L. Gierhart and Pinakin Gunvant Davey

Abstract

Diabetic retinopathy is the leading cause of blindness and visual disability globally among working-age adults. Until recently, diabetic eye disease is primarily regarded by its microvasculature complications largely characterized by progressive retinopathy and macular edema. However, a growing body of evidence suggests that hyperglycemia-induced oxidative stress and inflammation play an integral role in the early pathogenesis of diabetic retinopathy by potentiating retinal neurodegeneration. The onset of type 2 diabetes mellitus starts with insulin resistance leading to insulin deficiency, hyperglycemia, and dyslipidemia. Which in turn enhances the pro-oxidant and pro-inflammatory pathways. Additionally, various poor dietary behaviors along with obesity worsen physiological state in diabetics. However, decreased levels and depletion of the endogenous antioxidant defense system in the retina can be sufficiently augmented via carotenoid vitamin therapy. Therefore, dietary supplementation of antioxidant micronutrients particularly macular carotenoids lutein, zeaxanthin and *meso*-zeaxanthin that promote retinal health and optimal visual performance, may serve as an adjunctive therapy in the management of diabetic eye disease.

Keywords: carotenoids, macular pigment, macular pigment optical density, MPOD, lutein, zeaxanthin and meso-zeaxanthin, diabetes, diabetic eye disease, diabetic retinopathy

1. Introduction

The prevalence of diabetes is endemic in the United States and developed countries. According to the 2018 reports it is estimated that the United States has more than 31 million adults diagnosed with diabetes [1]. Diabetes prevalence remains underestimated with approximately one in four individuals that have diabetes are undiagnosed [1]. There are various forms of diabetes and individuals with Type 2 diabetes (T2DM) account for 90–95% of all cases of diabetes within the US [1]. The incidence of diabetes is also likely to increase with 88 million individuals are diagnosed to be pre-diabetic who have potential ongoing subclinical damage [1]. The prevalence of diabetes mellitus in the US is predicted to reach 36 million by the year 2045 and will continue to pose a significant global health problem [2].

Nearly half a billion people are currently living with diabetes globally, and the total number of cases is projected to surge by 25% (578 million) in 2030 [3, 4] and to 700 million by the year 2045 [3–5]. Diabetes is severely underdiagnosed condition with one in two people (50.1%) currently living with the condition are unaware [3, 4] . The International Diabetes Foundation estimates the socioeconomic burden of diabetes to be USD 760 billion and potentially increase to USD 845 billion by 2045 [2]. The global estimates of socioeconomic burden are predicted to rise in response to the increasing prevalence of diabetes, improved survival rates (longer life expectancy with the condition), and consequently prolonged duration of diabetes mellitus [3, 4, 6–8].

Diabetic retinopathy (DR) is characterized by the hallmark feature of retinal capillary degeneration that could lead to, significant visual impairment. The natural history of unmanaged or poorly managed diabetic retinopathy leads to proliferative retinopathy (PDR) and/or macular edema [9, 10]; contingent upon the disease-severity, these complications may arise individually or simultaneously. DR affects roughly one in three individuals with diabetes and its severity is closely linked to both the duration of diabetes and the glycemic load [5, 6, 11, 12]. It is estimated that 4.1 million individuals in the US are afflicted with DR, and 899,000 of which are affected by vision-threatening retinopathy [1]. The global prevalence of DR is estimated to affect 146 million adults and projected to reach 191 million by 2030 [3, 4, 8]. Currently, DR remains a leading cause of irreversible, yet preventable, vision loss among adults and is associated with a poorer quality of life, increased susceptibility for developing further complications, and considerable rise in healthcare expenditures [5, 12].

1.1 Diabetic retinopathy

Clinically, retinopathy is routinely graded upon its presenting clinical features during ophthalmic examination in accordance with the International Clinical Disease Severity Scale for DR [7, 10, 13–16]. The five-stage disease severity classification system (**Table 1**) was created using prior clinical trials: the Early Treatment Diabetic Retinopathy Study (ETDRS) and the Wisconsin Epidemiological Study of DR (WESDR) [14–17]. The stages of non-proliferative diabetic retinopathy (NPDR) are based on the severity of microvascular abnormalities limited to the surface of the retina; in addition to reflecting the patients' risk of developing more

Disease Severity Scale	Clinical Features
No apparent retinopathy	No fundus abnormalities
Mild NPDR	Microaneurysms only
Moderate NPDR	More than just MAs, but less than severe NPDR
Severe NPDR	Any of the following: (with no signs of PDR) extensive DBH in each of 4 quadrants (+20/quadrant), venous beading in at least 2 quadrants, and/or IRMA in at least 1 quadrant
PDR	One or more of the following: neovascularization, tractional retinal detachment, or vitreous/preretinal hemorrhage

NPDR = non-proliferative diabetic retinopathy; MA = microaneurysms; PDR = proliferative diabetic retinopathy; DBH = dot blot hemorrhages; IRMA = intraretinal microvascular abnormalities.

Table 1.
International clinical disease severity scale for diabetic retinopathy [14].

advanced, vision-threatening retinopathy. Examination of NPDR by ophthalmoscopy may reveal the presence of microaneurysms, hard exudates, intraretinal hemorrhages ("dot and blot" shaped), and intraretinal microvascular abnormalities (such as tortuous sinus shunt vessels) [14, 15, 17].

Progressive oxidative injury in NPDR is evident within the vasculature, by the presence of acellular capillaries and endothelial apoptosis. This injury is further exaggerated within local tissue by the onset of capillary nonperfusion and vascular occlusion that may develop in the disease [13, 18, 19]. The resultant retinal injury due to ischemia further exacerbate pro-oxidant and pro-inflammatory mechanisms by compromising oxygenation of the metabolically demanding retinal neurons. This in turn promotes angiogenesis through the release of vascular endothelial growth factor (VEGF) [13, 18–20]. The retinal neurodegeneration induced by hypoxia can be observed by the presence of abnormal fluffy white patches known as cotton wool spots, upon fundoscopic examination [19]. The ensuing retinal neovascularization indicates the clinical progression of NPDR into the advanced-stages of PDR. These aberrant new blood vessels are fragile and ineffective in restoring tissue perfusion because they grow from the retinal surface and towards the posterior pole of the vitreous cavity [7, 10, 13, 16]. Thus, subsequent risk of acute vision loss is evaluated on the extent of neovascular proliferations, particularly on/near the optic disc, which perniciously emanate from the steady vasculature of the retina.

Diabetic macular edema (DME) develops when fragile or damaged capillary beds leak and cause thickening of macula due to fluid accumulation. Alterations in the microvasculature such as endothelial cell proliferation and retinal pericyte necrobiosis gradually enhance the vascular permeability, which ultimately causes the breakdown of the blood-retinal barrier [13, 18]. The progressive deposition of fluid and proteins can amass on or under the macula which can be clinically examined by optical coherence tomography (OCT), identifying areas of diffuse retinal thickening or hard exudates, indicating the extent of focal leakage [21, 22]. Alternatively, onset of macular edema can occur during any stage of retinopathy (NPDR or PDR) leading to vision loss [6, 13].

Traditionally, diabetic eye disease has largely been considered to be a microvascular end-organ complication of diabetes mellitus. The severity of retinopathy correlates with the susceptibility of further complications such a peripheral neuropathy, nephropathy and cardiovascular disease [6, 11, 12, 23–25]. It is established that chronic hyperglycemia promotes oxidative injury in the highly-susceptible retina; in part due to high metabolic demands and constant light exposure [26, 27]. However, a growing body of evidence strongly implicates retinal neurodegeneration is potentiated by pro-oxidant and pro-inflammatory processes during the early pathogenesis of DR. Indications of retinal dysfunction that can be detected in diabetic patients even prior to manifestation of clinical signs of retinopathy [6, 12, 19, 25, 27–31]. Appropriately, the American Diabetes Association defines DR as a highly tissue-specific neurovascular complication and has identified several modalities of management of disease and its progression [7, 11, 28].

The body's inherent defense against oxidative damage, involving the neutralization of reactive oxygen species (ROS), relies upon the interplay between both endogenous and exogenous antioxidants to maintain redox homeostasis [27, 32]. The interdependence between hyperglycemia, oxidative stress, and changes in redox homeostasis are essential facets in the pathology of diabetic retinopathy [26, 32]. In particular, exogenous antioxidants such as vitamin C, vitamin E and xanthophyll carotenoids (including lutein, zeaxanthin and *meso*-zeaxanthin) possess significant antioxidant and anti-inflammatory effects on the retina [32]. Studies have demonstrated the clinical benefits in visual performance associated with dietary supplementation of carotenoids and antioxidants, such as the Age-Related Eye

Disease Study 2 (AREDS-2) and various other studies [33–36]. Despite similarities in pathogenesis of macular degeneration and diabetic retinopathy involving oxidative damage in the retina, only a limited number of studies have concentrated on the relationship between dietary carotenoids intake to influence pathophysiology in diabetes mellitus.

Recently, the onset of diabetes in experimental murine models consistently demonstrated a significant increase in pro-oxidant and pro-inflammatory molecules, such as malondialdehyde, oxidatively damaged DNA, and VEGF [37–45]. Importantly, administration of antioxidants including lutein and/or zeaxanthin was demonstrated to effectively prevent, and in some cases reverse, the hyperglycemia-induced changes in oxidative stress and inflammation [37–42, 45]. The beneficial effects of lutein and zeaxanthin were shown to augment the endogenous antioxidant defense system by improving retinal concentrations of glutathione (GSH) and glutathione peroxidase (GPx) [37–39, 42]. The antioxidant and anti-inflammatory effects of lutein and zeaxanthin were also shown to attenuate the microvascular abnormalities that characterize DR pathology, in addition to protecting the retina against accelerated vasoregression that may proceed alterations in the vasculature [37–44, 46].

To date, only a limited number of observational [26, 32, 47–53], and randomized-controlled trials [35, 54] have investigated the association of macular pigment optical density (MPOD) levels in diabetic eye disease. Generally, the evidence suggests that MPOD levels are lower in individuals with diabetes when compared to healthy controls [48, 51], and some studies indicate MPOD status may differ between types of diabetes (type 1 and type 2) [26, 32, 50]. MPOD depletion was also negatively correlated with the presence of retinopathy in T2DM [26, 32, 50] and may be attributed in part due to oxidative stress [49]. These findings are promising and begs for additional investigation to substantiate the beneficial role of carotenoid vitamin therapy in the management of diabetic eye disease.

2. Biomarkers and its importance in clinical care

Sensible, relatively inexpensive techniques to evaluate the status of macular carotenoids can serve as important biomarkers in monitoring retinal health in individuals with diabetes and increased risk of retinal neurodegeneration. Biomarkers serve as important tools with significant potential for innovating novel drugs and substantiating the safety and efficacy of available therapies [55, 56]; however, their application is not limited to clinical research and extends into improving clinical practice and establishing public health guidelines. The concept of biomarkers is delusively simple, with which a single biomarker may satisfy the criteria for several different purposes; therefore, it is critical to establish scientific justification how a particular biomarker will be defined according to its situation-specific application. Thus, several categories of biomarkers have been established by the FDA-NIH's "Biomarkers, EndpointS, and other Tools (BEST)" resource, described in more detail elsewhere [55, 57]. Moreover, by establishing the context of use, this directly expounds the nature, objective and methodology intended for utilizing a biomarker within a particular setting [55, 57, 58].

Advancements in retinal imaging modalities have allowed MPOD status to serve as a biomarker in multiple settings for diabetic retinal disease, including: (1) prognostic biomarker for screening individuals with sub-clinical disease with no overt retinopathy; (2) identification of surrogate biomarkers for the prediction of low MPOD in T2DM; and (3) monitoring biomarker for evaluating the efficacy of carotenoid supplementation on DR. The depletion of MPOD in diabetes has been consistently reported in a number of cross-sectional studies, and some suggest that low MPOD may be a potential clinical feature of T2DM [26, 32, 48–51]. Studies have demonstrated significant correlations between MPOD and central subfield thickness, retinal volume, and photoreceptor outer segment length in diabetic and healthy controls [59–61]; thus, clinical measurements of MPOD levels may serve an important role in early-detection of retinal neurodegeneration and prognosticating treatment outcomes. Furthermore, one study identified possible surrogate biomarkers including smoking status, hypertension, and vitamin D insufficiency, that may predict low MPOD in T2DM [32]. Alternatively, serial MPOD measurements have been used as a monitoring biomarker to assess the benefits of the antioxidant micronutrients on visual performance and features of NPDR in Type 1 (T1DM) and T2DM [35]. Based on the systematic review conducted MPOD is found to be a prognostic, surrogate and monitoring biomarker as defined by the FDA-NIH [55].

3. Role of MPOD in the management of diabetic eye disease

3.1 MPOD basics

The macular pigment is comprised of three lipid-soluble carotenoids: including lutein, zeaxanthin, and *meso*-zeaxanthin [62, 63]. They are responsible for the fovea's yellow pigmentation and are densely concentrated within the photoreceptor axons, the inner plexiform layer and the outer plexiform layer at the center of the macula [62–66]. The carotenoids, lutein and zeaxanthin, cannot be synthesized *de novo* within the eye, and can only be acquired through dietary intake; found primarily in leafy green vegetables, like spinach and kale, and egg yolks [63, 67–69]. A biochemical isomer of zeaxanthin called *meso*-zeaxanthin is found in the macula. *Meso*-zeaxanthin in the eye is a byproduct of conversion of lutein in the retinal pigment epithelium (RPE). Several studies have demonstrated that oral supplementation of these carotenoids can greatly improve their levels within the serum [63, 67, 70] and can be retained in the human retina for a sustained period of time [71].

Macular carotenoids are quantified by the macular pigment optical density (MPOD) and are associated with maintaining retinal health and optimal visual performance; suggesting that MPOD levels may serve as an important biomarker in health and diseased states [63, 65, 69, 72]. Research suggests that carotenoids serve to protect the retina, specifically the macula, via two proposed methods: 1) they act as a filter against blue light, and 2) they reduce oxidative stress and inflammation in the retinal tissue [63, 69, 72–76]. The macular pigment attenuates the amount of blue light that reaches the photoreceptor cells, due to the peak wavelength of MPOD's absorption spectrum (peak ~460 nm) which lies within the range of blue light on the visible light spectrum (400-500 nm); and may provide some preservation and improvement in visual function [62, 76, 77]. Short wavelengths of blue light are of high energy, which can prompt the formation of ROS and induce oxidative injury; causing damage to the lipid bilayer of cell membranes, proteins and DNA, and cause mitochondrial dysfunction leading to cellular necrosis [63, 74–78]. Thus, the neuroprotective capabilities of the macular carotenoids in the retina, namely MPOD levels, have led researchers to further investigate the role of MPOD levels and its depletion in various ocular diseases.

3.2 Measuring MPOD

Techniques to quantify MPOD levels may also serve as susceptibility/risk biomarkers for diabetic eye disease, prior to indications of retinopathy that become clinically evident. Meanwhile, more expensive and advanced imaging modalities such as OCT, can play a more significant role in prognosticating outcome or determining course of treatment [79]. Several methods have been described aiming to effectively quantify levels of MPOD non-invasively in clinical settings; categorized by either psychophysical (subjective) or objective techniques [65, 69, 80]. In brief, these techniques are differentiated by patient-response, or participation required from the individual being evaluated, and requiring minimal participant-involvement to collect measurements, respectively [65, 69, 80, 81].

The clinical measurements of MPOD levels are primarily heterochromatic flicker photometry (HFP) [65, 69, 80, 82–84]. HFP technology is based on a stimulus of light, alternating between two wavelengths, that differ according to the retinal absorption spectrum of macular pigments (400-540 nm); a short-wavelength blue light maximally absorbed by the pigments, and a longer-wavelength (green) stimuli with minimal absorption [65, 69, 81]. Briefly, current HFP devices collect measurements in the fovea by adjusting the intensity of the target-stimuli, which is perceived as flickering light, according to the participant's involvement indicating the appearance of flickering light; estimating the level of MPOD as the difference in responsive sensitivity (of blue- and green-wavelength flicker) required at the fovea [65, 69, 81, 83, 85–87]. Thus, individuals with higher MPOD would require greater intensity blue light (perceive less blue light) at foveal measurements as a result of higher concentrations of macular pigment in the fovea [65, 69, 81, 88].

Objective techniques such as reflectometry [89–94], fundus autofluorescence [95–97] and resonance Raman spectroscopy [66, 98, 99], are all non-invasive, *in vivo* imaging modalities that can quantitatively measure levels of macular pigment [69, 80]. Briefly, measurements collected by fundus reflectance can be performed with a digital fundus camera integrated with a reflection photometer or a spectrometer to quantify and analyze the light reflected from the retina and choroid [88, 90, 92, 93, 96, 100, 101]. Similarly, dual-wavelength confocal scanning laser ophthalmoscopy (cSLO) can collect measurements reliably by using the autofluorescence of lipofuscin deposits in the RPE as an indirect measure of MPOD, while concurrently generating a 3-D topographical map of the retina [22, 95–97, 101, 102]. The resonance Raman spectroscopy is an optical technique that elicits an extraordinarily, resonance-enhanced Raman spectra of the macular carotenoids, in a molecule-specific manner, upon excitation by blue (488 nm) argon laser [66, 99, 103, 104].

The topic of debate for more than three decades, each technique exhibits unique advantages along with clinical limitations that have been discussed in more detail elsewhere [80, 95, 96, 100, 102]. The heterochromatic flicker photometry is the current gold standard of MPOD measurement.

3.3 Procedure of systematic review on carotenoids and diabetic eye disease

A systematic review was performed and published articles on the topic were identified using database searches from PubMed and Web of Science indexes. We identified all relevant publications which reported on the association between diabetic retinopathy and MPOD/carotenoids (lutein and/or zeaxanthin and/or *meso*-zeaxanthin), from human and animal studies prior to 21 December 2020. The search query terms used include 'carotenoids', 'lutein', 'zeaxanthin', 'macular pigment', 'macular pigment optical density AND diabetic eye disease', 'macular pigment optical density AND diabetic retinopathy', and 'MPOD AND diabetes'. Initial entries were selected based on titles and abstracts available in English. Eligible full-text publications were scanned and retrieved in regard to carotenoid levels or supplementation and diabetic retinopathy. Clinical studies evaluating carotenoids levels in diabetes had to quantify either serum concentrations of lutein and/or zeaxanthin, or measure levels of MPOD using validated, repeatable measurement techniques. Studies were considered eligible only on diabetic retinopathy and diabetic macular edema. Other types of diabetic eye diseases were excluded.

3.4 Carotenoids in the management of diabetic eye disease (*Animal Studies*)

The therapeutic benefits of macular carotenoids have been documented in diabetic murine models, investigating the molecular mechanisms underlying the onset of hyperglycemia-linked retinopathy; in particular, the protective effects of lutein (L) and/or zeaxanthin (Z) on the progression of retinal neurodegeneration [37–45]. Data from these reports are consistent in providing further evidence that administration of L and Z may delay or prevent the onset of DR by counteracting the proposed causative factors including oxidative stress (by attenuating ROS production with a concomitant regeneration of endogenous antioxidants), in addition to ameliorating inflammation and augmenting neuroprotection of retinal tissue. Administration of the drug Alloxan or Streptozotocin (STZ), which are toxic glucose-analogs that preferentially amass within the pancreatic beta cells that produce insulin, are commonly used for inducing diabetes mellitus in mice and rats, which will later develop retinopathy [37–43, 105–107]. Genetic murine models, including the leptin-receptor deficient (db/db) mice, spontaneously develop hyperglycemia and obesity at 4–8 weeks of age [44, 45, 106, 107]. A summary of the experimental animal models evaluating the effects of carotenoids administration on diabetic eye disease is outlined in **Table 2**.

Hyperglycemia-induced oxidative damage has been strongly considered the causative factor in the onset and development of diabetic retinopathy; resulting from the proliferation of pro-oxidant stressors if left untreated. Following the onset of diabetes in mice and rats, there was a significant increase in retinal markers of oxidative stress including: malondialdehyde, lipid peroxide, oxidatively-modified DNA (8-hydroxy-2'deoxyguanosine, 8-OHdG), and nitrotyrosine [37–40, 42]. However, reports were consistent in demonstrating that administration of antioxidants (L and/or Z) ameliorated the diabetes-induced increase in these markers of oxidative stress, comparable to levels observed from control animals. Furthermore, one study evaluated the effects of an AREDS-based formula containing antioxidant micronutrients which were shown to attenuate the rise in expression of oxidative stress-related genes modulated by chronic hyperglycemia [38, 40, 108, 109].

Study	Design (DM induced by)	L and/or Z	Effect of L/Z on Outcomes
Arnal et al. [37]	Rats (STZ)	L	prevented loss of retinal thickness
Kowluru et al. [39]	Rats (STZ)	Z	ameliorated rise in 8-OHdG
Kowluru et al. [40]	Rats (STZ)	L and Z	significantly reduced total ROS levels
Muriach et al. [42]	Mice (A)	L	restored levels of GSH and GPx
Sasaki et al. [43]	Mice (STZ)	L	prevented cell loss in GCL & INL
Tang et al. [44]	Mice (db/db)	L and Z*	improved central retinal thickness
Yu et al. [45]	Mice (db/db)	L and Z*	enhanced mitochondrial biogenesis

DM = diabetes mellitus; L = lutein; Z = zeaxanthin; STZ = streptozotocin; A = Alloxan; db/db = leptin-receptor deficient; 8-OHdG = oxidatively modified DNA; ROS = reactive oxygen species; GSH = glutathione; GPx = glutathione peroxidase; GCL = ganglion cell layer; INL = inner nuclear layer.
** = Wolfberry.*

Table 2.
Effects of carotenoids lutein and/or zeaxanthin in experimental animal models for diabetic eye disease.

Similarly, two clinically distinct features of early-stage retinopathy, microvascular lesions and retinal capillary degeneration, were prevented following treatment with alpha-lipoic acid, a micronutrient with antioxidant properties commonly included in carotenoid supplements for clinical use, such as the EyePromise Diabetes Visual Function Supplement Study (DVS; DiVFuSS) formulation by ZeaVision (MO, USA) [33, 38, 110–112]. Supplementation treatment with L and Z prevented increase in total retinal ROS levels in rats, suggesting they may prevent the continuation of superoxide free radical production caused by hyperglycemia and subsequent progression of retinopathy [41, 108, 113].

The supplementation of L and Z also attenuates retinal expression of endoplasmic reticulum stress biomarkers like BiP (binding-immunoglobulin protein), PERK (protein kinase RNA-like ER kinase), ATF6 (activating transcription factor 6), and activate caspase-12, in diabetic mice [42, 44]. The administration of L and Z also prevented diabetes-induced dysfunction of the mitochondria and damage to mitochondrial DNA (mtDNA), which was confirmed by enhanced expression of mtDNA-encoded proteins of the electron transport chain [41]. Wolfberry, a traditional Asian fruit containing large amounts of diester forms of L and Z protected against mitochondrial stress and markedly enhanced retinal expression of proteins involved in mitochondrial biogenesis [44, 45, 114]. Thus, L and Z reduced oxidative injury on retinal mitochondria by possibly restoring the effective transfer of electrons during oxidative phosphorylation and attenuating mitochondrial dysfunction.

The metabolic correlates of diabetes, such as insulin resistance, insulin deficiency, hyperglycemia and hyperlipidemia have been linked with inhibition of the endogenous antioxidant defense system, caused by overwhelming generation of pro-oxidant stressors and compromised antioxidant capacity. Restoration of endogenous antioxidant levels, such as GSH, GPx and manganese superoxide-dismutase (MnSOD) are essential for nutrient metabolism, regulation of gene expression, free radical neutralization and inhibition of pro-inflammatory pathways [115–120]. In the diabetic retina, regeneration of GSH is compromised by reduced GPx activity and redox cycle [121, 122]; however, L and/or Z reversed the hyperglycemia-induced impairment in GSH and GPx activity in the retina [37–39, 42]. Similarly, diabetic impairment of total antioxidant capacity was sufficiently prevented with supplementation of L and Z [41] along with restoration of MnSOD activity and mRNA expression following administration of AREDS-based micronutrient formula [39, 40, 44].

Carotenoids may prevent the development of DR by suppressing pro-inflammatory pathways activated by overexpressed superoxide free radicals and oxidative injury which are significant contributors in this low-grade chronic inflammatory condition [115, 116, 118]. Metabolic and oxidative insults associated with hyperglycemia can promote induction of inflammation, and concurrently, inflammatory processes can induce oxidative stress. Administration of antioxidants (including L and Z) has been demonstrated to inhibit increased-activation of retinal redox-sensitive nuclear transcriptional factor-B (NF-kB), an important transcriptional regulator of cytokines and growth factors [38, 41, 42, 123–126]; in addition to suppression of pro-inflammatory cytokine, interleukin-1β [41, 124]. Increases in pro-angiogenic factors such as VEGF, which significantly contribute to the neovascularization of PDR, were effectively prevented by L and Z in both rats and mice [39, 41, 45, 126]. However, increased levels of VEGF also play a significant role in the early-stages of retinopathy, by enhancing cell permeability of vascular and non-vascular retinal cells [116, 118–120, 126, 127]. Impaired glutamate metabolism in glial cells, resulting from diabetes, may lead to vascular instability in adjacent blood vessels [128, 129]; these changes in glial cell permeability often occur rapidly as a result of hyperglycemia, contributing to neural degeneration and may result in DME [127–129]. Thus, the protective effects of L and Z are effectual in attenuating multiple inflammatory response pathways and may preserve the retina from adaptive changes in microvasculature.

Clinical findings of early-stage retinopathy are currently characterized by pathogenic alterations in retinal vasculature, represented by microvascular abnormalities like vasoregression, along with choroidal occlusion and leakage [127, 130]. However, there is growing evidence in animal models that alterations in non-vascular cells (such as Mullers, bipolar, amacrine, and photoreceptor cells) are evident prior to the development of vascular abnormalities [131, 132]. The effects of L in retinal ischemic/reperfusion injury, a clinical feature of PDR, demonstrated improvements in cell viability and enhanced survival of Muller glial cells [133, 134]. Meanwhile, accelerated decline of total retinal thickness, including the inner nuclear layer (INL), outer nuclear layer (ONL), inner plexiform layer (IPL) and ganglion cell layer (GCL; thickness and cell number) were sufficiently prevented by L and/or Z in experimental murine models [37, 43, 44]. Significant thinning of the photoreceptor layer (inner segment and outer segment) and structural abnormalities (nuclear distribution) of the ONL were prevented by L and Z (wolfberry) in db/db mice [44]. The alterations in retinal histology, caused by diabetes mellitus, are closely linked with apoptotic oxidative injury in vascular cells; observed in humans and animals. Prevention of capillary cell apoptosis, determined by terminal deoxyribonucleotide transferase-mediated dUTP nick-end labeling (TUNEL)-staining, and increases in degenerative (acellular) capillaries, was achieved by L and/or Z; regarded as a surrogate endpoint for DR-therapeutic development and hallmark sign of early-stage NPDR, respectively [37–41, 43, 111, 112]. Thus, the neuroprotective potential of L and Z in maintaining the retina, an integral part of the central nervous system, is essential in preventing neural degeneration and irreversible vision loss.

Visual performance dysfunction caused by retinal degeneration, observed by electroretinogram (ERG) in the inner retinal layers, show a decrease in oscillatory potentials (OPs; OP3 and total OPs) in diabetic mice [43]; similar functional impairment observed clinically in early-stage retinopathy [135–137]. Similarly, the neuroprotective effects of L and Z were observed in ERG recordings which indicated the preservation of b-wave latency and a-wave/b-wave amplitudes, restoring retinal dysfunction induced by diabetes [37, 41–43]. Synaptophysin, a synaptic vesicle protein that plays an important role in neuronal synaptic network activity, is also reduced in diabetic retina [43]; which is caused by chronic activation of pro-oxidant extracellular signal-regulated kinase (ERK) [138, 139]. In the retina of hyperglycemia-induced mice, administration of L preserved synaptophysin protein and suppressed ERK activation. This provides evidence of neuroprotective potential of L to help maintain synaptic activity [43, 137]. Furthermore, supplementation of L demonstrated enhanced preservation of neural activity by restoring expression levels of retinal neurotrophic factor, BDNF (brain-derived neuronal trophic factor) [43]; an important mediator of synaptic network activity and cell survival in the inner retinal and ganglion cell layers [140–143]. The neuroprotective benefits of L and Z observed in animal models may be explained by supporting cell survival and increased viability and thus, enhancing overall visual function.

There are some limitation to the findings from animal models. Briefly, lack of studies on the effects of L and Z in non-murine models, restricts the translative potential for clinical use due to species differences between humans and rodents; namely, absence of the macula in these animals [144, 145]. Retinal preservation and neuroprotection with L and/or Z were observed in some [38, 42–45] but not all [37, 39–41] studies, independent of any change in hyperglycemic status and thus, interpretation of these findings must be exercised with prudence. Moreover, the dosage of L and Z tested in experimental models is typically inflated to significantly higher amounts than those observed in clinical application to achieve a dose-dependent effect, which may prompt the necessity for renewed clinical trials to determine safety and toxicity of these carotenoids in larger amounts. It is not an exaggeration to conclude that these animal model experiments of diabetes provide substantial evidence in support of the putative anti-angiogenic and anti-inflammatory benefits of carotenoids lutein and zeaxanthin in protecting against retinal neurodegeneration.

3.5 Carotenoids in the management of diabetic eye disease (*Clinical Studies*)

To date, a limited number of studies have examined the complex association of macular carotenoids levels and diabetic eye disease in individuals with type 1 and type 2 diabetes [26, 32, 35, 47–54]. Studies evaluating the relationship between serum levels of L and Z and DR demonstrated that: (1) serum concentrations of L and Z were lower in patients with DR when compared to healthy controls; (2) higher plasma concentrations of non-pro-vitamin A carotenoids (including lycopene, L and Z) were associated with lower risk of developing or progression of retinopathy in T2DM, after adjusting for potential confounders; (3) supplementation with carotenoid vitamin therapy may improve visual function and features of macular edema in patients with DR [47, 54]. It is known that carotenoid levels in the plasma are positively correlated with concentrations in the macular pigment [71, 146]. However, there are limitations when measuring serum levels to evaluate the effects of L and Z on DR, namely that their concentrations are almost entirely dependent upon relatively-recent dietary-behaviors; fluctuations that can occur in response to dietary intake of high-glycemic index foods and/or sugar-sweetened beverages [147–150]. Moreover, these dietary habits, similar to those in the Western diet, have been attributed largely to the prevalence and onset of the metabolic syndrome [147–149, 151, 152].

Several studies investigated the putative role of L and Z in attenuating the pathogenesis of DR by evaluating levels of MPOD in cohorts that included both type 1 and type 2 diabetes [26, 32, 35, 48–53]. The findings from these reports suggest the following: (1) MPOD levels are lower in patients with diabetes, in particular T2DM, than healthy individuals; (2) in T2DM, MPOD was inversely associated with several behavioral, anthropometric, and novel serum biomarkers such as vitamin D insufficiency; (3) MPOD levels can be augmented with dietary supplementation in patients with diabetes (type 1 and 2) [26, 32, 47–53]. Generally, reports are consistent suggesting MPOD levels are significantly lower in individuals with diabetes, and a negative correlation has been indicated between severity of diabetic maculopathy and level of macular carotenoids [48, 49, 51]. The type of diabetes also had a statistically significant difference on MPOD when accounting for other covariates (including history of smoking, hypertension and bodyweight) [26, 32, 50]. Current smoking status and increased adiposity are potential predictors of low MPOD in diabetes [26, 32] and concomitantly, one study found low serum vitamin D ($\leq$50 nmol/L; $P = 0.006$) was significantly correlated with MPOD in T2DM after multivariate regression analysis [32]. The DiVFuSS study demonstrated that carotenoid supplementation, which included antioxidant micronutrients such as alpha-lipoic acid and vitamin D3, can significantly improve MPOD levels (mean increase of 27% in participants on active supplement) and measures of visual function in patients with diabetes (with no retinopathy) and those with mild to moderate NPDR [35, 109, 153].

Evidence suggests that the MPOD depletion may be a clinical feature of T2DM, however, the proposed causal mechanisms may elucidate distinct contributing factors in the development of diabetic retinopathy; mechanistic associations with MPOD status that may differ between type 1 and type 2. Metabolic comorbidities observed in T2DM including increased adiposity and dyslipidemia, primarily characterized by reduced high-density lipoprotein (HDL) and hypertriglyceridemia, may substantially compromise the bioavailability of dietary carotenoids. Thus, diminished transport and assimilation of serum L and Z into the macular pigment may be directly represented by low MPOD levels [154–161]. Not surprisingly, L and Z are regularly deposited into visceral and subcutaneous adipose tissue, major body sites for carotenoids, which may make them less available to retinal tissue. In fact, reports have demonstrated higher percentages of body fat and body mass index (BMI) are inversely associated with MPOD levels [155, 158, 162–164]. Adipose concentrations of macular carotenoids vary according to the body site, coordinated by the hormonally-regulated deposition and mobilization of fatty acids, with demonstrably elevated levels in abdominal fat [164–166]; which may also explain sex-based differences observed in MPOD levels [154, 161]. Metabolic correlates like dyslipidemia may further contribute to low MPOD in T2DM by compromising the transport of plasma carotenoids to the retina in consequence of increased serum triglycerides to HDL (TG/HDL) ratio concurrent with worsening insulin resistance [166–168]. Furthermore, evidence suggests that serum carotenoids are predominantly transported by HDL particles and retinal absorption of L and Z is mediated by a 'piggy-back' mechanism involving scavenger receptor class B type-1 (SR-1B) in the RPE [157, 159, 169].

The depletion of MPOD in T2DM or poorly controlled T1DM is likely dependent upon the complex interplay between the development of metabolic perturbations including increased adiposity, dyslipidemia, insulin deficiency and hyperglycemia and the oxidative stress and inflammation induced by diabetes mellitus. Traditionally, adipose tissue has mainly been considered in the context of energy storage, however, they produce a variety adipocytokines and inflammatory mediators and has been suggested to function like a metabolically-active immune organ [170, 171]. In fact, increased intra-abdominal fat is a crucial determinant of the atherogenic lipid profile in T2DM with obesity, and research indicates visceral adipose tissue may be the principal mediator of inflammation associated with diabetes [172–174]. Therefore, this chronic low-grade inflammatory disease in turn exacerbates oxidative injury, causing a positive feedback loop between oxidative stress and inflammation, which may lead to compounding depletion of macular pigment concentrations [35, 115, 152, 175–177]. The elevated serum concentrations of a marker for total systemic oxidative stress *in-vivo*, 8-OHdG, have been positively correlated with BMI in T2DM [173, 177]. It is suggested that the metabolic correlates and comorbidities frequently associated with T2DM (or poorly controlled T1DM) contribute significantly to the onset and progression of retinopathy into PDR.

Results from these [26, 32, 35, 48–53] clinical studies that have investigated the implications of MPOD on diabetic eye disease are promising, but not without limitations: (1) with one exception [26], individuals with T1DM and T2DM were evaluated and analyzed homogeneously in comparison to controls; (2) only a limited number of studies evaluated cohorts based on status of DR; (3) relatively small and unequal sample sizes (of individuals with diabetes and controls) in multiple studies; (4) with one exception [35], studies were only observational in nature. Additional research is necessary to further elucidate the potentially different associations that may exist between MPOD status and T1DM and T2DM.

4. Conclusions

Diabetic retinopathy is the most common microvascular complication of diabetes mellitus and DR remains the leading cause of preventable blindness in developed countries among working-age adults. It appears chronic hyperglycemia has significant deleterious effects on the endogenous defense systems, resulting in the depletion of macular carotenoids lutein, zeaxanthin and *meso*-zeaxanthin, in addition to other potent antioxidants that are pertinent for maintaining retinal health. Additionally, the metabolic correlates of diabetes negatively impact concentrations of macular pigments, however, carotenoid vitamin therapy has shown promising results in augmenting MPOD levels and visual performance. To this accord, regularly measuring MPOD may be well suited for monitoring retinal neurodegeneration brought on by diabetes and screening at-risk patients before clinical features of retinopathy become apparent. Meanwhile, routine management of established risk factors such as poor glycemic control, obesity and hypertension are critical in preventing or delaying the progression of DR. However, there is tremendous need for both timely and functional prophylactic measures that can be implemented before irreversible loss of vision begins. Finally, carotenoid vitamin therapy shows great promise with increasing evidence both in animal and human studies, further clinical investigations must be performed to assess its full potential in the management of diabetic eye disease.

Acknowledgements

The authors would like to thank the Assessment & Public Relations Librarian from Western University of Health Sciences, Rudy Barreras for his counsel in conducting the systematic review.

Conflict of interest

Drake W. Lem none. Dr. Pinakin Davey is a consultant and has received research grants from ZeaVision and Guardion Health Sciences. Dr. Dennis L. Gierhart is an Employee, Chief Scientific Officer for ZeaVision manufacturer of various nutritional supplements including the DVS.

Author details

Drake W. Lem[1†], Dennis L. Gierhart[2] and Pinakin Gunvant Davey[1*†]

1 College of Optometry, Western University of Health Sciences, Pomona, CA, USA

2 ZeaVision, LLC, Chesterfield, MO, USA

*Address all correspondence to: contact@pinakin-gunvant.com

† These authors contributed equally.

References

[1] Prevention, C.f.D.C.a. *National Diabetes Statistics Report 2020*. 2020.

[2] International Diabetes Federation, t.e. *IDF Diabetes Atlas*. 2019; 9th:[Available from: https://www.diabetesatlas.org/en/.

[3] Saeedi, P., et al., *Global and regional diabetes prevalence estimates for 2019 and projections for 2030 and 2045: Results from the International Diabetes Federation Diabetes Atlas, 9(th) edition.* Diabetes Res Clin Pract, 2019. **157**: p. 107843.

[4] Lin, X., et al., *Global, regional, and national burden and trend of diabetes in 195 countries and territories: an analysis from 1990 to 2025.* Sci Rep, 2020. **10**(1): p. 14790.

[5] Wong, T.Y. and C. Sabanayagam, *Strategies to Tackle the Global Burden of Diabetic Retinopathy: From Epidemiology to Artificial Intelligence.* Ophthalmologica, 2020. **243**(1): p. 9-20.

[6] Lee, R., T.Y. Wong, and C. Sabanayagam, *Epidemiology of diabetic retinopathy, diabetic macular edema and related vision loss.* Eye Vis (Lond), 2015. **2**: p. 17.

[7] Solomon, S.D., et al., *Diabetic Retinopathy: A Position Statement by the American Diabetes Association.* Diabetes Care, 2017. **40**(3): p. 412-418.

[8] WHO, W.H.O. *World report on vision 2019*. 2020.

[9] Antonetti, D.A., R. Klein, and T.W. Gardner, *Diabetic retinopathy.* N Engl J Med, 2012. **366**(13): p. 1227-39.

[10] Cheloni, R., et al., *Global prevalence of diabetic retinopathy: protocol for a systematic review and meta-analysis.* BMJ Open, 2019. **9**(3): p. e022188.

[11] Pearce, I., et al., *Association between diabetic eye disease and other complications of diabetes: Implications for care. A systematic review.* Diabetes Obes Metab, 2019. **21**(3): p. 467-478.

[12] Simo-Servat, O., C. Hernandez, and R. Simo, *Diabetic Retinopathy in the Context of Patients with Diabetes.* Ophthalmic Res, 2019. **62**(4): p. 211-217.

[13] Berco, E., et al., *Management of Diabetic Retinopathy and Other Ocular Complications in Type 1 Diabetes*, in *Major Topics in Type 1 Diabetes*. 2015, InTech.

[14] Wilkinson, C.P., et al., *Proposed international clinical diabetic retinopathy and diabetic macular edema disease severity scales.* Ophthalmology, 2003. **110**(9): p. 1677-82.

[15] Yonekawa, Y., et al., *American Society of Retina Specialists Clinical Practice Guidelines: Management of Nonproliferative and Proliferative Diabetic Retinopathy Without Diabetic Macular Edema.* Journal of VitreoRetinal Diseases, 2020. **4**(2): p. 125-135.

[16] Wu, L., et al., *Classification of diabetic retinopathy and diabetic macular edema.* World J Diabetes, 2013. **4**(6): p. 290-4.

[17] Group, E.T.D.R.S.R., *Grading diabetic retinopathy from stereoscopic color fundus photographs--an extension of the modified Airlie House classification. ETDRS report number 10. Early Treatment Diabetic Retinopathy Study Research Group.* Ophthalmology, 1991. **98**(5 Suppl): p. 786-806.

[18] Cheung, N., P. Mitchell, and T.Y. Wong, *Diabetic retinopathy.* Lancet, 2010. **376**(9735): p. 124-36.

[19] Duh, E.J., J.K. Sun, and A.W. Stitt, *Diabetic retinopathy: current understanding, mechanisms, and treatment strategies.* JCI Insight, 2017. **2**(14).

[20] Ishibazawa, A., et al., *Retinal Nonperfusion Relationship to Arteries or Veins Observed on Widefield Optical Coherence Tomography Angiography in Diabetic Retinopathy.* Invest Ophthalmol Vis Sci, 2019. **60**(13): p. 4310-4318.

[21] Acon, D. and L. Wu, *Multimodal Imaging in Diabetic Macular Edema.* Asia Pac J Ophthalmol (Phila), 2018. **7**(1): p. 22-27.

[22] You, Q.S., et al., *Reproducibility of Macular Pigment Optical Density Measurement by Two-Wavelength Autofluorescence in a Clinical Setting.* Retina, 2016. **36**(7): p. 1381-7.

[23] He, F., et al., *Diabetic retinopathy in predicting diabetic nephropathy in patients with type 2 diabetes and renal disease: a meta-analysis.* Diabetologia, 2013. **56**(3): p. 457-66.

[24] Kawasaki, R., et al., *Risk of cardiovascular diseases is increased even with mild diabetic retinopathy: the Japan Diabetes Complications Study.* Ophthalmology, 2013. **120**(3): p. 574-582.

[25] Tong, L., et al., *Association of macular involvement with proliferative retinopathy in Type 2 diabetes.* Diabet Med, 2001. **18**(5): p. 388-94.

[26] Scanlon, G., et al., *Macular Pigment Optical Density Is Lower in Type 2 Diabetes, Compared with Type 1 Diabetes and Normal Controls.* Retina, 2015. **35**(9): p. 1808-16.

[27] Kowluru, R.A. and P.S. Chan, *Oxidative stress and diabetic retinopathy.* Exp Diabetes Res, 2007. **2007**: p. 43603.

[28] Simo, R., A.W. Stitt, and T.W. Gardner, *Neurodegeneration in diabetic retinopathy: does it really matter?* Diabetologia, 2018. **61**(9): p. 1902-1912.

[29] Simo, R., C. Hernandez, and R. European Consortium for the Early Treatment of Diabetic, *Neurodegeneration in the diabetic eye: new insights and therapeutic perspectives.* Trends Endocrinol Metab, 2014. **25**(1): p. 23-33.

[30] Bek, T., *Diameter Changes of Retinal Vessels in Diabetic Retinopathy.* Curr Diab Rep, 2017. **17**(10): p. 82.

[31] Gardner, T.W. and J.R. Davila, *The neurovascular unit and the pathophysiologic basis of diabetic retinopathy.* Graefes Arch Clin Exp Ophthalmol, 2017. **255**(1): p. 1-6.

[32] Scanlon, G., et al., *Identification of Surrogate Biomarkers for the Prediction of Patients at Risk of Low Macular Pigment in Type 2 Diabetes.* Curr Eye Res, 2019. **44**(12): p. 1369-1380.

[33] Age-Related Eye Disease Study 2 Research, G., *Lutein + zeaxanthin and omega-3 fatty acids for age-related macular degeneration: the Age-Related Eye Disease Study 2 (AREDS2) randomized clinical trial.* JAMA, 2013. **309**(19): p. 2005-15.

[34] Age-Related Eye Disease Study Research, G., et al., *The relationship of dietary carotenoid and vitamin A, E, and C intake with age-related macular degeneration in a case-control study: AREDS Report No. 22.* Arch Ophthalmol, 2007. **125**(9): p. 1225-32.

[35] Chous, A.P., et al., *The Diabetes Visual Function Supplement Study (DiVFuSS).* Br J Ophthalmol, 2016. **100**(2): p. 227-34.

[36] Davey, P.G., et al., *Visual Function and Macular Carotenoid Changes in Eyes with Retinal Drusen-An Open Label Randomized Controlled Trial to Compare a Micronized Lipid-Based Carotenoid Liquid Supplementation and AREDS-2 Formula.* Nutrients, 2020. **12**(11).

[37] Arnal, E., et al., *Beneficial effect of docosahexanoic acid and lutein on retinal*

structural, metabolic, and functional abnormalities in diabetic rats. Curr Eye Res, 2009. **34**(11): p. 928-38.

[38] Kowluru, R.A. and S. Odenbach, *Effect of long-term administration of alpha-lipoic acid on retinal capillary cell death and the development of retinopathy in diabetic rats.* Diabetes, 2004. **53**(12): p. 3233-8.

[39] Kowluru, R.A., B. Menon, and D.L. Gierhart, *Beneficial effect of zeaxanthin on retinal metabolic abnormalities in diabetic rats.* Invest Ophthalmol Vis Sci, 2008. **49**(4): p. 1645-51.

[40] Kowluru, R.A., et al., *Inhibition of retinopathy and retinal metabolic abnormalities in diabetic rats with AREDS-based micronutrients.* Arch Ophthalmol, 2008. **126**(9): p. 1266-72.

[41] Kowluru, R.A., et al., *Beneficial effects of the nutritional supplements on the development of diabetic retinopathy.* Nutr Metab (Lond), 2014. **11**(1): p. 8.

[42] Muriach, M., et al., *Lutein effect on retina and hippocampus of diabetic mice.* Free Radic Biol Med, 2006. **41**(6): p. 979-84.

[43] Sasaki, M., et al., *Neurodegenerative influence of oxidative stress in the retina of a murine model of diabetes.* Diabetologia, 2010. **53**(5): p. 971-9.

[44] Tang, L., et al., *Dietary wolfberry ameliorates retinal structure abnormalities in db/db mice at the early stage of diabetes.* Exp Biol Med (Maywood), 2011. **236**(9): p. 1051-63.

[45] Yu, H., et al., *Dietary wolfberry upregulates carotenoid metabolic genes and enhances mitochondrial biogenesis in the retina of db/db diabetic mice.* Mol Nutr Food Res, 2013. **57**(7): p. 1158-69.

[46] Hammes, H.P., et al., *Diabetic retinopathy: targeting vasoregression.* Diabetes, 2011. **60**(1): p. 9-16.

[47] Brazionis, L., et al., *Plasma carotenoids and diabetic retinopathy.* Br J Nutr, 2009. **101**(2): p. 270-7.

[48] Cennamo, G., et al., *The Relationship between Macular Pigment and Vessel Density in Patients with Type 1 Diabetes Mellitus.* Ophthalmic Res, 2019. **61**(1): p. 19-25.

[49] Davies, N.P. and A.B. Morland, *Color matching in diabetes: optical density of the crystalline lens and macular pigments.* Invest Ophthalmol Vis Sci, 2002. **43**(1): p. 281-9.

[50] Lima, V.C., et al., *Macular pigment optical density measured by dual-wavelength autofluorescence imaging in diabetic and nondiabetic patients: a comparative study.* Invest Ophthalmol Vis Sci, 2010. **51**(11): p. 5840-5.

[51] Mares, J.A., et al., *Predictors of optical density of lutein and zeaxanthin in retinas of older women in the Carotenoids in Age-Related Eye Disease Study, an ancillary study of the Women's Health Initiative.* Am J Clin Nutr, 2006. **84**(5): p. 1107-22.

[52] She, C.Y., et al., *Association of macular pigment optical density with early stage of non-proliferative diabetic retinopathy in Chinese patients with type 2 diabetes mellitus.* Int J Ophthalmol, 2016. **9**(10): p. 1433-1438.

[53] Zagers, N.P., M.C. Pot, and D. van Norren, *Spectral and directional reflectance of the fovea in diabetes mellitus: photoreceptor integrity, macular pigment and lens.* Vision Res, 2005. **45**(13): p. 1745-53.

[54] Hu, B.J., et al., *Application of Lutein and Zeaxanthin in nonproliferative diabetic retinopathy.* Int J Ophthalmol, 2011. **4**(3): p. 303-6.

[55] Group, F.-N.B.W., *BEST (Biomarkers, EndpointS, and other Tools)*

Resource. Silver Spring (MD): Food and Drug Administration (US), 2016.

[56] Robb, M.A., P.M. McInnes, and R.M. Califf, *Biomarkers and Surrogate Endpoints: Developing Common Terminology and Definitions.* JAMA, 2016. **315**(11): p. 1107-8.

[57] Califf, R.M., *Biomarker definitions and their applications.* Exp Biol Med (Maywood), 2018. **243**(3): p. 213-221.

[58] Wickstrom, K. and J. Moseley, *Biomarkers and Surrogate Endpoints in Drug Development: A European Regulatory View.* Invest Ophthalmol Vis Sci, 2017. **58**(6): p. BIO27-BIO33.

[59] Nagai, N., et al., *Association of macular pigment optical density with serum concentration of oxidized low-density lipoprotein in healthy adults.* Retina, 2015. **35**(4): p. 820-6.

[60] Nagai, N., et al., *Macular Pigment Optical Density and Photoreceptor Outer Segment Length as Predisease Biomarkers for Age-Related Macular Degeneration.* J Clin Med, 2020. **9**(5): p. 10.

[61] Ozkaya, A., et al., *Thickness of the retinal photoreceptor outer segment layer in healthy volunteers and in patients with diabetes mellitus without retinopathy, diabetic retinopathy, or diabetic macular edema.* Saudi J Ophthalmol, 2017. **31**(2): p. 69-75.

[62] Bernstein, P.S., et al., *The value of measurement of macular carotenoid pigment optical densities and distributions in age-related macular degeneration and other retinal disorders.* Vision Res, 2010. **50**(7): p. 716-28.

[63] Gruszecki, W.I. and J. Sielewiesiuk, *Orientation of xanthophylls in phosphatidylcholine multibilayers.* Biochim Biophys Acta, 1990. **1023**(3): p. 405-12.

[64] de Kinkelder, R., et al., *Macular pigment optical density measurements: evaluation of a device using heterochromatic flicker photometry.* Eye (Lond), 2011. **25**(1): p. 105-12.

[65] Leung, I.Y., *Macular pigment: new clinical methods of detection and the role of carotenoids in age-related macular degeneration.* Optometry, 2008. **79**(5): p. 266-72.

[66] Li, B., et al., *Imaging lutein and zeaxanthin in the human retina with confocal resonance Raman microscopy.* Proc Natl Acad Sci U S A, 2020. **117**(22): p. 12352-12358.

[67] Bone, R.A., et al., *Stereochemistry of the human macular carotenoids.* Invest Ophthalmol Vis Sci, 1993. **34**(6): p. 2033-40.

[68] Scripsema, N.K., D.N. Hu, and R.B. Rosen, *Lutein, Zeaxanthin, and meso-Zeaxanthin in the Clinical Management of Eye Disease.* J Ophthalmol, 2015. **2015**: p. 865179.

[69] Howells, O., F. Eperjesi, and H. Bartlett, *Measuring macular pigment optical density in vivo: a review of techniques.* Graefes Arch Clin Exp Ophthalmol, 2011. **249**(3): p. 315-47.

[70] Bone, R.A., et al., *Macular pigment in donor eyes with and without AMD: a case-control study.* Invest Ophthalmol Vis Sci, 2001. **42**(1): p. 235-40.

[71] Landrum, J.T., et al., *A one year study of the macular pigment: the effect of 140 days of a lutein supplement.* Exp Eye Res, 1997. **65**(1): p. 57-62.

[72] Bone, R.A., et al., *Macular pigment response to a supplement containing meso-zeaxanthin, lutein and zeaxanthin.* Nutr Metab (Lond), 2007. **4**: p. 12.

[73] Howells, O., F. Eperjesi, and H. Bartlett, *Improving the repeatability of heterochromatic flicker photometry for measurement of macular pigment optical density.* Graefes Arch Clin Exp Ophthalmol, 2013. **251**(3): p. 871-80.

[74] Krinsky, N.I. and E.J. Johnson, *Carotenoid actions and their relation to health and disease.* Mol Aspects Med, 2005. **26**(6): p. 459-516.

[75] Junghans, A., H. Sies, and W. Stahl, *Macular pigments lutein and zeaxanthin as blue light filters studied in liposomes.* Arch Biochem Biophys, 2001. **391**(2): p. 160-4.

[76] Kijlstra, A., et al., *Lutein: more than just a filter for blue light.* Prog Retin Eye Res, 2012. **31**(4): p. 303-15.

[77] Landrum, J.T. and R.A. Bone, *Mechanistic Evidence for eye disease and carotenoids*. Carotenoids in Health and Disease. 2004, New York, NY, USA: CRC Press.

[78] Li, S.Y., Z.J. Fu, and A.C. Lo, *Hypoxia-induced oxidative stress in ischemic retinopathy.* Oxid Med Cell Longev, 2012. **2012**: p. 426769.

[79] Markan, A., et al., *Novel imaging biomarkers in diabetic retinopathy and diabetic macular edema.* Ther Adv Ophthalmol, 2020. **12**: p. 2515841420950513.

[80] Suarez-Berumen, K. and P.G. Davey, *Macular Pigments Optical Density: A Review of Techniques of Measurements and Factors Influencing their Levels.* JSM Ophthalmol, 2014. **3**(1022): p. 4.

[81] Bartlett, H., O. Howells, and F. Eperjesi, *The role of macular pigment assessment in clinical practice: a review.* Clin Exp Optom, 2010. **93**(5): p. 300-8.

[82] Bartlett, H. and F. Eperjesi, *Apparent motion photometry: evaluation and reliability of a novel method for the measurement of macular pigment.* Br J Ophthalmol, 2011. **95**(5): p. 662-5.

[83] Moreland, J.D., *Macular pigment assessment by motion photometry.* Arch Biochem Biophys, 2004. **430**(2): p. 143-8.

[84] Davey, P.G., S.D. Alvarez, and J.Y. Lee, *Macular pigment optical density: repeatability, intereye correlation, and effect of ocular dominance.* Clin Ophthalmol, 2016. **10**: p. 1671-8.

[85] Lee, B.B., P.R. Martin, and A. Valberg, *The physiological basis of heterochromatic flicker photometry demonstrated in the ganglion cells of the macaque retina.* J Physiol, 1988. **404**: p. 323-47.

[86] Bone, R.A. and A. Mukherjee, *Innovative Troxler-free Measurement of Macular Pigment and Lens Density with Correction of the Former for the Aging Lens.* Journal of Biomedical Optics, 2013. **18**(10): p. 9.

[87] Obana, A., et al., *Reliability of a commercially available heterochromatic flicker photometer, the MPS2, for measuring the macular pigment optical density of a Japanese population.* Jpn J Ophthalmol, 2018. **62**(4): p. 473-480.

[88] Christaras, D., et al., *Objective method for measuring the macular pigment optical density in the eye.* Biomed Opt Express, 2019. **10**(7): p. 3572-3583.

[89] Berendschot, T.T., et al., *Influence of lutein supplementation on macular pigment, assessed with two objective techniques.* Invest Ophthalmol Vis Sci, 2000. **41**(11): p. 3322-6.

[90] Berendschot, T.T. and D. van Norren, *Objective determination of the macular pigment optical density using fundus reflectance spectroscopy.* Arch Biochem Biophys, 2004. **430**(2): p. 149-55.

[91] Davey, P.G., et al., *Macular Pigment Reflectometry: Development and evaluation of a novel clinical device for rapid objective assessment of the macular carotenoids*, in *Ophthalmic Technologies Xxix*, F. Manns, P.G. Soderberg, and A. Ho, Editors. 2019, Spie-Int Soc Optical Engineering: Bellingham.

[92] Huang, H., et al., *Macular Pigment Optical Density Measured by a Single Wavelength Reflection Photometry with and without Mydriasis.* Curr Eye Res, 2019. **44**(3): p. 324-328.

[93] Kilbride, P.E., et al., *Human macular pigment assessed by imaging fundus reflectometry.* Vision Res, 1989. **29**(6): p. 663-74.

[94] Sanabria, J.C., et al., *Measurement of Carotenoids in Perifovea using the Macular Pigment Reflectometer.* J Vis Exp, 2020(155): p. 9.

[95] Delori, F.C., et al., *Macular pigment density measured by autofluorescence spectrometry: comparison with reflectometry and heterochromatic flicker photometry.* J Opt Soc Am A Opt Image Sci Vis, 2001. **18**(6): p. 1212-30.

[96] Dennison, J.L., et al., *Concordance of macular pigment measurements obtained using customized heterochromatic flicker photometry, dual-wavelength autofluorescence, and single-wavelength reflectance.* Exp Eye Res, 2013. **116**: p. 190-8.

[97] Delori, F.C., *Autofluorescence method to measure macular pigment optical densities fluorometry and autofluorescence imaging.* Arch Biochem Biophys, 2004. **430**(2): p. 156-62.

[98] Bernstein, P.S., et al., *Resonance Raman measurement of macular carotenoids in the living human eye.* Arch Biochem Biophys, 2004. **430**(2): p. 163-9.

[99] Gellermann, W., et al., *In vivo resonant Raman measurement of macular carotenoid pigments in the young and the aging human retina.* J Opt Soc Am A Opt Image Sci Vis, 2002. **19**(6): p. 1172-86.

[100] Lapierre-Landry, M., J. Carroll, and M.C. Skala, *Imaging retinal melanin: a review of current technologies.* J Biol Eng, 2018. **12**(1): p. 29.

[101] Bartlett, H. and F. Eperjesi, *Use of fundus imaging in quantification of age-related macular change.* Surv Ophthalmol, 2007. **52**(6): p. 655-71.

[102] Yung, M., M.A. Klufas, and D. Sarraf, *Clinical applications of fundus autofluorescence in retinal disease.* Int J Retina Vitreous, 2016. **2**(1): p. 12.

[103] Bernstein, P.S. and W. Gellermann, *Measurement of carotenoids in the living primate eye using resonance Raman spectroscopy.* Methods Mol Biol, 2002. **196**: p. 321-9.

[104] Neelam, K., et al., *Measurement of macular pigment: Raman spectroscopy versus heterochromatic flicker photometry.* Invest Ophthalmol Vis Sci, 2005. **46**(3): p. 1023-32.

[105] Rakieten, N., M.L. Rakieten, and M.R. Nadkarni, *Studies on the diabetogenic action of streptozotocin (NSC-37917).* Cancer Chemother Rep, 1963. **29**: p. 91-8.

[106] Olivares, A.M., et al., *Animal Models of Diabetic Retinopathy.* Curr Diab Rep, 2017. **17**(10): p. 93.

[107] Robinson, R., et al., *Update on animal models of diabetic retinopathy: from molecular approaches to mice and higher mammals.* Dis Model Mech, 2012. **5**(4): p. 444-56.

[108] Kanwar, M., et al., *Oxidative damage in the retinal mitochondria of diabetic mice: possible protection by superoxide dismutase.* Invest Ophthalmol Vis Sci, 2007. **48**(8): p. 3805-11.

[109] Brownlee, M., *The pathobiology of diabetic complications: a unifying mechanism.* Diabetes, 2005. **54**(6): p. 1615-25.

[110] ZeaVision. *EyePromise DVS*. 2020; Available from: http://www.eyepromise.com/doctors/products/eyepromise-dvs/?utm_

source=Website&utm_medium=Blog-Post&utm_campaign=Doctor-Blog&utm_content=Diabetes-Awareness-Series-3-Sept2018.

[111] Kern, T.S., et al., *Response of capillary cell death to aminoguanidine predicts the development of retinopathy: comparison of diabetes and galactosemia.* Invest Ophthalmol Vis Sci, 2000. **41**(12): p. 3972-8.

[112] Mizutani, M., T.S. Kern, and M. Lorenzi, *Accelerated death of retinal microvascular cells in human and experimental diabetic retinopathy.* J Clin Invest, 1996. **97**(12): p. 2883-90.

[113] Kowluru, R.A., et al., *Oxidative stress and epigenetic modifications in the pathogenesis of diabetic retinopathy.* Prog Retin Eye Res, 2015. **48**: p. 40-61.

[114] Inbaraj, B.S., et al., *Determination of carotenoids and their esters in fruits of Lycium barbarum Linnaeus by HPLC-DAD-APCI-MS.* J Pharm Biomed Anal, 2008. **47**(4-5): p. 812-8.

[115] Neelam, K., et al., *Putative protective role of lutein and zeaxanthin in diabetic retinopathy.* Br J Ophthalmol, 2017. **101**(5): p. 551-558.

[116] Izumi-Nagai, K., et al., *Macular pigment lutein is antiinflammatory in preventing choroidal neovascularization.* Arterioscler Thromb Vasc Biol, 2007. **27**(12): p. 2555-62.

[117] Sarıkaya, E. and S. Doğan, *Glutathione Peroxidase in Health and Diseases*, in *Glutathione System and Oxidative Stress in Health and Disease*. 2020, IntechOpen.

[118] Bian, Q., et al., *Lutein and zeaxanthin supplementation reduces photooxidative damage and modulates the expression of inflammation-related genes in retinal pigment epithelial cells.* Free Radic Biol Med, 2012. **53**(6): p. 1298-307.

[119] Feit-Leichman, R.A., et al., *Vascular damage in a mouse model of diabetic retinopathy: relation to neuronal and glial changes.* Invest Ophthalmol Vis Sci, 2005. **46**(11): p. 4281-7.

[120] Li, S.Y., et al., *Anti-inflammatory effects of lutein in retinal ischemic/hypoxic injury: in vivo and in vitro studies.* Invest Ophthalmol Vis Sci, 2012. **53**(10): p. 5976-84.

[121] Kowluru, R., T.S. Kern, and R.L. Engerman, *Abnormalities of retinal metabolism in diabetes or galactosemia. II. Comparison of gamma-glutamyl transpeptidase in retina and cerebral cortex, and effects of antioxidant therapy.* Curr Eye Res, 1994. **13**(12): p. 891-6.

[122] Kowluru, R.A., T.S. Kern, and R.L. Engerman, *Abnormalities of retinal metabolism in diabetes or experimental galactosemia. IV. Antioxidant defense system.* Free Radic Biol Med, 1997. **22**(4): p. 587-92.

[123] Chan, P.S., M. Kanwar, and R.A. Kowluru, *Resistance of retinal inflammatory mediators to suppress after reinstitution of good glycemic control: novel mechanism for metabolic memory.* J Diabetes Complications, 2010. **24**(1): p. 55-63.

[124] Kowluru, R.A. and S. Odenbach, *Role of interleukin-1beta in the development of retinopathy in rats: effect of antioxidants.* Invest Ophthalmol Vis Sci, 2004. **45**(11): p. 4161-6.

[125] Kowluru, R.A., et al., *Diabetes-induced activation of nuclear transcriptional factor in the retina, and its inhibition by antioxidants.* Free Radic Res, 2003. **37**(11): p. 1169-80.

[126] Abcouwer, S.F., *Angiogenic Factors and Cytokines in Diabetic Retinopathy.* J Clin Cell Immunol, 2013. **Suppl 1**(11).

[127] Kern, T.S., *Interrelationships between the Retinal Neuroglia and*

Vasculature in Diabetes. Diabetes Metab J, 2014. **38**(3): p. 163-70.

[128] Lieth, E., et al., *Diabetes reduces glutamate oxidation and glutamine synthesis in the retina. The Penn State Retina Research Group.* Exp Eye Res, 2000. **70**(6): p. 723-30.

[129] Mizutani, M., C. Gerhardinger, and M. Lorenzi, *Muller cell changes in human diabetic retinopathy.* Diabetes, 1998. **47**(3): p. 445-9.

[130] Curtis, T.M., T.A. Gardiner, and A.W. Stitt, *Microvascular lesions of diabetic retinopathy: clues towards understanding pathogenesis?* Eye (Lond), 2009. **23**(7): p. 1496-508.

[131] Kohzaki, K., A.J. Vingrys, and B.V. Bui, *Early inner retinal dysfunction in streptozotocin-induced diabetic rats.* Invest Ophthalmol Vis Sci, 2008. **49**(8): p. 3595-604.

[132] Zeng, X.X., Y.K. Ng, and E.A. Ling, *Neuronal and microglial response in the retina of streptozotocin-induced diabetic rats.* Vis Neurosci, 2000. **17**(3): p. 463-71.

[133] Fung, F.K., B.Y. Law, and A.C. Lo, *Lutein Attenuates Both Apoptosis and Autophagy upon Cobalt (II) Chloride-Induced Hypoxia in Rat Muller Cells.* PLoS One, 2016. **11**(12): p. e0167828.

[134] Li, S.Y., et al., *Effect of lutein on retinal neurons and oxidative stress in a model of acute retinal ischemia/reperfusion.* Invest Ophthalmol Vis Sci, 2009. **50**(2): p. 836-43.

[135] Kizawa, J., et al., *Changes of oscillatory potentials and photopic negative response in patients with early diabetic retinopathy.* Jpn J Ophthalmol, 2006. **50**(4): p. 367-373.

[136] Yonemura, D., K. Tsuzuki, and T. Aoki, *Clinical importance of the oscillatory potential in the human ERG.* Acta Ophthalmol Suppl, 1962. **Suppl 70**: p. 115-23.

[137] Ozawa, Y., et al., *Neuroprotective effects of lutein in the retina.* Curr Pharm Des, 2012. **18**(1): p. 51-6.

[138] Busik, J.V., S. Mohr, and M.B. Grant, *Hyperglycemia-induced reactive oxygen species toxicity to endothelial cells is dependent on paracrine mediators.* Diabetes, 2008. **57**(7): p. 1952-65.

[139] Kurihara, T., et al., *Angiotensin II type 1 receptor signaling contributes to synaptophysin degradation and neuronal dysfunction in the diabetic retina.* Diabetes, 2008. **57**(8): p. 2191-8.

[140] Binder, D.K. and H.E. Scharfman, *Brain-derived neurotrophic factor.* Growth Factors, 2004. **22**(3): p. 123-31.

[141] Martin, P.M., et al., *Death of retinal neurons in streptozotocin-induced diabetic mice.* Invest Ophthalmol Vis Sci, 2004. **45**(9): p. 3330-6.

[142] Kern, T.S. and A.J. Barber, *Retinal ganglion cells in diabetes.* J Physiol, 2008. **586**(18): p. 4401-8.

[143] Seki, M., et al., *Involvement of brain-derived neurotrophic factor in early retinal neuropathy of streptozotocin-induced diabetes in rats: therapeutic potential of brain-derived neurotrophic factor for dopaminergic amacrine cells.* Diabetes, 2004. **53**(9): p. 2412-9.

[144] Xue, C., et al., *Management of Ocular Diseases Using Lutein and Zeaxanthin: What Have We Learned from Experimental Animal Studies?* J Ophthalmol, 2015. **2015**: p. 523027.

[145] Michikawa, T., et al., *Serum antioxidants and age-related macular degeneration among older Japanese.* Asia Pac J Clin Nutr, 2009. **18**(1): p. 1-7.

[146] Bone, R.A., et al., *Efficacy of Commercially Available Nutritional*

Supplements: Analysis of Serum Uptake, Macular Pigment Optical Density and Visual Functional Response. Nutrients, 2020. **12**(5): p. 15.

[147] Ludwig, D.S., et al., *High glycemic index foods, overeating, and obesity.* Pediatrics, 1999. **103**(3): p. E26.

[148] Gross, L.S., et al., *Increased consumption of refined carbohydrates and the epidemic of type 2 diabetes in the United States: an ecologic assessment.* Am J Clin Nutr, 2004. **79**(5): p. 774-9.

[149] Bray, G.A., S.J. Nielsen, and B.M. Popkin, *Consumption of high-fructose corn syrup in beverages may play a role in the epidemic of obesity.* Am J Clin Nutr, 2004. **79**(4): p. 537-43.

[150] Marshall, J.A., R.F. Hamman, and J. Baxter, *High-fat, low-carbohydrate diet and the etiology of non-insulin-dependent diabetes mellitus: the San Luis Valley Diabetes Study.* Am J Epidemiol, 1991. **134**(6): p. 590-603.

[151] van Het Hof, K.H., et al., *Dietary factors that affect the bioavailability of carotenoids.* J Nutr, 2000. **130**(3): p. 503-6.

[152] Scanlon, G., et al., *A review of the putative causal mechanisms associated with lower macular pigment in diabetes mellitus.* Nutr Res Rev, 2019. **32**(2): p. 247-264.

[153] Kowluru, R.A. and Q. Zhong, *Beyond AREDS: is there a place for antioxidant therapy in the prevention/ treatment of eye disease?* Invest Ophthalmol Vis Sci, 2011. **52**(12): p. 8665-71.

[154] Johnson, E.J., et al., *Relation among serum and tissue concentrations of lutein and zeaxanthin and macular pigment density.* Am J Clin Nutr, 2000. **71**(6): p. 1555-62.

[155] Hammond, B.R., Jr., T.A. Ciulla, and D.M. Snodderly, *Macular pigment density is reduced in obese subjects.* Invest Ophthalmol Vis Sci, 2002. **43**(1): p. 47-50.

[156] Thomson, L.R., et al., *Elevated retinal zeaxanthin and prevention of light-induced photoreceptor cell death in quail.* Invest Ophthalmol Vis Sci, 2002. **43**(11): p. 3538-49.

[157] Connor, W.E., et al., *The prime role of HDL to transport lutein into the retina: evidence from HDL-deficient WHAM chicks having a mutant ABCA1 transporter.* Invest Ophthalmol Vis Sci, 2007. **48**(9): p. 4226-31.

[158] Nolan, J., et al., *Macular pigment and percentage of body fat.* Invest Ophthalmol Vis Sci, 2004. **45**(11): p. 3940-50.

[159] Wang, W., et al., *Effect of dietary lutein and zeaxanthin on plasma carotenoids and their transport in lipoproteins in age-related macular degeneration.* Am J Clin Nutr, 2007. **85**(3): p. 762-9.

[160] Lim, C., et al., *Preparation and characterization of a lutein loading nanoemulsion system for ophthalmic eye drops.* Journal of Drug Delivery Science and Technology, 2016. **36**: p. 168-174.

[161] Broekmans, W.M., et al., *Macular pigment density in relation to serum and adipose tissue concentrations of lutein and serum concentrations of zeaxanthin.* Am J Clin Nutr, 2002. **76**(3): p. 595-603.

[162] Seddon, J.M., et al., *Progression of age-related macular degeneration: association with body mass index, waist circumference, and waist-hip ratio.* Arch Ophthalmol, 2003. **121**(6): p. 785-92.

[163] Nolan, J.M., et al., *Education is positively associated with macular pigment: the Irish Longitudinal Study on Ageing (TILDA).* Invest Ophthalmol Vis Sci, 2012. **53**(12): p. 7855-61.

[164] Bovier, E.R., R.D. Lewis, and B.R. Hammond, Jr., *The relationship between lutein and zeaxanthin status and body fat.* Nutrients, 2013. **5**(3): p. 750-7.

[165] Chung, H.Y., et al., *Site-specific concentrations of carotenoids in adipose tissue: relations with dietary and serum carotenoid concentrations in healthy adults.* Am J Clin Nutr, 2009. **90**(3): p. 533-9.

[166] Frayn, K.N., et al., *Coordinated regulation of hormone-sensitive lipase and lipoprotein lipase in human adipose tissue in vivo: implications for the control of fat storage and fat mobilization.* Adv Enzyme Regul, 1995. **35**: p. 163-78.

[167] Loane, E., J.M. Nolan, and S. Beatty, *The respective relationships between lipoprotein profile, macular pigment optical density, and serum concentrations of lutein and zeaxanthin.* Invest Ophthalmol Vis Sci, 2010. **51**(11): p. 5897-905.

[168] Goldberg, I.J., *Clinical review 124: Diabetic dyslipidemia: causes and consequences.* J Clin Endocrinol Metab, 2001. **86**(3): p. 965-71.

[169] During, A., S. Doraiswamy, and E.H. Harrison, *Xanthophylls are preferentially taken up compared with beta-carotene by retinal cells via a SRBI-dependent mechanism.* J Lipid Res, 2008. **49**(8): p. 1715-24.

[170] Rosen, B.S., et al., *Adipsin and complement factor D activity: an immune-related defect in obesity.* Science, 1989. **244**(4911): p. 1483-7.

[171] Tilg, H. and A.R. Moschen, *Adipocytokines: mediators linking adipose tissue, inflammation and immunity.* Nat Rev Immunol, 2006. **6**(10): p. 772-83.

[172] Nieves, D.J., et al., *The atherogenic lipoprotein profile associated with obesity and insulin resistance is largely attributable to intra-abdominal fat.* Diabetes, 2003. **52**(1): p. 172-9.

[173] Al-Aubaidy, H.A. and H.F. Jelinek, *Oxidative DNA damage and obesity in type 2 diabetes mellitus.* Eur J Endocrinol, 2011. **164**(6): p. 899-904.

[174] Castro, A.M., L.E. Macedo-de la Concha, and C.A. Pantoja-Meléndez, *Low-grade inflammation and its relation to obesity and chronic degenerative diseases.* Revista Médica del Hospital General de México, 2017. **80**(2): p. 101-105.

[175] Fernandez-Sanchez, A., et al., *Inflammation, oxidative stress, and obesity.* Int J Mol Sci, 2011. **12**(5): p. 3117-32.

[176] Kwon, H. and J.E. Pessin, *Adipokines mediate inflammation and insulin resistance.* Front Endocrinol (Lausanne), 2013. **4**: p. 71.

[177] Savini, I., et al., *Obesity-associated oxidative stress: strategies finalized to improve redox state.* Int J Mol Sci, 2013. **14**(5): p. 10497-538.

Chapter 13

Antioxidant Activity: The Presence and Impact of Hydroxyl Groups in Small Molecules of Natural and Synthetic Origin

Mohammed Ali Al-Mamary and Ziad Moussa

Abstract

Polyhydroxylated natural phenolic compounds, especially those with low molecular weights, are characterized by their ability to eliminate free radicals as they act as strong antioxidants. The various types of phenolic compounds represent the most important natural antioxidants in addition to some vitamins. The chemical structures of these compounds is discussed in details with their action mechanisms to remove free radicals and prevent many incurable and malignant diseases. In addition to these natural compounds, the last two decades have witnessed increased attempts by many scientific groups and research centers to synthesize chemical compounds in large quantities to mimic these natural compounds, but at a lower cost and greater biological effectiveness. Herein, we conduct a chemical survey of relevant synthetic compounds containing the hydroxyl groups prepared in chemical laboratories and studied for their biological efficacies, such as their effectiveness as antioxidants, as well as the mechanism of elimination of free radicals.

Keywords: antioxidants, hydroxyl Groups, natural antioxidants, synthetic antioxidants, small-molecules antioxidants

1. Introduction

1.1 Free radicals

Free radicals are chemical species such as atoms or group of atoms with an odd (unpaired) number of electrons. They are produced due to splitting weak bonds. The biological free radicals, such as reactive oxygen species (ROS) and reactive nitrogen species (RNS), are usually produced in our bodies. It is known that free radicals are very reactive and may quickly react with other chemical entities (atoms or molecules) by capturing the required electron to gain stability. There are two types of biologically important reactive species. The first type contains oxygen and is known as reactive oxygen species (ROS), while the second type contains nitrogen and is known as reactive nitrogen species (RNS). Both ROS and RNS can be classified into radicals and non-radical species.

1.1.1 Reactive oxygen species (ROS)

ROS can be classified into two types, radical species and non-radical species. The most important ROS radicals are: superoxide anion radical ($O_2^{\cdot-}$), hydroxyl radical ($^{\cdot}OH$), alkoxyl radical ($RO^{\cdot}$), lipid peroxide radical ($ROO^{\cdot}$), and hydroperoxy radical ($HOO^{\cdot}$). While the non-radicals ROS are: hydrogen peroxide (H_2O_2), singlet oxygen ($^1O_2$), ozone (O_3), organic peroxide (ROOH), and hypochlorous acid (HOCl).

1.1.1.1 Superoxide anion radical

It is important to emphasize that the mitochondria is the main source of the most active biological ROS [1–5] such as superoxide anion radical ($O_2^{\cdot-}$), hydrogen peroxide (H_2O_2) and hydroxyl radical ($^{\cdot}OH$). Thus, the initial reactive oxygen species ($O_2^{\cdot-}$) is produced due to the reduction of free oxygen by some electrons leaking out from the electron transport chain during the process of oxidative phosphorylation. This particle is relatively stable intermediate and considered as the precursor for most important ROS. The reduction of free oxygen by electrons in mitochondria can be illustrated as follows: $O_2 + e^- \rightarrow O_2^{\cdot-}$. In addition, the superoxide anion radical may be produced in a process of oxygen reduction by enzymatic systems in mammalian cells as follows [6]:

$$O_2 + e^- + \text{NADPD} - \text{oxidase or xanthine oxidase or cytochrome P450} \rightarrow O_2^{\cdot-}. \quad (1)$$

The superoxide anion radical and hydrogen peroxide are formed in vivo, in the brain, and the central nervous system (CNS). It is known that several areas in the brain contain high amount of iron which stimulates free radical reactions.

1.1.1.2 Hydroxyl radical ($^{\cdot}OH$)

The superoxide anion and hydrogen peroxide can be converted rapidly to hydroxyl radical ($^{\cdot}OH$), which is known as the most reactive and destructive radical in biological system. This radical is quickly produced via Fenton [7] and Haber-Wiess reactions as follows [8, 9]:

$$H_2O_2 + Fe^{2+} \rightarrow {}^{\cdot}OH + OH^- + Fe^{3+} \text{ (Fenton reaction)} \quad (2)$$

$$O_2^{\cdot-} + H_2O_2 \rightarrow {}^{\cdot}OH + {}^{-}OH + O_2 \text{ (Haber – Weiss reaction)} \quad (3)$$

The reaction of H_2O_2 with Fe^{+2} and Cu^+ metal ions which are typically complexed with certain intracellular proteins such as ferritin and ceruloplasmin, respectively [7], occurs due to stress conditions, which means an excess of superoxide anion radical ($O_2^{\cdot-}$). This phenomenon releases free ions (Fe^{+2}) from ferritin which in turn reacts with H_2O_2 according to Fenton reaction to produce hydroxyl radical ($^{\cdot}OH$). This free radical can strongly react with biomolecules such as DNA, proteins, lipids, and carbohydrates and cause severe damage to the cells than any other ROS [10]. The. OH is the most destructive free radical and can more easily penetrate the phospholipid bilayer than $O_2^{\cdot-}$, which is negatively charged. When ·OH is generated by Fenton reaction, the extent of its formation is largely determined by the availability and location of the metal ion catalyst. One feature of ·OH is that it leads to the generation of another radical, so when it reacts with a molecule, a new free radical is generated. However, the new free radical usually has lower reactivity than the hydroxyl radical (·OH). The ·OH attacks all proteins, DNA, polyunsaturated fatty acids (PUFA) in membranes, and almost any biological molecule it encounters [10]. The hydroxyl radical (·OH) can be obtained by another reaction in neutrophils, where HOCl reacts with superoxide anion radical [11, 12] as follows:

$$HOCl + O_2^{\cdot-} \rightarrow {}^{\cdot}OH + O_2 + Cl^- \quad (4)$$

The hydroxyl radical ($^{\cdot}OH$) is the strongest oxidant produced in biological systems. It reacts very rapidly and indiscriminately with most biological targets present at its site of formation.

1.1.1.3 Lipid peroxide radical (ROO$^{\cdot}$) and alkoxyl radical (RO$^{\cdot}$)

Peroxy radicals (ROO$^{\cdot}$) and alkoxy radicals (RO$^{\cdot}$) are moderately strong oxidants. Lipid peroxidation starts with abstraction of H-atom by $^{\cdot}OH$, or by RO$^{\cdot}$ to form alkyl radical (R$^{\cdot}$), then oxygen (O_2) is added to alkyl radical to generate peroxyl radical (ROO$^{\cdot}$). Lipid peroxidation or the oxidative destruction of PUFA containing methylene groups (-CH_2-) comprise the main targets [13]. This process can be illustrated in three steps as follows:

$$RH + {}^{\cdot}OH \rightarrow R^{\cdot} + H_2O \text{ (Initiation step)} \quad (5)$$

$$R^{\cdot} + O_2 \rightarrow ROO^{\cdot} \quad (6)$$

Then, peroxyl radical reacts with another polyunsaturated fatty acid (RH) to remove H-atom:

$$RH + ROO^{\cdot} \rightarrow R^{\cdot} + ROOH \text{ (Propagation step)} \quad (7)$$

Finally, to terminate lipid peroxidation, the following reaction takes place:

$$ROO^{\cdot} + ROO^{\cdot} \rightarrow ROH + RO^{\cdot} + {}^1O_2 \text{ (Termination step)} \quad (8)$$

It is clear that lipid peroxidation leads to the formation of alkyl (R$^{\cdot}$), peroxyl (ROO$^{\cdot}$), and alkoxyl (RO$^{\cdot}$) radicals. Generally, lipid hydroperoxide (ROOH) is relatively stable, but in the presence of Fe and Cu ions, it causes the formation of alkoxy and peroxy radicals [14, 15].

$$ROOH + Fe^{3+} \rightarrow RO^{\cdot} + Fe^{2+} \quad (9)$$

$$ROOH + Fe^{2+} \rightarrow ROO^{\cdot} + Fe^{3+} \quad (10)$$

The reactivity of RO$^{\cdot}$ and ROO$^{\cdot}$ is related to the presence of substituents at the α-carbon. As a result, the presence of an electron-withdrawing group increases the reactivity, while the presence of an electron-donating group decreases it. Thus, aromatic ROO$^{\cdot}$ and RO$^{\cdot}$ must be less reactive because of single electron delocalization. These free radicals react with biomolecules by abstracting H-atom [16, 17].

1.1.1.4 Hydroperoxyl radical (HOO˙)

Hydroperoxyl radical, also known as perhydroxyl radical (HOO˙), is formed due to the reversible reaction occurring between superoxide anion radical and proton. This reaction takes place in cells as follows:

$$O_2^{\bullet -} + H^+ \leftrightarrow HOO^\bullet \qquad (11)$$

The pKa of this radical is 4.88 [18]. At pH 7.2 in the cytoplasm, a small amount of this radical (1% of $O_2^{\bullet -}$) exists as HOO˙ [19]. Perhaps for this reason, many researchers presumed that HOO• has little or no role in initiation of lipid peroxidation [20]. In comparison with other oxidants, $HOO^\bullet$ shows high specificity in reaction with PUFA, linoleic (C18:2), and linolenic (C18:3) acids [21].

1.1.2 Non-radicals of ROS

1.1.2.1 Singlet oxygen

The singlet oxygen ($^1O_2$) is a potent oxidizing agent, because it can react with different macromolecules such as DNA [22], and is responsible for lipid peroxidation of membrane and other tissues [23]. It is generated in cells, specifically in neutrophils and eosinophils [24, 23]. In addition, this particle can be formed by enzymatic reactions [25–27]. This reactive particle is produced due to the activation of molecular oxygen to two excited states. In the first excited state, oxygen has two electrons with opposite spins in the same π* orbital, while in the second excited state oxygen has one electron in each of two degenerate π* orbitals. However, singlet oxygen in the first excited state is extremely reactive in comparison with other excited states like the triplet state. Allen [28] suggested the mechanism for the production of singlet oxygen from H_2O_2 and Cl^- in the presence of the myeloperoxidase (MPO) enzyme as follows:

$$H_2O_2 + H^+ + Cl^- + MPO \rightarrow HOCl + H_2O \qquad (12)$$

$$H_2O_2 + HOCl \rightarrow H_2O + H^+ + Cl^- + {}^1O_2 \qquad (13)$$

1.1.2.2 Hydrogen peroxide (H_2O_2)

Hydrogen peroxide is generated via an enzymatic reaction where the reactive superoxide anion radical is rapidly converted by an antioxidant enzyme called superoxide dismutase (SOD). The new formed oxygen species H_2O_2 is less reactive. Thus, hydrogen peroxide is formed as follows by SOD:

$$2O_2^{\cdot -} + 2H^+ + SOD \rightarrow H_2O_2 + H_2O \qquad (14)$$

It is clear that, in the dismutation reaction (an oxidation–reduction process), two superoxide anion radicals are involved. In this reaction, one superoxide anion radical is oxidized to oxygen while the other is reduced to hydrogen peroxide [29]. The latter (H_2O_2) is relatively stable and membrane permeable so this non-radical species can diffuse inside the cell and can be removed by mitochondrial antioxidant enzymatic systems such as catalase (CAT) and glutathione peroxidase (GPx) [30, 31].

$$2H_2O_2 + cat \rightarrow O_2 + 2H_2O \quad (15)$$

$$2\,H_2O_2 + 2GSH + GP_x \rightarrow GSSG + 2H_2O \quad (16)$$

As illustrated, glutathione peroxidase (GPx) removes hydrogen peroxide (H_2O_2) by oxidizing two glutathione molecules (GSH) to produce oxidized glutathione disulfide (GSSG). It is clear that the three SOD, CAT, and GPx enzymes show synergistic effect in the scavenging of superoxide anion radical ($O_2^{\cdot -}$). The in vivo destruction effects of hydrogen peroxide (H_2O_2) result due to the presence of transition metals or enzymes, such as heme-peroxidase. The destruction of H_2O_2 leads to the formation of other more reactive oxidants such as·OH, NO·, and HOCl. Thus, reaction of hydrogen peroxide with Cu^{1+} and Fe^{2+} leads to the production of. OH. On the other hand, in phagocytic cells, myeloperoxidase uses its substrate H2O2 to generate HOCl. The release of MPO during phagocytosis may play an important role in microbial elimination [32].

1.1.2.3 Ozone (O_3)

Ozone gas (O_3) exists in polluted atmosphere and the inhalation of this gas by human may lead to lung injury and inflammation. In living organisms, ozone is thought to be formed due to oxidation of H_2O to H_2O_2 in the presence of antibodies [33]. Thus, antibodies use H_2O as an electron source, facilitating its addition to $^1O_2$ to generate dihydrogen trioxide (H_2O_3), which is converted to ozone [34].

$$H_2O + {}^1O_2 \rightarrow HOOOH \rightarrow O_3 + H_2O_2 \quad (17)$$

Ozone reacts with fatty acids, cholesterol, amino acids and DNA. The lung is the most affected organ due to exposure to ozone. The effect of ozone on tissues occurs via free radical mechanisms [35–37]. The ozone radical anion then reacts with a proton to form the hydroxyl radical and oxygen as follows [36].

$$O_3^{\cdot -} + H^+ \rightarrow HO^{\cdot} + O_2 \quad (18)$$

1.1.2.4 Hypochlorous acid (HOCl)

This species (HOCl) is generated in neutrophils by the reaction of Cl^- with H_2O_2, which is catalyzed by the enzyme myeloperoxidase [38]. It is illustrated as follows:

$$H_2O_2 + Cl^- + MPO \rightarrow HOCl + {}^{\cdot}OH \quad (19)$$

The hypochlorous acid is considered to be a very reactive oxidizing agent. So, it may affect different biomolecules and may destroy phagocytized pathogens by causing oxidative damage to their biomolecules which include proteins [39], DNA [40], and lipids [41]. On the other hand, the overproduction of HOCl can lead to many health problems such as atherosclerosis and cancer [42, 38].

1.1.3 Reactive nitrogen species (RNS)

Reactive nitrogen species (RNS) can be found in biological systems as free radical species and non-radical species. However, the most common RNS radical is nitric oxide radical ($NO^{\cdot}$) and nitrogen dioxide (NO_2). On the other side, the important non-radical RNS is peroxynitrite ion ($ONOO^-$). Generations of these reactive species is discussed below.

1.1.3.1 Nitric oxide ($NO^{\cdot}$)

Nitric oxide free radical ($NO^{\cdot}$) is an endogenous free radical synthesized in the presence of nitric oxide synthase (NOS) that oxidizes L-arginine to L-citrulline [43]. In this reaction, one of the guanidino nitrogen atoms is oxidized to form $NO^{\cdot}$. This process is shown below:

$$L-Arginine + O_2 + NADPH + NOS \rightarrow L-Citrullin + NO^{\cdot} + NADP^+ \quad (20)$$

The $NO^{\cdot}$ radical can diffuse easily and has the ability to reach many intracellular targets and cause biological damage [44]. The enzyme nitric oxide synthase (NOS) is found in different cells such as vascular endothelial cells, smooth muscle cells, platelets, neuronal cells, macrophages, and neutrophils [45]. In addition, this radical plays an important role in biological tissues such as vasodilation, memory, neuronal response, among others [46–50].

1.1.3.2 Peroxynitrite ($OONO^-$) and Other Reactive Nitrogen Species

This nitrogenous species is generated due to reaction of superoxide anion radical ($O_2^{-\cdot}$) with nitrogen oxide radical ($NO^{\cdot}$) radical as follows:

$$O_2^{-\cdot} + NO^{\cdot} \rightarrow ONOO^- \quad (21)$$

It is noted that at physiological pH (7.4), peroxynitrite exists in equilibrium with peroxynitrous acid, ONOOH [51].

$$ONOO^- + H^+ \leftrightarrow ONOOH \quad (22)$$

Then, peroxynitrous acid (ONOOH) is subjected to homolysis to produce hydroxyl radical ($OH^{\bullet}$) and nitrogen dioxide radical ($NO_2^{\cdot}$), which may rearrange to form nitrate (NO_3^-).

$$ONOO^- + H^+ \leftrightarrow ONOOH \leftrightarrow \left[HO^{\cdot} + NO_2^{\cdot}\right] \rightarrow NO_3^- + H^+ \quad (23)$$

The $ONOO^-$ is a very reactive anion, even more so than the particle ($NO^{\cdot}$ and $O_2^{\bullet-}$) from which it is formed [52–54]. The peroxynitrite anion can cross biological membranes and interact with most critical biomolecules [55]. Thus, it can cause oxidation of lipids, and proteins via oxidation of methionine and tyrosine residues and can oxidize DNA to generate nitroguanine [56]. Under most biological conditions, ONOO- and ONOOH exist in equilibrium [57]:

$$ONOO^- + H^+ \leftrightarrow ONOOH \quad (24)$$

Indeed, protonation weakens the O–O bond in ONOOH and leads to homolytic cleavage to generate hydroxyl radicals ($^{\cdot}OH$) and nitrogen dioxide ($^{\cdot}NO_2$), two strongly oxidizing/hydroxylating and nitrating species, respectively.

$$ONOOH \rightarrow {}^{\cdot}NO_2 + .OH \quad (25)$$

As a nucleophile, a central reaction of peroxynitrite in biology is the addition of the anion to carbon dioxide (CO_2) to yield a nitrosoperoxocarboxylate adduct ($ONOOCO_2$) that undergoes fast homolysis to NO_2 and [58–60].

$$ONOO^- + CO_2 \rightarrow ONOOCO_2^- \rightarrow {}^{\cdot}NO_2 + CO_3^- \quad (26)$$

1.2 Antioxidants

An antioxidant is any substance that has the ability to prevent, inhibit, or delay the oxidation of other substances. In biological systems, antioxidants play a very important roles in removing free radicals such as ROS and RNS, and consequently reduce oxidative stress. Antioxidant molecules can be classified based on the type of mechanistic defense they offer:

1.2.1 Antioxidants suppressing formation of free radicals

These are endogenous antioxidant enzymes like superoxide dismutase (SOD), catalase (CAT) and glutathione peroxidase (GPx). These enzymes efficiently suppress or prevent the formation of free radicals and other ROS in tissues. Thus, SOD removes superoxide anion radical as follows:

$$2O_2^{\cdot -} + 2H^+ + SOD \rightarrow H_2O_2 + H_2O \quad (27)$$

On the other hand, CAT reduces formed H_2O_2 to water and oxygen:

$$2\,H_2O_2 + cat \rightarrow O_2 + 2H_2O \quad (28)$$

The GPx enzyme system detoxifies H_2O_2 by catalyzing its reduction using glutathione (GSH) as a sacrificial reductant to produce one molecule of oxidized glutathione (GSSG). Thus, the enzymes SOD, CAT, and GPx, work collectively to prevent the effect of $O_2^{\cdot -}$.

$$2\,H_2O_2 + 2GSH + GP_x \rightarrow GSSG + 2H_2O \quad (29)$$

In addition, Fe and Cu ions are included to this type of defense, since these ions bind proteins such as transferrin and caeruloplasmin and prevent them from free radical formation. Generally, any chemical compound having two or more of the following functional groups: –OH, –SH, –COOH, $-PO_3H_2$, C=O, $-NR_2$, –S– and –O– may have chelating activity [61]. The mechanism of metal ion chelation with some natural phenolics such as protocatechuic acid and anthocyanins is shown in **Figure 1**.

Transition metal ions (Fe^{+2} and Cu^+) make complex species with different types of phenolic compounds such as flavonoids containing multiple hydroxyl groups (polyhydroxylated). The involvement of these ions in the formation of complexes prevents the Fenton reaction which leads to the formation of hydroxyl radical (${}^{\cdot}OH$) which is considered as the most dangerous ROS.

$$H_2O_2 + M^{+n} \rightarrow HO^- + HO^{\cdot} + M^{n+1}\,(M = Fe\,or\,Cu) \quad (30)$$

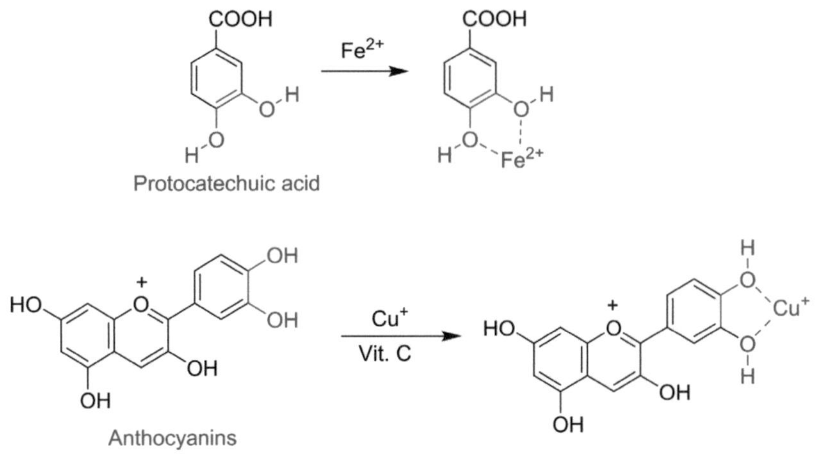

Figure 1.
Mechanism of metal ion chelation with some natural phenolics.

1.2.2 Antioxidants that repair damage resulting from the action of free radicals

This type of antioxidants are enzymes which are involved in repairing damage due to the effects of free radicals on biomolecules (DNA, proteins, lipids and carbohydrates). These enzymes prevent the accumulation of toxic substances resulting from destruction of biomolecules in body tissues. Examples of this type of enzymatic antioxidants include the DNA repair enzyme systems (polymerases, glycosylases and nucleases), and proteolytic enzymes (proteinases, proteases and peptidases) located in both, cytosol and mitochondria of mammalian cells.

1.2.3 Antioxidants that utilize signals for the formation of free radicals

This type of antioxidants use the signals, which are required for the formation of free radicals. As a result, the signal generated from the formed free radical causes the formation and transport of the appropriate antioxidant to the appropriate and required site [62].

1.2.4 Antioxidants scavenging free radicals

This type of scavenging antioxidants can directly neutralize free radicals by two mechanisms, either by donating a hydrogen free radical ($H^{\cdot}$) or donating an electron (e^-). These mechanisms can be illustrated as follows:

$$Ar-OH+R^{\cdot} \rightarrow Ar-O^{\cdot}+RH \tag{31}$$

In the preceding mechanism, the antioxidant donates a hydrogen free radical ($H^{\cdot}$) to scavenge free radicals, and the antioxidant (Ar-OH) itself becomes a free radical, though not as biologically harmful.

$$Ar-OH+R^{\cdot} \rightarrow Ar-OH^{+\cdot}+R^{-} \rightarrow Ar-O^{\cdot}+H^{+} \tag{32}$$

The second mechanism involves one-electron transfer where the antioxidant donates an electron to the free radical and becomes itself a radical cation. Generally, the new radicals are more stable and can be easily neutralized and made completely harmless and removed easily from biological systems. Many antioxidants such as ascorbic acid, uric acid, glutathione, vitamin E, and other natural compounds like polyhydroxyphenolic compounds belong to this class. This type of antioxidants are usually small molecules containing hydroxyl groups either of natural or synthetic origin. The importance of these compounds prompted us to review them in details.

2. Small antioxidant molecules containing hydroxyl groups

There are many studies that have shown the biological effectiveness of phenolic compounds as natural antioxidants. They play very important roles in the prevention of dangerous diseases such as cancers, heart diseases, diabetes and others. There is a need for simple molecules capable of neutralizing free radicals responsible for what is known as oxidative stress, the lead cause of dangerous diseases like cancers, heart disease, diabetes and others. Antioxidants play a critical role in biological systems in getting rid of free radicals and work to prevent the phenomenon of oxidative stress. The most available natural antioxidants exist in plants such as fruits, vegetables, and medicinal plants. Herein, we present an overview of the natural and synthetic phenolic compounds acting as antioxidants.

2.1 Natural antioxidants containing hydroxyl groups

2.1.1 Phenols

Simple phenols are known as compounds containing at least one hydroxyl group attached to an aromatic ring which comprises the basic skeleton. The most important compounds under this class are: phenol, catechol, resorcinol, and phloroglucinol. Generally, phenols are widely distributed in plants and play very important roles in human health because of their ability to neutralize free radicals due to their hydroxyl groups. It is considered that these simple phenols along with other phenolic compounds can inhibit and prevent cancer diseases in humans (**Figure 2**) [63].

The study by Spiegel et al. [64] has shown that the most active of simple natural phenols as antioxidants were those containing more than one hydroxyl group in the *ortho* position of the aromatic ring. This suggests that the most active antioxidant compound is catechol since it contains two hydroxyl groups in the ortho position. This could be attributed to the bond dissociation energy (BDE) of O-H which is typically used to evaluate the activity of an antioxidant to neutralize free radicals [65–67]. Thus, the weaker the O-H BDE, the faster the reaction of antioxidant with the free radical. In other words, the weaker the BDE of O-H in phenols, the easier it will be to transfer an H-radical to deactivate the free radical. The antioxidant activity of catechol and hydroquinone is illustrated as shown in **Figure 3**.

2.1.2 Phenolic acids: hydroxybenzoic and hydroxycinnamic acids

Phenolic acids are also known as phenol carboxylic acids (**Figure 4**). There are two important groups of natural phenolic acids which are hydroxybenzoic acids and hydroxycinnamic acids. These are derived from benzoic and cinnamic acid, respectively. The molecular structural features of phenolic acids, such as the numbers and positions of the hydroxyl groups in relation to the carboxyl functional group, esterification, and glycosylation great impacts their antioxidant properties. Many studies [68, 69] have shown that the antioxidant activity of phenolic acids and their esters was enhanced substantially when the number of hydroxyl (-OH) and methoxy ($-OCH_3$) groups increased. On the other hand, the carboxyl group has an electron

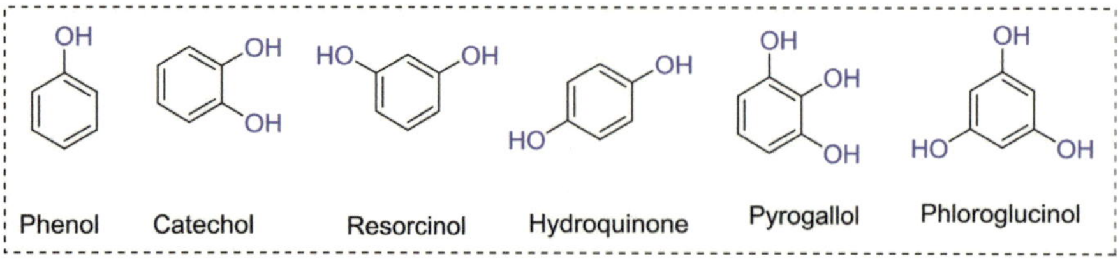

Figure 2.
Natural phenolic antioxidants containing hydroxyl groups.

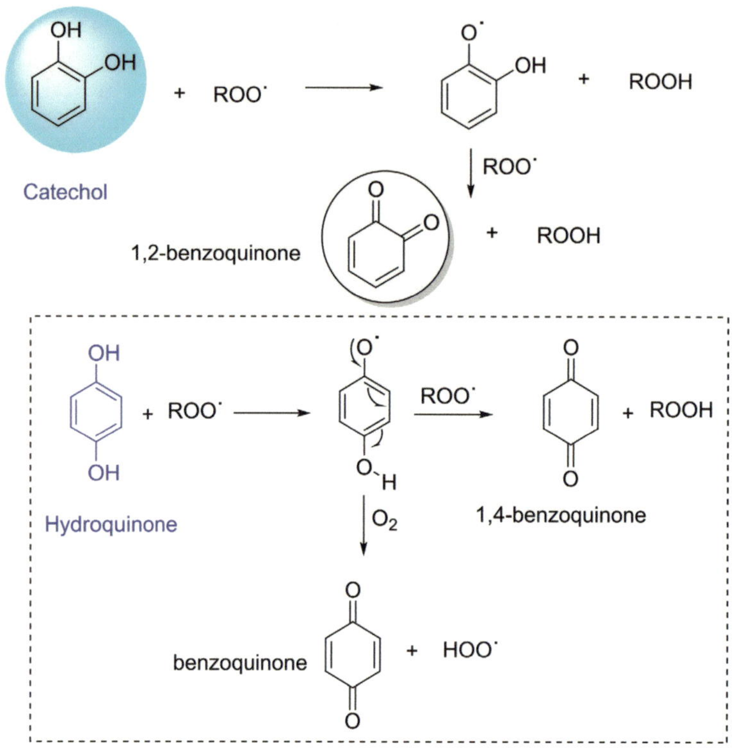

Figure 3.
Mechanism of action of natural phenolic antioxidants by transfer of hydrogen free radical (H•).

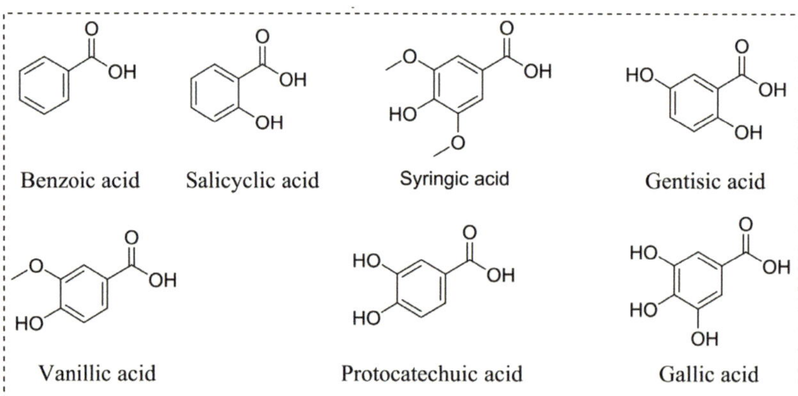

Figure 4.
Benzoic acid and the related hydroxybenzoic acids.

withdrawing effect, making the H-atom less available to be donated. However, the antioxidant activity of hydroxylated cinnamates are greater than that of benzoates [70–72]. The antioxidant activities of different hydroxybenzoic acids such as 4-hydroxybenzoic acid, 3,4-dihydroxybenzoic acid, and 3,4,5-trihydroxybenzoic acid were shown to be dependent on the number and position of attached hydroxyl groups to the aromatic ring [73]. Based on bond dissociation energy of O-H group, the dihydroxybenzoic acid has greater antioxidant activity than monohydroxybenzoic acid. It was observed that the BDE for -OH at 3-position is greater than the BDE of -OH at 4-position, as a result the abstraction of H-atom from the 4-position becomes easier than abstraction from the 3-position. Thus, it can be concluded that in 3,4-dihydroxybenzoic acid, the ability to abstract H-atom from the 4-position is easier than the 3-position. On the other hand, gallic acid (3,4,5-trihydroxybenzoic acid) showed lower antioxidant activity than that of 3,4-dihydroxybenzoic acid. This phenomenon could be attributed to the formation of a weak intramolecular H-bond between the -OH at 4-position and -OH at 5-position [74]. The obtained theoretical BDE of the -OH groups in gallic acid were in the order 4-OH $\leq$ 5-OH $<$ 3-OH, which indicates that the removal of H-atom is easier from 4-OH and 5-OH. Both of these values in gallic acid become lower than that of 4-hydroxybenzoic acid. Thus, the introduction of two hydroxyl groups at 3-position and 5-position significantly increases the antioxidant activity [73].

Similarly, the antioxidant activities of hydroxycinnamic acids (**Figure 5**) are related to their hydroxyl groups. The study of relationship between antioxidant activities and structures of hydroxycinnamic acids was carried out by Chen and Ho [74]. The BDE value of O-H group is a good indicator to evaluate the antioxidant activity of an antioxidant. Thus, the weaker the O-H bond, the greater the ability of an antioxidant to neutralize free radicals. In addition, phenolic molecules bearing two hydroxyl groups in *o*-position relative to one another showed high antioxidant activities [75–77] as observed with caffeic acid. On the other hand, replacement of one hydroxyl group by methoxy group as in ferulic acid leads to lower antioxidant activity [65–67, 75–80]. Therefore, the BDE value of O-H would be expected to follow the following order: caffeic acid $<$ ferulic acid $<$ p-coumaric acid. As a result, the antioxidant activities of these acids will be in the order: caffeic acid $>$ ferulic acid $>$ p-coumaric acid. However, it is important to remember that the removal of H-atom from caffeic acid could arise from *m*-OH and *p*-OH to form free radicals. Consequently, the resulting free radical due to removal of the H-atom from *p*-OH would be more stable because of resonance where the electron is delocalized over the whole molecule, but in the case of removal of the H-atom from *m*-OH, the unpaired electron cannot be delocalized over the whole molecule since it cannot cross the propenoic tether [81].

2.1.3 Flavonoids

The flavonoids consist of a large group of low-molecular weight polyphenolic substances, benzo-γ-pyrone derivatives (**Figure 5**). The basic structural feature of all flavonoids is the flavane (2-phenyl-benzo-γ-pyran) nucleus, a system of two benzene rings (A and B) linked by an oxygen-containing pyran ring (C). According to the degree of oxidation of the C ring, the hydroxylation pattern of the nucleus, and the substituent at carbon 3, flavonoids can be categorized into the following subclasses: flavones, isoflavones, flavanols (catechins), flavonols, flavanones, anthocyanins, and proanthocyanidins. Flavonols differ from flavanones by a hydroxyl group at the C3 position and by a C2–C3 double bond. Anthocyanidins differ from the other flavonoids by possessing a charged oxygen atom in the C ring (**Table 1**).

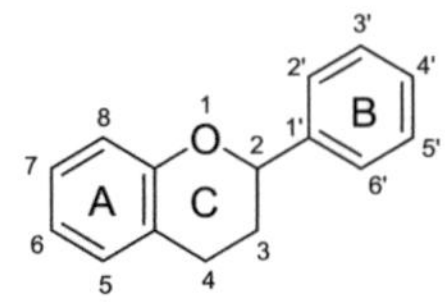

Entry	Types of flavonoids	Examples	
1	**Flavanone** 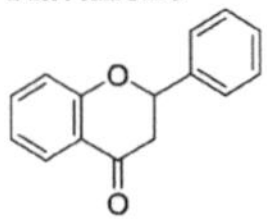	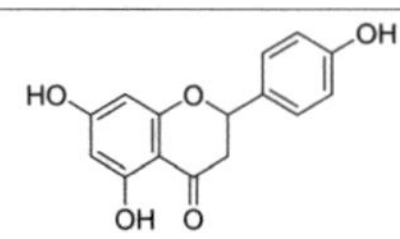 Naringenin	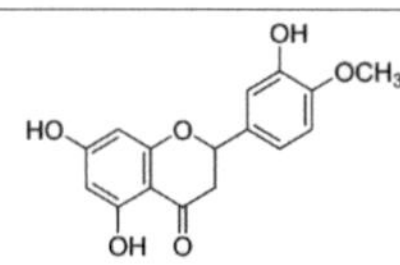 Hesperidin
2	**Flavan-3-ol** 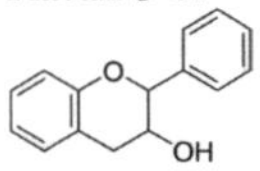	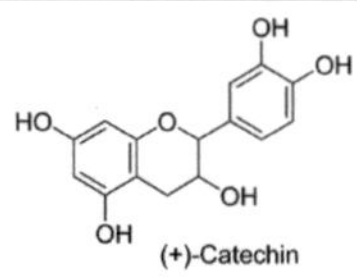 (+)-Catechin	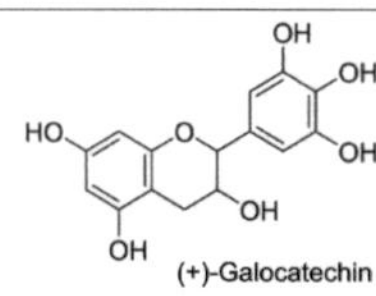 (+)-Galocatechin
3	**Flavone** 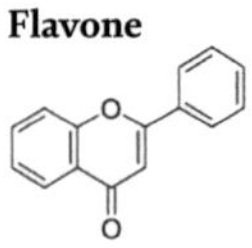	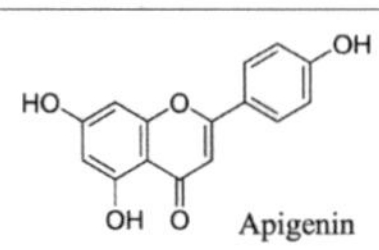 Apigenin	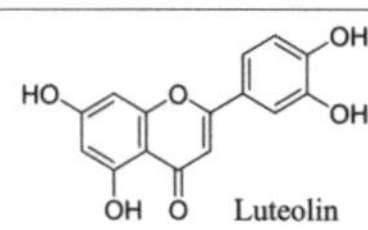 Luteolin
4	**Flavonol** 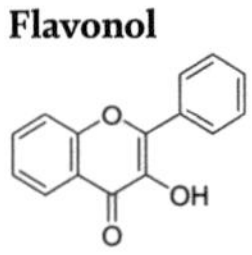	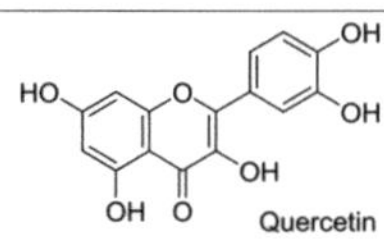 Quercetin	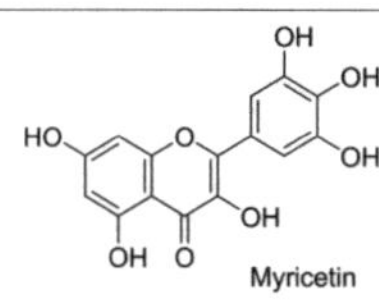 Myricetin
5	**Anthocyanidin** 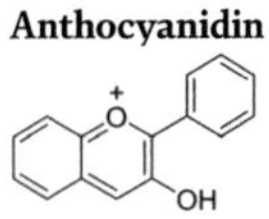	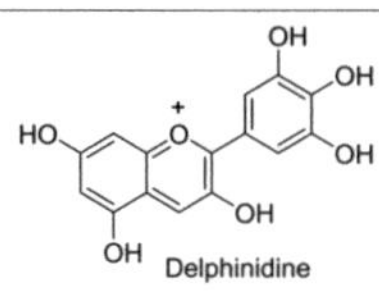 Delphinidine	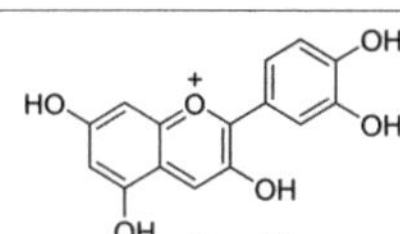 Cyanidin
6	**Isoflavone** 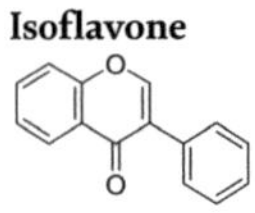	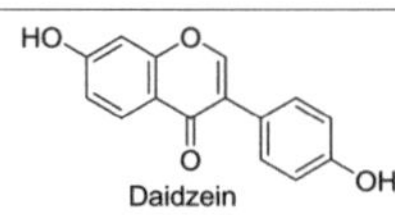 Daidzein	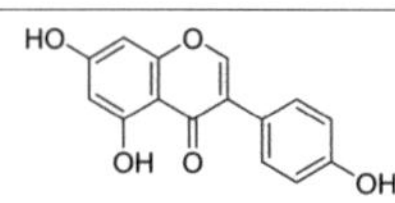 Genistein

Table 1.
Types of flavonoids.

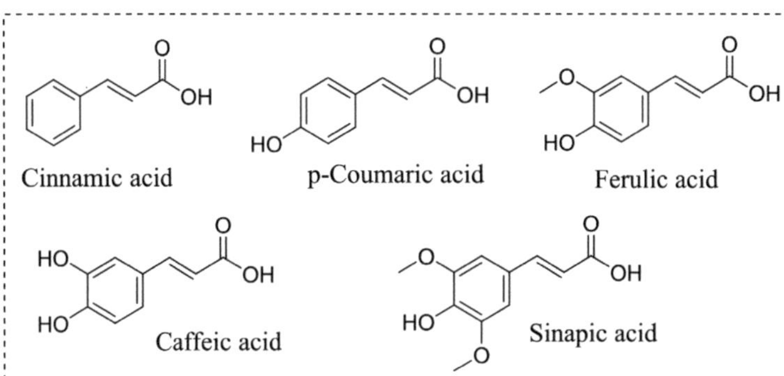

Figure 5.
Cinnamic acid and hydroxycinnamic acids.

Flavonoids are secondary metabolites and mainly distributed in the plant kingdom such as green and black tea, coffee, vegetables, fruits, olive oil, red wine, white wines, and chocolate [82–92]. They are consumed in milligrams per serving of these plant sources. Many researchers have shown that flavonoids possess different biological activities which include vasodilating, anti-allergenic, antiviral, and anti-inflammatory actions [93–95]. However, the antioxidant activity of these compounds attracted the most interest because, in addition to their ability to scavenge free radicals, they also reduce or prevent free radical formation.

The capability of antioxidant activities of flavonoids is mainly related to their chemical structures. Many previous investigations attributed the high antioxidant activities of these compounds to the presence and positions of hydroxyl groups attached to the A and B rings and/or to the $C_2 = C_3$ double bond in conjugation with the carbonyl group at 4-position, and the -OH group at 3-position [93, 94, 96]. On the other hand, the replacement of hydrogen atom by a saccharide at 3-position to form a glycosidic bond, the antioxidant activity decreases. The radical scavenging efficiency of flavonoids is related to their phenolic hydroxyl groups which follow the mechanism of H-atom transfer or the single electron transfer followed by sequential electron transfer-proton transfer (SETPT) [97–100]. As in the case of phenolic acids, the antioxidant activity of flavonoids, is based on the value of the dissociation energy of the O-H bond [67, 97, 101]. The study by Quan et al. [102] showed that the dissociation energy of C-H at 3-position in some flavonoids appeared to be lower than that of the dissociation energy of O-H. As a result, the antioxidant activity might be due the donation of H-atom from C-H at 3-position. However, the mechanism of antioxidant activity via H-atom transfer from the -OH group appeared to be the most significant [102]. Generally, flavonoids as antioxidants may act by different mechanisms such as hydrogen atom transfer, single electron transfer, and transition metal chelation. These mechanisms are shown below in **Figures 6–9**. **Figure 6** shows the proposed mechanism of radical scavenging activity of cyanidin by Nimse and Palb [103] following HAT mechanism.

2.1.3.1 -Hydrogen atom transfer (HAT)

The flavonoid quercetin is found in many plants and foods and in notable quantities especially in onions, red wine, green tea, apples, berries, and others.

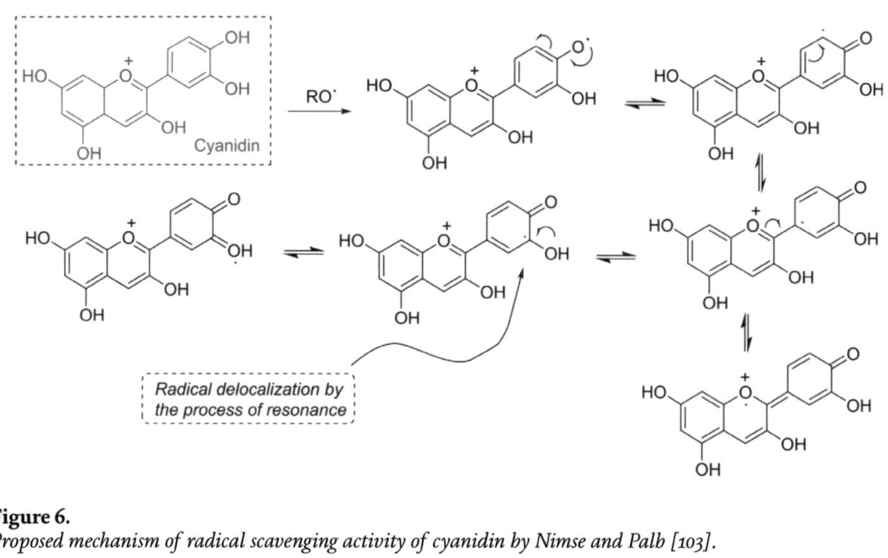

Figure 6.
Proposed mechanism of radical scavenging activity of cyanidin by Nimse and Palb [103].

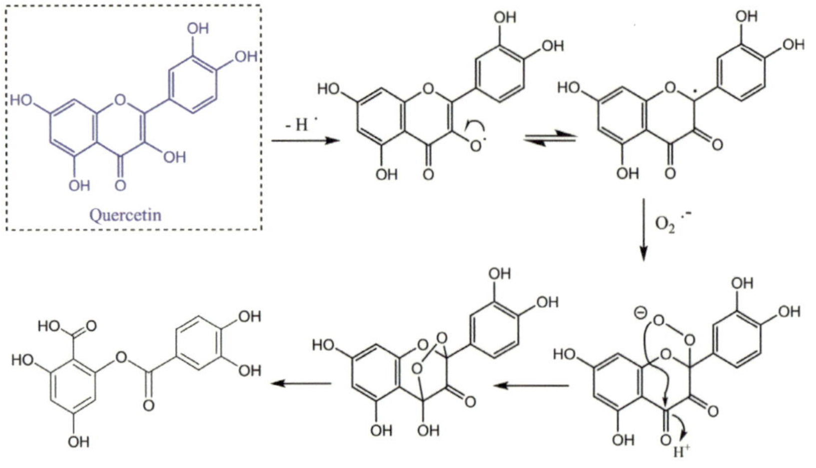

Figure 7.
Proposed mechanism of superoxide anion radical scavenging activity of quercetin by Nimse and Palb [103].

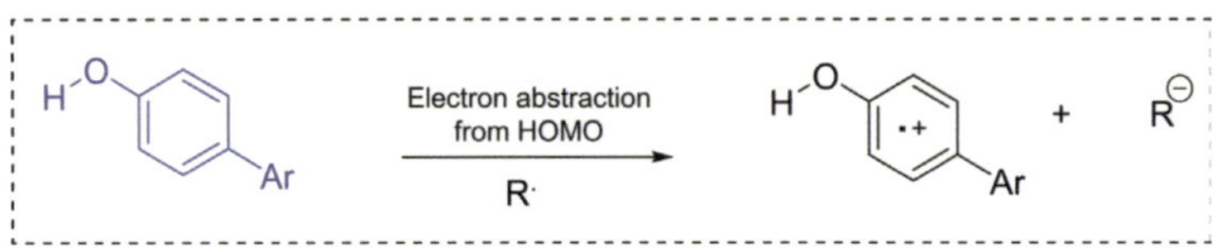

Figure 8.
Proposed mechanism of single electron transfer by Leopoldini et al. [104].

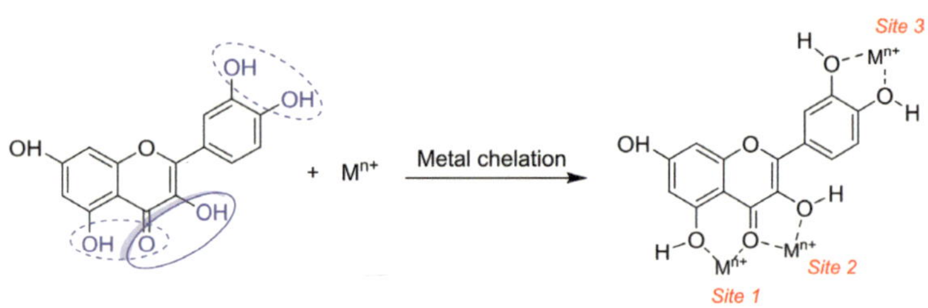

Figure 9.
Proposed metal–quercetin chelation by Leopoldinia et al. [104].

The proposed mechanism of superoxide anion radical scavenging activity of quercetin by Nimse and Palb [103] is shown in **Figure 7**.

The proposed mechanism of single electron transfer by Leopoldini et al. [104] for single electron transfer (SET) and transition metal chelation (TMC) are shown in **Figures 8** and **9**.

2.1.3.2 Single electron transfer (SET)

2.1.3.3 Transition metal chelation (TMC)

Flavonoids with their multiple hydroxyl groups and the carbonyl group at the 4 position on ring C may offer several available sites for metal chelation. The ability of flavonoids to chelate Fe and Cu ions is related to their indirect antioxidant activities. This property of flavonoids is attributed to their multiple hydroxyl groups and the carbonyl group at 4-position [104].

2.1.4 Stilbenes

The Stilbene family includes several compounds [105] among which resveratrol, pterostilbene, and piceatannol are the main representatives, characterized by a *trans* double bond connecting the phenolic rings (**Figure 10**).

Stilbene compounds are part of a group of natural polyphenols occurring in plant kingdom such as grapes [106], peanuts [107], and berries [108]. Resveratrol (3, 5, 4′-trihydroxy-trans-stilbene), which is found in grapes, showed different biological activities including antidiabetic, antiobesity, and neuroprotective properties against Alzheimer's disease (AD) [109]. In addition, other stilbenes have shown additional activities as antimicrobials and antioxidants [110]. Different studies have shown that piceatannol (4′, 5′, 3, 5-tetrahydroxystilbene) expresses a wide spectrum of biological activities: anti-inflammatory, anticarcinogenic, antiviral, antioxidative, neuroprotective and estrogenic properties, and antioxidant activities [111–117]. A study by Hussein [118] demonstrated the strong ability of resveratrol to scavenge free radicals using different tests. The mechanism of antioxidant activity of resveratrol was proposed to be as follows (**Figure 11**).

2.2 Synthetic antioxidants containing hydroxyl groups

Synthetic antioxidants are usually used as food preservatives to prevent lipid oxidation [119]. The well-known synthetic antioxidants are butylated hydroxyanisole (BHA), butylated hydroxytoluene (BHT), and *t*-butyl-hydroxyquinone

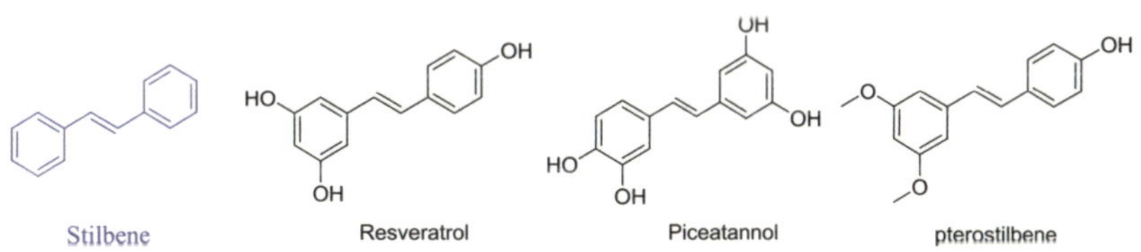

Figure 10.
Stilbene and its related polyphenolic derivatives.

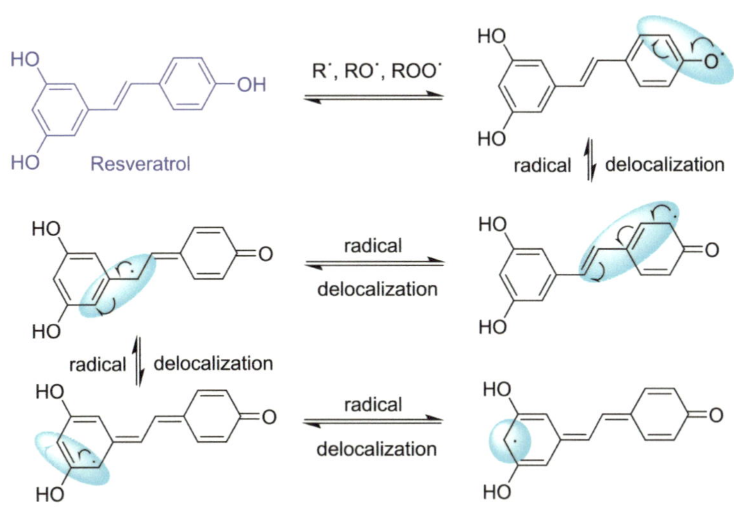

Figure 11.
Proposed mechanism of resveratrol antioxidant activity [118].

(TBHQ). These antioxidants stop the free radical chain of oxidative reactions via the donation of an H-atom radical from the phenolic -OH attached to the aromatic rings (**Figure 12**). The new formed radicals become stable and do not initiate or propagate further oxidation of lipids [120].

The progressively more sterically hindered BHT and the related BHA operated as radical terminators in a similar fashion to TBHQ (**Figure 13**).

Another type of radical quencher is shown in **Figure 14** where the generated phenoxy radical is stabilized by intramolecular hydrogen bond.

The presence of a bulky group introduces steric hindrance in proximity to the radical center, decreasing the rate of further propagation reactions. Another example which illustrates the increase in antioxidant activity is the presence of an extra hydroxyl group at the ortho or para position of the hydroxyl group of phenol. The stability of the phenoxy radical in this case is enhanced by the formation of an intramolecular hydrogen bond. Other studies [121–123] described the synthesis of different compounds like aromatic Schiff bases and aromatic hydrazones containing hydroxyl groups attached to different positions in the aromatic rings. These compounds were designed to mimic as much as possible natural phenolic compounds such as stilbene and chalcones. The number of hydroxyl groups and their locations in the aromatic rings play an important role in the antioxidant activity. The mechanism of antioxidant activity can be illustrated as follows and involves the donation of hydrogen radical (**Figure 15**).

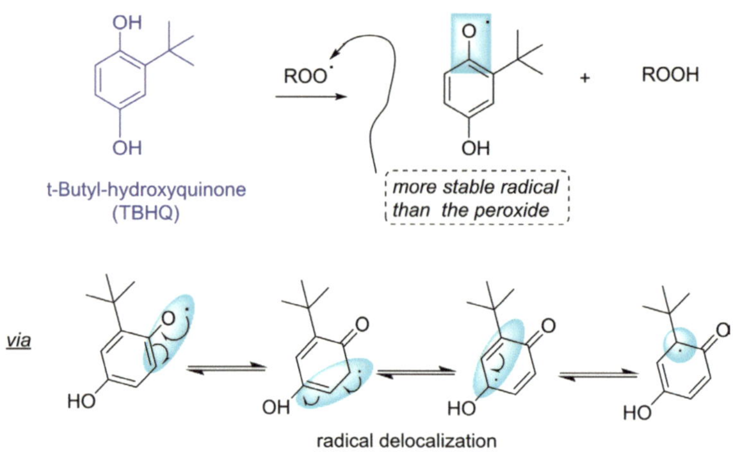

Figure 12.
Antioxidant action of t-butyl-hydroxyquinone as a radical terminator via the donation of a hydrogen radical and subsequent radical delocalization by resonance.

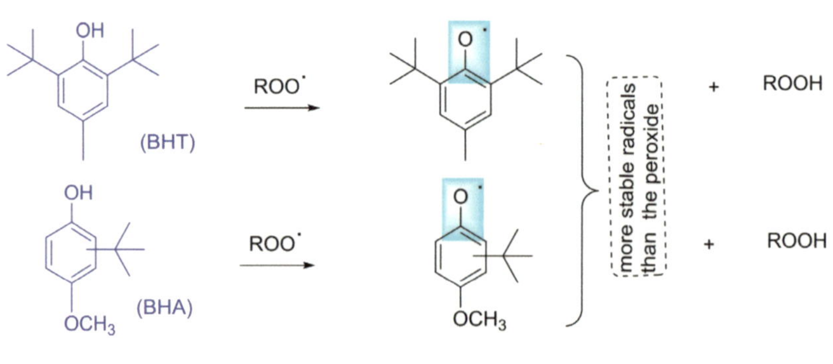

Figure 13.
Oxidation of BHT and BHA via donation of a hydrogen radical from a phenolic hydroxyl group.

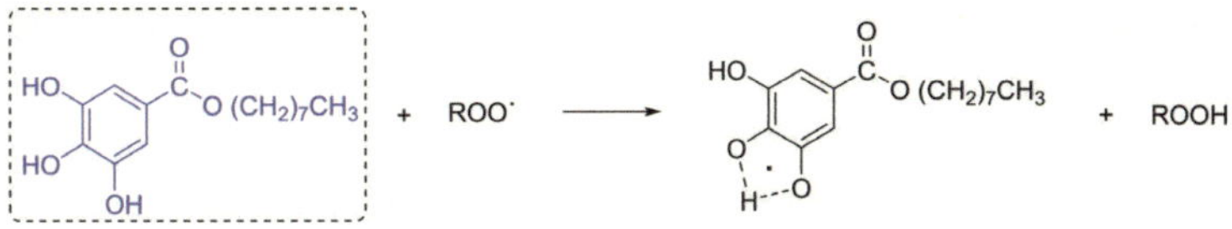

Figure 14.
Generation of a phenoxy radical with intramolecular hydrogen bond shown.

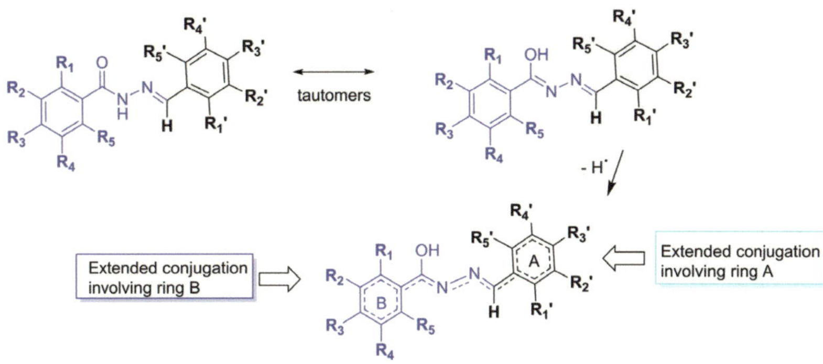

Figure 15.
Proposed mechanism for the action of aromatic hydrazones via H radical donation.

3. Oxidative stress

Oxidative stress is a phenomenon occurring in living systems and is related to the presence of free radicals (oxidants) and antioxidants (reductants). When we talk about free radicals in biological systems, we mean two types: reactive oxygen species (ROS) and reactive nitrogen species (RNS). Imbalance between free radicals and antioxidants (endogenous and exogenous) in biological systems creates a state know as oxidative stress. In this case, the present antioxidants cannot remove the ROS and RNS from living species. As a result, excess free radicals can negatively impact different biological processes, leading to the destruction of cell membrane, blocking pathways of major enzymes, stopping cell division, destruction of DNA, and halting energy production [124–126]. On the other hand, free radicals appear to be necessary for some processes in living organisms since they destroy bacteria by phagocytes (granulocytes and macrophages). In addition, ROS can be beneficial for the maintenance of homeostasis as well as other cellular functions [125, 127]. Again, it is important to remember that the primary free radicals are superoxide anion radicals $O_2^{\cdot -}$ and hydroxyl radical$^{\cdot}$ ^{O}H which are derived from molecular oxygen (O2). High levels of these radicals may cause different biological problems which may lead to cancer, stroke (Reuter et al., 2010) [126], myocardial infarction, diabetes, and other significant conditions [128].

It is not easy to avoid the exposure of free radicals and consequently oxidative stress. However, the increase of consumption of natural antioxidants through diet may help to decrease the production of free radicals. In other words, to prevent oxidative stress, it is highly recommended to consume enough amounts of vegetables, fruits, medicinal plants, and honey to ensure sufficient supplementation of natural antioxidants [129–133].

4. Conclusion

To maintain normal health and avoid incurable diseases such as cardiovascular disease, cancer diseases, diabetes, among other, it is necessary to protect the existing balance between free radicals and antioxidants in biological systems. Naturally the human body has means of internal defense to neutralize free radicals. These means of defense are represented by a group of biological molecules known as antioxidant enzymes. In addition, there are a number of small molecules such as urea, bilirubin, vitamin E, vitamin A, and others. These simple molecules play a positive role in eliminating free radicals. However, when the internal system fails to get rid of free radicals, a supply of external antioxidants, especially those from natural sources, is needed to remove excess free radicals. There are many antioxidants in nature especially those that contain hydroxyl groups such as phenolic compounds, such as phenolic acids (derivatives of hydroxybenzoic and hydroxy cinnamic acids), flavonoids, stilbenes, chalcones and others. These compounds are found in fruits, vegetables and medicinal herbs. There are some chemically prepared antioxidants in laboratories which use is almost limited to the food and pharmaceutical industries. However, there are many attempts to manufacture antioxidants that mimic those found in nature, especially those containing hydroxyl groups, in the hope of obtaining compounds at the lowest cost, safe to use, and in large quantities.

Acknowledgements

Dr. Ziad Moussa is grateful to the United Arab Emirates University (UAEU) of Al-Ain and to the Research Office for supporting the research developed in his laboratory (Grant no. G00003291/Fund no.31S401/Project #852).

Author details

Mohammed Ali Al-Mamary[1] and Ziad Moussa[2*]

1 Department of Chemistry, Faculty of Applied Science, Taiz University, Republic of Yemen-Taiz

2 Department of Chemistry, College of Science, United Arab Emirates University, Al Ain, United Arab Emirates

*Address all correspondence to: zmoussa@uaeu.ac.ae

References

[1] Li X, Fang P, Mai J, Choi ET, Wang H, Yang XF. Targeting mitochondrial reactive oxygen species as novel therapy for inflammatory diseases and cancers. J Hematol Oncol. 2013; 6 (19): 19. DOI: 10.1186/1756-8722-6-19

[2] Reichart G, Mayer J, Zehm C, Kirschstein T, Tokay T, Lange F, Baltrusch S, Tiedge M, Fuellen G, Ibrahim S, Köhling R. Mitochondrial complex IV mutation increases ROS production and reduces lifespan in aged mice. Acta Physiologica.2018; 225: e13214. DOI: 10.1111/apha.13214

[3] Maurel A., Hernandez C., Kunduzova O., Bompart G., Cambon C., Parini A., Francés F. Age-dependent increase in hydrogen peroxide production by cardiac monoamine oxidase A in rats. American Journal of Physiology; Heart and Circulatory Physiology. 2003; 84: 1460-1467. https://doi.org/10.1152/ajpheart.00700.2002

[4] Turrens JF: Mitochondrial formation of reactive oxygen species. J Physiol. 2003; 552: 335-344. https://doi.org/10.1111/j.1469-7793.2003.00335.x

[5] Cadenas E and Davies KJ: Mitochondrial free radical generation, oxidative stress, and aging. Free Radic Biol Med. 2000; 222-230. DOI: 10.1016/s0891-5849(00)00317-8

[6] Kuppusamy P, Zweier JL. Characterization of free radical generation by xanthine oxidase. Evidence for hydroxyl radical generation. J Biol Chem. 1989;264(17):9880-4.

[7] Fenton HJH. Oxidation of tartaric acid in the presence of iron. J Chem Soc Trans. 1894;65:899-910. https://doi.org/10.1039/CT8946500899

[8] Knight JA, in Free radicals, antioxidants, aging and disease, AACC Press, Washington, 1999.

[9] Haber F, Weiss J. The catalytic decomposition of hydrogen peroxide by iron salts. Proc R Soc London (A). 1934;147:332-51. DOI:10.1098/rspa.1934.0221

[10] Halliwell B. Oxidants and human disease: some new concepts. FASEB J. 1987;1(5):358-64. https://doi.org/10.1096/fasebj.1.5.2824268

[11] Cohen MS, Britigan BE, Hassett DJ, Rosen GM: Do human neutrophils form hydroxyl radical? Evaluation of an unresolved controversy. Free Radic Biol Med. 1988; 5:81. doi: 10.1016/0891-5849(88)90033-0

[12] Kettle AJ, Winterbourn CC: Superoxide-dependent hydroxylation by myeloperoxidase. J Biol Chem. 1994; 269:17146.

[13] Halliwell B, and Gutteridge JM. Oxygen toxicity, oxygen radicals, transition metals and disease. Biochem J. 1984; 219(1): 1-14. doi: 10.1042/bj2190001

[14] Repetto MG, Ferrarotti N, Boveris A. The involvement of transition metal ions on iron-dependent lipid peroxidation. Archives of Toxicology. 2010; 84(4):255-62. doi: 10.1007/s00204-009-0487-y

[15] Repetto MG, Semprine J, Boveris A. Lipid Peroxidation: Chemical Mechanism, Biological Implications and Analytical Determination. D.A. Catala (Ed.) Lipid Peroxidation (2012). InTechopen 2012: 1-30. DOI: 10.5772/45943

[16] Antunes F, Salvador A, Marinho HS, Alves R, Pinto RE. Lipid peroxidation in mitochondrial inner membranes.1.

An integrative kinetic model. *Free Radic Biol Med* 1996;21:917-43. doi: 10.1016/s0891-5849(96)00185-2

[17] Xu L, Davis TA, Porter NA. Rate constants for peroxidation of polyunsaturated fatty acids and sterols in solution and in liposomes. *J Am Chem Soc.* 2009;131:13037-44. https://doi.org/10.1021/ja9029076

[18] Bielski BHJ, Reevaluation of the spectral and kinetic properties of HO2 and O2-FREE radicals, Photochemistry and Photobiology. 1978; 28 (4-5): 645-649. DOI: 10.1111/j.1751-1097.1978.tb06986.x

[19] McCord JM, and Fridovich I. Superoxide dismutase. An enzymic function for erythrocuprein (hemocuprein), The Journal of Biological Chemistry. 1978; 244:6049-6055.

[20] Gutteridge JM, Lipid peroxidation and antioxidants as biomarkers of tissue damage, Clinical Chemistry. 1995; 41: 1819-28.

[21] Bielski BHJ, Arudi RL, Sutherland MW. A study of the reactivity of HO2/O2- with unsaturated fatty acids. The Journal of Biological Chemistry. 1983; 258 (8): 4759-4761.

[22] Sies H, Menck CF. Singlet oxygen induced DNA damage. Mutat Res. 1992;275:367-75. doi: 10.1016/0921-8734(92)90039-r

[23] Kanovasky JR. Singlet oxygen production by biological systems. Chem Biol Interact. 1989;70(1-2):1-28. doi: 10.1016/0009-2797(89)90059-8

[24] Hampton MB, Kettle AJ, Winterbourn CC. Inside the neutrophil phagosome: oxidants, myeloperoxidase, and bacterial killing. Blood. 1998;92(9):3007-17. https://doi.org/10.1182/blood.V92.9.3007

[25] Chan HWS. Singlet oxygen analogs in biological systems: coupled oxygenation of 1,3-dienes by soybean lipoxidase. J Am Chem Soc. 1971;93(9):2357-8. https://doi.org/10.1021/ja00738a064

[26] Hayaishi O, Nozaki M. Nature and mechanisms of oxygenases. Science. 1969;164:389-96. doi: 10.1126/science.164.3878.389

[27] Kanofsky JR. Singlet oxygen production by lactoperoxidase. J Biol Chem. 1983;258(10):5991-3.

[28] Allen R C. Halide dependence of the myeloperoxidase-mediated antimicrobial system of the polymorphonuclear leukocyte in the phenomenon of electronic excitation. *Biochem. Biophys. Res. Commun. 1975;* 63: 675-683. https://doi.org/10.1016/S0006-291X(75)80437-2

[29] Bielski BHJ, Cabelli BH, Arudi RL, Ross AB. Reactivity of RO2/O2. Radicals in aqueous solution. J Phys Chem Ref Data. 1985;14:1041-100. https://doi.org/10.1063/1.555739

[30] Vitale M, Di Matola T, Ďascoli F. Iodide excess induces apoptosis in thyroid cells trough a p53-independent mechanism involving oxidative stress. Endrocriology Scoeity. 2000;141:598-605. doi: 10.1210/endo.141.2.7291

[31] Fernandez V, Barrientos X, Kiperos K, Valenzuela A, Videla LA. Superoxide radical generation, NADPH oxidase activity and cytochrome P-450 content of rat liver microsomal fractions in an experimental hyperthyroid state: Relation to lipid peroxidation. Endocrinology. 1985;117:496-501. doi: 10.1210/endo-117-2-496.

[32] Klebanoff SJ. Oxygen metabolites from phagocytes. In: Gallin JI, Snyderman R, eds. *Inflammation: basic principles and clinical correlates.*

Philadelphia: Lippincott Williams & Wilkins; 1999:721-68.

[33] Wentworth PJr., McDunn JE, Wentworth AD, Takeuchi C, Nieva J, Teresa J. Evidence for Antibody-Catalyzed Ozone Formation in Bacterial Killing and Inflammation. *Science.* 2002; 298 (5601): 2195-2199. DOI: 10.1126/science.1077642

[34] Babior BM, Takeuchi C, Ruedi J, Gutierrez A, Wentworth PJr. (2003). Investigating antibody-catalyzed ozone generation by human neutrophils. Biochemistry. 2003; 100 (6): 3031-3034. doi: 10.1073/pnas.0530251100

[35] Mustafa, M.G., Biochemical Basis of Ozone Toxicity, *Free Radical Biol. Med. 1990; 9*:245-265. doi: 10.1016/0891-5849(90)90035-h

[36] Pryor WA. Mechanism of Radical Formation from Reactions of Ozone with Target Molecules in the Lung, *Ibid. 1994; 17*:451-465. DOI: 10.1016/0891-5849(94)90172-4

[37] Kanofsky, JR. and Sima P. Singlet Oxygen Production from the Reactions of Ozone with Biological Molecules, *J. Biol. Chem. 1991; 266*:9039-9042.

[38] Daugherty A., Dunn JL, Rateri, DL, Heinecke JW. Myeloperoxidase, a catalyst for lipoprotein oxidation, is expressed in human atherosclerotic lesions. *J. Clin. Invest.1994;* 94: 437-444. DOI: 10.1172/JCI117342

[39] Pullar JM, Vissers MC, Winterbourn CC. Living with a killer: the effects of hypochlorous acid on mammalian cells. IUBMB Life. 2000; 50: 259-266. doi: 10.1080/713803731

[40] Prütz WA. Hypochlorous acid interactions with thiols, nucleotides, DNA, and other biological substrates. Arch Biochem Biophys,, 1996;332(1):110-20. doi: 10.1006/abbi.1996.0322

[41] David AF. Lipid oxidation by hypochlorous acid: chlorinated lipids in atherosclerosis and myocardial ischemia. Clin Lipidol. 2010; 5(6): 835-852. doi: 10.2217/clp.10.68

[42] Heinecke J W. Cellular mechanisms for the oxidative modification of lipoproteins: implications for atherogenesis. *Coronary Artery Dis. 1994;* 5: 205-210.

[43] Andrew PJ, Mayer B. Enzymatic function of nitric oxide synthases. Cardiovasc Res. 1999;43(3):521-31. doi: 10.1016/s0008-6363(99)00115-7

[44] Mayer B, Hemmens B. Biosynthesis and action of nitric oxide in mammalian cells. Trends Biochem Sci. 1997;22:477-481. doi:10.1016/s0968-0004(97)01147-x

[45] Moncada S, Higgs EA. Endogenous nitric oxide: physiology, pathology and clinical relevance. *Eur J Clin Invest.* 1991;21:361-374. doi: 10.1111/j.1365-2362.1991.tb01383.x

[46] Coleman W. Nitric oxide in immunity and inflammation, International Immunopharmacology. 2001; 1 (8): 1397-1406. doi: 10.1016/s1567-5769(01)00086-8

[47] Furchgott RF. Endothelium-derived relaxing factor: discovery, early studies, and identification as nitric oxide, Bioscience Reports. 1999; 19 (4): 235-251. doi: 10.1023/a:1020537506008

[48] Garthwaite J. Concepts of neural nitric oxide-mediated transmission. European Journal of Neuroscience. 2008; 27 (11): 2783-2802. doi: 10.1111/j.1460-9568.2008.06285.x

[49] Steinert JR, Chernova T, Forsythe ID. Nitric oxide signaling in brain function, dysfunction, and dementia. Neuroscientist. 2010; 16 (4); 435-452. doi: 10.1177/1073858410366481

[50] Thomas DD, Ridnour LA, J. S. Isenberg JS, Flores-Santana W., Switzer CH., Donzelli S., Hussain P., Vecoli C., Paolocci N., Ambs S., Colton CA., Harris CC., Roberts DD., Wink DA. The chemical biology of nitric oxide: implications in cellular signaling. Free Radical Biology & Medicine. 2008; 45 (1): 18-31. DOI: 10.1016/j.freeradbiomed.2008.03.020

[51] Liu X, Miller MJS, Joshi MS, Thomas DD, Lancaster JR. Accelerated reaction of nitric oxide with O2 within the hydrophobic interior of biological membranes. *Proc Natl Acad Sci U S A*. 1998;95:2175-2179. doi: 10.1073/pnas.95.5.2175

[52] Beckman JS. Ischaemic injury mediator. Nature. 1990; 345:27-28. doi: 10.1038/345027b0

[53] Beckman JS, Beckman TW, Chen J, Marshall PA, Freeman BA. Apparent hydroxyl radical production by peroxynitrite: implications for endothelial injury from nitric oxide and superoxide. Proc Natl Acad Sci USA 1990;87:1620-1624. doi: 10.1073/pnas.87.4.1620

[54] Beckman JS, Koppenol WH. Nitric oxide, superoxide, and peroxynitrite: the good, the bad, and ugly. Am J Physiol Cell Physiol 1996;271:C1424–C1437. Beckman JS, Koppenol WH. Nitric oxide, superoxide, and peroxynitrite: the good, the bad, and ugly. Am J Physiol Cell Physiol 1996;271:C1424–C1437

[55] Pryor WA, Squadrito GL. The chemistry of peroxynitrite: a product from the reaction of nitric oxide with superoxide. Am J Physiol Lung Cell Mol Physiol 1995;268:L699–L722. doi: 10.1152/ajplung.1995.268.5.L699

[56] Douki H, Cadet J. Peroxynitrite mediated oxidation of purine bases of nucleosides and isolated DNA. Free Rad Res. 1996;24(5):369-80. doi: 10.3109/10715769609088035

[57] Ferrer-Sueta G., and Radi, R. Chemical biology of peroxynitrite: kinetics, diffusion, and radicals. ACS Chem. Biol. 2009; 4: 161-177. https://doi.org/10.1021/cb800279q

[58] Goldstein S., and Mere'nyi G. The chemistry of peroxynitrite: implications for biological activity. Methods Enzymol. 2008; 436: 49-61. doi: 10.1016/S0076-6879(08)36004-2

[59] Lymar, SV, and Hurst JK. Rapid reaction between peroxynitrite ion and carbon dioxide: implications for biological activity. J. Am. Chem. Soc. 1995; 117: 8867-8868. https://doi.org/10.1021/ja00139a027

[60] Denicola A., Freeman BA., Trujillo M, Radi R. Peroxynitrite reaction with carbon dioxide/bicarbonate: kinetics and influence on peroxynitrite-mediated oxidations. Arch. Biochem. Biophys. 1996; 333: 49-58. doi: 10.1006/abbi.1996.0363.

[61] Lindsay RC. Food additives. In O. R. Fennema (Ed.), Food chemistry, Marcel Dekker Inc. New York, USA, 1996; 778-780.

[62] Lobo V, Patil A, Phatak A, Chandra N . Free radicals, antioxidants and functional foods: Impact on human health. Pharmacogn Rev. 2010; 4(8): 118-126. doi: 10.4103/0973-7847.70902

[63] Preethi G. Anantharaju, Prathima C. Gowda, Manjunatha G. Vimalambike & SubbaRao V. Madhunapantula. An overview on the role of dietary phenolics for the treatment of cancers. Nutrition Journal. 2016; 15:99. https://doi.org/10.1186/s12937-016-0217-2

[64] Spiegel M, Kapusta K, Kołodziejczyk W, Saloni J, Zbikowska B, Hill GA, Sroka Z. Antioxidant Activity of Selected Phenolic Acids–Ferric

Reducing Antioxidant Power Assay and QSAR Analysis of the Structural Features. Molecules. 2020; 25: 3088. https://doi.org/10.3390/molecules25133088

[65] Galato D, Ckless K, Susin MF, Giacomelli C, Ribeiro-do-Valle RM, Spinelli A. Antioxidant capacity of phenolic and related compounds: correlation among electrochemical, visible spectroscopy methods and structure–antioxidant activity. Communications in Free Radical Research. 2001; 6 (4): 243-250. https://doi.org/10.1179/135100001101536391

[66] Ohkatsua Y, Ishikawab SI, Tobitab E. Consideration on the effect of ortho-substituents of phenols by semiempirical molecular orbital method MOPAC. Polym Degrad Stab. 2000; 67: 541-545.

[67] Wright JS., Johnson ER., DiLabio GA. Predicting the activity of phenolic antioxidants: Theoretical method, analysis of substituent effects, and application to major families of antioxidants. Journal of the American Chemical Society. 2001; 123(6): 1173-1183. https://doi.org/10.1021/ja002455u

[68] Dziedzic SZ, B. Hudson BJF. Food Chem. 1984; 12: 205. https://doi.org/10.1021/ja002455u

[69] Nardini M, D'Aquino M, Tmassi G, Gentili V, Di Felice M, Scaccini C. Inhibition of human low-density lipoprotein oxidation by caffeic acid and other hydroxycinnamic acid derivatives. Free Radic Biol Med 1995; 19:541-52. doi: 10.1016/0891-5849(95)00052-y

[70] Bors W, Heller W, Michel C, Saran M. Met. Flavonoids as antioxidants: determination of radical-scavenging efficienciesEnzymol. 1990; 186: 343. doi: 10.1016/0076-6879(90)86128-i

[71] Mansouri A, Makris DP, Kefalas P. Determination of hydrogen peroxide scavenging activity of cinnamic and benzoic acids employing a highly sensitive peroxyoxalate chemiluminescence-based assay: structure–activity relationships. J. Pharm. Biomed. Anal. 2005; 39: 22-6. doi: 10.1016/j.jpba.2005.03.044

[72] Andreasen MF, Landbo AK, Christensen LP, Hansen A, A. S. Meyer AS. Antioxidant Effects of Phenolic Rye (*Secale cereale* L.) Extracts, Monomeric Hydroxycinnamates, and Ferulic Acid Dehydrodimers on Human Low-Density Lipoproteins. J. Agric. Food Chem. 2001; 49: 4090-4096. doi: 10.1021/jf0101758

[73] Nsangou M, Dhaouadi Z, Jaidane N, Lakhdar ZB. J. Mol. Struc: THEOCHEM. DFT study of the structure of hydroxybenzoic acids and their reactions with OH and O2-radicals. 2008; 850: 135-143. https://doi.org/10.1016/j.theochem.2007.10.032

[74] Chen JH, and Ho CT. Antioxidant Activities of Caffeic Acid and Its Related Hydroxycinnamic Acid Compounds. J. Agric. Food Chem. 1997; 45 (7): 2374-2378. https://doi.org/10.1021/jf970055t

[75] Omar, HS, El-Beshbishy HA, Moussa Z, Taha K F, Singab ANB. Antioxidant Activity of *Artocarpus heterophyllus* Lam. (Jack Fruit) Leaf Extracts: Remarkable Attenuations of Hyperglycemia and Hyperlipidemia in Streptozotocin-Diabetic Rats. The Scientific World JOURNAL 2011; 11: 788-800. DOI: 10.1100/tsw.2011.71

[76] Back TG, Moussa Z. Remarkable activity of a novel cyclic seleninate ester as a glutathione peroxidase mimetic and its facile in situ generation from allyl 3-hydroxypropyl selenide. J Am Chem Soc 2002; 124: 12104-12105. https://doi.org/10.1021/ja028030k

[77] Back TG, Moussa Z. Diselenides and allyl selenides as glutathione peroxidase mimetics. remarkable activity of cyclic seleninates produced in situ by the oxidation of allyl ω-hydroxyalkyl selenides. J Am Chem Soc 2003; 125: 13455-13460. https://doi.org/10.1021/ja0357588

[78] Lien EJ, Ren S, Bui H, Wang R. Quantitative structure–activity relationship analysis of phenolic antioxidants. Free Radic Biol Med 1999; 26: 285-294. doi: 10.1016/s0891-5849(98)00190-7

[79] Zhang H, Ge N, Zhang Z. Theoretical elucidation of activity differences of five phenolic antioxidants. Acta Pharmacol Sin 1999; 20: 363-366.

[80] Castelluccio C, Paganga G, Melikian N, Bolwell GP., Pridham J., Sampson J., Rice-Evans C. Antioxidant potential of intermediates in phenylporpanoid metabolism in higher plants. FEBS Lett 1995; 368: 188-192. DOI: 10.1016/0014-5793(95)00639-q

[81] Leopoldini M, Marino T, Russo N, Toscano M. Antioxidant properties of phenolic compounds: H-atom versus electron transfer mechanism. J Phys Chem A 2004; 108: 4916-4922. https://doi.org/10.1021/jp037247d

[82] Gardner EJ, Ruxton CHS, Leeds AR. Black tea—Helpful or harmful? A review of the evidence. European Journal of Clinical Nutrition. 2007; 61: 3-18.

[83] Vinson JA. Flavonoids in foods as in vitro and in vivo antioxidants. Advances in Experimental Medicine and Biology. 1998; 439: 151-164. https://doi.org/10.1007/978-1-4615-5335-9_11

[84] Nardini M, Cirillo E, Natella F, Scaccini C. Absorption of phenolic acids in humans after coffee consumption. Journal of Agricultural and Food Chemistry. 2002; 50: 5735-5741. doi: 10.1021/jf0257547

[85] Vinson JA., Su X, Zubik L, Bose P. Phenol antioxidant quantity and quality in foods: Fruits. Journal of Agricultural and Food Chemistry. 2001; 49: 5315-5321. doi: 10.1021/jf0009293

[86] Mertens-Talcott SU, Jilma-Stohlawetz P, Rios J, Hingorani L, & Derendorf H. Absorption, metabolism, and antioxidant effects of pomegranate (*Punica granatum* L.) polyphenols after ingestion of a standardized extract in healthy human volunteers. Journal of Agricultural and Food Chemistry. 2006; 54: 8956-8961. DOI: 10.1021/jf061674h

[87] Seeram NP, Aviram M, Zhang Y, Henning SM, Feng L, Dreher M, Heber D. Comparison of antioxidant potency of commonly consumed polyphenol-rich beverages in the United States. Journal of Agricultural and Food Chemistry. 2008; 56: 1415-1422. DOI: 10.1021/jf073035s

[88] Gil MI, Tomás-Barberán FA., Hess-Pierce B, Holcroft DM, Kader AA. Antioxidant activity of pomegranate juice and its relationship with phenolic composition and processing. Journal of Agricultural and Food Chemistry. 2000; 48: 4581-4589. doi: 10.1021/jf000404a

[89] Oboh G., and Rocha JBT. Polyphenols in red pepper [*Capsicum annuum var. aviculare* (Tepin)] and their protective effect on some pro-oxidants induced lipid peroxidation in brain and liver. European Food Research and Technology. 2007; 225: 239-247. DOI: 10.1007/s00217-006-0410-1

[90] Visioli F., Bellomo G., Galli C. Free radical-scavenging properties of olive oil polyphenols. Biochemical and Biophysical Research Communications. 1998; 247: 60-64. doi: 10.1006/bbrc.1998.8735

[91] Lodovici M, Guglielmi F, Casalini C, Meoni M, Cheynier V, Dolara P. Antioxidant and radical scavenging properties in vitro of polyphenolic extracts from red wine. European Journal of Nutrition. 2001; 40: 74-77. https://doi.org/10.1007/PL00007386

[92] Vinson JA., Proch J, Zubik L. Phenol antioxidant quantity and quality in foods: Cocoa, dark chocolate, and milk chocolate. Journal of Agricultural and Food Chemistry. 1999; 47: 4821-4824. doi: 10.1021/jf990312p

[93] Wang TY, Li Q, Bi KS. Bioactive flavonoids in medicinal plants: Structure, activity and biological fate. Asian J. Pharm. Sci. 2018; 13: 12-23. doi: 10.1016/j.ajps.2017.08.004

[94] Heim KE, Tagliaferro AR, Bobilya DJ. Flavonoid antioxidants: chemistry, metabolism and structure-activity relationships. J. Nutr. Biochem. 2002; 13:572-584. doi: 10.1016/s0955-2863(02)00208-5

[95] Harborne JB, and Williams CA. Advances in flavonoid research since. Phytochemistry. 2000; 55: 481 504. doi: 10.1016/s0031-9422(00)00235-1

[96] Cai YZ, Sun M, Xing J, Luo Q, Corke H. Structure–radical scavenging activity relationships of phenolic compounds from traditional Chinese medicinal plants. Life Sci. 2006; 78:2872-2888. DOI: 10.1016/j.lfs.2005.11.004

[97] Back TG, Moussa Z, Parvez M. The exceptional glutathione peroxidase-like activity of di (3-hydroxypropyl) selenide and the unexpected role of a novel spirodioxaselenanonane intermediate in the catalytic cycle. Angew. Chem. Int. Ed. Engl 2004; 43: 1268-1270. https://doi.org/10.1002/ange.200353128

[98] Janeiro P, Brett AMO. Catechin electrochemical oxidation mechanisms. Anal. Chim. Acta. 2004; 518: 109-115. https://doi.org/10.1016/j.aca.2004.05.038

[99] Nakanishi I, Miyazaki K, Shimada T, Ohkubo K, Urano S, Ikota N, Ozawa T, Fukuzumi S, Fukuhara K. Effects of metal ions distinguishing between one-step hydrogen-and electron-transfer mechanisms for the radical-scavenging reaction of (+)-catechin. J. Phys. Chem. 2002; 106: 11123-11126. https://doi.org/10.1021/jp026190c

[100] Mahmoud MAA, Chedea VS, Detsi A, Kefalas P. Ascorbic acid modifies the free radical scavenging behaviour of catechin: An insight into the mechanism. Food Res. Inter. 2013; 51: 907-913. https://doi.org/10.1016/j.foodres.2013.02.023

[101] Rimarcík J, Lukes V, Klein E, Ilcin M. Study of the solvent effect on the enthalpies of homolytic and heterolytic N–H bond cleavage in p-phenylenediamine and tetracyano-p-phenylenediamine. J. Mol. Struct.: THEOCHEM. 2010; 952: 25-30. DOI:10.1016/J.THEOCHEM.2010.04.002

[102] Quan VVo, Nam PC, Thong NM, Trung NT, Cam-Tu DP, Mechler A. Antioxidant Motifs in Flavonoids: O–H versus C–H Bond. ACS Omega. 2019; 4: 8935-8942. https://doi.org/10.1021/acsomega.9b00677

[103] Nimse SB and Palb D. Free radicals, natural antioxidants, and their reaction mechanisms. RSC Adv. 2015; 5: 27986-28006. https://doi.org/10.1039/C4RA13315C

[104] Leopoldini M, Russo N, Toscano M. The molecular basis of working mechanism of natural polyphenolic antioxidants. Food Chemistry. 2011; 288-306. DOI: 10.1016/j.foodchem.2010.08.012

[105] Soleas GJ, Diamandis EP, Goldberg DM. Resveratrol: a molecule

whose time has come? And gone?. Clin Biochem. 1997; 30(2):91-113. doi: 10.1016/s0009-9120(96)00155-5

[106] Bavaresco L, Fregoni M, Trevisan M, Mattivi F, Vrhovsek U, Falchetti R . The occurrence of the stilbene piceatannol in grapes.Vitis. 2002; 41: 133-136.

[107] Ku KL, Chang PS, Cheng YC, Lien CY. Production of stilbenoids from the callusof *Arachis hypogaea*: A novel source of the anticancer compound piceatannol. Journal of Agricultural and Food Chemistry. 2005; 5: 33877-3881. https://doi.org/10.1021/jf050242o

[108] Rimando AM, Kalt W, Magee JB, Dewey J, Ballington JR (2004) Resveratrol, pterostilbene, and piceatannol in vaccinium berries. Journal of Agricultural and Food Chemistry. 2004; 52: 4713-4719. doi: 10.1021/jf040095e

[109] Chang J, Rimando A, M. Pallas M, Camins A, Porquet D, Reeves J, Shukitt-Hale B, Smith MA, Joseph JA, Gemma Casadesus G. Low-dose pterostilbene, but not resveratrol, is a potent neuromodulator in aging and Alzheimer's disease, Neurobiology of Aging. 2012; 33 (9): 2062-2071. DOI: 10.1016/j.neurobiolaging.2011.08.015

[110] Chong J, Poutaraud A, Hugueney P. Metabolism and roles of stilbenes in plants. Plant Science. 2009; 177 (3): 143-155, 2009. https://doi.org/10.1016/j.plantsci.2009.05.012

[111] Jang M, Cai L, Udeani GO, Slowing KV, Thomas CF, Beecher CWW, Fong HH, Farnsworth NR, Kinghorn AD, Mehta RG, Moon RC, Pezzuto JM. (1997) Cancer chemo-preventive activity of resveratrol, a natural product derived from grapes. Science. 1997; 275: 218-220. DOI: 10.1126/science.275.5297.218

[112] Stivala LA, Savio M, Carafoli F, Perucca P, Bianchi L, Maga G, Forti L, Pagnoni UM, Albini A, Prosperi E, Vannini V. (2001) Specific structural determinants are responsible for the antioxidant activity and the cell cycle effects of resveratrol. Journal of Biological Chemistry. 2001; 276: 22586-22594. DOI: 10.1074/jbc.M101846200

[113] Djoko B, Chiou RYY, Shee JJ, Liu YW. Characterization of immunological activities of peanut stilbenoids, arachidin-1, piceatannol, and resveratrol on lipopolysaccharide-induced inflammation of RAW264.7 macrophages. Journal of Agricultural and Food Chemistry. 2007; 55: 2376-2383. https://doi.org/10.1021/jf900612n

[114] Bastianetto S, Dumont Y, Han Y, Quirion R. Comparative neuroprotective properties of stilbene and catechin analogs: action via a plasma membrane receptor site? CNS Neuroscience & Therapeutics. 2009; 15: 76-83. DOI: 10.1111/j.1755-5949.2008.00074.x

[115] Murias M, Jager W, Handler N, Erker T, Horvath Z, Szekeres T, Nohl H, Gille L. (2005) Antioxidant, prooxidant and cytotoxic activity of hydroxylated resveratrol analogues: structure-activity relationship. Biochemical Pharmacology. 2005; 69: 903-912. DOI: 10.1016/j.bcp.2004.12.001

[116] Rhayem Y, Therond P, Camont L, Couturier M, Beaudeux JL, Legrand A, Jore D, Gardés-Albert M, Bonnefront-Rousselot D. Chain-breaking activity of resveratrol and piceatannol in a linoleate micellar model. Chemistry and Physics of Lipids. 2008; 155: 48-56. DOI: 10.1016/j.chemphyslip.2008.06.001

[117] Yang Lu, AiHua Wang, Peng Shi, Hui Zhang. A Theoretical Study on the Antioxidant Activity of Piceatannol and Isorhapontigenin Scavenging Nitric Oxide and Nitrogen Dioxide Radicals. PLOS ONE. 2017; 12(1):e0169773.

https://doi.org/10.1371/journal.pone.0169773

[118] Hussein MA. A Convenient Mechanism for the Free Radical Scavenging Activity of Resveratrol. International Journal of Phytomedicine. 2011; 3 (4): 459-469.

[119] Shahidi, F, Janitha, P.K, Wanasundara, P.D. (1992). Phenolic antioxidants. Critical Reviews in Food Science and Nutrition. 1992; 32: 67—103. https://doi.org/10.1080/10408399209527581

[120] Anderson K, Domingos I, Emir B, Saad I, Wellington W, D. Vechiatto D, Helena M. Wilhelm HM, Luiz P. Ramos LP. The influence of BHA, BHT and TBHQ on the oxidation stability of soybean oil ethyl esters (biodiesel). J. Braz. Chem. Soc. 2007; 18 (2): 416-423. https://doi.org/10.1590/S0103-50532007000200026

[121] Al-Mamary MA, Abdelwahab SI, Ali HM, Salma Ismail, Abdulla MA, Darvish P. Synthesis of Some Schiff Bases Containing Hydroxyl and Methoxy Groups: thier Antioxidant and Antibacterial Activities. Asian Journal of Chemistry. 2012; 24(10):4335-4339.

[122] Said MA, Hughes DL, Al-Mamary MA , Al-Kaff NS , Al-Harbi WS. Different Chemical Behaviors and Antioxidant Activity of Three Novel Schiff bases Containing Hydroxyl Groups. X-ray structure of CH2{cyclo-C6H10-NH=CH-(2-O-naphth)}2.H2O. Journal of Molecular Structure. 2018; 1165: 305-311. DOI: 10.1016/j.molstruc.2018.03.089

[123] Moussa Z, Al-Mamary MA, Al-Juhani S, Ahmed SA. Preparation and biological assessment of some aromatic hydrazones derived from hydrazides of phenolic acids and aromatic aldehydes. Heliyon. 2020; 6 (9): e05019. https://doi.org/10.1016/j.heliyon.2020.e05019

[124] Kurutas EB. The importance of antioxidants which play the role in cellular response against oxidative/nitrosative stress: current state. Nutrition Journal. 2016; 15:71. https://doi.org/10.1186/s12937-016-0186-5

[125] Finkel T and N J Holbrook NJ. Oxidants, oxidative stress and the biology of ageing. Nature. 2000; 408(6809):239-47. doi: 10.1038/35041687

[126] Reuter S, Gupta SC, Chaturvedi MM, Aggarwal BB. Oxidative stress, inflammation, and cancer: how are they linked?. Free Radic Biol Med. 2010; 49(11):1603-16. doi: 10.1016/j.freeradbiomed.2010.09.006

[127] Bhattacharyya A, Chattopadhyay R, Mitra S, Crowe SE. Oxidative stress: an essential factor in the pathogenesis of gastrointestinal mucosal diseases. Physiol Rev. 2014; 94(2):329-54. doi: 10.1152/physrev.00040.2012

[128] Padureanu R, Albu CV, Mititelu RR, Bacanoiu MV, Docea AO, Calina D, Padureanu V, Olaru G, Sandu RE, Malin RD, Buga AM. Oxidative Stress and Inflammation Interdependence in Multiple Sclerosis. J Clin Med. 2019; 8(11):1815. doi: 10.3390/jcm8111815

[129] Stanner SA, Hughes J, Kelly CNM, Buttriss J. A review of the epidemiological evidence for the 'antioxidant hypothesis'. Public Health Nutrition. 2004; 7 (3): 407-422. doi: 10.1079/phn2003543

[130] Cherubini A, Vigna GB, Zuliani G, Ruggiero C, Senin U, Fellin R. Role of antioxidants in atherosclerosis: epidemiological and clinical update, Current Pharmaceutical Design. 2005; 11 (16): 2017-2032, 2005. doi: 10.2174/1381612054065783

[131] Lotito SB and Frei B. Consumption of flavonoid-rich foods and increased

plasma antioxidant capacity in humans: cause, consequence, or epiphenomenon? Free Radical Biology and Medicine. 2006; 41 (12): 1727-1746, 2006. doi: 10.2174/1381612054065783

[132] Boeing H, Bechthold A, Bub A, Ellinger S, Haller D, Kroke A, Leschik-Bonnet E, Müller MJ, Oberritter H, Schulze M, Stehle P, Watzl B. Critical review: vegetables and fruit in the prevention of chronic diseases,European Journal of Nutrition. 2012; 51 (6): 637-663. doi: 10.1007/s00394-012-0380-y

[133] Crowe FL, Roddam AW, T. J. Key TJ et al. Fruit and vegetable intake and mortality from ischaemic heart disease: results from the European Prospective Investigation into Cancer and Nutrition (EPIC)-Heart study. European Heart Journal. 2011; 32 (10):1235-1243. doi: 10.1093/eurheartj/ehq465

Chapter 14

Vitamin C and Sepsis

Adriana Françozo de Melo, Giulia Oliveira Timo and Mauricio Homem-de-Mello

Abstract

Vitamin C is a supplement used orally by several people globally. It may help in many other conditions, like sepsis, which is caused by an infection that leads to an imbalanced immune response involving pro (e.g., TNF-α, IL-1, IL-2, IL-6) and anti-inflammatory (e.g., IL-10, IL-4, IL-7) cytokines. Ascorbic acid is an antioxidant and acts against reactive oxygen species. At the same time, this vitamin influences cellular immune signaling, avoiding exacerbated transcription of pro-inflammatory cytokines. Very high intravenous doses have already shown to be beneficial in septic patients. Some clinical trials are still running to evaluate the real impact of vitamin C in this condition. To the moment, the combination of low-dose corticosteroids, high-dose parenteral ascorbate, and thiamine seems to be the most effective supportive treatment that could help septic patients recover.

Keywords: vitamin C, sepsis, emergency, Intensive Care Unit

1. Introduction

Vitamin C is a well-known potent antioxidant essential to various biological processes such as carnitine synthesis, neurotransmitter synthesis, hormone synthesis, and tyrosine metabolism. Furthermore, it stabilizes collagen and acts in iron absorption on the intestinal tract. Nevertheless, much is still discussed on its role in common cold, pneumonia, stress-related disorders, metabolic syndrome, and sepsis. Sepsis is a dysregulated host response to an infection that triggers the release of both pro and anti-inflammatory cytokines throughout its course. This "cytokine storm" is responsible for systemic septic symptoms such as vasodilatation, which leads to hypotension and hypoxia. Also, there is the activation of the clotting cascade leading to disseminated intravascular coagulation (DIC). This hemodynamic instability associated with high immune response makes sepsis a deadly disease. Having such nonspecific symptoms, treating sepsis is also problematic. However, the great majority of protocols include antimicrobial and fluid therapy, vasopressors, and inotropic agents. Using anticoagulants and corticosteroids is debated and varies according to symptoms and local protocols. The use of vitamin C in sepsis treatment is also a highly discussed subject, and there are many clinical trials ongoing trying to associate a better outcome with the help of vitamin C in high doses. Considering that sepsis leads to a depletion in vitamin C because of the increased need for reactive oxygen species (ROS) and the elevated cytokine release, it is fair to assume that supplementing it in high doses might help improve septic symptoms since it scavenges those oxygen-free radicals.

All things considered, this chapter intends to shed light on the pathophysiology of sepsis, and its current treatments, vitamin C's biochemical and therapeutic properties, and the pieces of evidence from clinical trials that applied vitamin C to treat sepsis and its outcomes.

2. Sepsis

2.1 Pathophysiology, molecular pathways, and mediators of sepsis

Sepsis is an overreaction to infections, resulting in multiple organ failure and septic shock, frequently leading to death [1]. Sepsis is commonly associated with a super systemic inflammatory condition followed by an immunosuppression phase in which secondary infections typically occur [2]. First sepsis models were developed using animal experiments after confirmation in human volunteers. Bacterial debris can stimulate an acute rise of pro-inflammatory cytokines, implying that this was the cause of the sepsis-associated organ failure. Guided by these results, several different proposed therapies failed to achieve a substantial positive outcome [3, 4]. Following the overwhelming inflammatory process, an intense anti-inflammatory reply leads to a lack of immune response, lymphopenia, and a high propensity for developing infections [5]. This information had provided the basis of the suppositions that the initial hyperinflammatory condition advances to a following immunosuppression [2]. Pro-inflammatory (as IL-6 and TNF) and anti-inflammatory (as IL-10) cytokines are elevated and death-related in septic patients [6].

After innate recognition of conserved microbial patterns, a substantial inflammatory response begins. The recognition, usually through Toll-Like receptors, leads to the activation of cytokines, growth factors and chemokines [7]. After CD4 T cells activation (**Figure 1**), both pro and anti-inflammatory cytokines are released [4]. The reason why CD4 T cells response is pro (Th1) or anti (Th2) inflammatory is supposed to be related to the size of the bacterial inoculum, pathogen type, and

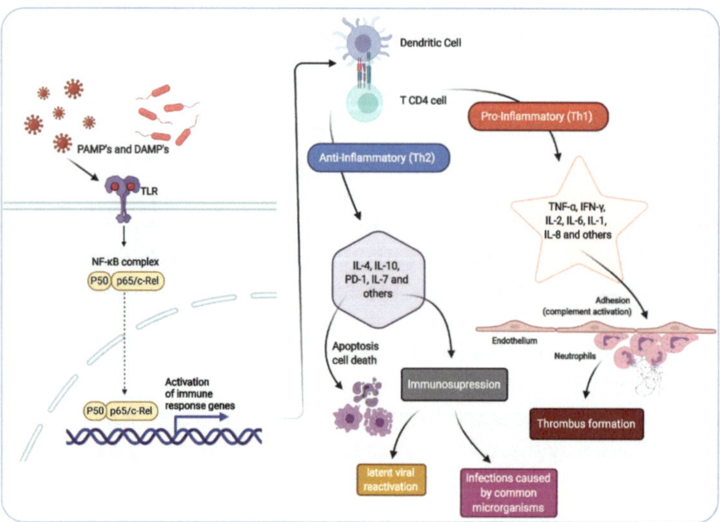

Figure 1.
Immune activation following microbial exposition or cellular damage. NF-κB: Nuclear Factor-κB; PAMP: Pathogen-associated molecular pattern; DAMP: Damage-associated molecular pattern; TLR: Toll-like Receptor; IL: Interleukin; TNF-α: Tumor Necrosis Factor-α; IFN-γ: Interferon-γ; PD-1: Programmed cell death protein 1.

the infected organ [8–11]. A more intense inflammatory response with higher cytokine levels is associated with severe sepsis situations. The spectrum of organic reactions is more intense, as well. General vasodilation, capillary leak, and lessened circulating fluid volume lead to blood clotting and multiple organ malfunction or failure [7].

2.2 Therapeutics of sepsis

The earlier the sepsis or septic shock diagnosis is achieved, the higher are the recovery chances. Broad-spectrum antibiotics (piperacillin/tazobactam, vancomycin, anidulafungin) are initiated while culture and antibiogram results are not available. Clindamycin associated with a β-lactam scheme can be recommended to avoid streptococcal toxic shock. Once the pathogen is identified and its susceptibility to antibiotics is defined, early interruption should be performed, depending on the patient's improvement [2, 12].

Supportive therapy is needed in virtually all cases. Fluid resuscitation, inotropic (e.g., dobutamine), and vasopressor agents (e.g., norepinephrine) are the most common, effective, and widespread therapies [13].

Other therapies have been studied over the years, but few or controversial results were obtained. Corticosteroids are frequently associated with septic shock therapy. Several randomized controlled trials focused on this issue, and some meta-analysis evaluated the outcomes. Considering all observed flaws of the trials (heterogeneity across studies, doses, the uncertainty of the statistical approach, time of observation, among others), the meta-analysis showed a small benefit using low doses of corticosteroids for a more extended period [14–20]. International Guidelines for Management of Sepsis and Septic Shock recommend corticosteroid therapy only if fluid resuscitation and vasopressor administration are not enough to restore patients' stability. Intravenous hydrocortisone (200 mg/day) and continuous evaluation of blood glucose and sodium (corticosteroids may induce hyperglycemia and hypernatremia) are the clinical guidance in those cases [12].

Anticoagulant therapy would be beneficial to oppose the disseminated intravascular coagulation that happens in sepsis conditions. However, antithrombin use did not show evidence to lower the mortality rate and was more prone to bleeding development [12, 21, 22]. On the other hand, thrombomodulin and heparin showed some positive effects on the mortality rate and reduced bleeding risk [23, 24].

Immunoglobulins are still controversial in sepsis. Studies using intravenous immunoglobulins could not show benefits on septic shock or sepsis conditions [25–29]. However, the majority of studies use a small sample size, so more extensive studies are still needed to evaluate its effectiveness [12, 29].

To the present, numerous researches are trying to achieve a satisfactory result for septic shock or sepsis. However, a long list of failures is along with all the tries. There is a rationale behind Vitamin C usage in these cases, and this chapter will then discuss what is already known and what still needs investigation.

3. Vitamin C

3.1 Redox potential

Vitamin C (VitC, ascorbate) is an antioxidant vitamin. This classification is based on the emission of solvated electrons in aqueous media. In organisms, this process can be enzymatically induced. VitC quickly loses electrons in aqueous media, forming ascorbate free radicals. This is why ascorbate is classified as a very potent electron donor. Peroxyl radicals may be formed under oxygenated conditions, by the reaction of solvated electrons with oxygen in aerated solutions [30].

Ascorbate can directly scavenge free radicals or restore other redox systems like α-tocopherol or glutathione (**Figure 2**). Simultaneously, it is vital to the activity of several iron and copper-dependent enzymes [31]. VitC and monodehydroascorbate radicals have low electron reduction potentials [32] to reduce more common radicals present in metabolic conditions.

It is well established that a severe dietary undersupply of vitamin C will result in scurvy. But vitamin C has also a role as a cofactor in several enzymes. It takes part in carnitine synthesis, which is essential for the transport of fatty acids into mitochondria for ATP generation [33, 34]; in the biosynthesis of norepinephrine from dopamine [35, 36], peptide hormones [37, 38], and tyrosine metabolism [39, 40]; in collagen synthesis, increasing its stability [41–43]; finally, it acts in nonheme iron absorption on the intestinal tract [44].

However, ascorbic acid's role in preventing or treating common and complex diseases is still uncertain. Even the widely held assumption that ascorbic acid is a significant biological antioxidant and has a prominent role in disease prevention has not been definitively validated [45, 46].

3.2 Evaluation of vitamin C therapeutic efficacy

Hundreds of studies have been published over the years on vitamin C's effects and its roles in preventing or treating several diseases. There have been many controversial outcomes from this association, whether they are positive or negative. **Table 1** presents the reviews that summarize those outcomes.

Nevertheless, when they are critically analyzed, one can realize they show many inconsistencies regarding the methodology. Recently, Lykkesfeldt interestingly analyzed some more expressive clinical trials and unraveled many of the study's limitations and flaws, as described below, which should be avoided in future researches in this field [59] (**Table 2**).

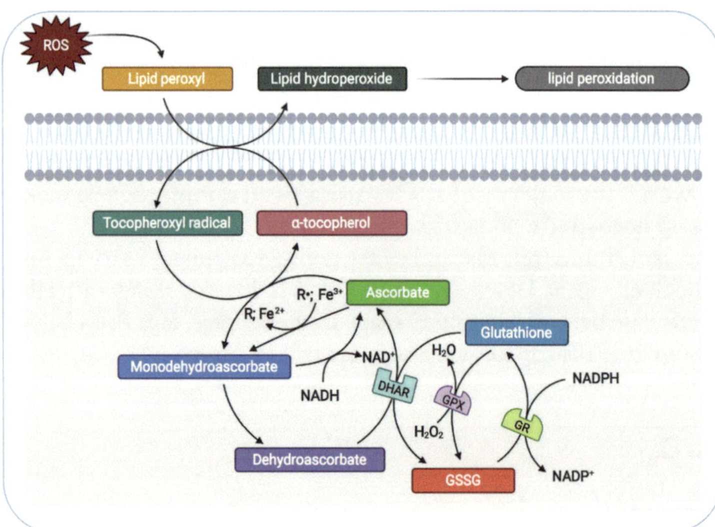

Figure 2.
Antioxidant network. Ascorbate plays a central role in the human antioxidant system. ROS: Reactive Oxygen Species; R·: Free Radical; DHAR: Dehydroascorbate Reductase; GPX: Glutathione Peroxidase; GSSG: Glutathione Disulfide; GR: Glutathione Reductase.

Effect	Conclusion of the study	Reference
Cardiovascular protection	Vitamin C deficiency is associated with a higher risk of cardiovascular disease (CVD) mortality.	[47]
	High vitamin C intake from supplements is associated with an increased risk of CVD mortality in postmenopausal women with diabetes.	[48]
	Population with optimal plasma levels of VitC has no benefit from supplementation. People with VitC deficiency have a higher risk of developing CVD.	[49]
Neurologic protection	Antiexcitotoxic, neuromodulator, and neurotrophic effects of ascorbic acid over the CNS are critical for neuroprotective strategies. Clinical trials have demonstrated that ascorbate supplementation produces beneficial results for depression and anxiety. More controlled clinical trials are still necessary to better understand the action mechanisms in stress-related disorders.	[50]
Metabolic syndrome	A direct positive effect of vitamin C alone on Metabolic syndrome needs to be confirmed in animals and human populations. Combination of vitamin C with other antioxidants may be worthwhile in managing Metabolic syndrome.	[51]
Common cold (CC) treatment and prevention	In adults, the duration of colds was reduced by 8% and in children by 14%. The severity of colds was also reduced by vitamin C administration during the cold process. No reliable effect of vitC was seen on the duration or severity of colds in the therapeutic trials.	[52]
	Regular supplementation has shown that ascorbate reduces the duration and severity of CC.	[53]
	Supplementation with vitamin C appears to be able to both prevent and treat respiratory and systemic infections.	[54]
Pneumonia treatment and prevention	Due to the small number of included studies and the low quality of the existing evidence, data is uncertain about the effect of vitamin C supplementation on preventing and treating pneumonia.	[55]
Exercise recovery	Vitamin C supplementation attenuates the oxidative stress (lipid peroxidation) and inflammatory response (IL-6) to a single exercise bout. No effects of vitamin C supplementation were found on creatine kinase (CK), C-reactive protein (CRP), cortisol levels, muscle soreness, and muscle strength.	[56]
Cancer treatment	Ascorbate can be positive as a pro-oxidative factor as well. VitC would promote the removal of 8-Oxo-2′-deoxyguanosine from DNA by upregulation of repair enzymes due to pro-oxidative properties. Vitamin C showed protection against radiation-induced cell damage.	[57]
	No clinically relevant positive effect of vitamin C in cancer patients on the overall survival, clinical status, quality of life, and performance status. The quality of the evaluated studies, however, is low. Small advantages were more associated to intravenous than oral administration.	[58]

Table 1.
Summary of reviews about therapeutic evidence associated with VitC.

Considering the lack of high-quality data to evaluate the efficacy of ascorbate in less severe or more chronic conditions, it is fair to assume that an acute and severe disease such as sepsis is a hard-to-evaluate condition. Vitamin C in sepsis has some particularities such as a diverse route of administration and a peculiar dose–response relationship. The scientific rationale behind this therapeutic proposal to sepsis is discussed in the rest of this chapter.

Concern	Trouble	Resolution
Measurement of Vit C intake vs. status	Focus on VitC intake rather than its status. Even large cohort studies used estimates of micronutrient intakes from self-reported questionnaires or diaries. Lack of precision due to recall error, loss of vitamin from storage and preparation, diet change over time, and possible different polymorphisms.	Retrieving blood samples from fasted individuals.
Lack of stability	Fasted blood samples can be obtained, but there are significant challenges in correlating vitamin C status to disease risk. This is due to the lability of ascorbate. Ascorbate is quickly oxidized ex vivo, and the resulting oxidation products are quickly degraded or metabolized	Process samples in a cold (4 °C) environment. Avoid hemolysis. Choose HPLC with electrochemical detection.
Study Design	Random Controlled Trials may require very long intervention periods to accumulate sufficient disease endpoints. This perspective is needed to observe an accumulated preventive potential of a lifelong VitC intake of both placebo and intervention groups up to the trial. This issue has been completely neglected in the available literature.	Perform multicentric randomized follow-up clinical trials.
Healthy Enrolee Effect	A tendency towards recruiting health-conscious, self-motivated subjects eating a healthy diet already rich in micronutrients, with higher exercise frequency and lower disease rate than the background population.	Work with more significant samples, baseline adjustment among groups, previous genetic evaluation

Table 2.
Concerns about clinical trials performed to evaluate ascorbate efficacy on diseases, according to Lykkesfeldt [59] (modified by the authors).

3.3 Dose-response in supplementation versus high dose

Sepsis is a condition associated with VitC deficiency because of its high consumption due to enhanced reactive oxygen species (ROS) production. Ascorbate supplementation is thus necessary, and the best results are thought to be achieved through high intravenous doses [60, 61]. The absorption, distribution, metabolism, and excretion (ADME) of vitC in humans are distinct from other small molecules.

3.3.1 Pharmacokinetics of vitamin C

3.3.1.1 Oral and intravenous administration

In biological systems, VitC exists in two main chemical forms (**Figure 3**), the reduced and predominant ascorbate anion and the oxidized dehydroascorbate (DHA). Due to the DHA reductase activity (**Figure 2**), virtually every cell can recycle DHA. Therefore, total ascorbate is considered the sum of VitC and DHA. The membrane transport can be performed by three possible mechanisms: passive or facilitated diffusion and active transport, the most relevant of the three [62].

Orally, VitC is absorbed by the saturable mucosal sodium-dependent Vitamin C transporter 1 (SVCT1) [60]. Ascorbate oral absorption is limited, achieving a plateau after 200-300 mg (**Figure 4**). SVCT transporters are widely distributed throughout organs and are responsible for most VitC passage across membranes, even against a concentration gradient [63–65].

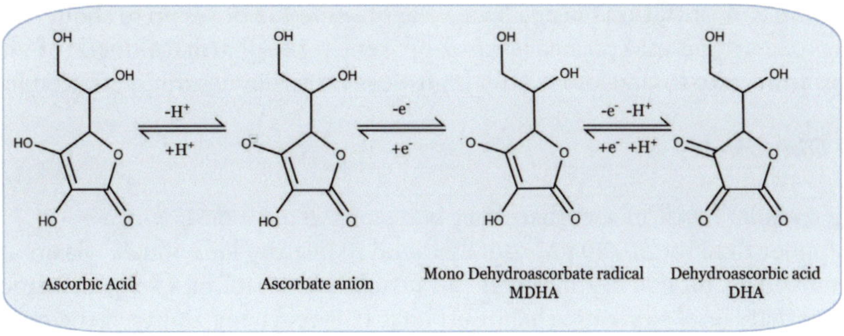

Figure 3.
VitC chemical forms in biological systems – Redox cycle. MDHA: Monodehydroascorbate radical. DHA: Dehydroascorbate.

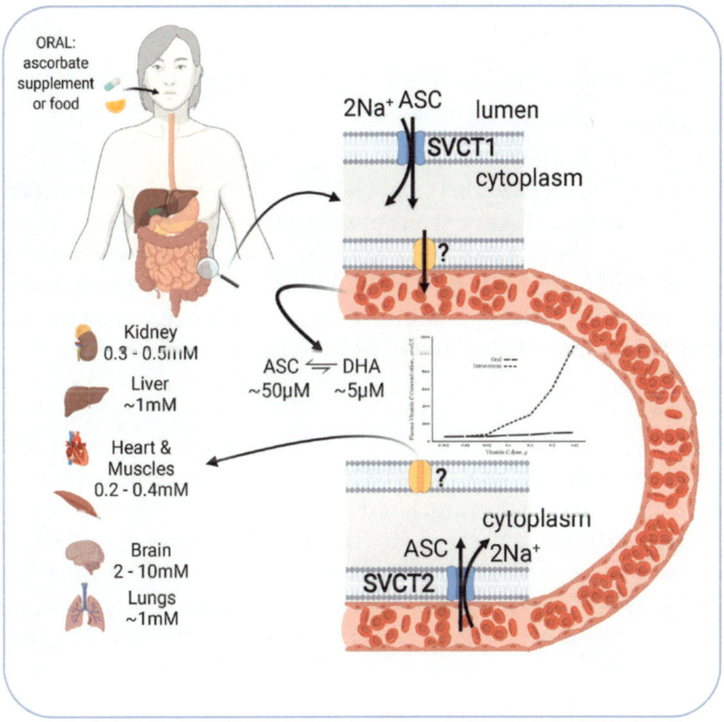

Figure 4.
VitC oral absorption and distribution. ASC: Ascorbate, SVCT1 and 2: sodium-dependent Vitamin C transporter 1 and 2, DHA: Dehydroascorbate.

Some SVCT polymorphisms have already been identified, which may be associated with a critical pharmacokinetic variation. Some of those SVCT alleles are supposed to lead to permanent ascorbate deficiency (plasma concentrations <23 μM) [62].

Humans do not synthesize vitC, so the oral ingestion of food is the primary source of vitC. There is enough ascorbate for healthy individuals in the average diets that contain food rich in it. However, pathologic conditions associated with low ascorbate levels may need supplementation to achieve the minimum plasma concentrations [62].

Intravenously, plasma levels of ascorbic acid continuously increase, producing plasma levels up to 70-fold higher than the maximum oral doses, achieving the millimolar concentration [66]. A linear relationship between dose and Cmax (maximum concentration plasma level) was observed in doses up to about 70 g/m^2, leading to nearly 50 mM plasma levels. Apparently, the pharmacokinetic of vitC changes from zero to first-order after high-dose intravenous administration [62].

3.3.1.2 Distribution

Intracellular levels of ascorbate vary between 0.5 to 10 mM, which is much higher than the 50–80 μM usually found in healthy individuals' plasma. Simultaneously, human erythrocytes can turn DHA to VitC and keep an intracellular ascorbate level similar to that of plasma. This recycling ability of the red blood cells is essential as an antioxidant reserve [62].

As it happens at the absorption phase, distribution depends on active transport as well. Ascorbate exits the bloodstream and crosses the organ's cell membranes through SVCT2 carriers (**Figure 4**). Yet, even in the steady-state achieved concentration after regular ascorbate dosage, different tissues present highly diverse concentrations. This may happen because of distinct levels of SVCT2 expression [62].

3.3.1.3 Metabolism

Metabolism of VitC is essentially associated with the redox cycle involved with the antioxidant function (**Figure 3**). As previously cited, ascorbate is an electron donor, and it can reduce free radicals (**Figure 2**) by oxidizing itself to the stable radical monodehydroascorbate (MDHA). This radical can react to another equal, providing an ascorbate molecule and the DHA metabolite that can be reduced, as mentioned before, to ascorbate through DHA reductase activity [62].

3.3.1.4 Excretion

VitC is a highly water-soluble (about 330 g/L) small molecule (about 8 Å large, 176.1 g/mol), it has a pKa of 4.2, and is almost insoluble in hydrophobic organic solvents [67]. Like other molecules with similar solubility, ascorbate is filtered through the glomerulus and is concentrated after water resorption. At this time, local pH drops to five, leading to an increase of the non-ionized ascorbic acid fraction. However, passive reabsorption does not occur because of the highly hydrophilic characteristic of the molecule. In the proximal tubules, the reuptake of ascorbate is controlled by the saturable active transporter SVCT1. In individuals with saturated plasma levels, supplemental vitC is excreted quantitatively [68].

After high-dose intravenous administration, vitC is rapidly eliminated through glomerular filtration. Reuptake is non-significant under this condition, and the half-life is constant, about two hours (after discontinuation of infusion), and first-order kinetic applies to this case. In about 16 h, physiological levels are back to normal [62, 69–71].

3.3.1.5 Pharmacokinetics in critically ill patients

Critically ill patients, such as those in septic shock conditions, have an increased ascorbate turnover, needing a dose many folds higher (oral or intravenous) than would be expected to saturate a healthy person. Systemic inflammation and severe pressure due to oxidative stress increase VitC consumption [61, 72, 73]. Mathematically predicted plasmatic ascorbate values are much higher than what is achieved in critically ill patients, suggesting that pharmacokinetics in this group of patients is changed.

3.4 Vitamin C in septic conditions

In sepsis conditions, the mitochondrial impairment may be a relevant route to cell death and organ collapse. Anomalies in the citric acid cycle and reduction of the fatty acid's beta-oxidation seem to be a characteristic aspect of this mitochondrial disorder [74].

While ascorbate is transported across membranes through SVCT's proteins, DHA can be transported by glucose transporters GLUT1, 3, and 4 [75]. DHA is transported into the mitochondria by GLUT1 and converted to ascorbate (**Figure 5**), where it works as an antioxidant, avoiding damage to the organelle [76]. Ascorbate can also act as a cofactor to the mitochondrial Trimethyllysine dioxygenase (TMLD) enzyme, responsible for the first L-carnitine synthesis, needed for the β-oxidation of fatty acids [77].

The heart is a vital organ that may be affected by sepsis. Proteolysis, mitochondrial injury, and calcium homeostasis dysfunction are expected consequences of the oxidative myocyte damage. Experimental models show that supplementation of the redox scavengers can diminish cardiac disorder [78]. Ascorbate can decrease apoptosis and improve mitochondrial integrity in myocytes through the blockage of the mitochondrial permeability transition pore opening, limiting calcium profusion [79].

VitC can achieve high concentrations in leukocytes, especially lymphocytes and macrophages. In other defense cells, VitC acts to improve chemotaxis, stimulating interferon expression, and promoting lymphocyte proliferation. In neutrophils, ascorbate increases phagocytic capacity and oxidative burst, and decreases NET (neutrophil-extracellular-trap) formation [61, 80].

VitC can mediate immune modulation. VitC inhibits nuclear Factor Kappa-B (NF-κB) activation. The mechanism that underlies this suppression involves the blockade of the TNFα-induced activation of NIK (NFκB-inducing kinase) and

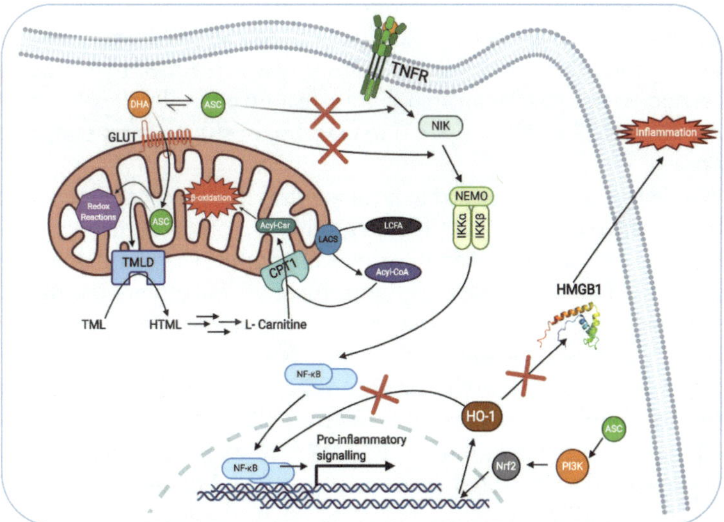

Figure 5.
Vitamin C multiple anti-inflammatory mechanisms. DHA: Dehydroascorbate, ASC: Ascorbate, GLUT: Glucose Transporter, (H)TML(D): (Hydroxy) Trimethyllysine (Dioxygenase), CPT1: Carnitine Palmitoyltransferase 1, LCFA: Long-Chain Fatty Acids; LACS: Long-Chain Acyl-CoA Synthetase, TNFR: Tumor Necrosis Factor Receptor, NF-κB: Nuclear Factor Kappa-light-chain-enhancer of activated B cells, NIK: NF-κB-Inducing Kinase, NEMO: NF-κB Essential Modulator, IKKα and β: IκBα and β kinases, PI3K: Phosphoinositide 3-Kinase, Nrf2: Nuclear Factor Erythroid 2-Related Factor 2, HO-1: Heme Oxygenase 1, HMGB1 - High Mobility Group Box 1.

IKKβ kinases (**Figure 5**) [81]. Further modulation is provided by the VitC induced decrease in the late pro-inflammatory cytokine HMGB1 (high mobility group box 1) secretion and through the lowering of histamine levels [82, 83].

3.4.1 Clinical trials: vitamin C and sepsis or other critically ill conditions

Table 1 shows studies that were performed to evaluate VitC efficacy in many pathological conditions. In critically ill patients, several clinical trials have already been completed or are still ongoing. Until December 2020, 39 studies involving ascorbate and some critically ill conditions were registered at the United States National Library of Medicine (NLM) databank clinicaltrials.gov. The list with all referred studies and links to the clinicaltrials.gov forms are available at the end of this chapter.

To the present date, 25 of the cited trials are already finished, 12 are ongoing, and two will begin in 2021. Twelve of these studies tested VitC alone, with no other experimental therapeutics except the usually applied in sepsis cases (i.e., antimicrobial and fluid therapy, vasopressors, and inotropic agents). Seventeen trials used a combination of hydrocortisone, ascorbate, and thiamine (HAT).

Ten studies experimented a combination of VitC with a corticosteroid only (2 trials) or VitC with VitB1 (5 trials) or VitC in combination with some other therapeutic agent (3 trials). Even if there is no consensus about intravenous doses to be used in critically ill patients, 23 of the 39 trials employed 6 g/day doses, mostly in a 6 h-interval regimen (1.5 g each). Five studies used doses below 6 g/day, and nine studies used doses above 6 g/day, mostly in a protocol of 200 mg/kg/day in a 6 h interval regimen (about 14 g/day to a 70 kg patient).

Sadly, from the 25 already finished trials, only 5 reported their results to clinicaltrials.gov or published them in a peer-reviewed journal. One of those was a pharmacokinetic study [84], so no outcomes were evaluated. The other four studies that reported results were called REDOXS [85], ORANGES [86], VITAMINS [87], and CITRIS-ALI [88].

REDOXS used ascorbate in 1.5 g/day dose administered enterally associated with glutamine and other antioxidants. The study was planned to evaluate glutamine associated with a pool of antioxidants effect on critically ill patients. Results reported no difference when compared to placebo for the primary endpoint (28-day mortality rate).

ORANGES was a study intended to evaluate the HAT protocol in septic patients. They evaluated almost 70 patients (in each group) in a protocol that involved 6 g/day ascorbate (1.5 g per dose) for a maximum of 4 days after ICU admission. The study concluded that HAT could decrease the duration of shock, but not the 28-day mortality rate in patients with sepsis, probably due to ascorbate administration (they had an arm of the study that received only corticosteroids).

VITAMINS used the same HAT and ascorbate dosage as described above. They evaluated about 100 patients (in each group). The difference between the ORANGES trial is the control group. While ORANGES intervention in control was essentially placebo, the VITAMINS used a corticoid and thiamine (when clinicians evaluated its need). VITAMINS results indicate that treatment with intravenous ascorbate, hydrocortisone, and thiamine, did not significantly improve the duration of mortality rate and discontinuation of vasopressor administration over seven days.

The CITRIS-ALI trial evaluated the administration of VitC alone in sepsis, associated with acute respiratory distress syndrome (ARDS) patients, in a dose of 200 mg/kg/day (about 14 g/day to a 70 kg patient). The primary outcome evaluated the change in the Sequential Sepsis Related Organ Failure Score (SOFA) and two plasma biomarkers (C-reactive protein and thrombomodulin). The study assessed groups of about 80 patients. Circa 65% of patients (from both control and treatment groups) received corticosteroids during the study, and the mortality rate was significantly lower in the VitC group. However, since this outcome was not a primary outcome, the authors did not consider it in this study. Authors concluded that patients with sepsis and ARDS did not have an improvement in organ dysfunction scores, nor did they have altered markers of inflammation and vascular injury after a 96-hour infusion of vitamin C compared with placebo.

Outside the clinicaltrial.gov, several studies have investigated the use of IV ascorbate in critically ill patients. Cases of trauma, severe burn, and septic shock were evaluated, in various dosage schemes, from 7 g until 110 g/day. No severe adverse effects related to the vitamin C infusion were reported in any of the studies. A decrease in the incidence of multiple system organ failure, trends to reduced mortality, and ICU stay length was the usual results achieved [89–91].

One of the most commented studies about the effects of the HAT approach, and maybe the reference for several of the clinical trials, was published by Dr. Marik from Eastern Virginia Medical School in 2017 [92]. This study proposed the early HAT protocol using ascorbate IV (1.5 g every 6 h for 4 days or until ICU discharge), hydrocortisone (50 mg every 6 h for 7 days or until ICU discharge), as well as IV thiamine (200 mg every 12 h for 4 days or until ICU discharge). VitC is administered as an infusion over 30 to 60 min and mixed in a 100 mL solution of either dextrose 5% in water or normal saline. Dr. Marik's results showed that early use of intravenous VitC, with hydrocortisone and thiamine, would be used effectively to prevent progressive organ impairment, including acute kidney damage, and reduce patients' mortality with severe sepsis and septic shock. However, the published work evaluated a small sample, and as the authors say at the end of the manuscript, additional studies are required to confirm their preliminary findings [92].

High doses of IV ascorbate, thiamine, and glucocorticoids can reduce pro-inflammatory mediators, ROS, and decrease immunosuppression. Thiamine is useful to energy production as a precursor of thiamine pyrophosphate and acts as an antioxidant. Thiamine is essential because ascorbate may cause oxalate accumulation in the kidneys, and the concomitant use can prevent it since thiamine pyrophosphate is a cofactor required for the oxidation of glyoxylate to carbon dioxide by the enzyme glyoxylate aminotransferase. Thiamine deficiency increases the conversion of glyoxylate to oxalate. At the same time, thiamine deficiency is common in septic patients and is associated with an increased risk of death [61, 93].

The VitC in critically ill patients is still a dilemma to be solved. There is a rationale behind its use that seems to be optimal. HAT therapy's premise is the use of a combination of drugs that aim at multiple sectors of the patient's response to an infectious agent, synergistically restoring the impaired immune system, avoid damage due to oxidants, and restore mitochondrial activity. However, to evaluate the clinical features and impact of this scheme, most of the studies performed were small, doses used between trials were highly different, and the risk of bias was usually uncertain or high. Secondary outcomes need bigger sample sizes, and so were yet harder to evaluate. The studies' duration was not uniform, so the follow-up and comparison analysis were possible only to the longest available time in each trial. Finally, the heterogeneity between treatment schemes made comparisons hard. Isolated analysis of VitC ignores any synergistic effects that could be seen with HAT therapy [94].

4. Conclusions

Vitamin C is a powerful antioxidant that takes part in many vital biological processes. Due to its properties, it has been proposed that VitC could improve sepsis and septic shock symptoms. Because of its pharmacokinetics, it is imperative that ascorbic acid is administered IV in high dosage to explore its full potential in sepsis. Furthermore, the inclusion of hydrocortisone and thiamine to compose the HAT protocol has shown to improve patients outcomes in some clinical trials. Nevertheless, there is still much debate on whether the HAT protocol can actually exert this improvement. To further investigate this proposal, trials should increase sample sizes and come to an agreement on treatment schemes so they can be accurately compared, in addition to sharing the results of the research on Clinical Trials.

Acknowledgements

JChem for Word was used for **Figure 3**, Product version 20.21.0.768, ChemAxon (https://www.chemaxon.com). All other images were created with BioRender.com

Conflict of interest

The authors declare no conflict of interest.

Appendix

Trial name	Internet link to the trial
High-dose Intravenous Vitamin C as an Adjunctive Treatment for Sepsis in Rwanda	https://clinicaltrials.gov/ct2/show/NCT04088591
Outcome Following Vitamin C Administration in Sepsis	https://clinicaltrials.gov/ct2/show/NCT01590303
VICTAS Vitamin C, Thiamine, and Steroids in Sepsis	https://clinicaltrials.gov/ct2/show/study/NCT03509350
Hydrocortisone, Vitamin C, and Thiamine for the Treatment of Sepsis and Septic Shock	https://clinicaltrials.gov/ct2/show/NCT03258684
Therapy With Hydrocortisone, Ascorbic Acid, Thamine in Patients With Sepsis	https://clinicaltrials.gov/ct2/show/NCT04160676
Vitamin C & Thiamine in Sepsis	https://clinicaltrials.gov/ct2/show/NCT03592277
Vitamin C Infusion for Treatment in Sepsis and Alcoholic Hepatitis	https://clinicaltrials.gov/ct2/show/NCT03829683
Vitamin C, Vitamin B1 and Steroid in Sepsis	https://clinicaltrials.gov/ct2/show/NCT04039815
Effect of Intravenous Vitamin Con SOFA Score Among Septic Patients	https://clinicaltrials.gov/ct2/show/NCT04137276
Ascorbic Acid, Corticosteroids, and Thiamine in Sepsis (ACTS) Trial	https://clinicaltrials.gov/ct2/show/NCT03389555
Pilot Study on the Use of Hydrocortisone, Vitamin c and Thiamine in Patient With Sepsis and Septic Shock	https://clinicaltrials.gov/ct2/show/NCT04111822
Vitamin C, Thiamine, Cyanocobalamine, Pyridoxine and Hydrocortisone in Sepsis	https://clinicaltrials.gov/ct2/show/NCT04197115

Trial name	Internet link to the trial
High Dose of Vitamin C on Mechanically Ventilated Septic Patients in Intensive Care Unit	https://clinicaltrials.gov/ct2/show/NCT04029675
Ascorbic Acid (Vitamin C) Infusion in Human Sepsis	https://clinicaltrials.gov/ct2/show/NCT01434121
The Effect of Vitamin C, Thiamine and Hydrocortisone on Clinical Course and Outcome in Patients With Severe Sepsis and Septic Shock	https://clinicaltrials.gov/ct2/show/NCT03335124
Effect of Anti-inflammatory and Anti-microbial Cosupplementations in Traumatic ICU Patients at High Risk of Sepsis	https://clinicaltrials.gov/ct2/show/NCT04216459
Ascorbic Acid and Thiamine Effect in Septic Shock	https://clinicaltrials.gov/ct2/show/NCT03756220
ASTER (Acetaminophen and Ascorbate in Sepsis: Targeted Therapy to Enhance Recovery)	https://clinicaltrials.gov/ct2/show/study/NCT04291508
ViCiS (Vitamin C to Reduce Vasopressor Dose in Septic Shock)	https://clinicaltrials.gov/ct2/show/NCT03835286
Vitamin C and Septic Shock	https://clinicaltrials.gov/ct2/show/NCT03338569
Comparative, Between Triple Therapy Regimen to Hydrocortisone Monotherapy in Reducing the MR in Septic Shock Patients	https://clinicaltrials.gov/ct2/show/study/NCT04508946
Outcomes of Septic Shock Patients Treated With a Metabolic Resuscitation Bundle Consisting of Intravenous Hydrocortisone, Ascorbic Acid and Thiamine	https://clinicaltrials.gov/ct2/show/NCT03913468
LOVIT (Lessening Organ Dysfunction With Vitamin C)	https://clinicaltrials.gov/ct2/show/NCT03680274
Vitamin C, Thiamine and Hydrocortisone for the Treatment of Septic Shock	https://clinicaltrials.gov/ct2/show/NCT03872011
CORVICTES (Vitamin C, Hydrocortisone and Thiamine for Septic Shock)	https://clinicaltrials.gov/ct2/show/NCT03592693
CORVICTES-YM (Vitamin C, Steroids, and Thiamine, and Cerebral Autoregulation and Functional Outcome in Septic Shock)	https://clinicaltrials.gov/ct2/show/NCT03649633
Effect of IV Vitamin C, Thiamine, and Steroids on Mortality of Septic Shock	https://clinicaltrials.gov/ct2/show/NCT03828929
Thiamine, Vitamin C and Hydrocortisone in the Treatment of Septic Shock	https://clinicaltrials.gov/ct2/show/NCT03540628
Effects of Glucocorticoid Combined With Vitamin C and Vitamin B1 on Microcirculation in Severe Septic Shock	https://clinicaltrials.gov/ct2/show/NCT03821714
Clinical Trial of Antioxidant Therapy in Patients With Septic Shock	https://clinicaltrials.gov/ct2/show/NCT03557229
STASIS (Steroids, Thiamine and Ascorbic Acid in Septic Shock)	https://clinicaltrials.gov/ct2/show/NCT04134403
HYVITS (Evaluation of Hydrocortisone, Vitamin C and Thiamine for the Treatment of Septic Shock)	https://clinicaltrials.gov/ct2/show/NCT0338050
AVoCaDO (Administration of Intravenous Vitamin C in Novel Coronavirus Infection (COVID-19) and Decreased Oxygenation)	https://clinicaltrials.gov/ct2/show/NCT04357782

Trial name	Internet link to the trial
REDOXS (Trial of Glutamine and Antioxidant Supplementation in Critically Ill Patients)	https://clinicaltrials.gov/ct2/show/study/NCT00133978
Pharmacokinetics of Two Different High-dose Regimens of Intravenous Vitamin C in Critically Ill Patients	https://clinicaltrials.gov/ct2/show/study/NCT02455180
High Dose Intravenous Ascorbic Acid in Severe Sepsis	https://clinicaltrials.gov/ct2/show/results/NCT02734147
ORANGES - Metabolic Resuscitation Using Ascorbic Acid, Thiamine, and Glucocorticoids in Sepsis.	https://clinicaltrials.gov/ct2/show/NCT03422159
VITAMINS The Vitamin C, Hydrocortisone and Thiamine in Patients With Septic Shock Trial	https://clinicaltrials.gov/ct2/show/NCT03333278
CITRIS-ALI Vitamin C Infusion for Treatment in Sepsis Induced Acute Lung Injury	https://clinicaltrials.gov/ct2/show/study/NCT02106975

Author details

Adriana Françozo de Melo, Giulia Oliveira Timo and Mauricio Homem-de-Mello*
inSiliTox, University of Brasilia, Brasilia, Brazil

*Address all correspondence to: mauriciohmello@unb.br

References

[1] WHO. Global report on the epidemiology and burden of sepsis: current evidence, identifying gaps and future directions. WHO. 2020. 56 p.

[2] Cecconi M, Evans L, Levy M, Rhodes A. Sepsis and septic shock. Lancet (London, England). 2018;392(10141):75-87. DOI: 10.1016/S0140-6736(18)30696-2

[3] Bone RC. Why sepsis trials fail. JAMA. 1996;276(7):565-566.

[4] Hotchkiss RS, Karl IE. The pathophysiology and treatment of sepsis. N Engl J Med. 2003;348(2):138-150. DOI: 10.1056/NEJMra021333

[5] Venet F, Chung C-S, Kherouf H, Geeraert A, Malcus C, Poitevin F, et al. Increased circulating regulatory T cells (CD4(+)CD25 (+)CD127 (−)) contribute to lymphocyte anergy in septic shock patients. Intensive Care Med. 2009;35(4):678-686. DOI: 10.1007/s00134-008-1337-8

[6] Kellum JA, Kong L, Fink MP, Weissfeld LA, Yealy DM, Pinsky MR, et al. Understanding the inflammatory cytokine response in pneumonia and sepsis: results of the Genetic and Inflammatory Markers of Sepsis (GenIMS) Study. Arch Intern Med. 2007;167(15):1655-1663. DOI: 10.1001/archinte.167.15.1655

[7] Boyd JH, Russell JA, Fjell CD. The meta-genome of sepsis: host genetics, pathogens and the acute immune response. J Innate Immun. 2014;6(3):272-283. DOI: 10.1159/000358835

[8] Abbas AK, Murphy KM, Sher A. Functional diversity of helper T lymphocytes. Nature. 1996;383(6603):787-793. DOI: 10.1038/383787a0

[9] Kim D-M, Jung S-I, Jang H-C, Lee CS, Lee SH, Yun NR, et al. Vibrio vulnificus DNA load and mortality. J Clin Microbiol. 2011;49(1):413-415. DOI: 10.1128/JCM.01913-09

[10] Darton T, Guiver M, Naylor S, Jack DL, Kaczmarski EB, Borrow R, et al. Severity of meningococcal disease associated with genomic bacterial load. Clin Infect Dis an Off Publ Infect Dis Soc Am. 2009;48(5):587-594. DOI: 10.1086/596707

[11] Hackett SJ, Guiver M, Marsh J, Sills JA, Thomson APJ, Kaczmarski EB, et al. Meningococcal bacterial DNA load at presentation correlates with disease severity. Arch Dis Child. 2002;86(1):44-46. DOI: 10.1136/adc.86.1.44

[12] Rhodes A, Evans LE, Alhazzani W, Levy MM, Antonelli M, Ferrer R, et al. Surviving Sepsis Campaign: International Guidelines for Management of Sepsis and Septic Shock: 2016. Intensive Care Med. 2017;43(3):304-377. DOI: 10.1007/s00134-017-4683-6

[13] Dugar S, Choudhary C, Duggal A. Sepsis and septic shock: Guideline-based management. Cleve Clin J Med. 2020;87(1):53-64. DOI: 10.3949/ccjm.87a.18143

[14] Annane D, Bellissant E, Bollaert PE, Briegel J, Keh D, Kupfer Y, et al. Corticosteroids for treating sepsis in children and adults. Cochrane database Syst Rev. 2019;12(12):CD002243. DOI: 10.1002/14651858.CD002243.pub4

[15] Rochwerg B, Oczkowski SJ, Siemieniuk RAC, Agoritsas T, Belley-Cote E, D'Aragon F, et al. Corticosteroids in Sepsis: An Updated Systematic Review and Meta-Analysis. Crit Care Med. 2018;46(9):1411-1420. DOI: 10.1097/CCM.0000000000003262

[16] Bollaert PE, Charpentier C, Levy B, Debouverie M, Audibert G, Larcan A. Reversal of late septic shock with supraphysiologic doses of hydrocortisone. Crit Care Med. 1998;26(4):645-650. DOI: 10.1097/00003246-199804000-00010

[17] Briegel J, Forst H, Haller M, Schelling G, Kilger E, Kuprat G, et al. Stress doses of hydrocortisone reverse hyperdynamic septic shock: a prospective, randomized, double-blind, single-center study. Crit Care Med. 1999;27(4):723-732. DOI: 10.1097/00003246-199904000-00025

[18] Sprung CL, Annane D, Keh D, Moreno R, Singer M, Freivogel K, et al. Hydrocortisone therapy for patients with septic shock. N Engl J Med. 2008;358(2):111-124. DOI: 10.1056/NEJMoa071366

[19] Sligl WI, Milner DAJ, Sundar S, Mphatswe W, Majumdar SR. Safety and efficacy of corticosteroids for the treatment of septic shock: A systematic review and meta-analysis. Clin Infect Dis an Off Publ Infect Dis Soc Am. 2009;49(1):93-101. DOI: 10.1086/599343

[20] Annane D, Bellissant E, Bollaert PE, Briegel J, Keh D, Kupfer Y. Corticosteroids for treating sepsis. Cochrane database Syst Rev. 2015;2015(12):CD002243. DOI: 10.1002/14651858.CD002243.pub3

[21] Warren BL, Eid A, Singer P, Pillay SS, Carl P, Novak I, et al. Caring for the critically ill patient. High-dose antithrombin III in severe sepsis: a randomized controlled trial. JAMA. 2001;286(15):1869-1878. DOI: 10.1001/jama.286.15.1869

[22] Allingstrup M, Wetterslev J, Ravn FB, Møller AM, Afshari A. Antithrombin III for critically ill patients: a systematic review with meta-analysis and trial sequential analysis. Intensive Care Med. 2016;42(4):505-520. DOI: 10.1007/s00134-016-4225-7

[23] Vincent J-L, Ramesh MK, Ernest D, LaRosa SP, Pachl J, Aikawa N, et al. A randomized, double-blind, placebo-controlled, Phase 2b study to evaluate the safety and efficacy of recombinant human soluble thrombomodulin, ART-123, in patients with sepsis and suspected disseminated intravascular coagulation. Crit Care Med. 2013;41(9):2069-2079. DOI: 10.1097/CCM.0b013e31828e9b03

[24] Zarychanski R, Abou-Setta AM, Kanji S, Turgeon AF, Kumar A, Houston DS, et al. The efficacy and safety of heparin in patients with sepsis: a systematic review and metaanalysis. Crit Care Med. 2015;43(3):511-518. DOI: 10.1097/CCM.0000000000000763

[25] Alejandria MM, Lansang MAD, Dans LF, Mantaring JB 3rd. Intravenous immunoglobulin for treating sepsis, severe sepsis and septic shock. Cochrane database Syst Rev. 2013;2013(9):CD001090. DOI: 10.1002/14651858.CD001090.pub2

[26] Laupland KB, Kirkpatrick AW, Delaney A. Polyclonal intravenous immunoglobulin for the treatment of severe sepsis and septic shock in critically ill adults: a systematic review and meta-analysis. Crit Care Med. 2007;35(12):2686-2692.

[27] Kreymann KG, de Heer G, Nierhaus A, Kluge S. Use of polyclonal immunoglobulins as adjunctive therapy for sepsis or septic shock. Crit Care Med. 2007;35(12):2677-2685.

[28] Soares MO, Welton NJ, Harrison DA, Peura P, Shankar- Hari M, Harvey SE, et al. An evaluation of the feasibility, cost and value of information of a multicentre randomised controlled trial of intravenous immunoglobulin for sepsis (severe sepsis and septic shock): incorporating a systematic review,

meta-analysis and value of informat. Health Technol Assess. 2012;16(7):1-186. DOI: 10.3310/hta16070

[29] Werdan K, Pilz G, Bujdoso O, Fraunberger P, Neeser G, Schmieder RE, et al. Score-based immunoglobulin G therapy of patients with sepsis: the SBITS study. Crit Care Med. 2007;35(12):2693-2701.

[30] Getoff N. Vitamin C: electron emission, free radicals and biological versatility. In Vivo. 2013;27(5):565-570.

[31] Marik PE. Hydrocortisone, Ascorbic Acid and Thiamine (HAT Therapy) for the Treatment of Sepsis. Focus on Ascorbic Acid. Nutrients. 2018;10(11). DOI: 10.3390/nu10111762

[32] Tur'yan YI, Kohen R. Formal redox potentials of the dehydro-l-ascorbic acid/l-ascorbic acid system. J Electroanal Chem. 1995;380(1):273-277. DOI: Https://doi.org/10.1016/0022-0728(94)03524-7

[33] Rebouche CJ. Ascorbic acid and carnitine biosynthesis. Am J Clin Nutr. 1991;54(6 Suppl):1147S–1152S. DOI: 10.1093/ajcn/54.6.1147s

[34] Dunn WA, Rettura G, Seifter E, Englard S. Carnitine biosynthesis from gamma-butyrobetaine and from exogenous protein-bound 6-N-trimethyl-L-lysine by the perfused guinea pig liver. Effect of ascorbate deficiency on the in situ activity of gamma-butyrobetaine hydroxylase. J Biol Chem. 1984;259(17):10764-10770.

[35] Levine M, Dhariwal KR, Washko P, Welch R, Wang YH, Cantilena CC, et al. Ascorbic acid and reaction kinetics in situ: a new approach to vitamin requirements. J Nutr Sci Vitaminol (Tokyo). 1992;Spec No:169-172. DOI: 10.3177/jnsv.38.special_169

[36] Kaufman S. Dopamine-beta-hydroxylase. J Psychiatr Res. 1974;11:303-316. DOI: 10.1016/0022-3956(74)90112-5

[37] Eipper BA, Milgram SL, Husten EJ, Yun HY, Mains RE. Peptidylglycine alpha-amidating monooxygenase: a multifunctional protein with catalytic, processing, and routing domains. Protein Sci. 1993;2(4):489-497. DOI: 10.1002/pro.5560020401

[38] Eipper BA, Stoffers DA, Mains RE. The biosynthesis of neuropeptides: peptide alpha-amidation. Annu Rev Neurosci. 1992;15:57-85. DOI: 10.1146/annurev.ne.15.030192.000421

[39] Englard S, Seifter S. The biochemical functions of ascorbic acid. Annu Rev Nutr. 1986;6:365-406. DOI: 10.1146/annurev.nu.06.070186.002053

[40] Lindblad B, Lindstedt G, Lindstedt S. The mechanism of enzymic formation of homogentisate from p-hydroxyphenylpyruvate. J Am Chem Soc. 1970;92(25):7446-7449. DOI: 10.1021/ja00728a032

[41] Prockop DJ, Kivirikko KI. Collagens: molecular biology, diseases, and potentials for therapy. Annu Rev Biochem. 1995;64:403-434. DOI: 10.1146/annurev.bi.64.070195.002155

[42] Peterkofsky B. Ascorbate requirement for hydroxylation and secretion of procollagen: relationship to inhibition of collagen synthesis in scurvy. Am J Clin Nutr. 1991;54(6 Suppl):1135S–1140S. DOI: 10.1093/ajcn/54.6.1135s

[43] Kivirikko KI, Myllylä R. Post-translational processing of procollagens. Ann N Y Acad Sci. 1985;460:187-201. DOI: 10.1111/j.1749-6632.1985.tb51167.x

[44] Hallberg L, Brune M, Rossander L. The role of vitamin C in iron absorption. Int J Vitam Nutr Res Suppl = Int Zeitschrift fur Vitamin- und

Ernahrungsforschung Suppl. 1989;30:103-108.

[45] Padayatty SJ, Katz A, Wang Y, Eck P, Kwon O, Lee J-H, et al. Vitamin C as an antioxidant: evaluation of its role in disease prevention. J Am Coll Nutr. 2003;22(1):18-35. DOI: 10.1080/07315724.2003.10719272

[46] Padayatty SJ, Levine M. Vitamin C: the known and the unknown and Goldilocks. Oral Dis. 2016;22(6):463-493. DOI: 10.1111/odi.12446

[47] Moser MA, Chun OK. Vitamin C and Heart Health: A Review Based on Findings from Epidemiologic Studies. Int J Mol Sci. 2016;17(8). DOI: 10.3390/ijms17081328

[48] Lee D-H, Folsom AR, Harnack L, Halliwell B, Jacobs DRJ. Does supplemental vitamin C increase cardiovascular disease risk in women with diabetes? Am J Clin Nutr. 2004;80(5):1194-1200. DOI: 10.1093/ajcn/80.5.1194

[49] Granger M, Eck P. Dietary Vitamin C in Human Health. Adv Food Nutr Res. 2018;83:281-310. DOI: 10.1016/bs.afnr.2017.11.006

[50] Moritz B, Schmitz AE, Rodrigues ALS, Dafre AL, Cunha MP. The role of vitamin C in stress-related disorders. J Nutr Biochem. 2020;85:108459. DOI: 10.1016/j.jnutbio.2020.108459

[51] Wong SK, Chin K-Y, Ima-Nirwana S. Vitamin C: A Review on its Role in the Management of Metabolic Syndrome. Int J Med Sci. 2020;17(11):1625-1638. DOI: 10.7150/ijms.47103

[52] Hemilä H, Chalker E. Vitamin C for preventing and treating the common cold. Cochrane database Syst Rev. 2013;(1):CD000980. DOI: 10.1002/14651858.CD000980.pub4

[53] Rondanelli M, Miccono A, Lamburghini S, Avanzato I, Riva A, Allegrini P, et al. Self-Care for Common Colds: The Pivotal Role of Vitamin D, Vitamin C, Zinc, and Echinacea in Three Main Immune Interactive Clusters (Physical Barriers, Innate and Adaptive Immunity) Involved during an Episode of Common Colds-Practical Advice on Dosages a. Evid Based Complement Alternat Med. 2018;2018:5813095. DOI: 10.1155/2018/5813095

[54] Carr AC, Maggini S. Vitamin C and Immune Function. Nutrients. 2017;9(11). DOI: 10.3390/nu9111211

[55] Padhani ZA, Moazzam Z, Ashraf A, Bilal H, Salam RA, Das JK, et al. Vitamin C supplementation for prevention and treatment of pneumonia. Cochrane database Syst Rev. 2020;4(4):CD013134. DOI: 10.1002/14651858.CD013134.pub2

[56] Righi NC, Schuch FB, De Nardi AT, Pippi CM, de Almeida Righi G, Puntel GO, et al. Effects of vitamin C on oxidative stress, inflammation, muscle soreness, and strength following acute exercise: meta-analyses of randomized clinical trials. Eur J Nutr. 2020;59(7):2827-2839. DOI: 10.1007/s00394-020-02215-2

[57] Kaźmierczak-Barańska J, Boguszewska K, Adamus-Grabicka A, Karwowski BT. Two Faces of Vitamin C-Antioxidative and Pro-Oxidative Agent. Nutrients. 2020;12(5). DOI: 10.3390/nu12051501

[58] van Gorkom GNY, Lookermans EL, Van Elssen CHMJ, Bos GMJ. The Effect of Vitamin C (Ascorbic Acid) in the Treatment of Patients with Cancer: A Systematic Review. Nutrients. 2019;11(5). DOI: 10.3390/nu11050977

[59] Lykkesfeldt J. On the effect of vitamin C intake on human health: How to (mis)interprete the clinical evidence. Redox Biol. 2020;34:101532. DOI: 10.1016/j.redox.2020.101532

[60] Spoelstra-de Man AME, Elbers PWG, Oudemans-Van Straaten HM. Vitamin C: should we supplement? Curr Opin Crit Care. 2018;24(4):248-255. DOI: 10.1097/MCC.0000000000000510

[61] Marik PE. Vitamin C for the treatment of sepsis: The scientific rationale. Pharmacol Ther. 2018;189:63-70. DOI: 10.1016/j.pharmthera.2018.04.007

[62] Lykkesfeldt J, Tveden-Nyborg P. The Pharmacokinetics of Vitamin C. Nutrients. 2019;11(10). DOI: 10.3390/nu11102412

[63] Tsukaguchi H, Tokui T, Mackenzie B, Berger U V, Chen XZ, Wang Y, et al. A family of mammalian Na+–dependent L-ascorbic acid transporters. Nature. 1999;399(6731):70-75. DOI: 10.1038/19986

[64] Lindblad M, Tveden-Nyborg P, Lykkesfeldt J. Regulation of vitamin C homeostasis during deficiency. Nutrients. 2013;5(8):2860-2879. DOI: 10.3390/nu5082860

[65] Wilson JX. Regulation of vitamin C transport. Annu Rev Nutr. 2005;25:105-125. DOI: 10.1146/annurev.nutr.25.050304.092647

[66] Padayatty SJ, Sun H, Wang Y, Riordan HD, Hewitt SM, Katz A, et al. Vitamin C pharmacokinetics: implications for oral and intravenous use. Ann Intern Med. 2004;140(7):533-537. DOI: 10.7326/0003-4819-140-7-200404060-00010

[67] Davies MB, Austin J, Partridge DA. Vitamin C: Its Chemistry and Biochemistry. Royal Society of Chemistry; 1991. 153 p.

[68] Levine M, Conry-Cantilena C, Wang Y, Welch RW, Washko PW, Dhariwal KR, et al. Vitamin C pharmacokinetics in healthy volunteers: evidence for a recommended dietary allowance. Proc Natl Acad Sci U S A. 1996;93(8):3704-3709. DOI: 10.1073/pnas.93.8.3704

[69] Nielsen TK, Højgaard M, Andersen JT, Poulsen HE, Lykkesfeldt J, Mikines KJ. Elimination of ascorbic acid after high-dose infusion in prostate cancer patients: a pharmacokinetic evaluation. Basic & Clin Pharmacol & Toxicol. 2015;116(4):343—348. DOI: 10.1111/bcpt.12323

[70] Stephenson CM, Levin RD, Spector T, Lis CG. Phase I clinical trial to evaluate the safety, tolerability, and pharmacokinetics of high-dose intravenous ascorbic acid in patients with advanced cancer. Cancer Chemother Pharmacol. 2013;72(1):139-146. DOI: 10.1007/s00280-013-2179-9

[71] Ou J, Zhu X, Lu Y, Zhao C, Zhang H, Wang X, et al. The safety and pharmacokinetics of high dose intravenous ascorbic acid synergy with modulated electrohyperthermia in Chinese patients with stage III-IV non-small cell lung cancer. Eur J Pharm Sci Off J Eur Fed Pharm Sci. 2017;109:412-418. DOI: 10.1016/j.ejps.2017.08.011

[72] Carr AC, Rosengrave PC, Bayer S, Chambers S, Mehrtens J, Shaw GM. Hypovitaminosis C and vitamin C deficiency in critically ill patients despite recommended enteral and parenteral intakes. Crit Care. 2017;21(1):300. DOI: 10.1186/s13054-017-1891-y

[73] Carr AC, Shaw GM, Fowler AA, Natarajan R. Ascorbate-dependent vasopressor synthesis: a rationale for vitamin C administration in severe sepsis and septic shock? Crit Care. 2015;19:418. DOI: 10.1186/s13054-015-1131-2

[74] Langley RJ, Tipper JL, Bruse S, Baron RM, Tsalik EL, Huntley J, et al.

Integrative "omic" analysis of experimental bacteremia identifies a metabolic signature that distinguishes human sepsis from systemic inflammatory response syndromes. Am J Respir Crit Care Med. 2014;190(4):445-455. DOI: 10.1164/rccm.201404-0624OC

[75] Rumsey SC, Kwon O, Xu GW, Burant CF, Simpson I, Levine M. Glucose transporter isoforms GLUT1 and GLUT3 transport dehydroascorbic acid. J Biol Chem. 1997;272(30):18982-18989. DOI: 10.1074/jbc.272.30.18982

[76] Lowes DA, Webster NR, Galley HF. Dehydroascorbic acid as pre-conditioner: protection from lipopolysaccharide induced mitochondrial damage. Free Radic Res. 2010;44(3):283-292. DOI: 10.3109/10715760903468766

[77] Langley RJ, Tsalik EL, van Velkinburgh JC, Glickman SW, Rice BJ, Wang C, et al. An integrated clinico-metabolomic model improves prediction of death in sepsis. Sci Transl Med. 2013;5(195):195ra95. DOI: 10.1126/scitranslmed.3005893

[78] Haileselassie B, Su E, Pozios I, Niño DF, Liu H, Lu D-Y, et al. Myocardial oxidative stress correlates with left ventricular dysfunction on strain echocardiography in a rodent model of sepsis. Intensive care Med Exp. 2017;5(1):21. DOI: 10.1186/s40635-017-0134-5

[79] Hao J, Li W-W, Du H, Zhao Z-F, Liu F, Lu J-C, et al. Role of Vitamin C in Cardioprotection of Ischemia/Reperfusion Injury by Activation of Mitochondrial KATP Channel. Chem Pharm Bull (Tokyo). 2016;64(6):548-557. DOI: 10.1248/cpb.c15-00693

[80] Fisher BJ, Kraskauskas D, Martin EJ, Farkas D, Puri P, Massey HD, et al. Attenuation of sepsis-induced organ injury in mice by vitamin C. JPEN J Parenter Enteral Nutr. 2014;38(7):825-839. DOI: 10.1177/0148607113497760

[81] Cárcamo JM, Pedraza A, Bórquez-Ojeda O, Golde DW. Vitamin C suppresses TNF alpha-induced NF kappa B activation by inhibiting I kappa B alpha phosphorylation. Biochemistry. 2002;41(43):12995-13002. DOI: 10.1021/bi0263210

[82] Kim SR, Ha YM, Kim YM, Park EJ, Kim JW, Park SW, et al. Ascorbic acid reduces HMGB1 secretion in lipopolysaccharide-activated RAW 264.7 cells and improves survival rate in septic mice by activation of Nrf2/HO-1 signals. Biochem Pharmacol. 2015;95(4):279-289. DOI: 10.1016/j.bcp.2015.04.007

[83] Hattori M, Yamazaki M, Ohashi W, Tanaka S, Hattori K, Todoroki K, et al. Critical role of endogenous histamine in promoting end-organ tissue injury in sepsis. Intensive care Med Exp. 2016;4(1):36. DOI: 10.1186/s40635-016-0109-y

[84] de Grooth H-J, Manubulu-Choo W-P, Zandvliet AS, Spoelstra-de Man AME, Girbes AR, Swart EL, et al. Vitamin C Pharmacokinetics in Critically Ill Patients: A Randomized Trial of Four IV Regimens. Chest. 2018;153(6):1368-1377. DOI: 10.1016/j.chest.2018.02.025

[85] Heyland D, Muscedere J, Wischmeyer PE, Cook D, Jones G, Albert M, et al. A randomized trial of glutamine and antioxidants in critically ill patients. N Engl J Med. 2013;368(16):1489-1497. DOI: 10.1056/NEJMoa1212722

[86] Iglesias J, Vassallo A V, Patel V V, Sullivan JB, Cavanaugh J, Elbaga Y. Outcomes of Metabolic Resuscitation Using Ascorbic Acid, Thiamine, and Glucocorticoids in the Early Treatment of Sepsis: The ORANGES Trial. Chest.

2020;158(1):164-173. DOI: 10.1016/j.chest.2020.02.049

[87] Fujii T, Luethi N, Young PJ, Frei DR, Eastwood GM, French CJ, et al. Effect of Vitamin C, Hydrocortisone, and Thiamine vs Hydrocortisone Alone on Time Alive and Free of Vasopressor Support Among Patients With Septic Shock: The VITAMINS Randomized Clinical Trial. JAMA. 2020;323(5):423-431. DOI: 10.1001/jama.2019.22176

[88] Fowler AA 3rd, Truwit JD, Hite RD, Morris PE, DeWilde C, Priday A, et al. Effect of Vitamin C Infusion on Organ Failure and Biomarkers of Inflammation and Vascular Injury in Patients With Sepsis and Severe Acute Respiratory Failure: The CITRIS-ALI Randomized Clinical Trial. JAMA. 2019;322(13):1261-1270. DOI: 10.1001/jama.2019.11825

[89] Nathens AB, Neff MJ, Jurkovich GJ, Klotz P, Farver K, Ruzinski JT, et al. Randomized, prospective trial of antioxidant supplementation in critically ill surgical patients. Ann Surg. 2002;236(6):814-822. DOI: 10.1097/00000658-200212000-00014

[90] Tanaka H, Matsuda T, Miyagantani Y, Yukioka T, Matsuda H, Shimazaki S. Reduction of resuscitation fluid volumes in severely burned patients using ascorbic acid administration: a randomized, prospective study. Arch Surg. 2000;135(3):326-331. DOI: 10.1001/archsurg.135.3.326

[91] Zabet MH, Mohammadi M, Ramezani M, Khalili H. Effect of high-dose Ascorbic acid on vasopressor's requirement in septic shock. J Res Pharm Pract. 2016;5(2):94-100. DOI: 10.4103/2279-042X.179569

[92] Marik PE, Khangoora V, Rivera R, Hooper MH, Catravas J. Hydrocortisone, Vitamin C, and Thiamine for the Treatment of Severe Sepsis and Septic Shock: A Retrospective Before-After Study. Chest. 2017;151(6):1229-1238. DOI: 10.1016/j.chest.2016.11.036

[93] Mitchell AB, Ryan TE, Gillion AR, Wells LD, Muthiah MP. Vitamin C and Thiamine for Sepsis and Septic Shock. Am J Med. 2020;133(5):635-638. DOI: 10.1016/j.amjmed.2019.07.054

[94] Zhang M, Jativa DF. Vitamin C supplementation in the critically ill: A systematic review and meta-analysis. SAGE open Med. 2018;6:2050312118807615. DOI: 10.1177/2050312118807615

Section 3

Phytochemical Antioxidants

Chapter 15

Phytochemical Antioxidants: Past, Present and Future

Yasuko Sakihama and Hideo Yamasaki

Abstract

Most diseases that are difficult to prevent and cure are "syndromes" that are governed by multiple components with complicated interactions. Whatever the cause of such diseases, overproduction of harmful reactive oxygen species (ROS) can often be observed in progression of the disease. Under such conditions, the cells may be challenged by "oxidative stress" due to excessively generated oxidants. Antioxidants can be defined as chemical compounds that scavenge ROS or free radicals over-produced in the cells under oxidative stress conditions. The plant pigments flavonoids and betalains, rich in fruits and vegetables, are reactive not only with ROS but also with reactive nitrogen species (RNS) and possibly with reactive sulfur species (RSS). Here, we provide an overview of updates on the antioxidative functions of the plant pigments along with some prospects for future research on phytochemical antioxidants.

Keywords: flavonoid, betalain, reactive oxygen species (ROS), reactive nitrogen species (RNS), reactive sulfur species (RSS)

1. Introduction

Fruits and vegetables are appreciated as "healthy foods" compared with beef or pork meat. Many epidemiological studies as well as clinical investigations have suggested that a vegetable-based diet is beneficial in preventing chronic diseases including cancer, coronary heart disease, stroke and hypertension [1, 2]. Meanwhile, traditional herbal medicines have used specific plant species that contain phytochemicals exhibiting pharmacological activities [3]. Novel compounds have been isolated from such plants and they have been chemically synthesized for pharmaceutical production [4]. Nobody doubts that edible plants are beneficial in human health.

In "western" medicine, a disease can be defined as dysfunction of a physiological mechanism. Based on this concept, a drug in general is presumed to act on a specific component of a physiological mechanism. In many cases, these are inhibitors of enzymes or transporters, showing the "one-to-one" relationship between drug and target molecule. While recent drug designs have drastically changed due to a rapid development of computer technology [5] as well as gene therapy [6], the hunt for novel bioactive compounds contained in plants is still active for new drug discovery.

The "one-to-one" philosophy in medicine and pharmacology works well, if the cause of a disease is ascribed to a single component such as a protein or an enzyme. However, most diseases that are difficult to prevent and cure are "syndromes" that are governed by multiple components with complicated interactions. Whatever the cause of such diseases, overproduction of harmful reactive oxygen species (ROS) can often be observed in progression of the disease. Under such conditions, the cells may be challenged by "oxidative stress" due to excessively generated oxidants. The oxidative stress potentially impairs cellular functions eventually leading to death [7, 8]. This is a common biological feature that can be seen in all living organisms including bacteria, fungi, plants and animals. Living organisms have evolved to cope with the oxidative stress induced by biotic (pathogen attack or biological interactions) and abiotic (or environmental) stresses. Thus, under stress conditions, living organisms need to control cellular ROS levels for their survival. In this context, antioxidant systems are essential in any living organisms. This is a biological rationale for the importance of antioxidants in prevention and cure of diseases in humans.

Plant antioxidant research shows a history of twists and turns. Some early studies had suggested concepts opposite to the present recognition. Plant antioxidants had sometimes even been considered to be toxic or carcinogenic to animals. Contradictory reports in the old literatures may lead non-specialists to a state of confusion. Thus, to follow the current state of research advances in phytochemical antioxidants, understanding its historical background is of help for non-specialists and new researchers. Highlighting the research progress of plant pigments flavonoids and betalains, here, we provide an overview of phytochemical antioxidants with some prospects for future research.

2. Historical perspective of plant antioxidants

2.1 The vitamin that prevents the disease of age of discovery

A retrospective of the history of research on plant antioxidants needs to go back to the age of discovery. When voyagers such as Magellan, Columbus, Vasco da Gam and Cook were sailing over the world's oceans, more than three times as many sailors died due to the mysterious disease "scurvy" as soldiers died in the American Civil War [9]. For hundreds of years, the cause of the disease had not been clarified and there had been no cure for this disease of sailors [10]. In 1747, James Lind working as a naval surgeon at sea on the HMS *Salisbury* conducted "clinical trials" of potential cures for the disorder. In *Treatise of the Scurvy* published in 1753, he reported that there was no effect with the potential remedies vinegar, mustard, garlic purges, elixir of vitriol, but citrus fruits (orange and lemon) showed a significant cure effect [11]. It is now known that scurvy is caused by a vitamin C (L-ascorbate) deficiency due to a lack of fresh fruits and vegetables.

Historically, antioxidant and vitamin studies have developed independently in chemistry and health science, respectively. In chemistry, antioxidants were defined as chemical compounds that can suppress oxidation reactions. In early studies, oxidation was observed as absorption of molecular oxygen in a reaction such as polymerization reaction of natural rubber. On the other hand, a vitamin (the name "vitamine, vital + amine" was the original proposal and it was later renamed to "vitamin") was defined as an organic nutrient that is essential for human health care. The major recognized vitamins are vitamin A, B1, B2, B3, B5, B6, B7, B9, B12, C, D, E, and K. The biochemical requirements of these vitamins were revealed after their chemical identifications. Among these vitamins, vitamin A, C and E have been highlighted again in the late 20th century due to their antioxidant activities that potentially reduce the oxygen toxicity.

2.2 The oxygen toxicity and ROS

Although molecular oxygen (O_2) is required for respiration in animals, a high concentration or high partial pressure of oxygen often damages the central nervous and pulmonary systems, which leads to disease or death. Oxygen toxicity in the central nervous system and that in pulmonary system had been referred to as the Paul Bert effect and the Lorrain Smith effect, respectively [12]. Although the toxicity of oxygen itself was implied by Joseph Priestley in 1774 (dephlogisticated air at that time) [13], the modern style of experimental science has been opened up by Bert (1833–1886), the Father of Aviation of Medicine [14, 15]. In his *La Pression Barometrique* (1878), Bert described that a high partial pressure of breathing oxygen (hyperoxia) can lead to death of animals, the first experimental demonstration for the toxicity of pure oxygen [14]. Since his pioneering discovery had not been appreciated for a long time, unfortunately, eye damage (retinopathy of prematurity) to premature infants frequently occurred due to the use of pure oxygen [16].

The biochemical basis of the oxygen toxicity is ascribed to overproduction of reactive oxygen species (ROS) in cells. The ROS firstly produced in cells is mostly superoxide radical (O_2^-), which is the reaction product of the one electron reduction of molecular oxygen (O_2) [17]. Whereas chemists have known the inorganic reaction that produces O_2^- from O_2, the biological relevance of the reaction had not been considered in biochemistry. At that time most biochemists were fascinated by the oxidative phosphorylation that is the final step of ATP synthesis in aerobic respiration. For mitochondrial ATP synthesis, the presence of O_2 is prerequisite to drive the respiratory electron transport. Therefore, the toxicity of O_2 had been overlooked. The discovery of the enzyme superoxide dismutase (SOD) that destroys O_2^- is a landmark in the research history of oxygen toxicity [18]. The discovery of the antioxidant enzyme SOD has drastically changed our recognition: O_2 might be toxic for living organisms.

To prevent oxygen toxicity, it has been revealed that antioxidant enzyme systems are essential for the survival of all living organisms, including humans. The ROS O_2^- and H_2O_2 can be removed by the enzymatic reactions of SOD and peroxidases, but other unstable ROS molecules, hydroxyl radicals (•OH) for example, cannot be destroyed by those enzymatic reactions. These molecules are scavenged by antioxidants. Vitamin A or carotenoid can scavenge singlet oxygen ($^1O_2$) that could be produced in the eyes or skin under ultraviolet (UV) light [19]. Vitamin E, or α- tocopherol, can react with the ROS radicals produced in lipophilic environments such as in lipid membranes. Vitamin C (ascorbate) serves as a universal reducing power to the antioxidant enzyme systems while the ascorbate molecule itself scavenges various types of ROS (except H_2O_2) by its spontaneous reactions [20]. It is important to note that humans need to acquire these essential antioxidant vitamins (A, C, E) from dietary foods, largely from fruits and vegetables.

2.3 Vitamin P concept and plant pigments

Historically, there was a short-lived Vitamin P concept. Albert Szent-Györgyi, a Nobel prize winner who isolated ascorbate, demonstrated that flavonoid glycosides rich in citrus fruits can behave similar to ascorbate in maintaining capillary permeability [21]. Based on his observations, Szent-Györgyi proposed that the plant flavonoids, as a group of plant pigments, are also essential nutrients and referred to them as vitamin P (permeability) [22]. However, this vitamin P concept did not gain broad acceptance due to the chemical diversity of flavonoids. More recently, his idea that flavonoids can complement the function of ascorbate has been renewed with the development of the antioxidant hypothesis.

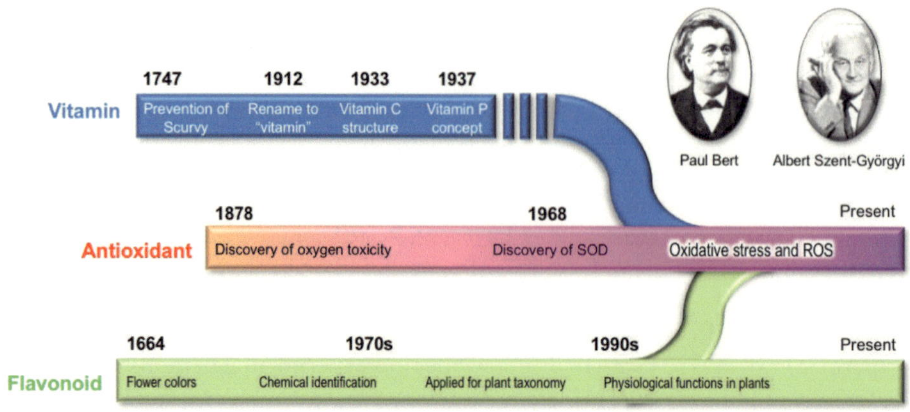

Figure 1.
A timeline of antioxidant research of phytochemicals. Flavonoids are major plant pigments that are widely appreciated as natural antioxidants. Historically, antioxidant studies, vitamin studies and flavonoid studies have independently progressed in health science, biochemistry and botany, respectively. These different lines of studies have been integrated into the present plant antioxidant studies.

Plant fruits and flowers display beautiful colorations ranging from blue to red. These plant colorations are produced with three major pigments i.e., chlorophylls, carotenoids and flavonoids. In plants, biological functions of chlorophylls and carotenoids have been known as the photosynthetic pigments that absorb light energy to drive photosynthesis. In contrast, only the visual attraction for flower pollinators such as bees or butterflies had been proposed as a biological function of colored flavonoids for a long time [23]. The chemical diversity of flavonoids found across plant species had made it difficult to consider common physiological or biochemical functions. Conversely, the huge chemical diversity of flavonoids was useful for plant taxonomy until amino acid or DNA sequence information available.

In 1990s, red anthocyanin, a flavonoid subgroup, was highlighted to account for the paradoxical epidemiological observation termed the "French paradox". French people have a relatively low incidence of coronary heart disease even though they consume a diet relatively rich in saturated fats [24]. Researchers were interested in anthocyanins and polyphenols contained in red wine that may suppress heart disease through their antioxidant activities [24]. Similarly, the longevity of Japanese people was explained by their daily consumption of green tea rich in catechin, another subgroup of flavonoid [25, 26]. These epidemiological reports have stimulated biochemical screening of natural antioxidants contained in plants.

To date, health science, biochemistry, botany and other different field of studies have been integrated into antioxidant research. A timeline for antioxidant research of phytochemicals is summarized in **Figure 1**.

3. Plant pigment flavonoid

3.1 Flavonoids in plants

Flavonoids are representative secondary metabolites of land plants. The pigments commonly accumulate in epidermal cells of the organs such as in flowers, leaves, stems, roots, seeds and fruits [27, 28]. Flavonoids are found as glycosidic forms (glycosides) and non-glycosidic forms (aglycones). Subcellular localization of the glycosides is largely confined to hydrophilic regions such as vacuoles and apoplasts. The aglycones are localized in lipophilic regions e.g., oil glands and waxy layers.

The term "flavonoid" originated from its yellow color (the *Latin* word *flavus* means yellow). Bioactive flavonoids such as flavones and flavonols are sometimes referred as to "bioflavonoids". **Figure 2** shows the basic structures of flavonoids. The general structure of flavonoids includes a C6-C3-C6 carbon skeleton with two phenyl rings (A- and B-rings) and a heterocyclic ring (C-ring). Based on the structure of the aglycones, flavonoids can be classified into subgroups: chalcone, flavanone, flavone, isoflavone, flavonol, and anthocyanidin (**Figure 3**). According to the IUPAC nomenclature, flavonoids are recommended to be subcategorized into flavonoids (bioflavonoids), isoflavonoids and neoflavonoids [29]. Since this classification has yet not been widely adopted, in this chapter, traditional phytochemical names and classifications are used to avoid confusions. Most of these subgroups show yellowish coloration while anthocyanins exhibit multiple colorations depending on the aglycone structure, the presence of metal, pH and conjugation with other molecules (**Figure 3**).

Common glycosylation positions are the 7-hydroxyl in flavones, isoflavones and dihydroflavones; the 3- and 7- hydroxyl in flavonols and dihydroflavones; the 3- and 5-hydroxyl in anthocyanidins [30]. The typical sugars involved in glycoside formation are glucose, galactose, rhamnose, xylose and arabinose. In addition to the glycosylation, methylation, isoprenylation and dimerization occur at those positions [30].

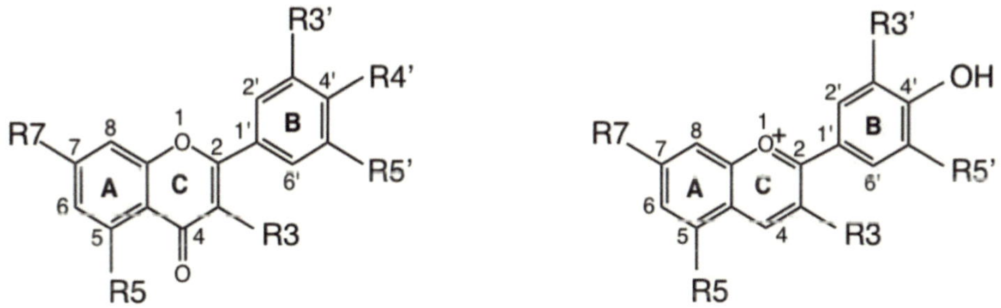

Figure 2.
Chemical structures of flavonoids. Chemical structures of flavonoids include a C6-C3-C6 carbon skeleton with two phenyl rings (A- and B-rings) and a heterocyclic ring (C-ring). Left, the basic structures of a flavone, isoflavone and flavonol. Right, the basic structures of anthocyanin. The –R on the rings can be replaced by other molecules including sugars to make a huge variety of chemical structures of flavonoids.

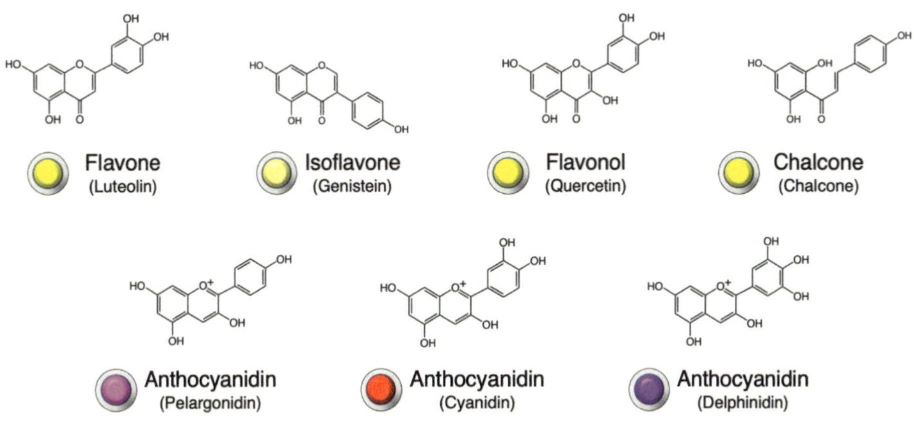

Figure 3.
Representative flavonoid subgroups. Based on the aglycone structures, flavonoids can be classified into flavone, isoflacone, flavonol, chalcone and anthocyanidin. Representative flavonoids with parenthesis along with apparent visual colorations are shown.

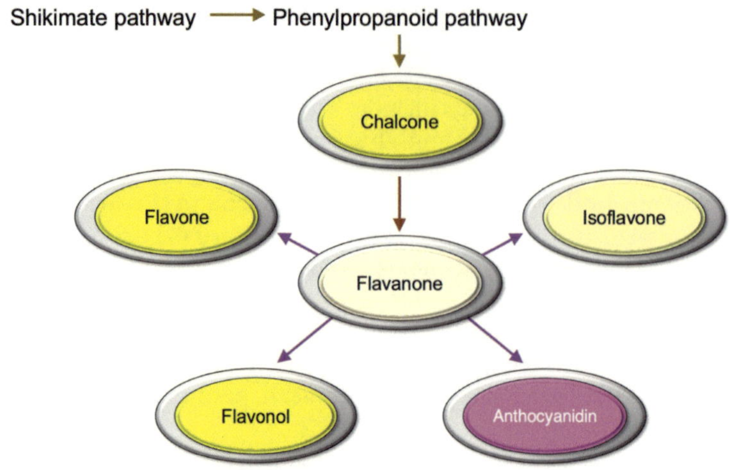

Figure 4.
An outline of flavonoid biosynthesis pathways in plants. The synthesis of the flower pigment anthocyanins requires multiple steps including the shikimate pathway, phenylpropanoid pathway, via chalone and flavanone. The number of required enzymatic steps reflects the evolutional order of the pigments.

These modifications produce a huge structural diversity of flavonoids. More than 9,000 chemical structures of flavonoids have been reported to date [31].

Enzymes and genes involved in flavonoid biosynthesis have been identified [27, 32–35]. **Figure 4** shows an outline of biosynthetic pathways of the major subclasses of flavonoids. Flavonoids are synthesized from phenylalanine, an aromatic amino acid produced in the shikimate pathway. Phenylalanine is sequentially metabolized by phenylalanine ammonia-lyase (PAL), cinnamate 4-hydroxylase, and 4-coumarate CoA ligase to 4-coumaroyl CoA. This 4-coumaroyl CoA and 3 molecules of malonyl CoA are condensed by chalcone synthase to form the flavonoid chalcone (yellow). Chalcone is isomerized to the flavanone naringenin (colorless) by chalcone isomerase. Naringenin is further converted to flavones (pale yellow) and isoflavone (pale yellow) catalyzed by flavone synthase and isoflavone synthase, respectively. Naringenin is hydroxylated to dihydroflavonol by flavanone 3-hydroxylase and further metabolized to flavonol (yellow) by flavonoid synthetase. Dihydroflavonol is converted to anthocyanidin (red, red-violet or blue-violet), an aglycone of anthocyanin, by dihydroflavonol 4-reductase and anthocyanidin synthase. Anthocyanidin is glycosylated by UDP-glycose-dependent glycosyltransferase. Manipulation of those genes has been challenged to change of flower or fruits coloration [28].

3.2 Antioxidant activity of flavonoids

Antioxidant activity or antioxidant capacity of flavonoids has been experimentally evaluated with either assays based on hydrogen atom transfer (HAT) reaction or assays based on electron transfer [36]. There are several protocols or assays that have been proposed. The ORAC (oxygen radical absorbance capacity), TRAP (total radical trapping antioxidant parameter) and crocin bleaching assays are based on HAT. TEAC (Torolox equivalent antioxidant capacity), ABTS (2,2′-azino-bis-(3-ethyl-benzthiazoline-6-sulfonic acid)) and DPPH (1,1-diphenyl-2-picryl-hydrazyl) assays are based on the electron transfer activity. Among these protocols, the DPPH assay has been widely used for plant materials because it is an easy and accurate method suitable for measuring antioxidant activity of fruits, vegetable juices or plant extracts [36]. Inhibition of the lipid peroxidation reaction is also a measure to assess the antioxidant activity of plant polyphenols [37].

In addition to the reactions with model radical substrates, it has been demonstrated that flavonoids can directly react with a various type of ROS. The flavonol quercetin was demonstrated to show quenching activity for the singlet oxygen ($^1O_2$), a non-radical ROS molecule [38]. The flavonol kaempferol [39] and the anthocyanidin cyanidin [40] *in vitro* were shown to scavenge superoxide radical (O_2^-). The flavonol quercetin was reported to scavenge hydroxyl radicals (•OH) produced by radiolysis of water [41, 42]. The flavonols rutin and quercetin were demonstrated to scavenge the hydroperoxide of linoleic acid (LOO•) to inhibit lipid peroxidation [43]. It is now evident that flavonoids are natural plant antioxidants contained in fruits and vegetables.

In principle, the OH groups on the aromatic rings of flavonoids are responsible for the antioxidant or free radical scavenging activity. Most antioxidant flavonoids share the catechol structure with two hydroxy groups (-OH) and/or the double bond between C2-C3 and carbonyl structure [44, 45]. Antioxidant flavonoids satisfying such criteria bear multiple hydroxy groups in a molecule, thereby the name of "polyphenols" being synonymously used for plant antioxidants by the public. It should be noted that polyphenol structure can be found not only in flavonoids but also in other plant phenolic compounds such as hydroxycinnamic acid [35].

When polyphenols scavenge ROS, either through a direct chemical reaction or as an electron donor for an enzymatic reaction, polyphenolic compounds are oxidized and phenoxyl radicals are generated [46]. The phenoxyl radicals are unstable, forming dimers or polymers as a result of spontaneous reaction. Tannin and lignin are the polymerization products of such phenoxyl radical reactions. In the presence of reductant such as ascorbate, the phenoxyl radicals produced are rapidly regenerated into their parent compounds [46]. The enzyme monodehydroascorbate reductase (MDAR) was demonstrated to regenerate flavonoids from their phenoxyl radicals, a possible recycling system of antioxidants [47]. In plants, it has been proposed that flavonoids complement the ascorbate antioxidant system [35].

4. Betalain in red beets and cactus

4.1 Structures and biosynthesis of betalains in plants

Plant coloration can be mostly attributed to spectral property of the colored flavonoids, i.e., anthocyanidins. The plant pigment betalains are exceptional. The term "betalain" comes from the *Latin* name of the common beet (*Beta vulgaris*) from which betalains were first extracted. Betalains are a class of tyrosine-derived pigments that are distributed in only 13 families of Caryophyllales order such as red beet (Amaranthaceae) and cactus (Cactaceae), and in some fungi [48], where they replace anthocyanin pigments [32]. To date, anthocyanins and betalains have never been detected jointly in plant tissues [48]. The biological meaning of the mutually exclusive relationship between betalains and anthocyanidins is still unknown [49, 50].

Betalains are immonium derivatives of betalamic acid [4-(2-oxoethylidene)-1,2,3,4-tetrahydropyridine-2,6-dicarboxylic acid] [48]. Betalains are classified into two groups: betacyanin (red-violet) and betaxanthin (yellow) as shown in **Figure 5**. Betacyanin is a conjugate with *cyclo*-dopa and its glycoside, while betaxanthin is a conjugate with amino acid or amine (**Figure 5**).

In contrast with flavonoids, biosynthetic pathway of betalains in plants has not been fully clarified [32, 50, 51]. Hydroxylation of tyrosine by tyrosinase or polyphenol oxidase produces L-dopa, which is catalyzed by 4,5-dopa dioxygenase

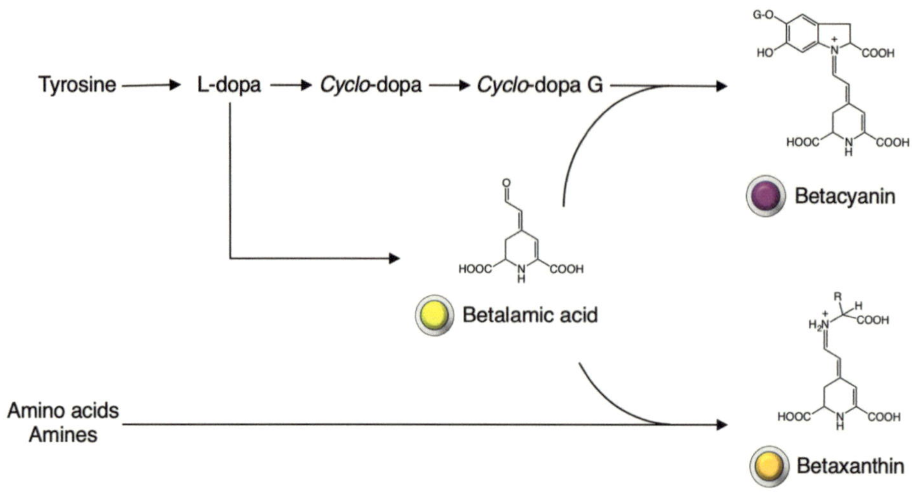

Figure 5.
Structures and biosynthesis pathways of betalains. Betalains are synthesized from L-tyrosine via L-dopa. The intermediate betalamic acid is condensed with cyclo-dopa glycoside or amino acid/amine to betacyanin and betaxanthin, respectively.

to form betalamic acid, the basic common skeleton of betalains. *Cyclo*-dopa, a component of betacyanin, had been considered to be formed by spontaneous chemical reaction after L-dopa is oxidized to dopaquinone by tyrosinase. Recently, the cytochrome P450 CYP76AD1 has been identified as the enzyme which catalyzes the conversion of L-dopa to *cyclo*-dopa, a novel biosynthesis route [52]. CYP76AD1 is a bifunctional enzyme that catalyzes tyrosine hydroxylation as well as *cyclo*-dopa synthesis. This P450 enzyme appears to play important roles not only in betacyanin synthesis but also in betalain synthesis. Furthermore, CYP76AD6 that catalyzes only tyrosine hydroxylation has also been reported [53]. No enzyme for condensing the obtained betalamic acid with a *cyclo*-dopa or an amino acid/amine has been found to date; instead, these condensations likely occur by a spontaneous reaction to form betacyanin or betaxanthin, respectively. Betacyanin usually accumulates as a glycoside, and two routes are estimated for glycosylation: *cyclo*-dopa being condensed with betalamic acid after it is glycosylated and *cyclo*-dopa and betalamic acid being condensed to be betacyanin and then glycosylated. Both are catalyzed by glucosyltransferases [54].

4.2 Antioxidant functions of betalains

Similar to flavonoids, betalains exhibit antioxidant or radical scavenging activity [55, 56]. In contrast with flavonoids, however, the chemistry of the antioxidant mechanism of betalains is less understood. It has been suggested that the common skeleton betalamic acid may contribute to their antioxidant activities [57–59]. Phenolic hydroxy group in *cyclo*-dopa moiety of betacyanin and the amino acid/amine portion of betaxanthin may increase the radical scavenging activities of betalamic acids [58]. Betalains can act as an electron donor for the enzyme peroxidases to detoxify hydrogen peroxide (H_2O_2) [60]. In food chemistry it has been suggested that the degradation of betalains during storage is suppressed in the presence of ascorbate, suggesting that betalain radicals formed by the oxidation might be reduced by ascorbate back to the parent molecules, similar to flavonoids.

5. Reactions of the phytochemicals with RNS and RSS

5.1 RNS and RSS

It is now evident that plant antioxidants remove ROS and free radicals that increase under oxidative stress conditions within cells. In addition to ROS, new players behaving similar to ROS have recently been identified, namely, reactive nitrogen species (RNS) and reactive sulfur species (RSS) [61]. As ROS refers to a group of reactive molecular species originating from molecular oxygen (O_2), RNS and RSS are named for the groups of reactive molecular species derived from nitric oxide (NO) and hydrogen sulfide (H_2S), respectively. Both NO and H_2S are simple gaseous molecules that had initially been appreciated within the life sciences only for their toxicity [62]. Recent investigations have confirmed that NO and H_2S are essential biomolecules synthesized in plants and animals. RNS and RSS are involved in the regulation of a variety of physiological processes. Along with carbon monoxide (CO), NO and H_2S are categorized as "gasotransmitters" [62]. Until recently, many enzymes that produce NO and H_2S have been identified in plants, animals and bacteria.

It is important to note that NO and H_2S are involved not only in physiological regulations (positive effect) but also in dysfunctions or disorders (negative effect). Similar to ROS, unregulated RNS and/or RSS production potentially causes dysfunction of metabolism under biotic as well as abiotic stress conditions, leading to sickness or death in humans [17]. Although a limited number of studies are available on anti-RNS and anti-RSS functions of phytochemicals, it has been reported that flavonoids and betalains could remove RNS and possibly RSS too.

NO reacts rapidly with O_2^- to produce the RNS peroxynitrite ($ONOO^-$) following the reaction:

$$O_2^- + NO \rightarrow ONOO^- \quad (1)$$

$ONOO^-$ at physiological pH is unstable and is in rapid equilibrium with its conjugate acid, peroxynitrous acid (ONOOH, pK_a 6.8) [63]. In early studies, NO was considered to act as an antioxidant because NO removes O_2^- from a solution as the consequence of the spontaneous reaction. However, this is half-side of a coin since the reaction product $ONOO^-$ attacks proteins and nucleic acids. The nitrated amino acid 3-nitrotyrosine (3-NO_2-Tyr) is produced when $ONOO^-$ reacts with tyrosine residues of proteins, which potentially disturbs enzyme activities that may lead dysfunction of metabolism, a situation referred as to "nitrosative stress" [64]. It is now widely accepted that $ONOO^-$ is a major cytotoxic agent of RNS.

H_2S is synthesized in plants and animals by multiple enzyme systems [62]. Biogenic H_2S production is involved in various physiological mechanisms as a signaling molecule [62]. Analogous to ROS and RNS, H_2S (or HS^-) produces many reactive molecular species such as persulfide, polysulfide, polysulfane and others [65]. These RSS modify thiol (-SH) groups of the cysteine residue of proteins and change enzymatic activities, resulting in both positive regulation and negative inhibition. Uncontrolled overproduction of RSS is a potential risk to damage the cells. Although there is yet little evidence to confirm that flavonoids and betalains scavenge RSS, results of epidemiological studies imply that dietary phytoantioxidants also contribute to reduce the cytotoxicity of RSS in humans [66].

5.2 Chemical reactions with RNS and RSS

Plant phenolic compounds, such as anthocyanin [67, 68] and *p*-hydroxybenzoic acid [69], have been reported to scavenge $ONOO^-$ [70]. Betalains also react with $ONOO^-$ [71, 72]. As the consequence of these reactions, the phytochemical antioxidants inhibit the $ONOO^-$-induced L-tyrosine nitration and DNA damage [35, 71]. In flavonoids, -OH group at the C3 position of the C-ring has been proposed to be involved in the $ONOO^-$ scavenging activity [69, 73]. As the result of the reaction with $ONOO^-$, the phytochemical antioxidants are nitrated [74]. These *in vitro* studies have suggested that flavonoids and betalains potentially protect the cells from the nitrosative stress that may induce disorders or mutations [75, 76].

Reactions of the phytochemicals that contribute to reduce the toxicity of RSS are largely unknown. The plant phenolic hydroxycinnamic acids are known to be sulfated by sulfotransferases highly expressed in the human liver and intestine [66]. Flavonoids act as inhibitors of the human sulfotransferases (SULTs) [66]. In plants, sulfate esters of flavonoids are rare compounds [77, 78] that are found in species occurring coastal and swampy areas as well as arid habitats [78]. Functions of sulfated flavonoids in plants and animals are not clear [79]. Sulfated flavonoids, such as quercetin 3-sulfate or quercetin persulfate, have been demonstrated with animals to show antioxidant activity, anti-inflammatory activity, antitumor activity and anticoagulant activity [80–83]. These different lines of studies may imply that sulfated phytochemicals might be associated with physiological regulations in stress tolerance or disease in plants and animals. Although, at present, it must be a speculation to consider specific reactions of flavonoids and betalains with RSS, it is promising that the future investigations of *S*-containing phytochemicals including sulfated flavonoids or sulfoflavonoids will open up a new research field in life sciences.

6. Antioxidant phytochemicals in human health

In modern science, a great number of studies have suggested health benefits of vegetable-based diets for humans. Many compounds identified from plants have been tested to evaluate their biochemical or pharmacological actions in prevention, mitigation and cure of diseases. According to the "one-to-one" principle, researchers have searched for novel bioactive phytochemicals that interact with specific target enzymes or molecules associated with disorders or diseases. The pharmacokinetic action of antioxidants, however, does not follow the "one-to-one" principle. The actual target is not a specific enzyme or protein but ROS. Since production of ROS is exclusively involved in any types of diseases including cancer, antioxidant activity of phytochemicals has attracted attention not only from researchers but also from the public due to their perceived "cure-all" actions. Nowadays, the antioxidant hypothesis described above has been accepted as the most probable explanation for the health benefits of vegetable-based diets.

Recent progress in medical science has clarified that unregulated RNS and RSS production are observed in many disorders or diseases, echoing findings from ROS research. Although a little is known how plants and animals might regulate RNS and RSS in the cells to achieve a fine balance, there is accumulating evidence to support the hypothesis that phytochemical antioxidants, such as flavonoids and betalains, also reduce the toxicity of RNS and RSS. The occurrence of nitrated flavonoids as well as sulfated flavonoids may imply the possible associations of the phytochemical antioxidants with RNS and/or RSS metabolisms in plants and animals. In this context, the term "antioxidant" for phytochemicals may need to be given a new name to reflect the latest research findings.

In 2020, more than million people died due to the coronavirus disease 2019 (COVID-19) pandemic. There is no promising specific drug or treatment (as of December 2020) for the severe hospitalized patients. A "cytokine storm" occurs in severe cases of COVID-19 and the anti-inflammatory steroid dexamethasone has been applied to lower mortality [84]. COVID-19 and the common "cold" both present a syndrome of disease states. It seems unrealistic to rely on a single drug or chemical to cure the disease. In prevention of the infection, ascorbate and vegetables appears to be effective. The antioxidant flavonoids can reduce inorganic nitrite (NO_2^-) to generate NO in an acidic solution [85]. The vegetable diets and beverages such as the beet juice have been reported to prevent hypertension probably because of increase in NO bioavailability due to nitrite-dependent NO production [2, 86]. It is likely that vegetable-based foods and beverages could prevent or mitigate COVID-19 through their phytochemical antioxidant activities along with their provision of nitrate/nitrite supplementation [84, 87].

7. Prospects for future research

Oxygen toxicity can be attributed ultimately to the biological evolution of oxygenic photosynthesis. In the ancient earth, H_2S and NO concentrations are considered to have been much higher than the present day due to active volcanism [62]. The concentration of these "old" gasses fell down following the evolutional development of oxygenic photosynthesis in cyanobacteria [62]. It is presumed that most living organisms that were dominant at that time went extinct but some of them successfully developed antioxidant systems to cope with new oxic environments. The survivors from the lethal environments are the ancestors of the present animals. Even for plants, a high partial pressure of O_2 made by photosynthesis is yet a great risk. To protect the photosynthetic apparatus, green plants have developed their unique antioxidant systems along with creation of many types of antioxidant molecules [88]. The left panel of **Figure 6** represents a conceptual illustration for ROS, RNS and RSS in biological evolution in the earth history from past to the

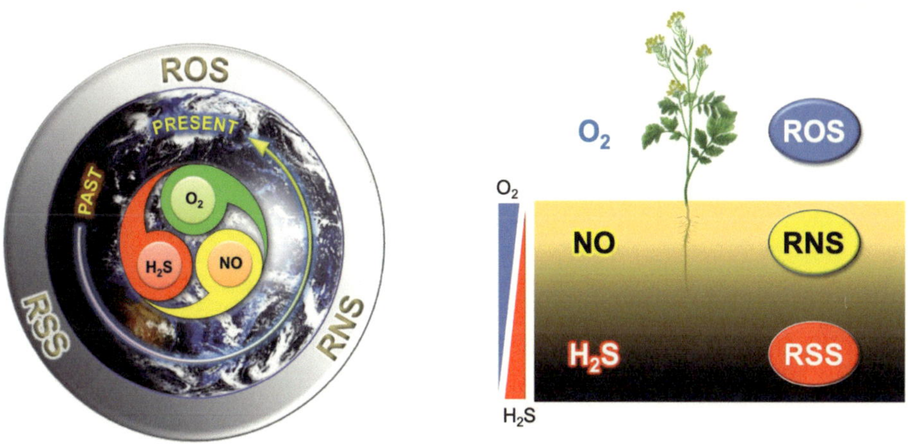

Figure 6.
The ONS gradient in evolution and habitats. In plants, antioxidants can be found abundantly in leaves where oxygenic photosynthesis occurs, with a risk of overproduction of ROS. If oxidative stress is defined as a condition of disturbance of the fine-tuned redox balance, knowing the interplays among ROS, RNS and RSS is important for understanding cellular homeostasis. Oxygen tension would alter the best balance for each living organism in the field where there is the ONS (O_2-NO-H_2S) gradient from surface to the deep in soils, which also reflects the order of their evolutional development (from ancient to the present) [54].

present. The order (ROS→RNS→RSS) can be found in ecological niches from surface to deep such as in soils (**Figure 6**, right). In the case of plants grown in the field, leaves are in oxic environments and roots are in hypoxic environments where there exists a gradient of O_2, NO and H_2S. Taking into account that sulfated plant phenolic compounds are found in plants inhabiting harsh environments, we consider it plausible that novel bioactive phytochemicals associated with RNS and RSS metabolisms might be found in the roots grown in such hypoxic environments [89].

8. Conclusions

Flavonoids and batalains are natural antioxidants that mitigate oxidative stress in plants and animals. In life sciences, oxidative stress can be defined as an imbalance of pro-oxidants and antioxidants in cells. Oxidative stress can be also defined as a disruption of redox signaling and control, emphasizing the importance of a dynamic but fine-tuned redox balance in cellular homeostasis [90]. According to this new definition, the ROS scavenging activity may be just a part of the pleiotropic functions of phytochemicals. Flavonoids and betalains could tune a fine redox balance through modulating the interplays among ROS, RNS and RSS. We are now entering into the next stage of plant "antioxidant" research.

Acknowledgements

We thank Dr. Michael Cohen at the Sonoma State University for his critical reading of the manuscript. This work was partly supported by JSPS KAKENHI Grant Number JP19K06339 to H.Y.

Conflict of interest

The authors declare no conflict of interest.

Author details

Yasuko Sakihama[1] and Hideo Yamasaki[2]*

1 Research Faculty of Agriculture, Hokkaido University, Sapporo, Japan

2 Faculty of Science, University of the Ryukyus, Okinawa, Japan

*Address all correspondence to: yamasaki@sci.u-ryukyu.ac.jp

References

[1] Van Duyn MAS, Pivonka E. Overview of the health benefits of fruit and vegetable consumption for the dietetics professional. Journal of the American Dietetic Association. 2000; 100 (12): 1511-1521. 10.1016/s0002-8223(00)00420-x

[2] Sundqvist ML, Larsen FJ, Carlstrom M, Bottai M, Pernow J, Hellenius ML, *et al.* A randomized clinical trial of the effects of leafy green vegetables and inorganic nitrate on blood pressure. American Journal of Clinical Nutrition. 2020; 111 (4): 749-756. 10.1093/ajcn/nqaa024

[3] Patwardhan B, Warude D, Pushpangadan P, Bhatt N. Ayurveda and traditional Chinese medicine: a comparative overview. Evidence-Based Complementary and Alternative Medicine. 2005; 2 (4): 465-473. 10.1093/ecam/neh140

[4] He M, Yan X, Zhou J, Xie G. Traditional Chinese medicine database and application on the web. Journal of Chemical Information and Computer Sciences. 2001; 41 (2): 273-277.

[5] Åqvist J, Medina C, Samuelsson J-E. A new method for predicting binding affinity in computer-aided drug design. Protein Engineering, Design and Selection. 1994; 7 (3): 385-391.

[6] Verma IM, Weitzman MD. Gene therapy: twenty-first century medicine. Annual Review of Biochemistry. 2005; 74: 711-738. 10.1146/annurev.biochem.74.050304.091637

[7] Sies H, Berndt C, Jones DP. Oxidative stress. Annual Review of Biochemistry. 2017; 86: 715-748.

[8] Finaud J, Lac G, Filaire E. Oxidative stress: Relationship with excerise and training. Sports Medicine. 2006; 36 (4): 327-358.

[9] Lamb J. Scurvy: The disease of discovery: Princeton University Press; 2018.

[10] Magiorkinis E, Beloukas A, Diamantis A. Scurvy: past, present and future. European Journal of Internal Medicine. 2011; 22 (2): 147-152.

[11] Bartholomew M. James Lind's treatise of the scurvy (1753). Postgraduate Medical Journal. 2002; 78 (925): 695-696.

[12] Morgan AP. The pulmonary toxicity of oxygen. Anesthesiology: The Journal of the American Society of Anesthesiologists. 1968; 29 (3): 570-578.

[13] Yamasaki H. Nitric oxide research in plant biology: its past and future. In: Magalhaes JR, Singh RP, Passos LP, editors. Nitric oxide signaling in higher plants. Houston: Studium Press; 2004. p. 1-23.

[14] Colin J. Paul Bert. NASA technical memorandum. 1978; NASA TM 75599.

[15] Johnson ME. The History and Development of Aviation Medicine. Journal of the National Medical Association. 1943; 35 (6): 194.

[16] Saugstad OD. Oxygen and retinopathy of prematurity. Journal of Perinatology. 2006; 26 (1): S46-S50.

[17] Valko M, Leibfritz D, Moncol J, Cronin MT, Mazur M, Telser J. Free radicals and antioxidants in normal physiological functions and human disease. The International Journal of Biochemistry & Cell Biology. 2007; 39 (1): 44-84.

[18] McCord JM, Fridovich I. Superoxide dismutase an enzymic function for erythrocuprein (hemocuprein). Journal of Biological Chemistry. 1969; 244 (22): 6049-6055.

[19] Baier J, Maisch T, Maier M, Landthaler M, Bäumler W. Direct detection of singlet oxygen generated by UVA irradiation in human cells and skin. Journal of Investigative Dermatology. 2007; 127 (6): 1498-1506.

[20] Arrigoni O, De Tullio MC. Ascorbic acid: much more than just an antioxidant. Biochimica et Biophysica Acta (BBA)-General Subjects. 2002; 1569 (1-3): 1-9.

[21] Bentsath A, Szent-Györgyi A. Vitamin P. Nature. 1937; 140 (3540): 426.

[22] Bentsath A, Szent-Györgyi A. Vitamin nature of flavones. Nature. 1936; 138 (3497): 798-798.

[23] Yamasaki H. A function of colour. Trends in Plant Science. 1997; 2 (1): 7-8. 10.1016/s1360-1385(97)82730-6

[24] Nijveldt RJ, van Nood E, van Hoorn DEC, Boelens PG, van Norren K, van Leeuwen PAM. Flavonoids: a review of probable mechanisms of action and potential applications. American Journal of Clinical Nutrition. 2001; 74 (4): 418-425.

[25] Kuriyama S, Hozawa A, Ohmori K, Shimazu T, Matsui T, Ebihara S, *et al.* Green tea consumption and cognitive function: a cross-sectional study from the Tsurugaya Project. The American Journal of Clinical Nutrition. 2006; 83 (2): 355-361.

[26] Kuriyama S, Shimazu T, Ohmori K, Kikuchi N, Nakaya N, Nishino Y, *et al.* Green tea consumption and mortality due to cardiovascular disease, cancer, and all causes in Japan: the Ohsaki study. JAMA. 2006; 296 (10): 1255-1265.

[27] Agati G, Azzarello E, Pollastri S, Tattini M. Flavonoids as antioxidants in plants: location and functional significance. Plant Science. 2012; 196: 67-76. 10.1016/j.plantsci.2012.07.014

[28] Crecelius AC, Hölscher D, Hoffmann T, Schneider B, Fischer TC, Hanke M-V, *et al.* Spatial and temporal localization of flavonoid metabolites in strawberry fruit (*Fragaria*× *ananassa*). Journal of Agricultural and Food Chemistry. 2017; 65 (17): 3559-3568.

[29] Chemistry IUoPaA. Flavonoids (isoflavonoids and neoflavonoids). IUPAC Compendium of Chemical Terminology2009. 10.1351/goldbook. F02424

[30] Rice Evans AC, Miller JN, Pagang G. Antioxidant properties of phenolic compounds. Trends in Plant Science. 1997; 2 (4): 152-159.

[31] Williams CA, Grayer RJ. Anthocyanins and other flavonoids. Natural Product Reports. 2004; 21 (4): 539-573. 10.1039/b311404j

[32] Tanaka Y, Sasaki N, Ohmiya A. Biosynthesis of plant pigments: anthocyanins, betalains and carotenoids. The Plant Journal. 2008; 54 (4): 733-749. 10.1111/j.1365-313X.2008.03447.x

[33] Shirley BW. Flavonoid biosynthesis:'new'functions for an 'old'pathway. Trends in plant science. 1996; 1 (11): 377-382.

[34] Winkel-Shirley B. Flavonoid biosynthesis. A colorful model for genetics, biochemistry, cell biology, and biotechnology. Plant Physiology. 2001; 126 (2): 485-493.

[35] Sakihama Y, Cohen MF, Grace SC, H. Y. Plant phenolic antioxidant and prooxidant activities: phenolics-induced oxidative damage mediated by metals in plants. Toxicology. 2002; 177: 67-80.

[36] Huang DJ, Ou BX, Prior RL. The chemistry behind antioxidant capacity assays. Journal of Agricultural and Food Chemistry. 2005; 53 (6): 1841-1856. 10.1021/jf030723c

[37] Fauconneau B, WaffoTeguo P, Huguet F, Barrier L, Decendit A, Merillon JM. Comparative study of radical scavenger and antioxidant properties of phenolic compounds from *Vitis vinifera* cell cultures using *in vitro* tests. Life Sciences. 1997; 61 (21): 2103-2110. 10.1016/s0024-3205(97)00883-7

[38] Matsuura T, Matsushima H, Nakashima R. Photoinduced reactions—XXXVI: Photosensitized oxygenation of 3-hydroxyflavones as a nonenzymatic model for quercetinase. Tetrahedron. 1970; 26 (2): 435-443.

[39] Takahama U. Oxidation products of kaempferol by superoxide anion radical. Plant and Cell Physiology. 1987; 28 (5): 953-957.

[40] Yamasaki H, Uefuji H, Sakihama Y. Bleaching of the red anthocyanin induced by superoxide radical. Archives of Biochemistry and Biophysics. 1996; 332 (1): 183-186. 10.1006/abbi.1996.0331

[41] Wang W, Luo J, Yao S, Lian Z, Zhang J, Lin N, *et al.* Interaction of phenolic antioxidants and hydroxyl radicals. Radiation Physics and Chemistry. 1993; 42 (4-6): 985-987.

[42] Patil SL, Mallaiah SH, Patil RK. Antioxidative and radioprotective potential of rutin and quercetin in Swiss albino mice exposed to gamma radiation. Journal of Medical Physics. 2013; 38 (2): 87.

[43] Afanas' ev IB, Dcrozhko AI, Brodskii AV, Kostyuk VA, Potapovitch AI. Chelating and free radical scavenging mechanisms of inhibitory action of rutin and quercetin in lipid peroxidation. Biochemical Pharmacology. 1989; 38 (11): 1763-1769.

[44] Bors W, Heller W, Michel C, Saran M. Flavonoids as antioxidants: Determination of radical-scavenging efficiencies. Methods in Enzymology. 1990; 186: 343-355. https://doi.org/10.1016/0076-6879(90)86128-I

[45] Rolt A, Cox LS. Structural basis of the anti-ageing effects of polyphenolics: mitigation of oxidative stress. BMC Chemistry. 2020; 14 (1): 50. 10.1186/s13065-020-00696-0

[46] Yamasaki H, Grace SC. EPR detection of phytophenoxyl radicals stabilized by zinc ions: evidence for the redox coupling of plant phenolics with ascorbate in the H2O2-peroxidase system. FEBS Letters. 1998; 422: 377-380.

[47] Sakihama Y, Mano J, Sano S, Asada K, Yamasaki H. Reduction of phenoxyl radicals mediated by monodehydroascorbate reductase. Biochemical Biophysical Research Communications. 2000; 279 (3): 949-954. 10.1006/bbrc.2000.4053

[48] Miguel MG. Betalains in Some Species of the Amaranthaceae Family: A Review. Antioxidants. 2018; 7 (4). 10.3390/antiox7040053

[49] Timoneda A, Feng T, Sheehan H, Walker-Hale N, Pucker B, Lopez-Nieves S, *et al.* The evolution of betalain biosynthesis in Caryophyllales. New Phytologist. 2019; 224 (1): 71-85.

[50] Li G, Meng X, Zhu M, Li Z. Research progress of betalain in response to adverse stresses and evolutionary relationship compared with anthocyanin. Molecules. 2019; 24 (17). 10.3390/molecules24173078

[51] Sheehan H, Feng T, Walker-Hale N, Lopez-Nieves S, Pucker B, Guo R, *et al.* Evolution of L-DOPA 4,5-dioxygenase activity allows for recurrent specialisation to betalain pigmentation in Caryophyllales. New Phytologist. 2020; 227 (3): 914-929. 10.1111/nph.16089

[52] Hatlestad GJ, Sunnadeniya RM, Akhavan NA, Gonzalez A, Goldman IL, McGrath JM, *et al.* The beet *R* locus encodes a new cytochrome P450 required for red betalain production. Nature Genetics. 2012; 44 (7): 816-820. 10.1038/ng.2297

[53] Sunnadeniya R, Bean A, Brown M, Akhavan N, Hatlestad G, Gonzalez A, *et al.* Tyrosine hydroxylation in betalain pigment biosynthesis is performed by cytochrome P450 enzymes in beets (*Beta vulgaris*). PLoS One. 2016; 11 (2): e0149417. 10.1371/journal.pone.0149417

[54] Gandia-Herrero F, Garcia-Carmona F. Biosynthesis of betalains: yellow and violet plant pigments. Trends in Plant Science. 2013; 18 (6): 334-343. 10.1016/j.tplants.2013.01.003

[55] Vieira Teixeira da Silva D, Dos Santos Baiao D, de Oliveira Silva F, Alves G, Perrone D, Mere Del Aguila E, *et al.* Betanin, a natural food additive: stability, bioavailability, antioxidant and preservative ability assessments. Molecules. 2019; 24 (3). 10.3390/molecules24030458

[56] Kanner J, Harel S, Granit R. Betalains - a new class of dietary cationized antioxidants. Journal of Agriculture and Food Chemistry. 2001; 49: 5178-5185.

[57] Tesoriere L, Allegra M, Gentile C, Livrea MA. Betacyanins as phenol antioxidants. Chemistry and mechanistic aspects of the lipoperoxyl radical-scavenging activity in solution and liposomes. Free Radical Research. 2009; 43 (8): 706-717. 10.1080/10715760903037681

[58] Gandı́a-Herrero F, Escribano J, F. Ga-C. The role of phenolic hydroxy groups in the free radical scavenging activity of betalains. Journal of Natural Products. 2009; 72: 1142-1146.

[59] Tutone M, Lauria A, Almerico AM. Theoretical determination of the pK a values of betalamic acid related to the free radical scavenger capacity: comparison between empirical and quantum chemical methods. Interdisciplinary Science. 2016; 8 (2): 177-185. 10.1007/s12539-015-0101-3

[60] Allegra M, Tesoriere L, Livrea MA. Betanin inhibits the myeloperoxidase/nitrite-induced oxidation of human low-density lipoproteins. Free Radical Research. 2007; 41 (3): 335-341. 10.1080/10715760601038783

[61] Yamasaki H. The NO world for plants: achieving balance in an open system. Plant Cell and Environment. 2005; 28 (1): 78-84. 10.1111/j.1365-3040.2005.01297.x

[62] Yamasaki H, Cohen MF. Biological consilience of hydrogen sulfide and nitric oxide in plants: Gases of primordial earth linking plant, microbial and animal physiologies. Nitric Oxide. 2016; 55-56: 91-100. 10.1016/j.niox.2016.04.002

[63] Yamasaki H. Nitrite-dependent nitric oxide production pathway: implications for involvement of active nitrogen species in photoinhibition *in vivo*. Philosophical Transactions of the Royal Society B-Biological Sciences. 2000; 355 (1402): 1477-1488. 10.1098/rstb.2000.0708

[64] Wink DA, Mitchell JB. Chemical biology of nitric oxide: Insights into regulatory, cytotoxic, and cytoprotective mechanisms of nitric oxide. Free Radical Biology and Medicine. 1998; 25 (4-5): 434-456. 10.1016/s0891-5849(98)00092-6

[65] Mishanina TV, Libiad M, Banerjee R. Biogenesis of reactive sulfur species for signaling by hydrogen sulfide oxidation pathways. Nature Chemical Biology. 2015; 11 (7): 457-464.

[66] Wong CC, Williamson G. Inhibition of hydroxycinnamic acid sulfation by flavonoids and their conjugated metabolites. Biofactors. 2013; 39 (6): 644-651. 10.1002/biof.1127

[67] Iacopini P, Baldi M, Storchi P, Sebastiani L. Catechin, epicatechin, quercetin, rutin and resveratrol in red grape: Content, in vitro antioxidant activity and interactions. Journal of Food Composition and Analysis. 2008; 21 (8): 589-598. 10.1016/j.jfca.2008.03.011

[68] Rahman MM, Ichiyanagi T, Komiyama T, Hatano Y, Konishi T. Superoxide radical- and peroxynitrite-scavenging activity of anthocyanins; structure-activity relationship and their synergism. Free Radical Research. 2006; 40 (9): 993-1002. 10.1080/10715760600815322

[69] Tsuda T, Kato Y, Osawa T. Mechanism for the peroxynitrite scavenging activity by anthocyanins. FEBS Letters. 2000; 484: 207-210.

[70] Ketsawatsakul U, Whiteman M, Halliwell B. A reevaluation of the peroxynitrite scavenging activity of some dietary phenolics. Biochemical and Biophysical Research Communications. 2000; 279 (2): 692-699. 10.1006/bbrc.2000.4014

[71] Sakihama Y, Maeda M, Hashimoto M, Tahara S, Hashidoko Y. Beetroot betalain inhibits peroxynitrite-mediated tyrosine nitration and DNA strand cleavage. Free Radical Research. 2012; 46 (1): 93-99. 10.3109/10715762.2011.641157

[72] Taira J, Tsuchida E, Katon MC, Uehara M, Ogi T. Antioxidant capacity of betacyanins as radical scavengers for peroxyl radical and nitric oxide. Food Chemistry. 2015; 166: 531-536. 10.1016/j.foodchem.2014.05.102

[73] Heijnen CGM, Haenen G, van Acker FAA, van der Vijgh WJF, Bast A. Flavonoids as peroxynitrite scavengers: the role of the hydroxyl groups. Toxicology in Vitro. 2001; 15 (1): 3-6. 10.1016/s0887-2333(00)00053-9

[74] Sakihama Y, Tamaki R, Shimoji H, Ichiba T, Fukushi Y, Tahara S, *et al.* Enzymatic nitration of phytophenolics: evidence for peroxynitrite-independent nitration of plant secondary metabolites. FEBS Letters. 2003; 553 (3): 377-380. 10.1016/s0014-5793(03)01059-7

[75] Khan MI. Plant betalains: safety, antioxidant activity, clinical efficacy, and bioavailability. Comprehensive Reviews in Food Science and Food Safety. 2016; 15 (2): 316-330. 10.1111/1541-4337.12185

[76] da Silva DVT, Pereira AD, Boaventura GT, Ribeiro RSA, Vericimo MA, Carvalho-Pinto CE, *et al.* Short-term betanin intake reduces oxidative stress in wistar rats. Nutrients. 2019; 11 (9): 1978. 10.3390/nu11091978

[77] Kleinenkuhnen N, Buchel F, Gerlich SC, Kopriva S, Metzger S. A novel method for identification and quantification of sulfated flavonoids in plants by neutral loss scan mass spectrometry. Frontiers in Plant Science. 2019; 10: 885. 10.3389/fpls.2019.00885

[78] Bylka W, Stobiecki M, Frański R. Sulphated flavonoid glycosides from leaves of Atriplex hortensis. Acta Physiologiae Plantarum. 2001; 23 (3): 285-290.

[79] Correia-da-Silva M, Sousa E, Pinto MM. Emerging sulfated flavonoids and other polyphenols as drugs: nature as an inspiration. Medical Research Reviews. 2014; 34 (2): 223-279. 10.1002/med.21282

[80] Bedair TM, Bedair HM, Ko KW, Park W, Joung YK, Han DK.

Persulfated flavonoids accelerated re-endothelialization and improved blood compatibility for vascular medical implants. Colloids and Surfaces B: Biointerfaces. 2019; 181: 174-184. 10.1016/j.colsurfb.2019.05.033

[81] Haraguchi H, Ohmi I, Sakai S, Fukuda A. Effect of *Polygonum hydropiper* sulfated flavonoids on lens aldose reductase and related enzymes. Journal of Natural Products. 1996; 59: 443-445.

[82] Ku SK, Kim TH, Bae JS. Anticoagulant activities of persicarin and isorhamnetin. Vascular Pharmacology. 2013; 58 (4): 272-279. 10.1016/j.vph.2013.01.005

[83] Yagi A, Uemura T, Okamura N, Haraguchi H, Imoto T, Hashimoto K. Antioxidative sulphated flavonoids in leaves of *Polygonum hydropiper*. Phytochemistry. 1994; 35 (4): 885-887.

[84] Yamasaki H. Blood nitrate and nitrite modulating nitric oxide bioavailability: Potential therapeutic functions in COVID-19. Nitric Oxide. 2020; 103: 29-30. 10.1016/j.niox.2020.07.005

[85] Lundberg JO, Weitzberg E, Gladwin MT. The nitrate-nitrite-nitric oxide pathway in physiology and therapeutics. Nature Review Drug Discovovery. 2008; 7 (2): 156-167. 10.1038/nrd2466

[86] Xi L. Beet juice as nutraceutical remedy for alleviating pulmonary arterial hypertension: searching for optimal treatment timing and nitrate dose. American Journal of Hypertension. 2019; 32 (2): 135-138. 10.1093/ajh/hpy181

[87] Volino-Souza M, de Oliveira GV, Conte-Junior CA, Alvares TS. Covid-19 quarantine: impact of lifestyle behaviors changes on endothelial function and possible protective effect of beetroot Juice. Frontiers in Nutrition. 2020; 7: 582210. 10.3389/fnut.2020.582210

[88] Mittler R. Oxidative stress, antioxidants and stress tolerance. Trends in Plant Science. 2002; 7 (9): 405-410. 10.1016/s1360-1385(02)02312-9

[89] Mukherjee PK, Mukherjee D, Maji AK, Rai S, Heinrich M. The sacred lotus (*Nelumbo nucifera*) - phytochemical and therapeutic profile. Journal of Pharmacy and Pharmacology. 2009; 61 (4): 407-422. 10.1211/jpp/61.04.0001

[90] Hunyadi A. The mechanism(s) of action of antioxidants: From scavenging reactive oxygen/nitrogen species to redox signaling and the generation of bioactive secondary metabolites. Medical Research Reviews. 2019; 39 (6): 2505-2533. 10.1002/med.21592

Chapter 16

Broad Efficacy of Scavenging Free Radicals: *Cordyceps* sp.

Loknath Deshmukh, Rajendra Singh and Sardul Singh Sandhu

Abstract

Scavenging free radical potency of cordycepin is the major bioactive segment extricated from *Cordyceps* species. In some new years, *Cordyceps* has gotten growing thought inferable from its distinctive restorative/pharmacological tests. This assessment reviews continuous explores on the counter oxidant impacts and the associated analyses of *Cordyceps* species. The results from our review show that *Cordyceps* of the cordycepin applies protective effects against hostile to oxidant injury for certain, afflictions including constant obstructive pneumonic infection (COPD), hepatitis, asthma, cerebral paralysis, Parkinson's illness (PD), coronary course sickness (CAD), Alzheimer illness, respiratory failure, malignancy infection, maturing, waterfalls, and mind brokenness. *Cordyceps* coordinates the NF-κB, RIP2/Caspase-1, Akt/GSK-3β/p70S6K, TGF-β/Smads, and Nrf2/HO-1 hailing pathways among others of cordycepin. A couple of assessments focusing in on *Cordyceps* auxiliaries were surveyed and found to down metabolic speed of *Cordyceps* and augmentation its bioavailability. In addition, cordycepin further developed opposition, prevented the duplication of viral RNA, and covered cytokine storms, therefore proposing its capacity to treat COVID-19 and other viral defilements. From the accumulated and assessed information, this article gives the speculative reason to the clinical usages of cordycepin and inspects the way for future assessments focusing in on expanding the restorative use of *Cordyceps* species. Cordycepin and its analogs show unfathomable potential as the accompanying new class of against oxidant specialists.

Keywords: *Cordyceps* species, anti-oxidant, cordycepin, oxidant diseases, fruiting body and secondary metabolite, pharmacodynamics

1. Introduction

Cordyceps species (Ascomycetes*genus*) is a bug parasitizing development; they are thusly entomopathogenic life forms. The name *Cordyceps* begins from the Latin words line and ceps, meaning 'club' and 'head', independently. From a genuine perspective "summer grass, winter worm", Chinese caterpillar development, is the Chinese name given to the complex of hatchlings and parasites [1–3] which this helpful mushroom has been found ordinarily at high heights of around 14,000 ft. in the Himalayan territories including Nepal, China, Bhutan, Thailand, Tibet, and India [4]. The *Cordyceps* as*genus*ment consolidates more than 400 species, among which *Cordyceps* species have been used generally for millennia in China as a food, tonic, and natural drug for various prosperity related issues, for instance, kidney and lung brokenness, weakness, and exhaustion [5, 6]. This development lives in

IntechOpen

a general sense on the highest point of the hatchling of one explicit *genus* of moth, Hepialus armoricanus, and yet is unexpectedly found creating on other moth species [7]. It is generally called 'Dong Chong Xia Cao' in Chinese and 'Tockukaso' in Japanese, implying 'winter-frightening little animal and summer-plant' because of the creating cycle: the development at first parasitizes the hatchling of specific species Hepiaidae, outlining a parasitic complex that includes the leftover pieces of the caterpillar and the stroma of the creature [8]. *Cordyceps* are a stunning cordycepin wellspring of bioactive metabolites that show various clinically asserted advantages for human prosperity. Since people have an inclination towards trademark/home grown medicines, the usage of *Cordyceps* as a trademark remedial mushroom is unpreventable [9]. The bio metabolite cordycepin was first isolates from the matured supply of the therapeutic mushroom *Cordyceps* militaris [10]. Which is an entomopathogen creature that grows parasitically on lepidopteron hatchlings and bug pupae. The family *Cordyceps* is prominent in standard Chinese medicine and shows a variety of clinical prosperity impacts including hostile to diabetic, immunomodulatory, against oxidant, against oxidant, anticancer, cardiovascular effects, against fibrotic, and against microbial exercises [11–13]. *Cordyceps* sp. has been represented to have a various extent of pharmacological effects of which, its antitumor, against angiogenic, and antagonistic to oxidative properties are for the most part examined [14, 15]. Growing considers showing that it applies solid malignant growth counteraction specialist exercises in different cell types including macrophages, chondrocytes, glial, and lung epithelial cells [16]. Then, at that point, against oxidant impacts are furthermore found in liver, and LPS-impelled exceptional lung injury, alcohol started Hyperlipidemia, ominously vulnerable asthma, doxorubicin-instigated, cardiotoxicity, irritation actuated osteoporosis, and cerebral ischemia–reperfusion injury when various animal mice models are used [17–19]. With a rising income in cordycepin, the usage of assistant changes to block the metabolic speed and augmentation efficiency has been explored [20]. There are as of now a gigantic number of studies zeroing in on its enemy of oxidant impacts; regardless, an aggregate and productive overview of composing is inadequate. In this review, we surveyed the late enemy of oxidant focuses on cordycepin to choose its future perspective as an enemy of oxidant drug and to clarify its critical enemy of oxidant systems of activity.

2. Oxidative stress and damage to nucleic acid, protein and lipids

Oxidative mischief to nucleic acid (DNA), proteins, and various macromolecules gathers with age and has been conjectured to be a major, yet by all record not the sole, sort of endogenous damage inciting developing [6, 21, 22]. Superoxide (0_2), hydrogen peroxide (H_20_2), and hydroxyl progressive (– OH), which are mutagens conveyed by radiation, are also results of normal processing [12, 23]. Endogenous oxidants similarly hurt proteins and lipids [24] have demonstrated that the activity of proteolytic mixtures that hydrolyze oxidized proteins isn't fit thwart an age-related augmentation of oxidized proteins. In two human diseases related with inauspicious developing, Werner issue, and progeria, oxidized proteins increase at tons higher rate than is common [25]. Lipid peroxidation offers to rise to mutagenic lipid epoxides, lipid hydro-peroxides, lipid alkoxyl and peroxyl fanatics, and enals (a,4-unsaturated aldehydes) [26]. Singlet oxygen, a high-energy and mutagenic sort of oxygen, are frequently conveyed by the move of energy from light, the respiratory burst from neutrophils, or lipid peroxidation [27]. Animals have different malignancy avoidance specialist securities, yet since these watchmen aren't incredible, some DNA is oxidized. Oxidatively hurt DNA is fixed by intensifies that remove the wounds, which are then released inside the pee. Strategies are made to take a gander several of those separated hurt bases inside the pee of model rodents and others [28], basically all of which show up on the grounds that the free base from a fix by glycosylases. We check that the quantity of oxidative hits to DNA per cell daily is around 100,000 inside the model rodents and around 10,000 inside the human. DNA-fix synthetics capably dispense with most, yet not all, of the wounds outlined [6, 29–31] for instance, the significant change repeat in human lymphocytes, of which the responsibility of oxidative DNA bruises is dark, is around numerous occasions more vital in elderly people than in youths [32]. Mitochondrial DNA (mtDNA) from rat liver has in more than numerous occasions the level of oxidative DNA hurt than does nuclear DNA from an indistinguishable tissue [16, 33]. This extension could be because of a shortfall of mtDNA fix proteins, a shortfall of histones getting mtDNA, and subsequently the closeness of mtDNA to oxidants delivered during natural cycle. The cell shields itself against this high speed of mischief by a uniform turnover of mitochondria, thusly presumably killing those hurt mitochondria that produce extended oxidants. Notwithstanding this turnover, oxidative wounds appear to gather with age in mtDNA at a preferable rate over in nuclear DNA [34, 35]. Fluorescent tones, which are accepted to be relied upon somewhat to crosslinks among protein and lipid peroxidation things, moreover increase with age [36]. The significance of oxidative DNA wounds in illness and developing is highlighted by the presence of express fix glycosylases that separate these injuries from DNA. Because of 8-oxo-2′- deoxy-guanosine, a physical issue molded from oxidative mischief to guanine stores in DNA, loss of a particular glycosylase development prompts a reasonable extension inside the unconstrained change rate [12, 20, 37, 38], exhibiting the trademark mutagenic ability of this DNA sore. Various other oxidative DNA injuries are probably going to be huge too [39].

3. Sources and effects of cordycepin

Cordyceps sp. cordycepin (3′-deoxyadenosine) prominent as purine or pyrimidine nucleobase adenosine, cytidine, and guanosine straightforward that have particular sort of bioactivities [40]. The cordycepin will be changed over into 5′-mono, di, and triphosphates and thusly obstruct the advancement of ribose-phosphate pyrophospho kinase and 5-phosphoribosyl-1-pyrophosphate amido-transferase in the again purines biosynthesis, just as the nucleic acids, mix causing the counter metastatic, antitumor and antimicrobial results [12, 41, 42]. Similarly, cordycepin with its enemy of leukemic limit normally get along with adenosine deaminase inhibitor and this will cause the inhibitory effect on happen which serves to analogs of 2′, 5′-oligoadenylate towards the human immunodeficiency contamination illness [43]. Immense degree refined of mycelial through designed can be used as another wellspring of cordycepin on account of its limited total in a typical source. Tow stage control of deteriorated oxygen or development of $NH4+$ to the brought down medium can help with working on the formation of cordycepin [44]. Despite creation using development advancement, cordycepin could be in like manner conveyed misleadingly. In any case, the manufactured blend has some hindrance, for instance, the trouble of the cycle and the utilization of gigantic volume of normal solvents which decrease the allure of this cycle [18, 45]. Exploration that the lifestyle created on xylose showed high creation yield of cordycepin on dry biomass. Standing out xylose from other carbon sources, a lot of essentially up-coordinated characteristics in xylose were progressed in pentose and glucoronate interconversion, and cordycepin biosynthesis [46]. The place of the current examination was to choose if cordycepin controls duplication, development, and angiogenesis in a

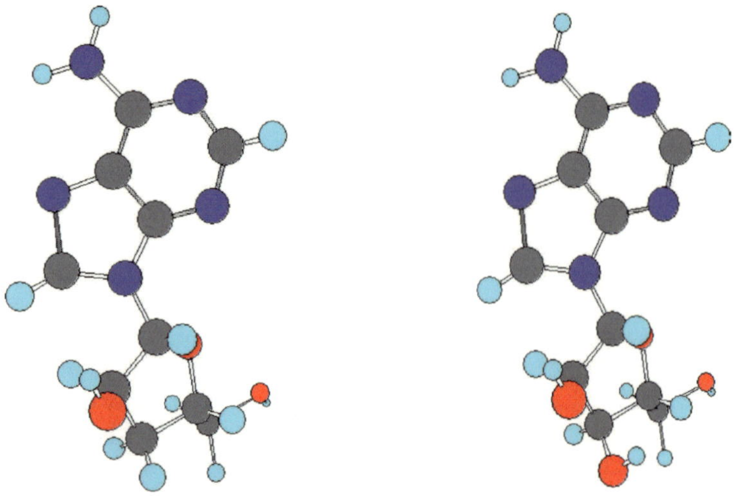

Figure 1.
Chemical structure of Cordycepin and Adenosine [40].

human umbilical vein endothelial (huve) cell line and in a hepatocellular carcinoma (hcc) cell line [47–49]. MTT was used to study cell development. Apoptosis was poor somewhere near stream cytometry (propidium iodide recoloring). Transwell and wound repairing measures were used to research the movement and interruption of hcc cell line and huve cells. Angiogenesis in huve cells was studied using a chamber advancement test. Cordycepin immovably smothered hcc cell line and huve cell increase in a dose- and time-dependent way. Cordycepin activated huve cell apoptosis in a dose-dependent way (2,000 μg/ml, 50.20 ± 1.55% versus 0 μg/ml, 2.62 ± 0.19%, $P < 0.01$) [50–53]. The genome-wide transcriptome assessment showed 8747 imparted characteristics in the glucose and sucrose social orders created under light-programming and faint conditions. Cordycepin curbed cell improvement and set off apoptosis in U87MG cells with wild-type p53, yet not in T98G cells with freak type p53 [54, 55] (**Figure 1**).

4. Fruiting body and secondary metabolites action

The entomopathogenic development *Cordyceps* species is a consumable mushroom with numerous drug/therapeutic properties. Numerous past research analyzed the cell reinforcement exercises that of the refined where refined fruiting collection of *Cordyceps sinensis* and *Cordyceps militaries* class [56, 57]. Methanolic concentrate of *Cordyceps* sp. was tasted when exercises for its antibacterial, cancer prevention agent, antifungal, and antiproliferative properties in different human cell lines. The methanolic concentrate of *Cordyceps* showed to thwart lipid peroxidation, have reducing force and search free radicals [58]. The assessment was coordinated under research facilities produce *Cordyceps* sp. improvement, with five Selenium (Se) different centers (μg g^{-1}) and three sorts of Selenium components like selenate. *Cordyceps* can hold inorganic component from the compound and overhaul it to normal Selenium blends in fruiting bodies [59–62]. As per Yamaguchi and partners the concentrates investigated, the high temperature water discrete (70°C for 5 min) demonstrated the best without oxygen extremist searching activity. Moreover, when low-thickness lipoprotein (LTL) was incubated with macrophages inside seeing copper dichloride (1 mM), the high temperature water eliminate demonstrated a strong inhibitory effect against lipid peroxidation in medium and resulting assortment of cholesteryl ester in macrophages [63–66]. As per the as of late examinations, the fruiting body tests were set up in four particular model plans, which were flawless fruiting bodies, cut fruiting bodies, dried powder, and dried unpleasant concentrate [67, 68]. The real proportion of the adenosine and cordycepin obsessions in fresh fruiting bodies was inspected by world class liquid chromatography [69]. These optimal models gave a coefficient of confirmation of assumption, standard botch of figure, inclination, and waiting farsighted deviation, which were independently 0.95, 16.60 mg kg^{-1}, −8.57 mg kg^{-1}, and 5.04 for adenosine conjecture, and 0.98, 181.56 mg kg^{-1}, −1.05 mg kg^{-1}, and 8.9 for cordycepin gauge by Singpoonga and partners [70].

There is uncommon potential for the creation of metabolites from *Cordyceps* species, this is one phase towards finding and depicting with the bounty of nuclear essential assortment in this genera. Presented here is the essential chromosome level social affair of a genome from the *Cordyceps* genera. This get-together and assessment has revealed that *Cordyceps* militaris has seven chromosomes containing a wealth of value bunches for optional metabolite creation that entomopathogenic sort. With this genome, further assessment and depiction of the discretionary metabolites conveyed by *Cordyceps* militaris might benefit from outside input through genome based procedures including heterologous explanation of value gatherings. Of the 36 quality gatherings recognized using the antiSMASH and SMURF computations, three gatherings are found to have a genuine degree of equivalence with bunches from various life frames that produce a known molecule [58, 62, 71, 72].

5. Anti-oxidant potency

5.1 Antioxidants secure against disease

Different affirmation parts inside the living being have advanced to restrict the degrees of open oxidants and the underhandedness they cause to the human body [73]. Among the protections are compounds, for example, glutathione peroxidase, catalase, and superoxide dismutase. The glutathione S-transferases inactivate responsive electrophilic mutagens, including the aldehyde delayed consequences of lipid peroxidation. There are also different partner guards, for example, sequestration of H202-production engineered substances in peroxisomes and chelation of any free iron or copper salts in transferrin and ferritin or ceruloplasmin to keep away from Fenton science. O_2, in any case, can pass on iron from ferritin [65, 74]. Oxidized DNA is fixed by a development of glycosylases that are unequivocal for express oxidized bases and perhaps by questionable extraction fix compounds. Without cell division, these oxidative wounds are discarded from DNA sensibly and the change rate is kept to a base [20, 75]. Oxidized proteins are destroyed by proteases. Lipid hydroperoxides are crushed by glutathione peroxidase. Basically these safeguards show up, clearly, to be inducible, as are most different sorts of watchmen i.e., the sums increment because of hurt. There is enormous making exhibiting that cells react to low degrees of radiation, and oxidative mutagen, by beginning infection aversion expert shields that help to promise them against change by gigantic levels of radiation [44, 68, 71]. In spite of the defensive impacts of endogenous enzymatic harm evasion expert safeguards, utilization of dietary cell fortresses shows up, evidently, to be fundamental. Food sources created all along, fundamental wellspring of cell fortresses in the eating schedule, are associated with a cut down hazard of degenerative issues [76]. Square and her associates have really inspected various numbers amasses in the epidemiological forming that relate, with unimaginable consistency, the deficit of good use of verdant food assortments to destructive advancement rate. The quarter of everybody with low dietary affirmation of food assortments created beginning from the soonest stage twofold the infection rate for most kinds of hurtful turn of events (lung, larynx, oral melancholy, throat, stomach, colon and rectum, bladder, pancreas, cervix, and ovary) when stuck out and the quarter from high attestation [14, 40, 77]. Information on the genus of perilous improvement known to be associated with compound levels are not as reliable and show less affirmation by food sources created beginning from the most punctual stage: chest disease the defensive impact was about 30% [78]. The expense of after effects of the soil is an immense factor in agitating use. Less fortunate individuals spend a more raised level of their remuneration on food, eat less consequences of the soil, and have more confined future than all the more wealthy individuals [79]. A basic partner of thriving in this century was made pesticides, which very diminished the expense of food creation and guaranteed that by a wide margin the vast majority of the harvests planted would be eaten by people as opposed to bugs [80]. Planned pesticide stores don't show up in everybody to be a huge defense compromising turn of events.

5.2 Birth defects, childhood tumour and oxidation

Oxidative stresses in sperm DNA are extended products number when levels of dietary ascorbate are insufficient to keep unique fluid ascorbate at an adequate level [81]. A sizable level of the few country people ingests lacking levels of dietary ascorbate, particularly single folks, destitute individuals, and smokers [82]. The oxidants in tobacco smoke channel the cell fortifications in plasma. Smokers should eat 2–3 times more ascorbate than non-smokers to achieve a comparable level of ascorbate in the blood [83], nonetheless, they only sometimes do. In assessments of sperm from smokers and non-smokers [84] the amount of sperm and the degree of motile sperm decay basically in smokers, and this reducing was dependent upon the part and term of smoking. Paternal smoking, explicitly, appears to in-wrinkle the peril of birth distortions and youth threatening development in successors [85, 86]. One expects, and discovers, much greater obligation to the germ-line change rate from the father than from the mother, with the age of the father being a huge peril factor [87, 88]. As such, inadequate eating regimens (and smoking) of fathers appear to achieve hurt not only to their own DNA yet moreover to the DNA of their sperm, an effect that may resonate down individuals later on and new age [81, 89, 90].

5.3 Cardiovascular system diseases

Coronary vein illness (CAD) is a condition reliant upon various factors or causes diligent vascular provocative bruises that lead to the start of cardiovascular framework infections [91]. Atherosclerotic coronary illness related irritation is mediated by great for combustible cytokines, provocative hailing pathways, bioactive lipids, and bond particles [92]. Extended extension and development of cardio vascular smooth muscle cells also intercede in the beginning and development of CAD [93]. *Cordyceps* controls the duplication of aortic smooth muscle cells (RatAOSMCs) in the carotid stock course of inflatable hurt Sprague–Dawley rodent model. In addition, in collagen type I-incited RatAOSMCs, Cordycepin (3′- deoxyadenosine) famously controls the inception of MMP-2 and - 9 and the surge of particles [94]. Myocardial ischemia–reperfusion (I/R) injury is a cardiovascular sickness caused in view of an outrageous prevention in coronary blood adaptability. It can provoke tissue hypoxia, cell decay, organ brokenness, and even apoptosis in outrageous conditions [95]. 3′- deoxyadenosine applies cardio-defensive effects against I/R-started rat heart injury; its arrangement of action can be credited to the obstacle of Bax, isolated caspase-3 enunciation, the ascent of Bcl-2 verbalization, and activation of the Akt/GSK-3β/p70S6K hailing pathways. Plus, *Cordyceps* sp. in like manner grows the affirmation of the disease anticipation specialist protein HO-1 [93, 96]. In a mouse cardiovascular exchange model, *Cordyceps* 3′- deoxyadenosine got together with ECDI-SPs has an immense effect in lessening the production of good for combustible cytokines including IL-1β, IL-6, IL-17, and TNF-α, growing the release of quieting cytokines IL-10 and TGF-β, and upsetting Th17 and progressing Tregs, then, at that point ECDI-SPs monotherapy alone [92]. All things considered, *Cordyceps* could ease up disturbance activated by CAD through impeding the extension and development of smooth muscle cells similarly as tweaking diverse related cytokines and chemokines and the assertion of record factors. Additionally, *Cordyceps* applies therapeutic ramifications for myocardial ischemia–reperfusion (I/R) injury by obstructing cell apoptosis, lessening the making of positive for red hot cytokines, and overseeing safe cell limits [97].

5.4 Central nervous system diseases

Parkinson's affliction is a neurodegenerative disease that shows as an improvement issue, in which degeneration and loss of dopaminergic neurons of the substantia nigra are the brand name features. Oxidative pressing factor and neuro-aggravation accept critical parts in the pathogenic frameworks of Parkinson's disorder [98–100]. In a continuous report, cordycepin is found to direct the motor issues in MPTP-treated Parkinsonism rodents and seemed to apply neuroprotective effects through easing up bothering and oxidative pressing factor response. Likewise, such neuroprotective effects may be connected with the limitation of the TLR/NF κB hailing pathway in MPTP-started Parkinson's disorder rodents and LPS-incited BV2 cells [101]. Stroke is perhaps the most notable ailments in cerebrovascular affliction and can be clinically isolated into two genuss: ischemic and hemorrhagic. Extreme ischemic stroke is responsible for 80%, in light of everything, and the fundamental wellspring of failure and end from one side of the planet to the other. Recovery of circulation system (reperfusion) and contravention of cell injury (neuroprotection) are two potential treatment frameworks got in the organization of strokes [102, 103]. Extending evidence suggests that a blazing response is related with stroke and contributes by and large to mind injury [104]. In a MCAO-started preliminary frontal cortex injury model with pathogenesis taking after that of human ischemic stroke, cordycepin applies neuroprotective effects by preventing the outpouring of MMP-3, lessening glutamate and aspartate levels, working on the development of SOD, and reducing MDA levels [105]. The standardized *Cordyceps* in improved concentrate of *C. militaris*, which contains 8.2% (w/w) cordycepin, on a very basic level reduces the attack of ED-1-and MPO-positive searing cells into ischemic wounds, diminishes infarct volume, and debilitates cerebral edema and blood–mind limit hurts in MCAO rodents [102, 105, 106]. Likewise, cordycepin quite eases up frontal cortex edema, neurological lacks, and perihematomal tissue hurt after ICH, joined by an immense decline in the statement of HMGB1. Foolishly, cordycepin applies a neuroprotective effect in ICH models possibly through the prevention of NLRP3 inflammasome commencement [107]. Another assessment shows that cordycepin can enough get BBB genuineness by recovery of tight crossing point proteins, relief of close by exacerbation, and restriction of NOX activity [108].

Different sclerosis is a provocative demyelinating disease of the central tangible framework depicted by motor brokenness, neuro-aggravation, glial-cell institution, loss of foster oligodendrocytes, and axonal injury [109]. The CPZ-prompted demyelination model has been by and large used to assessment MS, especially in investigating de-and re-myelination in the corpus callosum. Cordycepin mitigates CPZ-prompted incidental effects in mice by protecting motor brokenness, propelling re-myelination, stifling glial-cell incitation, lessening the outpouring of the steady of combustible cytokines, IL-1β and IL-6, and growing the levels of the quieting cytokine IL-4 [101, 106, 110]. All around, cordycepin is useful in Parkinson's infection and applies its possessions generally by reducing oxidative pressing factor and against oxidant bothering through the TLR/NF-κB hailing pathway. Besides, cordycepin could further develop stroke by diminishing the infarct volume, reducing cerebral edema, controlling the levels of the connected cytokines, and obstructing the commencement of the NLRP3 inflammasome. Additionally, cordycepin applies impacts on MS through protecting motor brokenness, propelling re-myelination, stifling glial-cell incitation, and dealing with the steady of and against oxidant cytokines [111].

5.5 Dietary antioxidants

The effect of dietary affirmation of the malignant growth anticipation specialist's ascorbate, tocopherol, and carotenoids is difficult to disentangle by epidemiological assessments from other critical supplements and trimmings in verdant food sources [112, 113]. Taking everything into account, a couple of conflicts suggest that the disease avoidance specialist content of results of the dirt is a critical ally of their protective effect. Biochemical data, discussed above, show that oxidative damage is gigantic and is likely going to be the major endogenous mischief to DNA, proteins, and lipids [114]. Oxidative damage to sperm DNA is extended when dietary ascorbate is inadequate. Epidemiological assessments and intervention fundamentals on neutralization of harmful development and cardiovascular disease in people taking malignancy counteraction specialist supplements are interesting, notwithstanding, greater examinations ought to be done [115]. Clinical starters using disease anticipation specialists will be the essential test for an enormous number of considerations inspected here [116]. Studies on oxidative instruments and the investigation of infection transmission on malignant growth anticipation specialist protection for individual degenerative ailments are discussed underneath. Little particle dietary disease counteraction specialists [112, 117], for instance, supplement C (ascorbate), supplement E (tocopherol), and carotenoids have made explicit interest as adversaries of malignancy causing specialists and as shields against degenerative sicknesses [118]. Most carotenoids have cell support development, particularly against singlet oxygen, and many, including/ - carotene, can be utilized to supplement A (retinal) [119]. Earlier papers have called attention to different as of late dismissed physiological cell fortifications, including urate, bilirubin, carnosine, and ubiquinol [120]. Ubiquinone (CoQ1o), for example, is the fundamental little molecule for delivery electrons in mitochondria for the period of energy [121]. Its reduced construction, ubiquinol, is an amazing disease counteraction specialist in films [122]. Optimal levels of dietary ubiquinone/ubiquinol could be of importance in an enormous number of degenerative contaminations.

5.6 Respiratory system diseases

Cordyceps has been seemed to apply against oxidant impacts in exploratory models of avionics course provocative contaminations including extremely touchy asthma and intense lung injury [123]. Ominously vulnerable asthma is a continuous provocative sickness of the flight course divider that is depicted by means of aeronautics course aggravation, flying course divider overhauling, organic liquid hypersecretion, and avionics course hyper-responsiveness [12, 124]. It is credited to the infiltration of leukocytes including lymphocytes, eosinophils and neutrophils into the lungs. Also, the tallness of Th2 cytokines, for instance, IL-4, IL-5, and

IL-13, and extended levels of IgE are watched [38, 123, 125]. T accomplice type 2 (Th2) cells and the cytokines conveyed by them are clinically associated with the presentation of a wide range of asthma and are the fundamental drivers of extremely touchy asthma. The Th2 cytokine pathway is one of the rule centers in developing new prescriptions for asthma [126]. *Cordyceps* sp. has been all around archived by different assessment social affairs and is known to have expected therapeutic properties for the treatment of ominously defenseless asthma [127].

Cordycepin concedes the release of allergen-unequivocal IgE, eotaxin, and ICAM-1, decreases the BAL fluid Th2 cytokines IL-4, IL-5, and IL-13 levels, and tightens ovalbumin-driven cup cell hyperplasia, organic liquid hypersecretion, and AHR in a bit subordinate way in the ovalbumin-incited mouse exploratory easily affected asthma model [128]. Carelessly, cordycepin has against asthmatic properties including the deterrent of Th2-type responses, no doubt through interfering with the MAPKs and NF-κB hailing course pathways. In another assessment, cordycepin is appeared to basically subdue an ovalbumin-affected augmentation in eosinophil check; it smothers IL-17A and fabricates IL-10 cytokine levels in the BALF, and supports [129]. Treg responses and covers Th17 responses in ovalbumin-honed mice [130]. In an ovalbumin-started rat model of steady asthma, cordycepin tightens immunoglobulin IgE, eases up the avionics course divider thickness, and reduces eosinophils and neutrophils in the BALF. Noticeably, cordycepin decreases the upregulation of IL-5, IL-13, and TNF-α in the BALF, and controls the development of A2AAR mRNA and the decay of TGF-β1 explanation. Besides, *Cordyceps* when co-controlled with glucocorticoids shows synergistically huge feasibility in quelling avionics course remodeling [123, 131]. From these results it might be derived that cordycepin applies medicinal effects in negatively powerless asthma by upsetting eotaxin verbalization, conveying cytokines, and dealing with the Th1/Th2 balance. The ideal for combustible cytokines TNF-α, IL–1β, IL-6, IL-8, and IL-18 are among the most reassuring biomarkers for predicting bleakness and mortality [132]. LPS-impelled ALI models resemble certain features of human ALI; *Cordyceps* is found to exceptionally decrease neutrophil gathering and MPO activity in lung tissues, decay the production of provocative cytokines including TNF-α, IL-6, and IL-1β, and debilitate lung disturbance in this model apparently by the sanctioning of Nrf2 and upregulation of HO-1 verbalization [133]. The inhibitory effect of cordycepin on TNF-α and IL-6 emanation is debilitated by before association of SnPP, an amazing HO-1 inhibitor, including that cordycepin gives protection against ALI through inception of HO-1. Extraordinarily, cordycepin treatment constructs the combination of IL-10, which insistently oversees disturbance [126, 130, 132]. These examinations suggest that cordycepin can ease up ALI by lessening the social affair of neutrophils and the production of strong of red hot cytokines. SARS-CoV-2, the causative microorganism of Coronavirus Disease 2019 (COVID-19), has caused a pandemic of respiratory infirmity all throughout the planet. The quick famous replication is fundamentally associated with gigantic provocative cell entrance and raised strong of combustible cytokine/chemokine responses. Raised levels of the cytokines GCSF, IP10, MCP1, MIP1A, and TNF-α, are perceived in the plasma of patients who test positive for COVID-19, showing the cytokine storm that is connected with contamination earnestness [134]. Adenosine is an amazing regulator of disturbance, which intervenes its effects on cells by interfacing with four particular receptor subtypes, explicitly, A1, A2A, A2B, and A3 [135]. In particular, the impelling of adenosine receptors A2A and A3 could cause quieting impacts, which are intervened by the covering of steady of combustible cytokines [136]. These revelations showed the capacity of cordycepin in the treatment of COVID-19, hence, it was invaluable to moreover research its enemy of oxidant component activity.

5.7 Cataracts and antioxidants

Cararacts departure is the most generally perceived action in the overall around (65.5 million consistently) with expenses of more than 98.45 billion dollars [137, 138], has actually investigated the imperative confirmation that Cataract have an oxidative etiology and that dietary cell fortifications can prevent their game plan in individuals [139]. Five epidemiological examinations that have investigated the effect of dietary cell fortifications on Cataract show strong insurance effects of ascorbate, tocopherol, and carotenoids [140, 141]. Those individuals taking regular upgrades of ascorbate or tocopherol had around 33% the risk of making Cataract. Smoking, a genuine oxidative pressing factor, is a huge peril factor for Cataract, and radiation, an oxidative mutagen, is striking to cause Cataract [142]. Eye proteins show an extended level of methionine sulfoxide with age, and proteins in human Cataract have >60% of their methionine stores oxidized [143]. Pregnant mice depleted of glutathione, the essential sulfhydryl disease avoidance specialist in cells, produce any kind of future family with Cataract [144]. The most reassuring hindrance framework against Cataract radiates an impression of being to extend dietary malignancy anticipation specialists (cell reinforcement specialists) and to lessen smoking [145].

5.8 Brain dysfunction and antioxidants

Biochemical assessments recommend that oxidation may be huge in different brain pathologies [146]. A few epidemiological assessments are dependable with a guarded effect of verdant food varieties or cell fortifications [147] in different neurological pathologies, including mind ischemia, Parkinson disease, and familial amyotrophic level sclerosis (Lou Gehrig's disorder), a degenerative issue of motor neurons [148, 149]. Ischemic scenes free iron, a critical stimulus in reactions forming oxygen progressives; iron chelators diminish neuron incident after this injury [150]. In individuals encountering Parkinson's ailment, oxidative DNA hurt is raised inside mind districts rich in dopaminergic neurons (E. Overvik, J. Sanchez-Ramos, and B.N.A., unpublished work) [151]. The most convincing confirmation so far for an association between neurological issues and oxygen progressive improvement is the strong alliance found between familial amyotrophic sidelong sclerosis and changes in the Cu/Zn superoxide dismutase quality, suggesting that oxygen progressives might be obligated for the specific degeneration of motor neurons occurring in this deadly sickness [152–155]. The cautious piece of superoxide dismutase against frontal cortex injury due to ischemia is maintained by the finding that its overproduction is guarded in a transgenic mouse model [156]. Considering the similar cautious effects against ischemia-activated brain injury by limitation of NO turn of events, and the continuous evidence involving these two radical species in cytotoxicity of neuronal cells [157, 158], without a doubt peroxynitrite, a historic oxidant molded from the mix of Oj and NO (1%), expects a huge capacity in neuronal injury following ischemia and reperfusion [159].

6. Lack of side effects

Cordyceps containing bioactive compounds with lower health risk. A month after oral association of *Cordyceps* (5 mg/kg), the hematology, blood science, and hypochondriac changes of the rodents show no basic changes are comparable to those of the conventional rodents. Furthermore, the Ames test exhibits that *Cordyceps* is a non-mutagenic compound [160, 161]. Another report in mice shows that *Cordyceps* shows slight destructiveness when controlled at oral doses of 20 mg/kg for 21 days

[162]. *Cordyceps* is found to apply unsafe effects when controlled at a part of 8 mg/kg for 3 days. Signs of toxicity, for instance, wasting and detachment of the guts are not seen when *Cordyceps* is overseen at a bit of 2 mg/kg or lower [163]. What's more, following 3 days of intravenous imbuements association of *Cordyceps* (20 mg/kg) in beagle canines, *Cordyceps* shows no prescription related toxic substance levels, displaying the security profile of *Cordyceps* [164]. *Cordyceps* is noxious just to hurtful threat cells and doesn't show cytotoxicity toward strong cells, subsequently showing it's anything but a foe of infection expert [165, 166]. In any case, a previous report communicates that *Cordyceps* shows toxicity toward sound erythrocytes and maybe starts feebleness in patients with harm when used in chemotherapy [167]. Despite these promising prosperity profiles, comprehensive preclinical toxicological assessments on *Cordyceps* ought to be coordinated and further checked for their effects.

7. Pharmacodynamics

Being a *Cordyceps* species simple, physiologic and biochemical impacts of medications (specifically, drug tranquilizes), the metabolic and pharmacodynamics profiles of *Cordyceps* cordycepin resemble those of adenosine. In vivo breaks down recommend that *Cordyceps* can be utilized to 30-deoxyinosine coming about in light of the fast deamination by Adenosine deaminase, or may go through phosphorylation by adenosine kinase to be changed over into 30-deoxyadenosine mono-, di-, and triphosphate [168]. It has been suggested ahead of time that 30-deoxyinosine is an inactive metabolite, while 30-deoxyadenosine triphosphate is the powerful moiety at risk for the accommodating effects of *Cordyceps* [169]. A continuous report shows that 30-deoxyinosine can be changed over to the unique moiety, 30-deoxyadenosine triphosphate, in mammalian cells [170]. In addition, the pharmacokinetics and bioavailability examinations of *Cordyceps* show that it is held and released rapidly in rodents. *Cordyceps* has a short removal half-life ($t1/2$) of 1.6 min at a bit of 10 mg/kg when overseen intravenously. In the meantime, the region under the curve, most noteworthy obsession, and the opportunity of *Cordyceps* have been made plans to be 38.5 ± 10.3 min μg/ml, 3.1 ± 0.9 μg/l and 2.1 ± 1.2 L/min/kg, independently [171]. In a biopharmaceutical assessment study, *Cordyceps* is seemed to have low protein official, high plasma breathing space, low vulnerability, and high hepatic first-pass sway in vitro, which can explain the shortfall of its oral bioavailability [172].

8. Conclusion and future perspectives

As a working fragment of customary Chinese drug, *Cordyceps* species has been seen to have expansive enemy of oxidant and safe managerial effects of cordycepin. The sensitive rule of provocative safe response is another course for the improvement of imaginative meds for the treatment of resistant framework ailments. *Cordyceps* species has shown its probable accommodating motivating force in various red hot contamination models, for instance, asthma, Parkinson's, rheumatoid joint torment, atherosclerosis, pneumonia, hepatitis, and atopic dermatitis. Many hailing pathways including MAPKs, TGF-β/Smads, and NF-κB, Nrf2/HO-1, and Akt/GSK-3β/p70S6K check out the disturbance cycle in various afflictions/infections [173]. As of late investigations, RNA-seq demonstrated 1088 differentially imparted characteristics among CMsA and CMsB social events. Furthermore, oxidative phosphorylation-related Gene reasoning terms were up-overseen in CMsB social affairs. Additionally, the eventual outcomes of fundamental examination (FTIR range, monosaccharide sythesis, periodate oxidation) and bioactivity appraisal guessed that *C. militaris* polysaccharides had higher β-(1 → 6)- glucan substance and malignancy counteraction specialist practices in CMsB social occasions [174]. Similarly, the water remove (CW) contained the on a very basic level most significant substance of cordycepin, phenolics, and flavonoids, which were at risk for cell support activity. CW was the most grounded disease avoidance specialist. CW had for all intents and purposes indistinguishable 2,2′-diphenyl-1-picrylhydrazyl progressive looking through activity and lipid peroxidation restriction to l-ascorbic corrosive (96.9 ± 3.1%) and alpha-tocopherol (87.2 ± 1.0%). worked on the adequacy of CW, had no cytotoxicity sway and no skin irritation, conveyed the most CW (0.9 ± 0.0% w/w after 24 h), and passed on the most raised CW into the skin layer (33.5 ± 0.7% w/w) by Marsup and colleagus [175].

As indicated by zhu and associates examined the cell support activity related with the polysaccharides from *Cordyceps* cicadae (CP). To moreover research which of the division of CP had the best strength, in here, the in vitro cell support and in vivo against developing activities of the parts CP30–CP80 of CP were evaluated. The in vitro malignancy avoidance specialist development results revealed that every one of the divisions (for instance CP30–CP80) were incredible with CP70 as the most grounded. Conspicuously, CP70 postponed the future of Drosophila ($P < 0.05$), extended the activities of catalase (CAT) and glutathione peroxidase (GSH-Px) ($P < 0.01$), and subdued the plan of malondialdehyde (MDA) ($P < 0.01$). Also, CP70 upregulated the enunciation level of cell support related characteristics CAT, SOD1 and MTH in Drosophila ($P < 0.05$). These results showed that CP70 may draw out the future of Drosophila through the up-rule of the verbalization level of cell support related characteristics CAT, SOD1 and MTH in Drosophila. Thusly, polysaccharides from *Cordyceps* cicadae have gigantic malignant growth anticipation specialist and threatening to developing activities, and could be examined as another dietary upgrade to ruin the developing cycle [176].

In this assessment, the NBW-liquid maturing system was first settled to evaluate the effects of NBW on mycelia of *Cordyceps* militaris. The most raised mycelium center (3.90 mg/mL) and crude polysaccharides extraction yield (12.76%) were obtained in 25%-NBW (v/v) gathering. The malignancy counteraction specialist activities of mycelia were on a very basic level progressed after supplementation with NBW. The polysaccharides from 25%-NBW, 75%-NBW, and half NBW bundles showed the most grounded DPPH progressive, ABTS radical scrounging works out, and diminishing power, independently, achieving the most raised progressive looking through rate (practically 100% at 1.2 mg/mL), the least IC50 regard (1.09 mg/mL) and the most raised OD regard (2.13 at 2.0 mg/mL) [177].

In any case, there are still some data openings and limitations in energy research. First thing, most assessments revolve around the cell level; accordingly, more in vivo assessments in various animal models that appear as though human fanatical conditions and clinical applications are expected to support the sufficiency of *Cordyceps* in treating diverse blazing diseases and clarifying its nuclear parts. Second, a couple of examinations show that *Cordyceps* has staggering enemy of oxidant and safe authoritative contacts with less outcomes. Regardless, broad preclinical toxicological screens and clinical security research on *Cordyceps* are at this point inadequate. Accordingly, construct more productive assessments to survey the effects of its estimations on pharmacological activity and choose destructiveness so it will in general be used safely. Likewise, pharmacodynamics and active analyzes show that *Cordyceps* has a short half-life and vulnerable oral bioavailability generally in view of the quick deamination by adenosine deaminase (ADA), which confines its applications in affliction countering and treatment. Along these lines, the impediment of cordycepin to ADA addresses a basic issue which ought to be tended to in future assessment. Lately, this issue has been tended to through the mix of cordycepin and

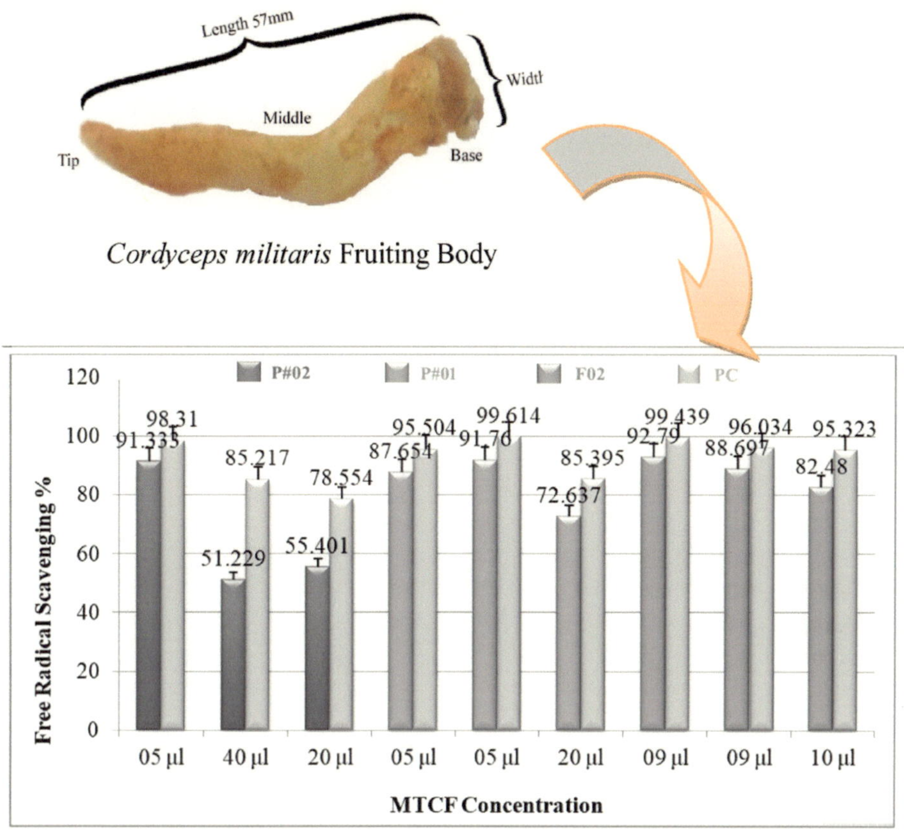

Figure 2.
Showing research output: Cordyceps militaris have broad spectrum free radical scavenging activity with their improved strains (P#01, P#02, F02).

ADA inhibitors to design ADA-safe cordycepin subordinates using nanotechnology or scaled down atom movement systems to fight ADA-resistance. These systems may be important for growing the oral bioavailability of cordycepin. Essential change is a promising system for procuring cordycepin auxiliaries with a respectable accommodating effect and high bioavailability. Appropriately, the insightful arrangement of new *Cordyceps* auxiliaries is of unfathomable vitality for the headway of new meds later on. With everything taken into account, more assessments are relied upon to progress cordycepin bioavailability and accomplish an amicability between its toxicological security and remedial practicality. This review intends to plot the medicinal potential and possible frameworks of *Cordyceps* in various provocative ailments and to give the reason to its use in the incredible treatment of searing issues (**Figure 2**).

Acknowledgements

The authors are obliged to Vice Chancellor, R.D. University, Jabalpur and interminable thankfulness to Director, Bio-Design Innovation Centre, R.D. University, Jabalpur (M.P.), for finishing this review & to avail in words for publication.

Conflict of interest

The authors declare no conflict of interest.

Author details

Loknath Deshmukh[1]*, Rajendra Singh[2] and Sardul Singh Sandhu[1]

1 Department of Biological Science, Bio-Design Innovation Centre, R.D. University, Jabalpur, M.P., India

2 Department of Biological Science, Fungal Biotechnology and Invertebrate Pathology Laboratory, R.D. University, Jabalpur, M.P., India

*Address all correspondence to: loknath.deshmukh3108@gmail.com

References

[1] Zhu JS et al. The scientific rediscovery of an ancient Chinese herbal medicine: *Cordyceps sinensis*: part I. J Altern Complement Med. 1998; 4: 289-303.

[2] Meena H, Mohsin M, Pandey HK, Negi PS, Ahmed Z. Estimation of cordycepin by improved HPLC method in the natural and cultured mycelia of high medicinal value Himalayan entomogenous fungus *Cordyceps sinensis*. EJEAF Che. 2010;9: 1598-603.

[3] Deshmukh, L., Agrawal, D., Sandhu, S.S., 2019. Development of Marker in the Soft Gold Mushroom *Cordyceps* spp. for Strain Improvement. In: Kundu R, Narila R. Advance in plant & microbial biotechnology. Springer Nature, Singapore; 2019.p.33-39.

[4] Pegler DN. The Chinese 'caterpillar fungus'. Mycologist. 1994; 8: 3-5.

[5] Mizuno T. Medicinal effects and utilization of *Cordyceps* (Fr.) Link (Ascomycetes) and Isaria Fr. (Mitosporic Fungi) Chinese caterpillar fungi, 'Tochukaso' (review). Int J Med Mushrooms. 1999; 1: 251-261.

[6] Hardeep S. Tuli, Anil K. Sharma, Sardul S. Sandhu, and Dharambir Kashyap. Cordycepin: A bioactive metabolite with therapeutic potential Life Sciences. 2013; 93:863-869.

[7] Sung GH, Hywel-Jones NL, Sung JM, Luangsa-ard JJ, Shrestha B, Spatafora JW. Phylogenetic classification of *Cordyceps* and the clavicipitaceous fungi. Stud Mycol. 2007; 57:5-59.

[8] Cunningham KG, Manson W, Spring FS, Hutchinson SA. Cordycepin, a metabolic product isolated from cultures of *Cordyceps militaris* (Linn.) link. Nature. 1950; 166:949-54.

[9] Li, N., Song, J.G., Liu, J.Y. and Zhang, H. Compared chemical composition between *Cordyceps militaris* and *Cordycpes sinensis*. Journal of Jilin Agriculture University. 1995; 17: 80-83. (in Chinese).

[10] Hur H. Chemical ingredients of *Cordyceps militaris*. Mycobiology. 2008; 36:233-5.

[11] Liu Y, Wang J, Wang W, Zhang H, Zhang X, Han C. The chemical constituents and pharmacological actions of *Cordyceps sinensis*. Evid Based Complement Alternat Med 2015;2015: 575063.

[12] Tuli HS, Sandhu SS, Sharma AK. Pharmacological and therapeutic potential of *Cordyceps* with special reference to cordycepin. Biotechnology. 2013;3. http://dx.doi.org/10.1007/s13205-013-0121-9.

[13] Lu H, Li X, Zhang J, Shi H, Zhu X, He X. Effects of cordycepin on HepG2 and EA. hy926 cells: potential antiproliferative, antimetastatic and anti-angiogenic effects on hepatocellular carcinoma. Oncol Lett. 2014; 7: 1556-1562.

[14] Kodama EN, McCaffrey RP, Yusa K and Mitsuya H: Antileukemic activity and mechanism of action of cordycepin against terminal deoxynucleotidyl transferasepositive (TdT+) leukemic cells. Biochem Pharmacol. 2000; 59:273-281.

[15] Rong Wu, Jian-Ping Gao, Hui-Lin Wang, Yan Gao, Qian Wu, Xiao-Hua Cui. Effects of fermented *Cordyceps sinensis* on oxidative stress in doxorubicin treated rats. 2015; 11, 44: 724-731.

[16] Shengli Yanga, Xi Yanga and Hui Zhangb. Extracellular polysaccharide biosynthesis in *Cordyceps*. 2020. https://doi.org/10.1080/1040841X.2020.1794788.

[17] Jian-Hui Xiao, Dai-Min Xiao, Dai-Xiong Chen, Yu Xiao, Zong-Qi Liang, and Jian-Jiang Zhong. Polysaccharides from the Medicinal Mushroom *Cordyceps* taii Show Antioxidant and Immunoenhancing Activities in aD-Galactose-Induced Aging Mouse Model. Evidence-Based Complementary and Alternative Medicine. 2012, Article ID 273435, 15 pages doi:10.1155/2012/273435.

[18] Park, E. S., Kang, D. H., Yang, M. K., Kang, J. C., Jang, Y. C., Park, J. S., Shin, H. S. Cordycepin, 30-deoxyadenosine, prevents rat hearts from ischemia/reperfusion injury via activation of Akt/GSK- 3β/p70S6K signaling pathway and HO-1 expression. Cardiovascular Toxicology. 2014; 14(1), 1-9. https://doi.org/10.1007/s12012-013-9232-0.

[19] Lei, J., Wei, Y., Song, P., Li, Y., Zhang, T., Feng, Q., & Xu, G. Cordycepin inhibits LPS-induced acute lung injury by inhibiting inflammation and oxidative stress. European Journal of Pharmacology. 2018; 818:110-114. https://doi.org/10.1016/j.ejphar.2017.10.029.

[20] Deshmukh, L., Singh, R., Sandhu, S.S. Far ranging antimicrobial and free radical scavenging activity of Himalayan soft gold mushroom; *Cordyceps sp*. Biotechnology and Biological Sciences. 2019; pp. 297-302. DOI: 10.1201/9781003001614-50.

[21] Hui Mei Yu, Bor-Sen Wang, Shiow Chyn Huang, and Pin-Der Duh. Comparison of Protective Effects between Cultured *Cordyceps* militaris and Natural *Cordyceps sinensis* against Oxidative Damage. J. Agric. Food Chem. 2006; 54:8,3132-3138 https://doi.org/10.1021/jf053111w.

[22] Deng-Bo Ji, Jia Ye, Chang-Ling Li, Yu-Hua Wang, Jiong Zhao and Shao-Qing Cai. Antiaging effect of *Cordyceps sinensis* extract. 2008. https://doi.org/10.1002/ptr.2576.

[23] Opeyemi J. Olatunji, Yan Fenga, Oyenike O. Olatunji, Jian Tanga, Yuan Wei a, Zhen Ouyanga, and Zhaoliang Suc. Polysaccharides purified from *Cordyceps cicadae* protects PC12 cells against glutamate-induced oxidative damage. Carbohydrate Polymers, 2016; 153, 187-195. doi:10.1016/j.carbpol.2016.06.108.

[24] Shen, W., Song, D., Wu, J., & Zhang, W. Protective effect of a polysaccharide isolated from a cultivated *Cordyceps* mycelia on hydrogen peroxide-induced oxidative damage in PC12 cells. Phytother. Res. 2010;25: 675-680. DOI: 10.1002/ptr.3320.

[25] Mei Tong He, Ah Young Lee, Chan Hum Park, and Eun Ju Cho. Protective effect of *Cordyceps militaris* against hydrogen peroxide-induced oxidative stress *in vitro.* Nutr Res Pract. 2019; 13(4): 279-285. doi: 10.4162/nrp.2019.13.4.279.

[26] Singh, M., Tulsawani, R., Koganti, P., Chauhan, A., Manickam, M., & Misra, K. *Cordyceps sinensis* Increases Hypoxia Tolerance by Inducing Heme Oxygenase-1 and Metallothione in via Nrf2 Activation in Human Lung Epithelial Cells. BioMed Research International. 2013; 1-13. doi:10.1155/2013/569206.

[27] Li, S. P., Zhao, K. J., Ji, Z. N., Song, Z. H., Dong, T. T.., Lo, C. K., Tsim, K. W. A polysaccharide isolated from *Cordyceps sinensis*, a traditional Chinese medicine, protects PC12 cells against hydrogen peroxide-induced injury. Life Sciences. 2003; 73(19), 2503-2513. doi:10.1016/s0024-3205(03)00652-0.

[28] Zhang, L., Wu, T., Olatunji, O. J., Tang, J., Wei, Y., & Ouyang, Z. N6-(2-hydroxyethyl)-adenosine from *Cordyceps cicadae* attenuates hydrogen peroxide induced oxidative toxicity in PC12 cells. Metabolic Brain Disease. 2019. doi:10.1007/s11011-019-00440-1.

[29] Liu, H., Cao, D., Liu, H., Liu, X., Mai, W., Lan, H., ... Zheng, Q. The Herbal Medicine *Cordyceps sinensis* Protects Pancreatic Beta Cells from Streptozotocin-Induced Endoplasmic Reticulum Stress. Canadian Journal of Diabetes. 2016; 40(4), 329-335. Doi:10.1016/j.jcjd.2016.02.001.

[30] Xiao, Y., Zhang, Q., Miao, J., Rui, X., Li, T., & Dong, M. (2015). Antioxidant activity and DNA damage protection of mung beans processed by solid state fermentation with *Cordyceps militaris* SN-18. Innovative Food Science & Emerging Technologies, 31, 216-225. doi:10.1016/j.ifset.2015.06.006.

[31] Li, Z., Zhang, Z., Zhang, J., Jia, J., Ding, J., Luo, R., & Liu, Z. *Cordyceps militaris* Extract Attenuates D-Galactose-Induced Memory Impairment in Mice. Journal of Medicinal Food. 2012; 15(12), 1057-1063. doi:10.1089/jmf.2011.2105.

[32] Wang, J., Chen, C., Jiang, Z., Wang, M., Jiang, H., & Zhang, X. Protective effect of *Cordyceps militaris* extract against bisphenol A induced reproductive damage. Systems Biology in Reproductive Medicine. 2016; 62(4),249-257. doi:10.1080/19396368.2016.1182234.

[33] Karbownik M and Reiter RJ. Antioxidative effects of melatonin in protection against cellular damage caused by ionizing radiation. Proc Soc Exp Biol Med. 2000; 225:9-22.

[34] Chen C, Luo SS, Li Y, Sun YJ and Zhang CK: Study on antioxidant activity of three *Cordyceps sp*. by chemiluminescence Shanghai. J Trad Chinese Med. 2004; 38:53-55.

[35] Yu HM, Wang BS, Huang SC and Duh PD. Comparison of protective effects between cultured *Cordyceps militaris* and natural *Cordyceps sinesis* against oxidative damage. J Agric Food Chem. 2006; 54:3132-3138.

[36] Ogawa Y, Kobayashi T, Nishioka A, et al. Radiation-induced reactive oxygen species (ROS) formation prior to oxidative DNA damage in human peripheral T cells. Int J Mol Med. 2003; 11:149-152.

[37] Chu HL, Chien JC and Duh PD. Protective effect of *Cordyceps militaris* against high glucose-induced oxidative stress in human umbilical vein endothelial cells. Food Chem. 2011; 129:871-876.

[38] Li SP, Zhang GH, Zeng Q, et al. Hypoglycemic activity of polysaccharide, with antioxidation, isolated from cultured *Cordyceps* mycelia. Phytomedicine. 2006; 13:428-33.

[39] Yan, F., Wang, B., & Zhang, Y. Polysaccharides from *Cordyceps sinensis* mycelium ameliorate exhaustive swimming exercise-induced oxidative stress. Pharmaceutical Biology. 2013; 52(2), 157-161. doi:10.3109/13880209.2013.820197.

[40] Overgaard-Hansen, K. The inhibition of 5-phosphoribosyl-1-pyrophosphate formation by cordycepin triphosphate in extracts of Ehrlich ascites tumor cells. Biochimica et Biophysica Acta (BBA) - Specialized Section on Nucleic Acids and Related Subjects. 1964; 80(3), 504-507. doi:10.1016/0926-6550(64)90154-9.

[41] Deshmukh, L., Sharma, A. K., & Sandhu, S. S. Contrive Himalayan Soft Gold *Cordyceps Species*: a Lineage of Eumycota Bestowing Tremendous Pharmacological and Therapeutic Potential. Current Pharmacology Reports. 2020. doi:10.1007/s40495-020-00223-8.

[42] Robins, M. J., & Robins, R. K. The Synthesis of 2′,3′-Dideoxyadenosine from 2′-Deoxyadenosine. Journal of the American Chemical Society. 1964; 86(17), 3585-3586. doi:10.1021/ja01071a055.

[43] Ota, T., Suzuki, Y., Nishikawa, T., Otsuki, T., Sugiyama, T., Irie, R., Nagai, K. Complete sequencing and characterization of 21,243 full-length human cDNAs. Nature Genetics. 2003; 36(1), 40-45. doi:10.1038/ng1285.

[44] Rottman, F., & Guarino, A. J. The inhibition of purine biosynthesis De novo in *Bacillus subtilis* by cordycepin. Biochimica et Biophysica Acta (BBA) - Specialized Section on Nucleic Acids and Related Subjects. 1964; 80(4), 640-647. doi:10.1016/0926 -6550(64)90308-1.

[45] S. Katayama et al. Antisense Transcription in the Mammalian Transcriptome. Science, (2005). 309(5740), 1564-1566. doi:10.1126/ science.1112009.

[46] Yi Liu, Jihui Wang, Wei Wang, Hanyue Zhang, Xuelan Zhang, and Chunchao Han. The Chemical Constituents and Pharmacological Actions of *Cordyceps sinensis.* Evidence-Based Complementary and Alternative Medicine. 2015; Article ID 575063, 12 pages http://dx.doi. org/10.1155/2015/575063.

[47] Liyang Yang, Guilan Li, Zhi Chai, Qiang Gong, Jianquan Guo. Synthesis of cordycepin: current scenario and future perspectives. Fungal Genetics and Biology. 2020; S1087-1845(20)30122-5. DOI: https://doi.org/10.1016/j. fgb.2020.103431.

[48] Ahn Y. J, Park S. J, Lee S. G, Shin S. C, Choi D. H. Cordycepin: Selective growth inhibitor derived from liquidculture of *Cordyceps militaris* against *Clostridium spp.* J Agric Food Chem. 2000;48:2744-8.

[49] Balon T. W, Jasman A. P, Zhu J. S. A fermentation product of *Cordyceps sinensis* increases whole-body insulinsensitivity in rats. J Altern Complement Med. 2002; 8:315-23.

[50] Xian-Bing Mao, Jian-Jiang Zhong. Significant effect of NH4+ on cordycepin production by submerged cultivation of medicinal mushroom *Cordyceps militaris.* Enzyme and Microbial Technology. 2006; 38:343-350. doi:10.1016/j. enzmictec.2004.10.010.

[51] M. Soltani, R. A. Malek, N. A. Elmarzugi, M. F. Mahomoodally, D. Uy, O. M. Leng, and H. A. El-Enshasy. Cordycepin: A Biotherapeutic Molecule from Medicinal Mushroom. Biology of Macrofungi, Fungal Biology, 2018; 319-349. https://doi. org/10.1007/978-3-030-02622-6_16.

[52] Ji-Sue Baik, Seo-Won Mun, Kyoung-Sook Kim, Shin-Ji Park, Hyun-Kyoung Yoon, Dong-Hyun Kim, Min-Kyu Park, Cheorl-Ho Kim, and Young-Choon Lee. Apoptotic Effects of Cordycepin Through the Extrinsic Pathway and p38 MAPK Activation in Human Glioblastoma U87MG Cells. J. Microbiol. Biotechnol. 2016; 26(2), 309-314. http:// dx.doi.org/10.4014/jmb.1507.07090.

[53] Boontariga Wongsaa, Nachon Raethongb, Pramote Chumnanpuena,c, Jirasak Wong-ekkabutc,d, Kobkul Laotenge, Wanwipa Vongsangnak. Alternative metabolic routes in channeling xylose to cordycepin production of *Cordyceps militaris* identified by comparative transcriptome analysis. Genomics. 2019. https://doi. org/10.1016/j.ygeno.2019.04.015.

[54] Roypim Thananusak, Kobkul Laoteng, Nachon Raethong, Yu Zhang and Wanwipa Vongsangnak. Metabolic Responses of Carotenoid and Cordycepin Biosynthetic Pathways in *Cordyceps militaris* under Light-Programming Exposure through Genome-Wide Transcriptional Analysis. Biology 2020, 9, 242. doi:10.3390/ biology9090242.

[55] Haisheng lu, Xiting li, Jianying zhang, Hui shi, Xiaofeng zhu and

Xiaoshun he. Effects of cordycepin on HepG2 and EA.hy926 cells: Potential antiproliferative, antimetastatic and anti-angiogenic effects on hepatocellular carcinoma, oncology letters. 2014; 7: 1556-1562. DOI: 10.3892/ol.2014.1965.

[56] Dong, J. Z., Ding, J., Yu, P. Z., Lei, C., Zheng, X. J., & Wang, Y. Composition and distribution of the main active components in selenium-enriched fruit bodies of *Cordyceps militaris* link. Food Chemistry. 2013; 137(1-4), 164-167. doi:10.1016/j.foodchem.2012.10.021.

[57] Hu, T., Liang, Y., Zhao, G. *et al.* Selenium Biofortification and Antioxidant Activity in *Cordyceps militaris* Supplied with Selenate, Selenite, or Selenomethionine. Biol Trace Elem Res. 2019; 187, 553-561. https://doi.org/10.1007/s12011-018-1386-y.

[58] Song, J., Wang, Y., Teng, M., Cai, G., Xu, H., Guo, H., Teng, L. Studies on the Antifatigue Activities of *Cordyceps militaris* Fruit Body Extract in Mouse Model. Evidence-Based Complementary and Alternative Medicine. 2015; 1-15. doi:10.1155/2015/174616.

[59] Shin, K. H., Lim, S. S., Lee, S. H., Lee, Y. S., & Cho, S. Y. Antioxidant and Immunostimulating Activities of the Fruiting Bodies of Paecilomyces japonica, a New Type of *Cordyceps sp.* Annals of the New York Academy of Sciences. 2006; 928(1), 261-273. doi:10.1111/j.1749-6632.2001.tb05655.x.

[60] Yamaguchi, Y., Kagota, S., Nakamura, K., Shinozuka, K., & Kunitomo, M. Inhibitory effects of water extracts from fruiting bodies of cultured *Cordyceps sinensis* on raised serum lipid peroxide levels and aortic cholesterol deposition in atherosclerotic mice. Phytotherapy Research. 2000; 14(8), 650-652. doi:10.1002/1099-1573(200012)14:8<650::aid-ptr675>3.0.co;2-0.

[61] N. Singpoonga, R. Rittiron, B. Seang-on, and P. Chaiprasart, Determination of Adenosine and Cordycepin Concentrations in *Cordyceps militaris* Fruiting Bodies Using Near-Infrared spectroscopy. ACS Omega. 2020; 5, 27235–27244. https://dx.doi.org/10.1021/acsomega.0c03403.

[62] Lin, R., Liu, H., Wu, S., Pang, L., Jia, M., Fan, K., ... Jia, L. Production and in vitro antioxidant activity of exopolysaccharide by a mutant, *Cordyceps militaris* SU5-08. International Journal of Biological Macromolecules. 2012; 51(1-2), 153-157. doi:10.1016/j.ijbiomac.2012.04.011.

[63] Li, Y., Yang, H., Yang, H. *et al.* Assessment of drying methods on the physiochemical property and antioxidant activity of *Cordyceps militaris*. Food Measure. 2019; 13, 513-520. https://doi.org/10.1007/s11694-018-9965-3.

[64] Leung, P. H., Zhao, S., Ho, K. P., & Wu, J. Y. Chemical properties and antioxidant activity of exopolysaccharides from mycelial culture of *Cordyceps sinensis* fungus Cs-HK1. Food Chemistry. 2009; 114(4), 1251-1256. doi:10.1016/j.foodchem.2008.10.081.

[65] Won, S.-Y., & Park, E.-H. Anti-inflammatory and related pharmacological activities of cultured mycelia and fruiting bodies of *Cordyceps militaris*. Journal of Ethnopharmacology. 2005; 96(3), 555-561. doi:10.1016/j.jep.2004.10.009.

[66] Yang, T., Guo, M., Yang, H. et al. The blue-light receptor CmWC-1 mediates fruit body development and secondary metabolism in *Cordyceps militaris*. Appl Microbiol Biotechnol. 2016; 100, 743-755 (2016). https://doi.org/10.1007/s00253-015-7047-6.

[67] Kramer, G.J., Nodwell, J.R. Chromosome level assembly and

secondary metabolite potential of the parasitic fungus *Cordyceps militaris*. BMC Genomics 2017; 18, 912. https://doi.org/10.1186/s12864-017-4307-0.

[68] Woolley, V. C., Teakle, G. R., Prince, G., de Moor, C. H., & Chandler, D. Cordycepin, a metabolite of *Cordyceps militaris*, reduces immune-related gene expression in insects. Journal of Invertebrate Pathology. 2020; 107480. doi:10.1016/j.jip.2020.107480.

[69] Lu, Y., Luo, F., Cen, K., Xiao, G., Yin, Y., Li, C., Wang, C. Omics data reveal the unusual asexual-fruiting nature and secondary metabolic potentials of the medicinal fungus *Cordyceps cicadae*. BMC Genomics. 2017; 18(1). doi:10.1186/s12864-017-4060-4.

[70] Yang, T., Guo, M., Yang, H., Guo, S., & Dong, C. The blue-light receptor CmWC-1 mediates fruit body development and secondary metabolism in *Cordyceps* militaris. Applied Microbiology and Biotechnology. 2015; 100(2), 743-755. doi:10.1007/s00253-015-7047-6.

[71] Kramer, G. J., & Nodwell, J. R. Chromosome level assembly and secondary metabolite potential of the parasitic fungus *Cordyceps* militaris. BMC Genomics. 2017; 18(1). doi:10.1186/s12864-017-4307-0.

[72] Jiaojiao, Z., Fen, W., Kuanbo, L. *et al.* Heat and light stresses affect metabolite production in the fruit body of the medicinal mushroom *Cordyceps militaris*. Appl Microbiol Biotechnol. 2018; 102, 4523-4533. https://doi.org/10.1007/s00253-018-8899-3.

[73] Yu, H. M., Wang, B.-S., Huang, S. C., & Duh, P.-D. Comparison of Protective Effects between Cultured *Cordyceps militaris* and Natural *Cordyceps sinensis* against Oxidative Damage. Journal of Agricultural and Food Chemistry. 2006; 54(8), 3132-3138. doi:10.1021/jf053111w.

[74] Ashraf, S. A., Elkhalifa, A. E. O., Siddiqui, A. J., Patel, M., Awadelkareem, A. M., Snoussi, M., ... Hadi, S. Cordycepin for Health and Wellbeing: A Potent Bioactive Metabolite of an Entomopathogenic Medicinal Fungus *Cordyceps* with Its Nutraceutical and Therapeutic Potential. Molecules. 2020; 25(12), 2735. doi:10.3390/molecules25122735.

[75] Buenz, E. J., Weaver, J. G., Bauer, B. A., Chalpin, S. D., & Badley, A. D. *Cordyceps sinensis* extracts do not prevent Fas-receptor and hydrogen peroxide-induced T-cell apoptosis. Journal of Ethnopharmacology. 2004; 90(1), 57-62. doi:10.1016/j.jep.2003.09.025.

[76] Dong, C.-H., & Yao, Y.-J. In vitro evaluation of antioxidant activities of aqueous extracts from natural and cultured mycelia of *Cordyceps sinensis*. LWT - Food Science and Technology. 2008; 41(4), 669-677. doi:10.1016/j.lwt.2007.05.002.

[77] Yan, J.-K., Wang, W.-Q., & Wu, J.-Y. Recent advances in *Cordyceps sinensis* polysaccharides: Mycelial fermentation, isolation, structure, and bioactivities: A review. Journal of Functional Foods. 2014; 6, 33-47. doi:10.1016/j.jff.2013.11.024.

[78] Jin, LQ., Xu, ZW., Zhang, B. *et al.* Genome sequencing and analysis of fungus Hirsutella *sinensis* isolated from *OphioCordyceps sinensis*. AMB Expr. 2020;10, 105. https://doi.org/10.1186/s13568-020-01039-x.

[79] Buranrat B, Sangdee K, Thammawat S, Sangdee A. Mechanisms of crude protein from medicinal mushroom *Ophiocordyceps sobolifera* against human breast MCF-7 cancer cells. Biologia. 2020. https://doi.org/10.2478/s11756-020-00482-2.

[80] Zhang, Z., Lv, G., Pan, H., Fan, L., Soccol, C. R., & Pandey, A. Production

of powerful antioxidant supplements via solid-state fermentation of wheat (*Triticum aestivum* Linn.) by *Cordyceps militaris*. Food Technology and Biotechnology. 2012; 50(1), 32-39.

[81] Kang, H. J., Baik, H. W., Kim, S. J., Lee, S. G., Ahn, H. Y., Park, J. S., ... Lee, S. M. *Cordyceps militaris* Enhances Cell-Mediated Immunity in Healthy Korean Men. Journal of Medicinal Food. 2015; 18(10), 1164-1172. doi:10.1089/jmf.2014.3350.

[82] Jin, J., Kang, W., Zhong, C., Qin, Y., Zhou, R., Liu, H., ... Zhang, S. (2018). The pharmacological properties of *OphioCordyceps xuefengensis* revealed by transcriptome analysis. Journal of Ethnopharmacology. 2018; 219, 195-201. doi:10.1016/j.jep.2018.02.007.

[83] Qin, Y., Zhou, R., Jin, J., Xie, J., Liu, H., Cai, P., ... Zhang, S. UPLC-ESI-Q-TOF-MS/MS analysis of anticancer fractions from *OphioCordyceps xuefengensis* and *OphioCordyceps sinensis*. Biomedical Chromatography. 2020; e4841. doi:10.1002/bmc.4841.

[84] Ng, T. B., & Wang, H. X. Pharmacological actions of *Cordyceps*, a prized folk medicine. Journal of Pharmacy and Pharmacology. 2005; 57(12), 1509-1519. doi:10.1211/jpp.57.12.0001.

[85] Quan, X., Kwak, B. S., Lee, J.-Y., Park, J. H., Lee, A., Kim, T. H., & Park, S. *Cordyceps militaris* Induces Immunogenic Cell Death and Enhances Antitumor Immunogenic Response in Breast Cancer. Evidence-Based Complementary and Alternative Medicine, 2020, 1-11. doi:10.1155/2020/9053274.

[86] Das, S. K., Masuda, M., Sakurai, A., & Sakakibara, M. Medicinal uses of the mushroom *Cordyceps militaris*: Current state and prospects. Fitoterapia. 2010; 81(8), 961-968. doi:10.1016/j.fitote.2010.07.010.

[87] Kuo, H.-C., Su, Y.-L., Yang, H.-L., & Chen, T.-Y. Identification of Chinese Medicinal Fungus *Cordyceps sinensis* by PCR-Single-Stranded Conformation Polymorphism and Phylogenetic Relationship. Journal of Agricultural and Food Chemistry. 2005; 53(10), 3963-3968. doi:10.1021/jf0482562.

[88] Jo, E., Jang, H.-J., Shen, L., Yang, K. E., Jang, M. S., Huh, Y. H., ... Park, S. J. *Cordyceps militaris* Exerts Anticancer Effect on Non–Small Cell Lung Cancer by Inhibiting Hedgehog Signaling via Suppression of TCTN3. Integrative Cancer Therapies. 2020; 19, 153473542092375. doi:10.1177/1534735420923756.

[89] Yue, K., Ye, M., Zhou, Z., Sun, W., & Lin, X. The genus *Cordyceps*: a chemical and pharmacological review. Journal of Pharmacy and Pharmacology. 2012; 65(4), 474-493. doi:10.1111/j.2042-7158.2012.01601.x .

[90] Xu, G., Yuan, G., Lu, X., An, L., Sheng, Y., & Du, P. Study on the effect of regulation of *Cordyceps* militaris polypeptide on the immune function of mice based on a transcription factor regulatory network. Food & Function. 2020. doi:10.1039/d0fo01043j.

[91] Won, S.-Y., & Park, E.-H. Anti-inflammatory and related pharmacological activities of cultured mycelia and fruiting bodies of *Cordyceps militaris*. Journal of Ethnopharmacology. 2005; 96(3), 555-561. doi:10.1016/j.jep.2004.10.009.

[92] Marchbank, T., Ojobo, E., Playford, C. J., & Playford, R. J. Reparative properties of the traditional Chinese medicine *Cordyceps sinensis* (Chinese caterpillar mushroom) using HT29 cell culture and rat gastric damage models of injury. British Journal of Nutrition. 2011; 105(09), 1303-1310. doi:10.1017/s0007114510005118.

[93] Pirinccioglu AG, Gökalp D, Pirinccioglu M, Kizil G, Kizil M.

Malondialdehyde (MDA) and protein carbonyl (PCO) levels as biomarkers of oxidative stress in subjects with familial hypercholesterolemia. Clin Biochem. 2010; 43:1220-4.

[94] Zhang J, Yu Y, Zhang Z, Ding Y, Dai X, Li Y. Effect of polysaccharide from cultured *Cordyceps sinensis* on immune function and anti-oxidation activity of mice exposed to 60Co. Int Immunopharmacol. 2011; 11:2251-7.

[95] Takemura G, Fujiwara H. Doxorubicin-induced cardiomyopathy from the cardiotoxic mechanisms to management. Prog Cardiovasc Dis. 2007; 49:330-52.

[96] Rong Wu, Jian-Ping Gao, Hui-Lin Wang, Yan Gao, Qian Wu, and Xiao-Hua Cui. Effects of fermented *Cordyceps sinensis* on oxidative stress in doxorubicin treated rats. Pharmacogn Mag. 2015, 11(44): 724-731.doi: 10.4103/0973-1296.165562.

[97] Eunhyun Choi, Junsang Oh & Gi-Ho Sung. Antithrombotic and Antiplatelet Effects of *Cordyceps militaris*. Mycobiology. 2020; 48:3, 228-232, DOI:1 0.1080/12298093.2020.1763115.

[98] Buenz, E. J., Bauer, B. A., Osmundson, T. W., & Motley, T. J. The traditional Chinese medicine *Cordyceps sinensis* and its effects on apoptotic homeostasis. Journal of Ethnopharmacology. 2005; 96(1-2), 19-29. doi:10.1016/j.jep.2004.09.029.

[99] Wang, J., Liu, Y.-M., Cao, W., Yao, K.-W., Liu, Z.-Q., & Guo, J.-Y. Anti-inflammation and antioxidant effect of Cordymin, a peptide purified from the medicinal mushroom *Cordyceps sinensis*, in middle cerebral artery occlusion-induced focal cerebral ischemia in rats. Metabolic Brain Disease. 2012; 27(2), 159-165. doi:10.1007/s11011-012-9282-1.

[100] Onasanwo, S. A., Oyagbemi, A. A., & Saba, A. B. Anti-inflammatory and analgesic properties of the ethanolic extract of *Cnidoscolus aconitifolius* in rats and mice. Journal of Basic and Clinical Physiology and Pharmacology. 2011; 22(1-2). doi:10.1515/jbcpp.2011.010.

[101] Min Yin, Na Li, Emmanuel Ayobami Makinde, Opeyemi Joshua Olatunji & Ziyuan Ni. N6 -2-hydroxyethyl-adenosine ameliorate cisplatin induced acute kidney injury in mice, All Life. 2020; 13:1, 244-251, DOI: 10.1080/26895293.2020.1760149.

[102] Yang, N.-N., Jiang, N., Ma, Q.-Y., Kong, F.-D., Xie, Q.-Y., Zhou, L.-M., ... Zhao, Y.-X. Chemical study of the strain *Cordyceps spp.* from cell fusion between *Cordyceps militaris* and *Cordyceps cicadae*. Journal of Asian Natural Products Research. 2018; 1-7. doi:10.108 0/10286020.2018.1451518.

[103] Thongchai, S., Sangdee, K. & Sangdee, A. Antibacterial activity of crude protein and development of species-specific molecular marker for fungus *OphioCordyceps sobolifera*. Biologia. 2020. https://doi.org/10.2478/ s11756-020-00589-6.

[104] Xiao, Y., Zhang, Q., Miao, J., Rui, X., Li, T., & Dong, M. Antioxidant activity and DNA damage protection of mung beans processed by solid state fermentation with *Cordyceps militaris* SN-18. Innovative Food Science & Emerging Technologies. 2015; 31, 216-225. doi:10.1016/j.ifset.2015.06.006.

[105] Yadav, R. Entomopathogenic Mushroom (*Cordyceps sp.*) as Immunity Booster. Biotica Research Today. 2020; 2, 7 (Jul. 2020), 690-692.

[106] Yao, L.-H., Li, C.-H., Yan, W.-W., Huang, J.-N., Liu, W.-X., & Xiao, P. Cordycepin decreases activity of hippocampal CA1 pyramidal neuron through membrane hyperpolarization. Neuroscience Letters. 2011; 503(3), 256-260. doi:10.1016/j. neulet.2011.08.048.

[107] Cheng, C., & Zhu, X. Cordycepin mitigates MPTP-induced Parkinson's disease through inhibiting TLR/NF-κB signaling pathway. Life Sciences. 2019. doi:10.1016/j.lfs.2019.02.037.

[108] Ying Sun, Wen-min Huang, Pei-chen Tang, Xin Zhang, Xiao-yan Zhang, Bo cheng Yu, Yi-Yun Fan, Xiao-qun Ge, Xiao-Ling Zhang. Neuroprotective effects of natural cordycepin on LPS-induced Parkinson's disease through suppressing TLR4/NF-κB/NLRP3-mediated pyroptosis. Journal of Functional Foods. 2020; 104274 https://doi.org/10.1016/j.jff.2020.104274.

[109] Olatunji, O. J., Feng, Y., Olatunji, O. O., Tang, J., Ouyang, Z., & Su, Z. Cordycepin protects PC12 cells against 6-hydroxydopamine induced neurotoxicity via its antioxidant properties. Biomedicine & Pharmacotherapy. 2016; 81, 7-14. doi:10.1016/j.biopha.2016.03.009

[110] He, M.T., Lee, A.Y., Kim, J.H. et al. Protective role of *Cordyceps militaris* in $A\beta_{1-42}$-induced Alzheimer's disease in vivo. Food Sci Biotechnol. 2019; 28, 865-872. https://doi.org/10.1007/s10068-018-0521-z.

[111] He, M. T., Lee, A. Y., Kim, J. H., Park, C. H., Shin, Y. S., & Cho, E. J. Protective role of *Cordyceps militaris* in Aβ1-42-induced Alzheimer's disease in vivo. Food Science and Biotechnology. 2018. doi:10.1007/s10068-018-0521-z.

[112] Yang, H.-Y., Leu, S.-F., Wang, Y.-K., Wu, C.-S., & Huang, B.-M. *Cordyceps sinensis* mycelium induces MA-10 mouse leydig tumor cell apoptosis by activating the caspase-8 pathway and suppressing the NF-κB pathway. Archives of Andrology. 2006; 52(2), 103-110. doi:10.1080/01485010500315818.

[113] Qian, G., Pan, G.-F., & Guo, J.-Y. Anti-inflammatory and antinociceptive effects of cordymin, a peptide purified from the medicinal mushroom *Cordyceps sinensis*. Natural Product Research. 2012; 26(24), 2358-2362. doi:10.1080/14786419.2012.658800.

[114] Au, D., Wang, L., Yang, D., Mok, D. K. W., Chan, A. S. C., & Xu, H. Application of microscopy in authentication of valuable Chinese medicine i-*Cordyceps sinensis*, its counterfeits, and related products. Microscopy Research and Technique. 2012; 75(1), 54-64. doi:10.1002/jemt.21024.

[115] Long, H., Qiu, X., Cao, L., Liu, G., Rao, Z., Han, R., Toxicological safety evaluation of the cultivated Chinese *Cordyceps*, Journal of Ethnopharmacology. 2020. https://doi.org/10.1016/ j.jep.2020.113600.

[116] Neeranjini Nallathamby, Sri Nurestri Abd Malek, Sharmili Vidyadaran, Chia-Wei Phan, Vikineswary Sabaratnam. Lipids in an Ethyl Acetate Fraction of Caterpillar Medicinal Mushroom, *Cordyceps militaris* (Ascomycetes), Reduce Nitric Oxide Production in BV2 Cells via Nrf2 and NF-? B Pathways. DOI: 10.1615/IntJMedMushrooms.2020037001.

[117] Wang, L., He, Y., Li, Y., Pei, C., Olatunji, O. J., Tang, J., ... Yan, B. Protective effects of nucleosides-rich extract from *Cordyceps cicadae* against cisplatin induced testicular damage. Chemistry & Biodiversity. 2020. doi:10.1002/cbdv.202000671.

[118] Eunhyun Choi, Junsang Oh & Gi-Ho Sung. Beneficial Effect of *Cordyceps militaris* on Exercise Performance via Promoting Cellular Energy Production, Mycobiology. 2020; 48:6, 512-517, DOI: 10.1080/12298093.2020.1831135.

[119] Xiong C, Xia Y, Zheng P et al. Increasing oxidative stress tolerance and subculturing stability of *Cordyceps militaris* by overexpression of a

glutathione peroxidase gene. Appl Microbiol Biotechnol. 2013; 97(5):2009-2015.

[120] Rintu Das, Silpak Biswas and Ena Ray Banerjee. Nutraceutical-prophylactic and Therapeutic Role of Functional Food in Health. J Nutr Food Sci. 2016; 6:4. http://dx.doi.org/10.4172/2155-9600.1000527.

[121] Zhang Y, Xu L, Zhang S, et al. Genetic diversity of *OphioCordyceps sinensis*, a medicinal fungus endemic to the Tibetan Plateau: implications for its evolution and conservation. BMC Evol Biol. 2009; 9(1):290.

[122] Qin, P.; Wang, Z.; Lu, D.; Kang, H.; Li, G.; Guo, R.; Zhao, Y.; Han, R.; Ji, B.; Zeng, Y. Neutral Lipid Content in Lipid Droplets: Potential Biomarker of Cordycepin Accumulation in Cordycepin-Producing Fungi. *Molecules.* 2019; *24*, 3363.

[123] Wang, Ningqun; Li, Jie; Huang, Xiaobo; Chen, Wenqiang; Chen, Yujing. Herbal Medicine (*Cordyceps sinensis*) Improves Health-Related Quality of Life in Moderate-to-Severe Asthma. Evidence-Based Complementary and Alternative Medicine. 2016; 1-8. doi:10.1155/2016/6134593.

[124] Patel, V. J., Biswas Roy, S., Mehta, H. J., Joo, M., & Sadikot, R. T. (2018). Alternative and Natural Therapies for Acute Lung Injury and Acute Respiratory Distress Syndrome. BioMed Research International. 2018; 1-9. doi:10.1155/2018/2476824.

[125] X. Yang, Y. Li, Y. He et al., Cordycepin alleviates airway hyperreactivity in a murine model of asthma by attenuating the inflammatory process. International Immunopharmacology. 2015; 26: 2, 401-408.

[126] J. C. Heo, S. H. Nam, D. Y. Nam, J. G. Kim, K. G. Lee, and J. H. Yeo. Anti-asthmatic activities in mycelial extract and culture filtrate of *Cordyceps* sphecocephala J201. International Journal of Molecular Medicine. 2010; 26:3, 351-356.

[127] K. Samitas, V. Delimpoura, E. Zervas, and M. Gaga. Anti-IgE treatment, airway inflammation and remodelling in severe allergic asthma: current knowledge and future perspectives. European Respiratory Review. 2015; 24:138, 594-601.

[128] Yue-Qin, C., Ning, W., Hui, Z., & Liang-Hu, Q. Differentiation of Medicinal *Cordyceps species* by rDNA ITS Sequence Analysis. Planta Medica. 2002; 68(7), *635-639.* doi:10.1055/s-2002-32892.

[129] Liu, Y.-N., Liu, B.-Y., Ma, Y.-C., Yang, H.-L., & Liu, G.-Q. (2020). Analysis of reference genes stability and histidine kinase expression under cold stress in *Cordyceps militaris.* Plos one. 2020; 15(8) e0236898. doi:10.1371/journal.pone.0236898.

[130] Shrestha B, Zhang W, Zhang Y, Liu X. What is the Chinese caterpillar fungus *OphioCordyceps sinensis* (Ophiocordycipitaceae)? Mycol. Int J Fungal Biol. 2010; 1:228-236. https://doi.org/10.1080/21501203.2010.536791.

[131] Sangdee A, Sangdee K. Isolation, identification, culture and production of adenosine and cordycepin from cicada larva infected with entomopathogenic fungi in Thailand. Afr J Microbiol Res. 2013; 7(2):137-146. https://doi.org/10.5897/AJMR12.1038.

[132] Y.-C. Kuo, W.-J. Tsai, J.-Y. Wang, S.-C. Chang, C.-Y. Lin, and M.-S. Shiao. Regulation of Broncho alveolar lavage fluids cell function by the immunomodulatory agents from *Cordyceps sinensis*. Life Sciences. 2001; 68:9, 1067-1082.

[133] Peng XX, Chai YQ, Zhu BC, Jin YW, Li XL, Yu LS. The protective

effects of N6-(2-hydroxyethyl)-adenosine extracted from *OphioCordyceps sobolifera* on renal ischemia reperfusion injury (IRI) in mice. Mycosystema. 2015; 34:311-320. http://jtp.cnki.net/bilingual/detail/html/JWXT201502016.

[134] Chen, G.-S., Huang, K.-F., Huang, C.-C., & Wang, J.-Y. Thaliporphine Derivative Improves Acute Lung Injury after Traumatic Brain Injury. BioMed Research International. 2015; 1-10. doi:10.1155/2015/729831.

[135] Chyau CC, Chen CC, Chen JC, Yang TC, Shu KH, Cheng CH. Mycelia glycoproteins from *Cordyceps sobolifera* ameliorate cyclosporine-induced renal tubule dysfunction in rats. J Ethnopharmacol. 2014; 153:650-658. https://doi.org/10.1016/j.jep.2014.03.020.

[136] Huo, M., Cui, X., Xue, J., Chi, G., Gao, R., Deng, X., ... Wang, D. Anti-inflammatory effects of linalool in RAW 264.7 macrophages and lipopolysaccharide-induced lung injury model. Journal of Surgical Research. 2013; 180(1), e47–e54. doi: 10.1016/j.jss.2012.10.050.

[137] Sperduto, R. D. The Linxian Cataract Studies. Archives of Ophthalmology. 1993; 111(9), 1246. doi:10.1001/archopht.1993.01090090098027.

[138] Flaxman SR, Bourne RR, Resnikoff S, Ackland P, Braithwaite T, Cicinelli MV, Das A, Jonas JB, Keeffe J, Kempen JH, Leasher J, Limburg H, Naidoo K, et al. Vision Loss Expert Group of the Global Burden of Disease Study. Global causes of blindness and distance vision impairment 1990-2020: a systematic review and meta-analysis. Lancet Glob Health. 2017; 5:e1221-34. https://doi.org/10.1016/S2214-109X(17)30393-5.

[139] Shuqi Liang, Shengqian Dou, Wenfeng Li, and Yusen Huang. Profiling of circular RNAs in age-related cataract reveals circ ZNF292 as an antioxidant by sponging miR-23b-3p. Aging. 2020; 12:17:17271-17287.

[140] Li, L., Li, S., Wang, S., Xing, X., Zhang, Y., Su, L., ... Gong, X. Antioxidant and anti-glycated TAT-modified platinum nanoclusters as eye drops for non-invasive and painless relief of diabetic cataract in rats. Chemical Engineering Journal. 2020; 398, 125436. doi:10.1016/j.cej.2020.125436.

[141] Heidari, N., Jabbari, M., Babashahi, M., Nabie, R., Asghari Jafarabadi, M. and Arefhosseini, S.R. The association between healthy eating index and serum antioxidant indices in patients with different degrees of cataract compared to healthy subjects: a case-control study. Nutrition & Food Science. 2020. https://doi.org/10.1108/NFS-04-2020-0153.

[142] Shuqi Liang, Shengqian Dou, Wenfeng Li,Yusen Huang. Profiling of circular RNAs in age-related cataract reveals circZNF292 as an antioxidant by sponging miR-23b-3p. Aging. 2020; 12:17. doi: 10.18632/aging.103683.

[143] Ling, X., Jarubula, R. Synthesis of Negatively Charged CeO_2 NPs and in Vitro Cytotoxicity Human Lens Epithelial (HLE) Cell Lines—Investigation for New Therapy for Cataract Treatment. J Inorg Organomet Polym. 2020. https://doi.org/10.1007/s10904-020-01793-2.

[144] Roupas, Peter; Keogh, Jennifer; Noakes, Manny; Margetts, Christine; Taylor, Pennie. The role of edible mushrooms in health: Evaluation of the evidence. Journal of Functional Foods. 2012; 4(4), 687-709. doi:10.1016/j.jff.2012.05.003.

[145] Spector A. Oxidative stress-induced cataract: mechanism of action. FASEB J. 1995; 9:1173-82. https://doi.org/10.1096/fasebj.9.12.7672510.

[146] Ravindran Kalathil Veena, Eluvathingal Joy Carme, Haridas Ramya, Thekkuttuparambil Ananthanarayanan Ajith, Solomon P Wasser, Kainoor K Janardhanan. Caterpillar Medicinal Mushroom, *Cordyceps militaris* (Ascomycetes) Mycelia Attenuates Doxorubicin-Induced Oxidative Stress and up Regulates Krebs Cycle Dehydrogenases Activity and ATP Level in Rat Brain. Janardhanan. 2020. DOI:10.1615/IntJMedMushrooms.2020035093.

[147] W. A. Elkhateeb and G. M. Daba. The endless nutritional and pharmaceutical benefits of the Himalayan gold, *Cordyceps*; Current knowledge and prospective potentials. Biofarmasi J nat prod biochem. 2020; 18,70-77. DOI: 10.13057/biofar/f180204.

[148] Hong T, Cui LK, Wen J et al. *Cordycepin* protects podocytes from injury mediated by complements complex C5b-9. Sichuan Da Xue Xue Bao Yi Xue Ban. 2015; 46(2):173-178. 227.

[149] Cheng, Y., Wei, Y., Yang, W. *et al.* Cordycepin confers neuroprotection in mice models of intracerebral hemorrhage via suppressing NLRP3 inflammasome activation. Metab Brain Dis. 2017; 32, 1133-1145. https://doi.org/10.1007/s11011-017-0003-7.

[150] Hwang, S., Cho, G.-S., Ryu, S., Kim, H. J., Song, H. Y., Yune, T. Y., ... Kim, W.-K. Post-ischemic treatment of WIB801C, standardized *Cordyceps* extract, reduces cerebral ischemic injury via inhibition of inflammatory cell migration. Journal of Ethnopharmacology. 2016; 186, 169-180. doi:10.1016/j.jep.2016.03.052.

[151] Jin, M. L., Park, S. Y., Kim, Y. H., Oh, J.-I., Lee, S. J., & Park, G. The neuroprotective effects of cordycepin inhibit glutamate-induced oxidative and ER stress-associated apoptosis in hippocampal HT22 cells. Neuro Toxicology. 2014; 41, 102-111. doi:10.1016/j.neuro.2014.01.005.

[152] Liu, Z., Li, P., Zhao, D. *et al.* Protective effect of extract of *Cordyceps sinensis* in middle cerebral artery occlusion-induced focal cerebral ischemia in rats. Behav Brain Funct. 2010; 6, 61. https://doi.org/10.1186/1744-9081-6-61..

[153] Chaicharoenaudomrung, N., Jaroonwitchawan, T., & Noisa, P. Cordycepin induces apoptotic cell death of human brain cancer through the modulation of autophagy. Toxicology in Vitro. 2018; 46, 113-121. doi:10.1016/j.tiv.2017.10.002.

[154] Yuan, J., Wang, A., He, Y., Si, Z., Xu, S., Zhang, S., ... Liu, Y. (2016). Cordycepin attenuates traumatic brain injury-induced impairments of blood-brain barrier integrity in rats. Brain Research Bulletin, 127, 171-176. doi:10.1016/j.brainresbull.2016.09.010.

[155] Jeong, J.-W., Jin, C.-Y., Kim, G.-Y., Lee, J.-D., Park, C., Kim, G.-D., ... Choi, Y. H. Anti-inflammatory effects of cordycepin via suppression of inflammatory mediators in BV2 microglial cells. International Immunopharmacology. 2010; 10(12), 1580-1586. doi:10.1016/j.intimp.2010.09.011.

[156] Sang-Hak Lee, Il-Gyu Ko, Sung-Eun Kim, Lakkyong Hwang, Jun-Jang Jin, Hyun-Hee Choi, Chang-Ju Kim. Aqueous extract of *Cordyceps* alleviates cerebral ischemia-induced short-term memory impairment in gerbils. Journal of Exercise Rehabilitation. 2016; 12(2): 69-78. DOI: https://doi.org/10.12965/jer.1632586.293

[157] He, X., Tian, Y., Lei, L., Zhi, Q., Zhao, J., & Ming, J. Protective effects of *Coreopsis tinctoria* buds extract against cognitive impairment and brain aging induced by d-galactose. Journal of Functional Foods. 2020; 73, 104089. doi:10.1016/j.jff.2020.104089.

[158] W. Li, P. Li, Q. Hua, J. Hou, J. Wang, H. Du, H. Tang, Y. Xu. The

impact of paracrine signaling in brain microvascular endothelial cells on the survival of neurons, Brain Res. 2009; 1287 (10): 28-38, https://doi.org/1.1016/j.brainres.2009.06.057.

[159] Bai, X., Tan, T.-Y., Li, Y.-X., Li, Y., Chen, Y.-F., Ma, R., ... Liu, Z.-Q. The protective effect of *Cordyceps sinensis* extract on cerebral ischemic injury via modulating the mitochondrial respiratory chain and inhibiting the mitochondrial apoptotic pathway. Biomedicine & Pharmacotherapy. 2020; 124, 109834. doi:10.1016/j.biopha.2020.109834.

[160] Hayden, M., West, A. & Ghosh, S. NF-κB and the immune response. Oncogene. 2006; 25, 6758-6780. https://doi.org/10.1038/sj.onc.1209943.

[161] Qin, P.; Li, X.; Yang, H.; Wang, Z.-Y.; Lu, D. Therapeutic Potential and Biological Applications of Cordycepin and Metabolic Mechanisms in Cordycepin-Producing Fungi. *Molecules*. 2019; *24*, 2231.

[162] Chen, B., Sun, Y., Luo, F., & Wang, C. Bioactive Metabolites and Potential Mycotoxins Produced by *Cordyceps* Fungi: A Review of Safety. Toxins. 2020; 12(6), 410. doi:10.3390/toxins12060410.

[163] Cai, Z. L., Wang, C. Y., Jiang, Z. J., Li, H. H., Liu, W. X., Gong, L. W., Li, C. H. Effects of cordycepin on Y-maze learning task in mice. European Journal of Pharmacology. 2013; 714(1-3), 249-253. https://doi.org/10.1016/j.ejphar.2013.05.049.

[164] Ren, Y., Sun, P., Li, H., & Zhu, Z. Effects of Na2SeO3 on growth, metabolism, antioxidase and enzymes involved in polysaccharide synthesis of *Cordyceps militaris*. Process Biochemistry. 2020. doi:10.1016/j.procbio.2020.06.018.

[165] Durán-Aranguren, D., Chiriví-Salomón, J. S., Anaya, L., Durán-Sequeda, D., Cruz, L. J., Serrano, J. D., Sierra, R. Effect of bioactive compounds extracted from *Cordyceps nidus* ANDES-F1080 on laccase activity of Pleurotus ostreatus ANDES-F515. Biotechnology Reports. 2020; 26, e00466. doi:10.1016/j.btre.2020.e00466.

[166] Rottenberg, M. E., Masocha, W., Ferella, M., Petitto-Assis, F., Goto, H., Kristensson, K., ... Wigzell, H. Treatment of African trypanosomiasis with cordycepin and adenosine deaminase inhibitors in a mouse model. Journal of Infectious Diseases. 2005; 192(9), 1658-1665.

[167] Lui, J.C.K., Wong, J.W.Y., Suen, Y.K. *et al.* Cordycepin induced eryptosis in mouse erythrocytes through a Ca^{2+}-dependent pathway without caspase-3 activation. Arch Toxicol. 2007; 81, 859-865. https://doi.org/10.1007/s00204-007-0214-5.

[168] Sornchaithawatwong, C., Kunthakudee, N., Sunsandee, N., & Ramakul, P. Selective extraction of cordycepin from *Cordyceps militaris* – optimisation, kinetics and equilibrium studies. Indian Chemical Engineer. 2020; 1-13. doi:10.1080/00194506.2020.1776163.

[169] Tsai, Y.-S., Hsu, J.-H., Lin, D. P.-C., Chang, H.-H., Chang, W.-J., Chen, Y.-L., & Chen, C.-C. Safety Assessment of HEA-Enriched *Cordyceps cicadae* Mycelium: A Randomized Clinical Trial. Journal of the American College of Nutrition. 2020; 1-6. doi:10.1080/07315724.2020.1743211.

[170] Chen, B.; Sun, Y.; Luo, F.; Wang, C. Bioactive Metabolites and Potential Mycotoxins Produced by *Cordyceps* Fungi: A Review of Safety. *Toxins* 2020; *12*:410.

[171] Zheng, P., Xia, Y., Zhang, S. *et al.* Genetics of *Cordyceps* and related fungi. Appl Microbiol Biotechnol. 2013; 97, 2797-2804. https://doi.org/10.1007/s00253-013-4771-7.

[172] Li, B., Hou, Y., Zhu, M., Bao, H., Nie, J., Zhang, G. Y., ... Du, J. 3'-Deoxyadenosine (Cordycepin) Produces a Rapid and Robust Antidepressant Effect via Enhancing Prefrontal AMPA Receptor Signaling Pathway. International Journal of Neuropsycho pharmacology. 2015; 19(4), pyv112. doi:10.1093/ijnp/pyv112.

[173] Tan, L., Song, X., Ren, Y., Wang, M., Guo, C., Guo, D., Deng, Y. Anti-inflammatory effects of cordycepin: A review. Phytotherapy Research. 2020. doi:10.1002/ptr.6890.

[174] Liu, Y., Li, Y., Zhang, H., Li, C., Zhang, Z., Liu, A., ... Wu, W. Polysaccharides from *Cordyceps miltaris* cultured at different pH: Sugar composition and antioxidant activity. International Journal of Biological Macromolecules. 2020. doi:10.1016/j.ijbiomac.2020.06.182.

[175] Marsup, P. Yeerong, K. Neimkhum, W. Sirithunyalug, J. Anuchapreeda, S. To-anun, C. Chaiyana, W. Enhancement of Chemical Stability and Dermal Delivery of *Cordyceps militaris* Extracts by Nanoemulsion. N*anomaterials.* 2020; *10*:1565.

[176] Zhu, Y., Yu, X., Ge, Q., Li, J., Wang, D., Wei, Y., & Ouyang, Z. Antioxidant and anti-aging activities of polysaccharides from *Cordyceps cicadae*. International Journal of Biological Macromolecules. 2020. doi:10.1016/j.ijbiomac.2020.04.163.

[177] Xiao, L., Sun, S., Li, K., Lei, Z., Shimizu, K., Zhang, Z., & Adachi, Y. Effects of nanobubble water supplementation on biomass accumulation during mycelium cultivation of *Cordyceps militaris* and the antioxidant activities of extracted polysaccharides. Bioresource Technology Reports. 2020; 12, 100600. doi:10.1016/j.biteb.2020.100600.

Chapter 17

One Health and the Positive Effects of Alaskan Blueberries

Vincent F. Lembo and Cheryl A. Frye

Abstract

One Health is a principle that takes into account the interactions of humans, animals, the surrounding environment, and how they affect each other. In order to examine this concept in an experimental paradigm, the effects and benefits of wild Alaskan blueberries were compared to those from the continental United States (Lower-48 states) in human and animal studies. Blueberries have been hailed as a superfood for years now due to their high antioxidant levels and the positive effects they have on cardiovascular health and overall health and well-being. We hypothesize that although they are both beneficial, wild Alaskan blueberries have a greater positive effect on health and well-being than those from the lower 48. First, teachers and staff at the Anne Wien Elementary School in Fairbanks Alaska were provided with Alaskan and Lower-48 blueberries and asked to log the effects each coded sample had on their mental and physical health compared to a 5-day control period without blueberries. There was a significant stepwise positive effect of respondents reporting higher self-ratings of well-being overall. Alaskan blueberries significantly improved self-ratings of well-being compared to those from Lower-48 blueberries, albeit those blueberries did improve well-being compared to no blueberries. This experiment was replicated at a control site contemporaneously. The following year it was also replicated by participating teachers and staff at William S. Hackett Middle School in Albany, New York, as well as a control site. Further, lab rats, whose diets were supplemented with with Alaskan blueberries, performed better in exploratory and cognitive tests than did rats whose diets were supplemented with Lower-48 blueberries (who, similar to the previous trials, performed better than rats whose diets had not been supplemented at all). These findings suggest that blueberries have an overall positive effect on self-rated wellness in people and cognitive performance in lab rats and that Alaskan blueberries have a particularly greater and more beneficial effect. Whether this is due to greater antioxidant effects associated with higher altitude or fewer endocrine-disrupting contaminants in Alaska compared to the Lower-48 States is unknown and subject to ongoing investigation.

Keywords: antioxidants, cholesterol, triglycerides, low density liposaccharides, high blood pressure, hypercholesterolemia, cognitive decline, neurosteroids

1. Introduction

Consumption of fruits and vegetables is often correlated with brain and heart health and cancer prevention. One way that fruits and vegetables have beneficial effects on health is through their antioxidant actions. Not all fruits and vegetables are the same in terms of their antioxidant actions. When scientists tested 143

IntechOpen

different plants for their antioxidant power: blueberries scored 4669 > cherries were 3747 and prune juice came in at 2036; avocado was at 1922; grapefruit had a power score of 1640, spinach was 1513 and raw broccoli was 1510 and pineapple was a low 385. These results on an ORAC scale compare items among food groups that show relative antioxidant activity. ORAC is a measure of water-soluble antioxidant levels and does not distinguish among those antioxidants that have benefits to humans and those that do not. It is simply an overall estimate of antioxidant activity in a particular experiment. Due to the limited utility of this index, the USDA's Nutrient Data Laboratory (NDL) removed the ORAC database from the NDL website [1].

Wild berries contain an impressive array of bioactive phytochemical compounds, which collectively present a range of biological activities targeting key mechanisms involved in healthy tissue development and aging [2, 3]. The human health-relevant bioactive properties of wild berries can be primarily attributed to their considerable diversity of polyphenolic constituents, typically exhibiting antioxidant, anti-inflammatory, and antimicrobial capabilities [4, 5]. The Nurses' Health Study evaluated 16,000 participants regarding cognitive decline and consumption of berries over a 20-year period. Greater intakes of flavonoids particularly from strawberries and blueberries were associated with slower cognitive decline in older adults [6]. This again supports the beneficial effects of blueberries.

Wild blueberries (*Vaccinium angustifolium*) are rich sources of polyphenols (e.g. flavonols, phenolic acids, anthocyanins) and decrease the risk of cardiovascular and degenerative diseases [7]. Memory function and mood in older adults with memory decline was improved by regular consumption of wild blueberries [8].

Various wild berry species endemic to Alaska and the circumpolar North that exhibit unique medicinal properties have long been appreciated by indigenous Arctic communities. Berry picking is a cherished tradition among all Alaskans that provides important physical and recreational activities for young and old alike. It has been an integral part of subsistence activities for thousands of years. Alaska is rich in wild edible berries that provide essential nutrients, especially vitamin C, and antioxidants for northern climates.

Interspecific differences, as well as environmental factors, such as geographic location and climatic variation, substantially influence the accumulation of berry phytochemicals and thus likely alter their profile of health-related bioactivities [9–11].

These experiments were designed to test the hypotheses that (1) wild blueberries would have beneficial short-term effects effect on healthy individuals (2) blueberries from Alaska would be more effective than those from the lower 48 (3) these effects would be seen across groups and species.

2. Methods

The protocol for Experiment 1 was approved by the Principal of Anne Wien Elementary School. All participants were volunteers and signed an informed consent indicating that they would comply with the guidelines of the experiment. At any time, volunteers could drop out as non-participants and their data would not be included.

2.1 Comparing effects of wild Alaskan blueberries to those from the lower 48 for effects on stress, mood, and affective function in people in Fairbanks, Alaska

The Native Alaskan blueberries used in this experiment were hand-picked by the authors, and their associates, the summer before the experiment began, and frozen at −20 degrees Fahrenheit. These were low bush blueberries of large size, which are known to have high antioxidant value. The store-bought blueberries were purchased fresh from the local grocery store (Fred Meyers, Fairbanks, Alaska) around the same time. Half cup portions were prepackaged and labeled (A or B) and then placed in a refrigerator in the faculty lounge in the experimental locations.

2.1.1 Procedures for examining effects of blueberries

Experiment 1: In the first experiment, teachers and staff members at Anne Wien Elementary School (https://www.k12northstar.org/annewien) were provided with two samples of blueberries: hand-picked Alaskan blueberries, labeled A, and store-bought blueberries, labeled B, and surveys (see **Figure 1**) for them to answer after consuming the blueberries for 5 days or no blueberries control. This experiment was three weeks long. Participants consumed ½ a cup of one type of blueberries every day for one work week, repeated that process the next week with the other type of blueberries, and completed another survey after a third control week where no blueberries were consumed. Participants were allowed to use any sample any given week, so long as they only used that sample (or no sample) for the full work week and completed the other two sample weeks in the remaining time.

Custom surveys were created to enable participants to fully document the effects, positive, negative, or lack thereof, of the blueberries on their mental and physical health and well-being. Datasheets were turned in to the research supervisor at each site each week. There were 7 participants from Anne Wien Elementary (Fairbanks, AK) and 6 from an alternate site in Fairbanks (https://www.uafarc.com/overview), as well as 7 more from Hackett Middle School (Albany, NY) and 5 more from an alternate site in Albany later on for replication in the lower 48 States. (Experiment 2).

The protocol for Experiment 2 was approved by the principal of Hackett Middle School, all participants were volunteers and signed an informed consent indicating that they would comply with the guidelines of the experiment. At any time, volunteers could drop out as non-participants and their data would not be included.

Experiment 2: Comparing Effects of Wild Alaskan Blueberries to those from the Lower 48 for effects on Stress, Mood, and Affective Function in People in Albany, New York.

Experiment 2 was identical in procedure to experiment 1, the difference was the population that was tested. Experiment 2 took place at Hackett Middle School (https://www.albanyschools.org/schools/hackett/index) in Albany, New York about a year after experiment 1.

Experiment 3: Comparing Effects of Wild Alaskan Blueberries to those from the Lower 48 for effects on Stress, Mood, and Affective Function in Long-Evans Rats.

The University of Alaska Fairbanks Institutional Animal Care and Use Committee approved the animal care and experimental procedures (IACUC assurance number 497513).

2.2 Rats

2.2.1 Husbandry

Long-Evans rats were housed in polypropylene cages with wood shavings in a temperature (22 ± 1°C) and humidity (60–80%) controlled room of the Biological Research and Diagnostics (BiRD) Facility vivarium on a reversed 12:12 h dark-light cycle. Pups were weaned at 19–21 days of age and housed with same-sex littermates until the end of all experiments. Food (Purina Mills, Rat Diet, St. Louis, MO) and water were available *ad libitum*. Rats were also provided ½ cup blueberries from

[SURVEY PREVIEW MODE] Blueberry AWES Survey 1/26/2014

Blueberry AWES

We are asking for your help with Vincent Lembo's (5th grade) science fair project, which we are conducting as a family.

All we ask you to do is eat blueberries and answer a few questions at the end of the week!

Over the next three school weeks, please spend one week snacking from each of the bags, "A" and "B", and complete one survey for the week. On one of the weeks, please just answer the survey.

A "snack" should be at least 1/2 a cup a day. Please eat from the same bag all week. On one of the weeks, please don't eat any blueberries (as a control), but answer the survey. It's your choice which weeks you eat which blueberries.

You can complete the survey on paper or on-line (https://www.surveymonkey.com/s/V37KPMH). Please return any paper surveys to Vincent Lembo in Mrs. Hedgecock's class.

Thank you!

*** 1. Which bag of blueberries did you eat from this week?**

○ Bag A ○ Bag B ○ None

2. How stressed do you feel right now?

Not stressed at all ○ ○ ○ ○ ○ ○ ○ Very stressed

3. Which adjective(s) best describe how you feel right now? (Choose all that apply.)

☐ Happy	☐ Sad	☐ Surprised
☐ Overwhelmed	☐ Angry	☐ Excited
☐ Confused	☐ Scared	☐ Content
☐ Hurt	☐ Tired	☐ Sick

4. In the last week, how often have you ... ?

	Never	Almost Never	Sometimes	Fairly Often	Very Often
...felt nervous and stressed?	○	○	○	○	○
...felt well-balanced physically and mentally?	○	○	○	○	○
...been able to control irritations in your life?	○	○	○	○	○
...felt that you were on top of things?	○	○	○	○	○
...felt cognitive impairments?	○	○	○	○	○

5. What is your age?

○ 18 to 24 ○ 25 to 34 ○ 35 to 44 ○ 45 to 54 ○ 55 to 64 ○ 65 to 74 ○ 75 +

6. What is your gender?

○ Female ○ Male

*** 7. Please create a unique, anonymous personal identifier and enter it here:**

Please remember the unique identifier you just created and use it on all subsequent surveys.

Your participation implies informed consent. All data will be treated in a confidential manner and presented with anonymity of the participants. Thank you for your participation!

http://www.surveymonkey.com/s.aspx?PREVIEW_MODE=DO_NOT_USE_THIS_LINK_FOR_COLLECTION&sm=%2f6c3l62B%2f4uMw1Ya2FjegNmS%2bSf7Zc7p4jldA8%2bcgc%3d 1 / 2

Figure 1.
This figure depicts the survey used by the participants of each trial to record the effects (or lack of effects) that each sample of blueberries, as well as no blueberries, has had on them. This survey was completed at the end of each trial week by each participant and is completely anonymous. Several measures were provided for the user to describe and show how they felt after each trial week including a list of pronouns that the participant could choose best reflects them that week and survey questions that would help identify if blueberries were having a positive or negative effect on the participant. Demographic information was also collected for each participant.

Alaska or the lower 48 or none (as a control) each day for 4–5 days leading up to their anticipated 5th day of proestrus when they were tested.

2.2.2 Estrous cycle

Female rats in proestrus were used for the study. The proestrus stage was determined daily by both visual and vaginal cytology methods. Vaginal cytology was performed on those females that showed visual signs of proestrus. The females for which proestrus was confirmed through cytology were subjected to behavioral testing the same day. This procedure was conducted daily until the desired sample sizes were achieved for a specific test. When the females cycled to their next proestrus, which was typically on the 4th or the 5th day, they were subjected to the next behavioral test in the schedule and this cycle was continued until all behavioral tests were completed. Typically, the no blueberry control week was the interval washout period between tests 1 and 3, which were randomized to blueberry condition.

2.2.3 Experimental design

All female rats were at least 60 days old at the start of the experiment. All behavioral tests were done in the dark phase of the light–dark cycle. For females, behavioral tests were conducted every 4–5 days depending on their cycle stage. All females underwent behavioral tests once every 5–10 days: open field (on day 5 or 10) and novel object recognition (on day 15 or 20). A minimum gap of 5 days for females between the two behavioral tests minimized the behaviors interfering with each other. An observer blind to the conditions of experimental animals and the hypothesized outcome of the study collected all data.

2.2.4 Open field

Behavior in the open field is used as a measure of exploration, anxiety, and locomotor behavior [12, 13]. The open field (76 cm x 57 cm x 35 cm) has a 48-square grid floor (6 x 8 squares, 9.5 cm/side): there is an overhead light illuminating the central squares (all but the 24 perimeter squares were considered central). Behavior was recorded by the ANYMaze video-tracking program (Stoelting Co., IL, USA). The apparatus was cleaned before and after each test. Per previous methods, rats were placed in the open field and the path of their exploration was recorded for five minutes. The number of squares entered by rats in the center or periphery of the grid was calculated and these data were added together to yield the total number of squares entered. Prior reports indicate that total square entries in this task are robustly modulated by the hormonal status of female rats and by steroid-sensitive manipulations [14–16]. Because the current study utilized a sample of female rats that were all matched on the phase of estrous cycle, motor differences were expected to be minimized. Thus, central square entries were utilized as an index of anti-anxiety, and total square entries as an index of thigmotaxis, and motor behavior. Additionally, engaging in this task provides habituation for object recognition, which occurs in the same box on the following days.

2.2.5 Object recognition

The object recognition task is a working memory task that primarily relies on cortical functioning and, to a lesser extent, hippocampal functioning [17–19]. This task was used as modified from previously published methods [20–22]. During training, rats are placed in a white open field (76 cm x 57 cm x 35 cm) in a brightly-lit testing room. Rats are allowed 3 min to explore the open field, which contains two identical objects in adjacent corners. These objects were colored spherical shapes (plastic toys in the shape of oranges). The time spent investigating the two identical objects (plastic toys) within a 5 cm distance in the open field arena was recorded for 3 min with the ANYMaze video tracking program (Stoelting.co, Chicago, IL). Rats were then taken out of the arena and returned to their holding cages for 4 hrs. After 4 hrs., one of the objects was replaced with a novel object of different shape and size, and animals were then reintroduced into the arena and allowed to explore the objects for 3 min. Time spent exploring the familiar and novel objects were recorded. The preference of one object over another was assessed through the Recognition

Percentage, which is the time spent on the novel object relative to the time spent on both novel and familiar objects: [RI = TN/(TN + TF) x 100] where TN is time spent on the novel object and TF is time spent on the familiar object). A greater percentage of time spent exploring the novel object as a function of the total amount of time spent exploring both objects during testing (duration spent with novel object/ (duration spent with novel object + duration spent with familiar object) Å x 100) is considered an index of enhanced cognitive performance in these tasks.

2.2.6 Statistical analyses: one-way repeated measure analyses of variance was utilized to examine the effects of the condition (Blueberries) on self ratings

Post hoc analyses to determine group differences consisted of repeated t-tests with Bonferroni-corrections. Results are only reported for effects where the overall ANOVAs were significant, at the alpha level of 0.05, which was the case for each experiment. Overall effects and specific group differences are described below and in the tables and figures and their legends.

3. Results

Experiment 1a: Self-reports of health and wellness of middle-aged elementary school teachers in Fairbanks, Alaska were significantly greater following 5 days of consumption of Alaskan blueberries compared to blueberries from the Lower-48, which still had a beneficial effect compared to no blueberry consumption.

Self-reports of beneficial effects on stress, anxiety, and cognition are reported among women participants in Fairbanks, Alaska (demographics in **Table 1** left side, far) after 5 days of consumption of Alaskan blueberries > Lower-48 blueberries > no blueberries. Repeated measures analysis of variance revealed that there was an overall interaction between the type of blueberries and effects on self-ratings. *Post hoc* analyses revealed consumption of Alaskan berries resulted in higher ratings overall than did berries from the Lower-48 or no consumption of berries. This effect was seen for ratings of calmness, feelings of being well-balanced, and ability to maintain control and stay on top of things. Notably, self-reports of cognitive benefits of blueberries from Alaska, as well as the Lower-48, were not different but were significantly higher than the consumption of no berries among the participants at Anne Wien Elementary School. See **Figure 2**.

Experiment 1b: Demographics are described in **Table 1** (left center). Self-reports of health and wellness of young adult lab workers in Fairbanks, Alaska were significantly greater following 5 days of consumption of Alaskan blueberries compared to blueberries from the Lower-48, which still had a beneficial effect compared to no blueberry consumption.

To confirm and extend these findings, the experiment was replicated at an alternative site in Fairbanks (see **Table 1**, left middle, for demographics). There were even greater statistically significant interactions between types of blueberries and effects on self-reports at this alternative site than at Anne Wien Elementary School. Ratings for weeks following consumption of Alaskan blueberries > Lower-48 blueberries >no blueberries for self-reports of feelings of calmness, being well-balanced, in control, on top of things, cognitive benefits. Thus, women in Alaska who consumed blueberries for 5 days experienced beneficial effects as per their self-ratings. The magnitude of these effects was greater at the alternative site. See **Figure 3**.

	Fairbanks, AK		Albany, NY	
Location	**Anne-Wien Eiementary School**	**Alternate site**	**Hackett Middle School Albany, NY**	**Alternate site**
n = of participants	7	8	6	5
Age (avg. years)	42.3	33.6	40.0	48.7
Education (avg. years)	15.3	14.7	16.0	15.4
Ethnicity	5 Caucasian 2 Native Alaskan	3 Caucasian 2 Native Alaskan 2 Biracial 1 African American	2 Caucasian 2 African American 2 Latina	3 Caucasian 1 African American 1 Native Alaskan 1 Native American

Table 1.
The mean average demographics obtained from the Anne-Wien elementary school and the alternative site in Fairbanks (Byrd animal facility staff at U Alaska Fairbanks) on the left side. On the right side are the demographics for the Hackett middle School in Albany and the alternative site in Albany, NY (Comprehensive Neuropsychological Services).

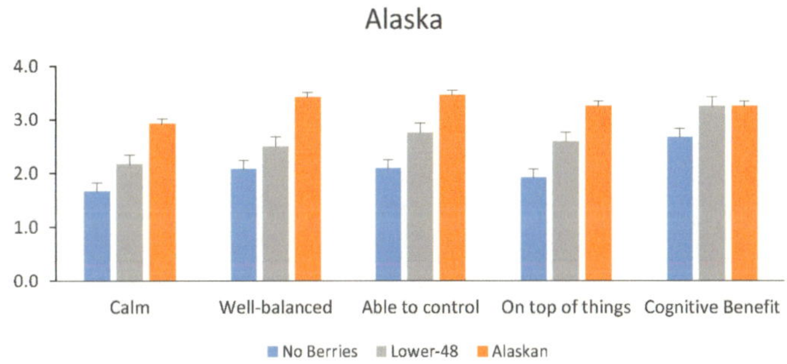

Figure 2.
This figure represents the mean + standard error of the mean of self-ratings in several categories by each participant in Fairbanks, Alaska at Anne-Wien Elementary School. This figure shows a significant overall effect of treatment (blueberries) to increase ratings of calm, a sense of well-balanced and ability to control surroundings and stay on top of things, except for self-ratings of cognitive benefit compared to consumption of no blueberries. Furthermore, consumption of wild Alaskan blueberries (orange) increased the participant's rating in each of the aforementioned categories compared to Lower-48 berries (gray) or no berries (blue).

Experiment 2a: Self-reports of health and wellness of middle-aged middle school teachers in Albany, New York were significantly greater following 5 days of consumption of Alaskan blueberries compared to blueberries from the Lower-48, which still had a beneficial effect compared to no blueberry consumption.

Self-reports of beneficial effects on stress, anxiety, and cognition are reported among women participants in Albany, New York after 5 days of consumption of Alaskan blueberries > Lower-48 blueberries > no blueberries. One-way, repeated analysis of variance revealed that there were overall interactions between the type of blueberries and effects on self-ratings. Some of the same patterns were observed among the participants at Hackett Middle School (Albany, NY) that were previously seen at Anne Wien Elementary (Fairbanks, AK). In particular, self-reports of feeling well-balanced, as well as in control and on top of things were higher in participants when they consumed Alaskan blueberries for a week compared to when they consumed Lower-48 blueberries or no blueberries. Demographics are reported in **Table 1** center-right. See **Figure 3** for results.

Experiment 2b: Self-reports of health and wellness of middle-aged office workers in Albany, New York were significantly greater following 5 days of consumption of Alaskan blueberries, compared to blueberries from the Lower-48.

There were even greater statistically significant interactions between types of blueberries and effects on self-reports at this alternative site than at Hackett Middle School in Albany, NY. Ratings for weeks following consumption of Alaskan blueberries > Lower-48 blueberries ≥ no blueberries for self-ratings of feelings of calmness, well-balanced. See demographics in **Table 1** and ratings in **Table 2**.

Experiment 3: Female Long-Evans rats whose diets were supplemented by Alaskan blueberries > Lower-48 blueberries > no supplement (control) were significantly more active, less anxious, and performed better in a novel object recognition task.

There were 8 female Long-Evans rats in each of the 3 trial groups. Those who had 5 days of access to Alaskan blueberries made more total entries (245 entries) into the brightly lit open field than did those with access to blueberries from the Lower-48 (223 entries), as well as those with no blueberry supplementation (196 entries) in a

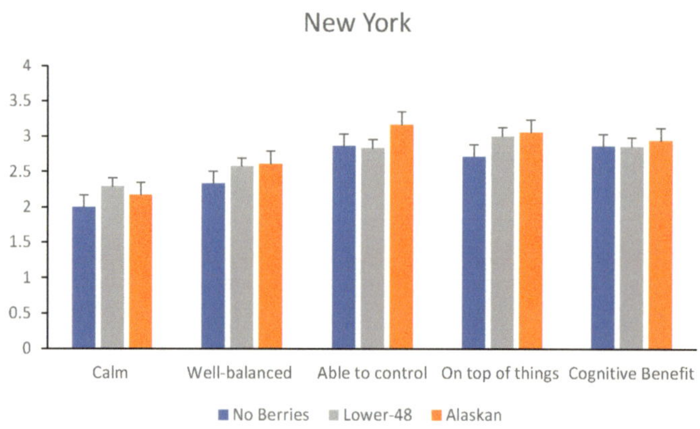

Figure 3.
This figure represents the mean + standard error of the mean of self-ratings in several categories by each participant in Albany, New York at Hackett Middle School. This figure shows a significant overall effect of treatment (blueberries) to increase ratings wild Alaskan blueberries (orange) to overall increase participant's rating in each of the aforementioned categories compared to Lower-48 berries (gray) or no berries (blue).

Self-ratings-alternative sites						
	Fairbanks-bird animal facility UAlaska			**Albany-comprehensive neuropsychological services**		
Blueberry Source	**None**	**Lower 48**	**Alaskan**	**none**	**Lower 48**	**Alaskan**
Self-Ratings						
Calmness	2.1	3.3	4.2	1.5	2.3	3.6
Well Balanced	1.6	2.5	3.6	1.8	2.9	4.3
Able to Control	1.5	2.3	3.8	1.3	2.4	2.7
On Top of Things	2.5	3.5	4.5	1.9	2.7	3.5
Cognitive Benefit	2.9	4.2	5.4	2.4	3.2	3.9

Table 2.
The mean average self-ratings obtained from the Fairbanks (n = 8) and Albany sites alternative site (n = 5) after 5 days of no consumption blueberries, lower 48 or Alaskan blueberries.

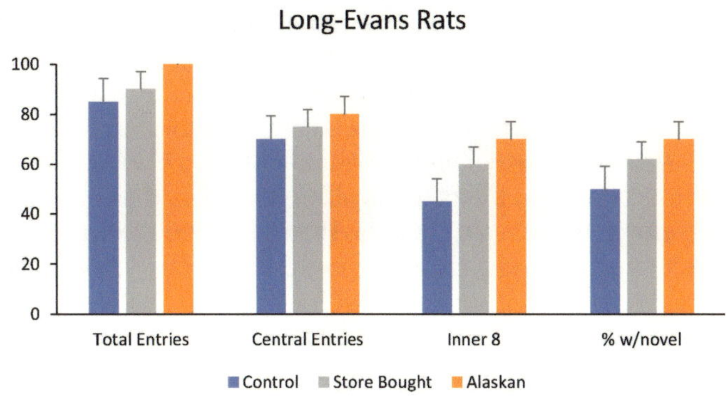

Figure 4.
This figure represents the scores in several tasks by Long-Evans laboratory rats at the BiRD Animal Research and Development facility at UAF as their diets were supplemented with Lower-48 or Alaskan blueberries, or no berries at all similar to human participants in the first trials. This figure shows that blueberries increase the number of total entries as well as central entries, Inner8 entries, and time spent with a novel object compared to consumption of no blueberries. Furthermore, consumption of wild Alaskan blueberries (orange) increased the rat's scores in each of the aforementioned categories compared to Lower-48 berries (gray) or no berries (blue).

5-minute period. The number of central entries (all but peripheral squares) during this 5-minute task was also greater for rats with access to Alaskan blueberries (120 entries) than rats whose diets were supplemented with blueberries from the Lower-48 (113 entries) as well as rats whose diets were not supplemented (93 entries). The number of inner 8 entries (central squares of open field) during this 5-minute task was greater for rats with access to Alaskan blueberries (25 entries) compared to rats whose diets were supplemented with blueberries from the Lower-48 (19 entries), as well as rats whose diets were not supplemented (13 entries). When rats were tested in the novel object recognition task, those consuming Alaskan berries spent 70% of their time than the novel object, whereas rats consuming Lower-48 berries spent only 61% of their time with the object. Rats whose diets were not supplemented spent the least amount of time, 51% (no greater than chance levels), with the novel object during testing (See **Figure 4**).

4. Discussion

The results of these experiments were consistent with the proposed hypotheses. First, blueberry consumption had beneficial short-term effects on healthy individuals. Blueberries had positive effects on the Alaskan participants' health and well-being after 5 days of consumption. This was also observed in the Albany cohorts. Participants consuming blueberries rated their levels of calm, well-balanced, ability to control themselves, and stay on top of things, and cognitive benefit, higher than when they consumed no berries. Second, this effect was seen more obviously when participants consumed Alaskan blueberries. They rated themselves even higher in the aforementioned categories than when they consumed Lower-48 blueberries. This effect was not identical; however, in New York, data from participants show an effect of blueberries but not a statistically significant difference between Alaskan blueberries and berries from the Lower-48. Third, blueberries had similar patterns of effects in rats. Notably, in more global tasks, such as total entries and central entries in an open field, there was an effect of blueberries, irrespective of their source, to improve performance among rats. However, in more challenging tasks, such as the Inner 8 entries and the percent of time with novel object, consumption of Alaskan blueberries had a greater effect than did those from the lower-48. In summary, short term consumption of blueberries can have beneficial effects among some individuals. Further, the consumption of blueberries from Alaska had a more amplified effect than did berries from the Lower-48. Among Long Evans laboratory rats, Lower-48 or Alaskan blueberries increased motor activity and central entries (all non-peripheral squares) compared to control rats that did not consume any blueberries. However, rats consuming Alaskan blueberries made more Inner-8 entries, indicating that they were significantly bolder than rats that consumed Lower-48 blueberries or none at all. They also showed greater recollection and memory skills in the object recognition task than did those that consumed Lower-48 blueberries or none.

As mentioned in previous studies, blueberries as well as other fruits and vegetables have been linked to improving memory function as well as mood in older adults [23–25]. Our findings confirm and extend previous findings that blueberries can be beneficial to staving off cardiovascular disease, cognitive decline, and other age-related deleterious effects when consumed as part of a lifestyle. Here we show that short-term consumption of blueberries, 5 days of consumption, has perceived cognitive benefit among women age 30–55. Our participants' self-ratings of their perceived cognitive benefit from short term consumption of blueberries, as well as high ratings in other categories, such as their ability to remain calm and well-balanced, show that short term consumption of blueberries has the ability to improve mood and mental well-being among women age 30–55. Further, in our third experiment, healthy adult rats' performances benefited from blueberry consumption to have enhanced motor function, exploratory behavior, anti-anxiety effects, and learning. These latter findings are clearly objective, as they are not self-ratings and they demonstrate cross-species performance effects. Together, these findings confirm and extend the previous literature that older individuals can benefit from blueberry consumption as part of their lifestyle to indicate that short-term consumption of blueberries improves self-ratings of neurotypical women age 30–55 as well as objective effects on performance in rats. Another explanation may be that people in Alaska have greater access and exposure to foods with higher antioxidant levels than do people from the Lower 48 [26].

Consumption of Alaskan blueberries seemed to have a greater effect among participants in Alaska compared to participants in New York. An important question to ask is, what underlies this effect? One explanation could be that experiment 1 was conducted in Fairbanks, Alaska at the end of the winter season. This time of year in Alaska is also known as breakup and is associated with higher rates of suicide. There is tension in communities throughout Alaska caused by long harsh winters, and fresh blueberries may have had a greater effect on the moods and mental well-being of consumers during this sensitive time. Experiment 2 was conducted almost a full year later in Albany, New York, where the winters are much less harsh and dark. There may be some confounding variables due to these time frames. For example, the wild Alaskan blueberries had to be frozen for a longer period of time between experiments, 8 months for Experiment 1, versus 20 months, which may have caused a depletion in the potency of the Alaskan berries.

Another interesting finding relating to group differences was that the Alaskan blueberries had a greater effect among the office workers controls compared to the teachers in both control cohorts in Fairbanks and Albany. A likely explanation for this is that the office workers had a much calmer work environment than did the schoolteachers. They had greater control over their scope of work and when they engaged in their work activities, compared to being on a rigorous schedule with a limited break time that was preset and absolute. Further, office workers were not responsible for or surrounded by 20–30 children each day. They had a much quieter work environment. As such, the blueberries may have had a greater effect on individuals who were in a position to feel greater effects of the blueberries because they could engage in other behaviors to enhance their wellbeing (such as listening to music, while at work engaging in brief meditation activities, having time for self-care).

All experiments have limitations, one possible limitation of this experiment was that the pool of participants was small, only 6–8 participants in each experiment. However, the fact that significant results were observed and replicated across multiple domains indicates the power and consistency of the effects shown in all 5 experiments. This limitation was out of our control because all participants were volunteers, and some participant's data were excluded because they did not participate in all 3 trial weeks. Another limitation is that a large majority of the participants in both trials were women, and mostly fell into the 30–55-year-old age range. A more diverse population next time might verify the results and show that the consumption of blueberries, especially wild Alaskan berries, are beneficial to everyone, and not just these populations. The notion that beneficial effects were seen in male rats suggests that this is a highly conserved effect and could be replicated on other populations. Another factor considered in this study is that living in Alaska is much closer to the earth and people in Alaska are much more affected by their environment. Experiences such as having 20 hours of sunlight each day in the summer and 20 hours of darkness in the winter have significant effects on mental and cognitive health and well-being. Also, the food that they eat is more likely to directly affect them; many Alaskans do not eat a strictly market diet but consume fish, game, and berries.

Blueberries are known to have a number of phytochemicals that contain several bioactive compounds that cause different physiological effects. One phytochemical are flavanols that contain the bioactive compounds *Epicatechin-gallates, Procyanidins*, and *Catechin* [27–30]. The physiological and pharmacological effects of these compounds include activities of antioxidants that increase free-radical scavenging, decrease the hypothalamic inflammation of microglia overactivation in the brain, and improve cognition. Further, other phytochemical effects include activities at phenolic acids, including the bioactive compounds phenolic acid and ferulic acid, which can have antioxidant and anti-inflammatory properties, as well as improve cognition and stave off neurodegeneration [31]. Blueberries are considered a functional food, which is defined as one that has clinically proven health benefits. Bioactive compounds such as flavonoids can suppress the release of cytokines such as IL-1beta and TNF-alpha from activated microglia. Flavonoids also affect nitric oxide synthase, inhibit activation of NADPH-oxidase, and down-regulate pro-inflammatory transcription factors including NF-kappa B which plays a role in intestinal responses through caffeic acid. NF-kappa B influences intestinal inflammatory responses through flavonoids' actions in part involving caffeic acid which inhibits the expression of TNF-alpha, IL-beta, CO-2, INOS, and other inflammatory factors [32–34].

An important question is how do blueberries have beneficial effects through the mechanisms described above? Particularly relevant to this study are Vitamins D, A, E, and K (fat-soluble vitamins). Vitamin D is considered a (neuro) steroid that has effects on calcium, metabolism, and absorption of calcium and phosphorus from the intestine. Vitamin D exerts many other biological effects including processes involved in brain development and neuronal activity [35]. Deficiency in Vitamin D is considered a risk factor for neuropsychiatric disorders, including post partum depression, major depression and schizophrenia [36–39]. It causes alterations in brain structure and in dopamine and glutamate signaling, which are hallmarks of depression, anxiety, drug abuse and schizoaffective disorders. Functional foods rich in micronutrients that have the ability to stimulate PPAR, in addition to exert important anti-inflammatory actions may also induce significant mood- elevating properties, although the underlying mechanisms are not fully understood. PPAR might work in synergism with stimulation of neurosteroid biosynthesis to exert their beneficial effects by decreasing inflammation and relieving mood symptoms.

In summary, these experiments revealed that five days of blueberry consumption has beneficial effects on middle-aged women in Fairbanks, Alaska, as well as Albany, New York. The initial study in Fairbanks, Alaska (during "breakup season"), revealed a greater sensitivity and responsiveness to Alaskan blueberries than those from the Lower-48. Albeit, the second experiment, conducted in Albany, New York, showed a beneficial effect of blueberry consumption but not a differential effect between wild Alaskan and store-bought berries from the Lower-48. This may be due to the decomposition of antioxidants, flavonoids, and other important health factors caused by freezer storage for a full year. Our third experiment, using an animal model, conducted over the summer between the two human experiments, revealed beneficial effects of both Alaskan and Lower-48 blueberries when given as a supplement to male Long Evans rats. The rats that consumed blueberries had improved motor skills and exploratory behavior, irrespective of the source of blueberries. However, in more challenging tasks, such as entries into the Inner 8 squares in an open field (an anti-anxiety measure) and performance on the object recognition task, Alaskan blueberries had a greater effect on performance than did berries from the Lower-48 or no berries. To address the mechanism underlying these effects, we will be extracting the bioactive compounds and creating an Alaskan elixir to reassess their relative efficacy of Alaskan blueberries versus those from the Lower-48 on people as well as animal subjects.

5. Conclusion

In conclusion, it seems that blueberries can have short term effects as functional foods when consumed by individuals over a 5-day period. The precise mechanisms underlying these effects are unclear, however, differences between Fairbanks and Albany suggest that blueberries from a higher altitude may be more effective because they contain more flavonoids and more antioxidant effects. The beneficial effects of flavonoids may be mediated in part through actions of neurosteroids, such as Vitamin-D, allopregnanolone, 3α diol, which can inhibit deleterious effects of activation of PPAR and other physiological and pharmacological effects [34].

Acknowledgements

Research herein was supported in part by grants National Institute of Mental Health (MH06769801, RMH067698B) and the National Institute of General Medical Sciences of the National Institutes of Health (P20GM103395). The content is solely the responsibility of the authors and does not necessarily represent the official views of the National Institutes of Health. Assistance in the studies described herein provided by members of the laboratory, past, and present, is greatly appreciated.

Author details

Vincent F. Lembo and Cheryl A. Frye*
Alaska INBRE Program, University of Alaska Fairbanks, Fairbanks, AK, USA

*Address all correspondence to: cherylafrye@gmail.com

References

[1] Oxygen radical absorbance capacity (ORAC) of selected foods, release 2. 2010. [cited 2012 Oct 10] US Department of Agriculture Agricultural Research Service. http://www.ars.usda.gov/Services/docs.htm?docid=15866.

[2] Paredes-Lopez O., Cervantes-Ceja M. L., Vigna-Perez M., Hernandez-Perez T. (2010). Berries: improving human health and healthy aging and promoting quality life—a review. Plant Foods Hum. Nutr. 65 (3), 299-308. 10.1007/s11130-010-0177-1

[3] Li Y., Zhang J. J., Xu D. P., Zhou T., Zhou Y., Li S., et al. (2016). Bioactivities and health benefits of wild fruits. Int. J. Mol. Sci. 17 (8), 1258. 10.3390/ijms17081258

[4] Seeram N. P. (2008). Berry fruits: compositional elements, biochemical activities, and the impact of their intake on human health, performance, and disease. J. Agric. Food Chem. 56 (3), 627-629. 10.1021/jf071988k

[5] Nile S. H., Park S. W. (2014). Edible berries: bioactive components and their effect on human health. Nutrition 30 (2), 134-144. 10.1016/j.nut.2013.04.007

[6] Devore EE, Kang JH, Breteler MM, Grodstein F. Dietary intakes of berries and flavonoids in relation to cognitive decline. Ann Neurol. 2012;72:135-43. doi: 10.1002/ana.23594.

[7] Michenaud-Rague A, Robinson S, Landsberger S. Trace elements in 11 fruits widely-consumed in the USA as determined by neutron activation analysis. J Radioanal Nucl Chem. 2012;291:237-40. doi: 10.1007/s10967-011-1266-9.

[8] Krikorian R, Schidler MD, Nash TA, Kalt W, Vinqvist-Tymchuk MR, Shukitt-Hale B, et al. Blueberry supplementation improves memory in older adults. J Agric Food Chem. 2010;58:3996-4000.

[9] Howard L. R., Clark J. R., Brownmiller C. (2003). Antioxidant capacity and phenolic content in blueberries as affected by genotype and growing season. J. Sci. Food Agric. 83 (12), 1238-1247. 10.1002/jsfa.1532

[10] Lila M. A. (2006). The nature-versus-nurture debate on bioactive phytochemicals: the genome versus terroir. J. Sci. Food Agric. 86 (15), 2510-2515. 10.1002/jsfa.2677

[11] Karppinen K., Zoratti L., Nguyenquynh N., Haggman H., Jaakola L. (2016). On the developmental and environmental regulation of secondary metabolism in Vaccinium spp. berries. Front. Plant Sci. 7, 655. 10.3389/fpls.2016.00655

[12] Blunt MJ, Blizard PJ. Recall and retrieval of anatomical knowledge. Br J Med Educ. 1975;9(4):252-263.

[13] Frye CA, Petralia SM, Rhodes ME. Estrous cycle and sex differences in performance on anxiety tasks coincide with increases in hippocampal progesterone and 3alpha,5alpha-THP. Pharmacol Biochem Behav. 2000;67(3):587-596. doi:10.1016/s0091-3057(00)00392-0

[14] Birke LI, Archer J. Open-field behaviour of oestrous and dioestrous rats: evidence against an 'emotionality' interpretation. Anim Behav. 1975;23(3):509-512. doi:10.1016/0003-3472(75)90127-x

[15] Frye CA, Paris JJ, Rhodes ME. Increasing 3alpha,5alpha-THP following inhibition of neurosteroid biosynthesis in the ventral tegmental area reinstates anti-anxiety, social, and sexual

behavior of naturally receptive rats. Reproduction. 2009;137(1):119-128. doi:10.1530/REP-08-0250

[16] Walf AA, Frye CA. The use of the elevated plus maze as an assay of anxiety-related behavior in rodents. Nat Protoc. 2007;2(2):322-328. doi:10.1038/nprot.2007.44

[17] Ennaceur A, Neave N, Aggleton JP. Spontaneous object recognition and object location memory in rats: the effects of lesions in the cingulate cortices, the medial prefrontal cortex, the cingulum bundle and the fornix. Exp Brain Res. 1997;113(3):509-519. doi:10.1007/pl00005603

[18] Broadbent JM, Thomson WM. Re: Diverse components of the oral environment in attention-deficit hyperactivity disorder (ADHD) make it difficult to establish whether ADHD is a risk factor for dental caries. JEBD 2005;5:39-40-review of Broadbent et al (2004). J Evid Based Dent Pract. 2006;6(3):250-252. doi:10.1016/j.jebdp.2006.06.001

[19] Akirav I, Maroun M. Ventromedial prefrontal cortex is obligatory for consolidation and reconsolidation of object recognition memory. Cereb Cortex. 2006;16(12):1759-1765. doi:10.1093/cercor/bhj114

[20] Ennaceur A, Delacour J. A new one-trial test for neurobiological studies of memory in rats. 1: Behavioral data. Behav Brain Res. 1988;31(1):47-59. doi:10.1016/0166-4328(88)90157-x

[21] Frye CA, Lacey EH. Posttraining androgens' enhancement of cognitive performance is temporally distinct from androgens' increases in affective behavior. Cogn Affect Behav Neurosci. 2001;1(2):172-182. doi:10.3758/cabn.1.2.172

[22] Luine VN, Jacome LF, Maclusky NJ. Rapid enhancement of visual and place memory by estrogens in rats. *Endocrinology*. 2003;144(7):2836-2844. doi:10.1210/en.2003-0004

[23] Popa-Wagner A, Dumitrascu DI, Capitanescu B, et al. Dietary habits, lifestyle factors and neurodegenerative diseases. Neural Regen Res. 2020;15(3):394-400. doi:10.4103/1673-5374.266045

[24] Giacalone M, Di Sacco F, Traupe I, Topini R, Forfori F, Giunta F. Antioxidant and neuroprotective properties of blueberry polyphenols: a critical review. Nutr Neurosci. 2011;14(3):119-125. doi:10.1179/14768305 11Y.0000000007

[25] Wood E , Hein S , Heiss C , Williams C , Rodriguez-Mateos A . Blueberries and cardiovascular disease prevention. Food Funct. 2019;10(12):7621-7633. doi:10.1039/c9fo02291k

[26] Dinstel RR, Cascio J, Koukel S. The antioxidant level of Alaska's wild berries: high, higher and highest. Int J Circumpolar Health. 2013;72:10.3402/ijch.v72i0.21188. Published 2013 Aug 5. doi:10.3402/ijch.v72i0.21188

[27] L. Wang, B. Waltenberger, E.M.Pferschy-Wenzig, M. Blunder, X. Liu, C. Malainer, *et al.*Natural product agonists of peroxisome proliferator-activated receptor gamma (PPARγ): a review Biochem. Pharmacol., 92 (2014), pp. 73-89

[28] M. Botta, M. Audano, A. Sahebkar, C.R. Sirtori, N. Mitro, M. RuscicaPPAR agonists and metabolic syndrome: an established role? Int. J. Mol. Sci., 19 (4) (2018)

[29] D. Mozaffarian, J.H.Y. WuFlavonoids, dairy foods, and cardiovascular and metabolic health: a review of emerging biologic pathways. Circ. Res., 122 (2) (2018), pp. 369-384

[30] A.B. Ward, H. Mir, N. Kapur, D.N.Gales, P.P. Carriere, S. SinghQuercetin inhibits prostate cancer by attenuating cell survival and inhibiting anti-apoptotic pathways. World J. Surg. Oncol., 16 (1) (2018), p. 108

[31] Mallik S.B., Mudgal J., Nampoothiri M., Hall S., Anoopkumar-Dukie S., Grant G. Caffeic acid attenuates lipopolysaccharide-induced sickness behaviour and neuroinflammation in mice. Neurosci. Lett. 2016;632:218-223.

[32] Ward et al., 2018 A.B. Ward, H. Mir, N. Kapur, D.N. Gales, P.P. Carriere, S. Singh Quercetin inhibits prostate cancer by attenuating cell survival and inhibiting anti-apoptotic pathwaysWorld J. Surg. Oncol., 16 (1) (2018),

[33] Wang et al., 2018J. Wang, P. Um, B.A. Dickerman, J. Liu Zinc, magnesium, selenium and depression: a review of the evidence, potential mechanisms and implications Nutrients, 10 (5) (2018)

[34] Matrisciano F, Pinna G. PPAR and functional foods: Rationale for natural neurosteroid-based interventions for postpartum depression. Neurobiol Stress. 2020 Apr 19;12:100222. doi: 10.1016/j.ynstr.2020.100222. PMID: 32426424; PMCID: PMC7226878.

[35] D. Eyles, T. Burne, J. McGrath Vitamin D in fetal brain development. Semin. Cell Dev. Biol., 22 (6) (2011), pp. 629-636

[36] S. Amini, R. Amani, S. Jafarirad, B.Cheraghian, M. Sayyah, A.A. HemmatiThe effect of vitamin D and calcium supplementation on inflammatory biomarkers, estradiol levels and severity of symptoms in women with postpartum depression: a randomized double-blind clinical trial Nutr. Neurosci., 3 (2020), pp. 1-11

[37] M.J. SzpunarAssociation of antepartum vitamin D deficiency with postpartum depression: a clinical perspective Publ. Health Nutr. (2019), pp. 1-6

[38] D.M. Zhu, W. Zhao, B. Zhang, Y. Zhang, Y. Yang, C. Zhang, et al.The relationship between serum concentration of vitamin D, total intracranial volume, and severity of depressive symptoms in patients with major depressive disorder Front. Psychiatr., 10 (2019), p. 322

[39] J.J. McGrath, D.W. Eyles, C.B.Pedersen, C. Anderson, P. Ko, T.H.Burne, et al.Neonatal vitamin D status and risk of schizophrenia: a population-based case-control study Arch. Gen. Psychiatr., 67 (2010), pp. 889-894

Chapter 18

Antioxidant Properties of Alpine Plant

Vijay Laxmi Trivedi and Mohan Chandra Nautiyal

Abstract

Alpines are the exceptional regions of the world's biomes. They have unique climatic and topographic conditions; they are the habitat of some of the highly specialized flora and fauna. The harsh environmental conditions and extreme fluctuations in them on a seasonal and diurnal basis created extremely stressful situations for the alpine plants. Such stress causes damage to biochemical structures and compounds of the plant cells leads to the production of free radicals, *i.e.* reactive oxygen species (ROS), which can further damage the plant cells or tissues. Alpine plants protect themselves from those ROS efficiently by their highly competent enzymatic and non-enzymatic antioxidant system. In general, this protection increases in alpine plants with altitudes; however, some exceptions are also reported. Antioxidant compounds *viz.* ascorbic acid, tocopherol, glutathione, carotenoids found in alpine flora in higher concentrations as compared to low land plants. Phenolic compounds protected the alpine plants from UV induced ROS by screening the UV radiations and blocking their entries in the cell's mesophyll. This higher antioxidant potential of the alpine plants is highly beneficial for the human being as most alpine plants are the sources of some life-saving drugs.

Keywords: enzymes, non-enzymatic compounds, UV radiation, medicinal plants, freeze–thaw cycles, flavonoids

1. Introduction

Alpine biomes of the world are characterized by their unique features and usually lie between an altitude of about 10,000 feet (3,000 meters) and where the snow line of a mountain begins. The Alpine and Arctic biomes cover 16% of the earth's surface area. Testolin *et al.* [1], based on regional tree line models, estimated their extent to 3.56 Mkm^2, corresponding to 2.64% of the total land area outside Antarctica. Asia hosts almost three-fourths of the global alpine area with 2.59 Mkm^2, followed by South America (15%; 0.55 Mkm^2), North America (9%; 0.32 Mkm^2), and Europe (2%; 0.08 Mkm^2), while Oceania and Africa together contribute to only 1% of the global alpine area. The climate of the alpine regions is dynamic and changes as you move above the lower to higher elevations. The most prominent environmental factor, *i.e.* the temperature normally drops by about 10 °C for every 1000 meters as we go up a mountain. The alpine regions experience a long and cold winter season that lasts about nine months in some alpine areas of the world from around October to May. Temperatures in summer normally ranges from 40 to 60 °F and may last from June to September. Temperature shows very high fluctuations and can normally drop from warm to freezing within a day. The alpine biome is usually dry, with an average precipitation of 12 inches (30 cm) each year. Topographical specialization such as physical gradients, rough terrain, and relative isolation, mountains created attitudinally segregated life zones, and harsh climatic factors of the regions make them very special and unique habitats of some wonderful floras around the world. However, to grow in such a harsh environment, they must have to cope up with the related constraints, including reduced O_2 and CO_2, strong winds, high solar irradiance, shallow rocky soils, low temperatures, and low water and nutrient contents, UV radiation, large temperature variations, *etc.* [2]. Combinations of high-altitude environmental stress lead to increased reactive oxygen species (ROS) production, which increases the risk of oxidative damages in the alpine floras. For performing the vital life functions, alpine flora must quench those ROS. Thus, the alpine flora showed specific adaptations such as accumulation of the secondary metabolites (SMs). Several enzymes such as ascorbate peroxidase, catalase, superoxide dismutase, and glutathione reductase, *etc.*, and other specific molecules such as carotenoids, xanthophylls, *etc.*, play an important role in the protection of alpine flora from the ROS. In this chapter, we will adress the challenges related to ROS production and protection from them in alpine plants.

2. Challenges of alpine habitats that leads to ROS production

Reduced or lower partial pressures of physiological gases (Atmospheric pressure is reduced from sea level values of c. 1000 h Pa (1 bar) by c. 10% for every 1000 m in elevation.), and other associated factors, for example, lower temperatures, correspondingly more precipitation falling as snow, and less atmospheric attenuation of radiation affected the life processes of the alpine plants. Temperature directly affects the plant metabolism by affecting them at the molecular *viz.* DNA, proteins or supramolecular *viz.* membranes, chromosomal structures [3]. The chilling temperature causes decreased activities of several enzymes, including the kinases, carboxylases, *etc.* involved in respiration and photosynthetic processes. Further lowering of the temperature beyond the freezing point leads to the cessation of the vascular functions. Other cytosolic damages involve the complications like the formation of embolisms or cavitation in the xylem and injury to cell membranes.

Along with this alpine region experiences unusually higher diurnal temperature fluctuations, the temperature may range from 0–18 °C from dawn to dusk, on these conditions, leaf temperatures might increase up to 35 °C and lower up to –7 °C to 28 °C. The freeze–thaw cycles operated in plants due to fluctuating diurnal and seasonal temperature may inactivate the PS II and catalase [4] and can enhance the ROS formation in the alpine flora. Radiations affect the alpine environments positively and negatively; for example, positive longwave radiation balance warms leaves in the cool alpine, but the more common negative longwave balance cools minimum temperatures in an already cool environment. Visible shortwave (solar) radiation drives photosynthesis and warms leaves but can also cause photochemical problems [5]. The most destructive radiations in the alpine region are ultraviolet radiation that may cause photochemical damage and other somatic and molecular damages in the alpine flora. High irradiation coupled with low temperature and other stresses leads to the photosynthesis machinery's photoinhibition and halts in synthesis, transport, and storage of the resources. Desiccation is also a profound problem in the alpine plants that are experienced by the plants either in winters due to the freezing lead complications in the plants *viz.* root damage, loss of xylem conductivity, ice formation inside the plants, and in the summer when warmer temperatures can intensify the leaf-to-air vapor deficit and further stimulated the desiccation stress [6]. All the above factors lead to the formation of the ROS that may lead to damage to the general cellular structure and loss of function and block of basic metabolism and repair processes [7], and control of ROS formation and ROS detoxification might be of key importance for the survival of alpine plants.

3. ROS protection in alpine plants

Plants operated several mechanisms to quench the ROS based on the enzymes and several other compounds, including several primary and secondary metabolites. Antioxidative enzymes enhanced their activities, and other lipid and water-soluble compounds, which serve as antioxidants, increase the tolerance in plants to several stresses responsible for ROS productions [8, 9]. Alpine plants also adopted numerous biochemical strategies to quench the ROS that may damage the lipid membrane generated during the physiological process. These strategies included oxidation of superoxide by cascades of enzymatic reactions and accumulation of the compounds like carotenoids, a-tocopherol, ascorbic acid, glutathione, flavonoids, *etc.* [10–12]. Mostly high altitudinal ecotypes consisted of higher antioxidants than their lower altitudinal counterparts mainly due to combined effect and higher light intensities and lower temperature as compared to lower elevations [13, 14].

3.1 Enzymatic antioxidant protection in alpine plants

The enzymatic antioxidative defense system is the cascade of the many enzymes; some of them catalyzes the ROS degradation [superoxide dismutase (SOD, EC 1.15.1.1), catalase (CAT, EC 1.11.1.6), guaiacol peroxidase (POX, EC 1.11.1.7), glutathione peroxidase (GPX, EC 1.11.1.9), *etc.*] and other's regenerated the soluble antioxidants [ascorbate peroxidase (APX, EC 1.1.11.1), monodehydro ascorbate reductase (MDAR, EC 1.6.5.4), dehydroascorbate reductase (DHAR, EC 1.8.5.1), and glutathione reductase (GR, EC 1.8.1.7)] [15]. Alpine flora showed an increase in many of these enzymes, such as CAT, SOD, APX, DHAR, GR [16, 17] but some plants also showed a contradictory pattern. For example, the SOD, GR, and CAT activities were higher in the leaves of *Soldanella alpina* but lower in leaves of *Ranunculus glacialis* [18]. Other plants also showed the range of the variations in antioxidant enzyme activities; for example, extremely higher antioxidant enzyme activities were found in high altitudinal ecotypes of *Soldanella pusilla* moderate in *Poa laxa*, *Carex curvula* and lower in *Taraxacum alpinum, Dryas octopetala,* and some other species [6, 18, 19]. For example, *Polygonum viviparum* showed increased antioxidant enzyme's activities as the altitude increases in the Tianshsan Mountain [20]. During the winter acclimation and spring rewarming, the role of the antioxidant enzymes becomes more prominent, especially in the perennial plants where roots also efficiently takes part in ROS quenching as found in roots of perennial grasses *Poa sphyondylodes, Bromus inermis, Bromus sinensis, Elymus nutans* [21]. In alpine plants, antioxidant enzymes are also involved in the freezing resistance [22] and protected the plants from the ROS produced due to the freeze–thaw cycles of the alpine habitats.

3.2 Non-enzymatic antioxidant

Non-enzymatic antioxidant comprises the major cellular redox buffers which interact with various cellular constituents includes the compounds like ascorbic acid (AA), glutathione (γ-glutamyl-cysteinyl-glycine, GSH), tocopherol, carotenoids, and phenolic compounds. These commands also served as the cofactors of the various enzymes involved in ROS quenching [23]; along with this, these compounds also participate in UV protection.

3.2.1 Ascorbic acid

L-ascorbic acid (L-AA or vitamin C) is the most important antioxidant found in the plants that also takes part in various physiological and developmental processes in the plants protected critical macromolecules from the ROS. Alpine plants are very specific about the L-AA, and some contain extremely high L-AA content. For example in the young leaves of *Soldanella alpina* [12] and *Polygonum viviparum* [20] reported a very high L-AA range. In few alpine species, ascorbate/L-AA is the major C metabolite after sucrose; for example, in the leaves of *S. alpina* [12] in such plant species majority of L-AA found outside the chloroplasts [18]. Although in some alpine flora relatively lower level of L-AA was reported, such as in *Ranuculus glacialis* and *Homogyne alpina,* and most of their L-AA content was reported to present in the chloroplasts. The importance of ascorbic acid in antioxidant protection was determined by Wildi and Lutz [19]. They found an increasing level of antioxidant content in some alpine plant species as the altitude increases. The role of the ascorbic acid is most prominent in this increase where they correlated this increase to increase in light intensity as altitude increases. The concentration of L-AA within an alpine plant species also reflected the diurnal variations. The rhythm of L-AA concentration was reported to go along with light intensity; hence the lowest L-AA was observed at the time of lowest light intensities and lowest temperature in some alpine plants [19].

3.2.2 Glutathione

Glutathione is a tripeptide (γ-glutamyl-cysteinyl-glycine; γ-Glu-Cys-Gly) with long hydrophilic groups and a key low molecular weight non-protein thiol compound known to play a crucial role as an antioxidant [24]. Glutathione also helps in the regeneration of other antioxidants, ascorbic acid and tocopherol, it is the substrate of dehydroascorbate reductase that catalyzes the regeneration of reduced ascorbate, which is the substrate for ascorbate peroxidase regenerated α-tocopherol while detoxifying of H_2O_2 and arresting lipid peroxidation reactions [25, 26]. Potentially higher glutathione synthesis was observed in many plant species in stress conditions, especially in high light intensities, chilling, or freezing temperatures, as reviewed by Tausz [27] and Hasanuzzaman *et al.* [28]. Alpine plants did not show uniformity in the presence of glutathione concentrations; for example, it was higher in *Taraxacum alpinum* and *Soldanella alpina* and comparatively lower in the *Homogyne alpina* and *Ranunculus glacialis*. In general, the alpine plant showed an increase in glutathione concentrations with increasing altitudinal gradients [19], as found in *S. alpina* and *R. glacialis* [26]. Diurnal variations were also observed in studied alpine flora where with increased glutathione concentrations during the morning and maximum during the mid-day and the concentration decline continuously in the afternoon and reached a minimum in the night [19]. Wildi and Lutz [19] also reported the diurnal fluctuations in the glutathione concentration in the alpine plant-like *T. alpinum* and *H. alpina,* which depend on the light intensities and the temperature differences. Glutathione plays an important role in the chilling and freezing protection along with other antioxidants from low temperature in the non-acclimatized plants as well as the acclimatized [29, 30]. Glutathione also plays an important role in increasing the alternative antioxidative scavenging by ascorbate and enzymes like catalase [26], and the glutathione status also acts as a signal or modulator for stress response in the plants [25, 31].

3.2.3 Tocopherols and tocotrienols

Tocopherols and tocotrienols, collectively termed tocochromanols are lipid-soluble molecules with a polar chromanol ring and a hydrophobic polyprenyl side chain [32]. They are synthesized in the shikimate and 1-deoxy-D-xylulose 5-phosphate (DOXP) pathways. The tocopherols are the tocochromanols having a fully saturated side chain. In contrast, tocotrienols are with an unsaturated side chain, and the naturally occurring form of tocopherols *viz.* α, β, γ, and δ is determined by the number of methyl groups in the chromanol ring. Tocochromanols participate in the quenching of peroxyl radicals and other ROS [33] and an important thylakoid-bound radical scavenger. The levels of tocopherols are generally high in some alpine and arctic plants; however, some exceptions are also present, for example, leaves of *Ranunculus glacialis* in which it is extremely low [19]. However, range of the variations was also observed in the tocopherols in the alpine plants [12, 18, 19] for example, Sickel *et al.* [34] showed the range of concentrations of the tocopherols in the dominants fodder species of the alpine pastures of the Norwegian alpine region from 2 to 664 $\mu g\ g^{-1}$ DW as the lowest level in *Avenella flexuosa* and tocopherol pool in all studied species was dominated by α-tocopherol. However, *Vaccinium myrtillus* showed relatively higher γ-tocopherol [34]. Tocopherol concentration also showed the diurnal rhythm in alpine plants. That was light and temperature-dependent in the study of the Wildi and Leutz [19], in which midday was represented by higher tocopherol concentrations and lower during the night. The fluctuations in the a-tocopherol content may be due to the rapid turnover of this compound. The plants react with rapid changes in the level of tocopherols to the slight differences in the environment (e.g., shading and chilling) [19, 35]. Light conditions affected the levels of tocopherols in the plants, and plants are grown in higher light exposer generally have higher tocopherol levels than plants from shady habitats. Concentrations of tocopherols increase typically with increasing altitudes in alpine plants as found in *Soldanella alpina* leaves in which a-tocopherol content showed a 2-fold increase at 2000 m as compared to 1000 m [19]. Tocopherol plays an important role in cold hardening, chilling, and freezing resistance in the various plants, including the alpine flora, as reported in Scots pine, where cold acclimatized older needles contain higher a-tocopherol levels than younger ones [36]. γ-tocopherol may also play an important role as an antioxidant in tissue that exhibits desiccation stress and an indicator of senescence and senescence-related changes.

3.2.4 Carotenoids

Carotenoids are lipophilic pigment and antioxidants which can quench the ROS like toxic oxygen and hydroxyl radicals [37] and broadly classified as hydrocarbon carotenes (included α-carotene, β-carotene, γ-carotene, lycopene, phytoene, and phytofluene) and oxygenated xanthophyll (lutein, zeaxanthin, β-cryptoxanthin, astaxanthin, and fucoxanthin) [38, 39]. Carotenoids are the parts of the light-harvesting complexes (LHC) and play a prominent role as photo-protectant by harvesting light efficiently along with chlorophyll [40] and quench the ROS before these species initiate the oxidative damage. The carotenoids quench the excess light energy and subsequently the ROS production via active non-photochemical quenching (NPQ) or by the dissipation of heat [40, 41]. Singlet oxygen formation at the PSII may damage the D1 protein of the PSII during photo-inhibition and initiate the lipid peroxidation in the chloroplast and carotenoids along with tocopherol protect chloroplast from this peroxidation [41, 42] and among all the carotenoids zeaxanthin reported to have the higher antioxidant capacity [43]. Singlet oxygen produced due to the low temperature-induced photoinhibition is reported either efficiently scavenged or its formation is avoided, which have a high implication on the alpine plants due to their low-temperature habitat. Under high light intensities, ROS production increases at PSI, including hydrogen peroxide (H_2O_2) and singlet oxygen at the PSII in the chloroplast [41]. Alpine plants are exposed to very high light intensities in their habitats. In that scenario role of carotenoids became most prominent from ROS protection in such high light intensities and, along with other antioxidants, carotenoids such as zeaxanthin, neoxanthin, and lutein [43] efficiently quenching ROS in alpine plants. That's why sun-exposed plants of higher altitude are characterized by the higher ratio of Chl a/b and b-carotene/xanthophyll accompanied and a lower ratio of Chl/Car, which results mainly from higher contents of xanthophylls and is interpreted as a higher capacity for non-radiative dissipation of excitation energy and antioxidative protection by carotenoids [6]. ROS are highly reactive and therefore accelerate photoinhibition through direct oxidative damage to PS II. However, the highly variable carotenoid content, especially the zeaxanthin contents reported in alpine plants, for example, a study by Streb *et al.* [18], reported a very high level of carotenoids and xanthophyll cycle pigments in leaves of *Soldanella alpine* and *Homogyne alpina* as compared to *Ranunculus glacialis* leaves. Oncel *et al* [44], in their study also reported the presence of the high b-carotene and xanthophyll in the alpine plants, and among the various alpine plant forms the higher b-carotene content was reported in tree and brush as compared to the herbaceous plants. The diurnal variations observed in the pigment content and carotenoids in alpine plants represented a light-dependent control study by Wildi and Leutz [19], showed all carotenoids except lutein and neoxanthin were showed diurnal rhythm in selected high alpine plant species. An increase in carotenoid content, especially the xanthophyll cycle pigments, also reported in the alpine plants as reported by Wildi and Leutz [19]. However, no effect of altitude in *R. glacialis*, and even decrease in some species such as in *Dryas octopelata* was reported. Seasonal variations also observed in the carotenoid content as reported by Gonzalez *et al.* [45] in *Polylepis tarapacana* where carotenoids content increase with altitude and exhibited seasonal variations, and the highest value recorded in winter. Hence increased carotenoids content in alpine and high altitudinal plants as a safety valve venting the excessive PAR energy before it can damage the photosynthetic system [46] against the large amounts of solar energy coupled with a low temperature in the alpine habitats [43, 47] along with their role in photosynthesis.

3.2.5 Phenolic compounds

Phenolics or polyphenols are the compounds found in plants that belong to secondary metabolites of the plants. Plant phenolics mainly belong to aromatic metabolites with one or more acidic phenolic hydroxyl groups. Their structure ranges from simple phenols such as salicylic acid to complex polymers such as suberin and lignin. Phenolics in plants included hydroxycinnamic acids (HCAs), flavonoids, anthocyanins, and tannins that are widely distributed in the plant kingdom to the classes that are limited taxonomic distribution such as isoflavones, stilbenes, coumarins, furanocoumarins, and styrylpyrones [48]. Phenolics have several functions in plants; they are an integral part of some structural components of the plants, component of plant–animal interactions, plant–plant interactions, act as signaling molecules, screening of highly visible and UV light, pathogens defenses, and general protection against oxidative stress [49, 50]. The role of phenolic compounds in the alpine became most important, especially for protecting against the harmful UV- radiations that are abundant in alpine regions and increase with elevation [51]. Mostly higher content of phenolic compounds was reported in alpine plants than the plants of the lower altitudes, and the reason for this was sighted there need to adapt to the harsh changing environment [52]. The phenolic compounds may also compensate for the lowering of the radical scavenging activity when temperatures become very low in alpine habitats [53]. Phenolic compounds showed great diversity in the interspecies and intra-species level; such variations were reported by Lefebvre *et al.* [54] on three alpine species *Dryas octopetala, Rhododendron ferrugineum,* and *Vaccinium myrtillus*, where flavonoid content and its diversity is very high in *Rhododendron ferrugineum*. *In vitro* evaluation of the phenolic content in extracts of several alpine plants represented their high antioxidant protection, such as in *Potentilla fulgens* [55]. A study in *Gaultheria trichophylla* an alpine Himalayan plant showed a positive correlation between the altitude with total phenolics, tannins, flavonoids, and flavonols, and a direct relationship with the antioxidant potential of the extract prepared from the species [56]. Seasonal variation in total phenolics in *Acorus calamus* and antioxidant activity was reported by Bahukhandi *et al.* [57]. This high phenolic content and diversity may be responsible for medicinal properties of some of the high valued plants of alpine areas such as *Nardostachys jatamansi, Aconetum, Picroriza Kurroa, Rheum* sp., *Hippophae* sp., etc. [58]

4. Freeze and thaw cycle, ROS production and antioxidant protection in alpine plants

Alpine plants have to cope with the phase shifts that are frequent events in the alpine regions, mainly the freeze–thaw cycles that can happen daily during the late winter to early spring. The freezing–thawing cycle (FTC) is a phenomenon in which the soil undergoes repeated freezing and melting due to seasonal or diurnal temperature change [59]. Alpine habitats are represented by the various growth forms such as small prostrate woody shrubs, grasses, sedges, tussocks, herbaceous perennials and annuals, cushion plants, etc. Some of them experienced the diurnal freeze–thaw cycles, and some escaped the seasonal cycle, mainly the herbaceous annuals. Still, almost all of them faced the diurnal freeze–thaw as well as freeze–thawing cycles in spring or autumn [52]. In the alpine regions the most important environmental phenomenon that enflunces the vegetation growth and survival is the freeze–thaw cycle. This cycling causes major complications in plants, such as injuries due to the leakage of cellular solutes [physico-molecular perturbations in cell membranes, and oxidative injury to macromolecules due to cellular accumulation of reactive oxygen species (ROS; e.g., superoxide, singlet oxygen, etc.)] [60]. In the alpine areas, plants mostly experienced two kinds of freeze–thaw moments. One is due to extreme day-night temperature variation, mainly during September–October. The other occurs from November to April, where the temperature is freezing in November and increasing in April [21]. Zhou *et al.* [21] analyzed four grass species from the alpine region for seasonal fluctuation in ROS and antioxidant protection. They found that this freeze–thaw cycle in the autumn destroyed the aerial part of those grasses due to the membrane damage, loss of membrane integrity, and higher electrolyte and lipid peroxidation [21]. This lipid peroxidation resulted due to the decrease in the antioxidant enzyme activities assayed in their work and leads to senescing process. Although roots of those perennial grasses resistant to such freeze–thaw cycle induced ROS with the help of their highly efficient antioxidant enzyme system. Most of the alpine herbaceous perennial plants survived winter with rhizomes, stolons, or other underground storage organs. Those organs may have high antioxidant enzyme activities; besides this, they are rich in secondary metabolites, which also ensures antioxidant protection to them. Complications of the freeze–thaw cycles are more challenging for the alpine woody shrubs, where roots and evergreen leaves have to experience and overcome these freeze–thaw cycles. The diurnal freeze–thaw cycle can also affect the reproductive shoots of several woody and herbaceous plants [61]. Somehow, natural antioxidant protection, either enzymatic or non-enzymatic, is genetically or environmentally induced in the alpine plants to protect them from diurnal and seasonal freeze–thaw cycles. However, the climate changing scenario disturbing this protection, such as unusual late spring frosts, early fall frosts events, a warmer- fall than normal, leaves the alpine plants in the vulnerable stages and subjected them to recurrent freeze–thaw conditions leads to more damage to plants due to more ROS production and little antioxidant protection.

5. Ultraviolet radiations ROS production and antioxidants in alpine plants

High ultraviolet radiations are the characteristic feature of the alpine regions [62]. That can be quite stressful to the alpine lives because of shade-devoid environments and high albedo due to the snow. Increasing UV doses affected the vital processes in plants such as productivity, carbon assimilation, stomatal function, etc. [63] that becomes more relevant when the ozone layer is depleting continuously. Exposure to higher UV radiations leads to the production of free radicals or ROS and other chemically active harmful molecules in the cells that can bring damage to the membrane lipids, nucleic acids proteins including enzymes, etc. [47, 64]. However, alpine plants are protected naturally from the UV radiation's harmful impact with its enzymatic and non-enzymatic equipment. Accumulation of the phenolic compounds such as flavonoids and derivatives of the phenylpropanoid, induction of photo-repair system either prevent the UV from penetrating the cells or help to cells to overcome all the UV driven difficulties. An increase in UV-B absorbing compounds such as pigments like carotenoids, chlorophylls, flavonoids contents was observed in alpine plants with increasing altitude as well as in different seasons [65]. Chanishvili [65] screened various alpine plants, for example, *Tripholium pratense, Plantago major Taraxacum officinale, Achillea millefolium, Polygonum aviculare* for antioxidant compounds content for different altitudes with different level of UV radiations and concluded that the numbers of stress factors in the alpine interacted with UV radiation stress with these plants and the mechanisms of these plant to adapt in such conditions are species-specific [65]. An antioxidant like glutathione, ascorbic acid, phenolic compounds efficiently protect these plants from UV induced ROS, but the protection mechanism or level was species-specific. In the comparison of the herbaceous species, other alpine or subalpine life forms generally have a higher screening capacity of UV radiations [66] leads to more ROS formation in herbaceous plants due to increased penetration of the UV radiations in the underlying mesophyll [67]. In an artificial UV simulation experiment, it was observed that in some alpine plants such as *Carex firma, Dryas octopetala, Ranunculus alpestris, Salix retusa* several striking changes were observed, such as the reduction in glutathione content in most of the studied species. In contrast, other antioxidants such as ascorbic acids, tocopherols, flavonoids seemed to remain unaffected, which means alpine plants are genetically fixed to cope up with such conditions [68].

6. Alpine plants antioxidant and medicinal importance

The alpine plants are packed with antioxidants, and enzymatic as well as non-enzymatic antioxidant makes them quench the ROS produced due to the stressful conditions. Human utilizes this potential of these unique floras for their purposes like food and medicines. The popularity of antioxidants as food and nutraceuticals is increasing globally, and there is a continuous spike in the research on plant-based antioxidants and their medicinal potentials. Several alpine plants were used in various traditional and modern health care systems for their antioxidant activities, which comprises their other properties such as anti-cancerous, immune-modulatory, anti-stress, etc. A range of studies are available on the alpine plants' antioxidant potential [56, 57, 58, 69] and revived by Bhatt *et al.* [70]. Alpine plants from the Himalayan region are most remarkable for their medicinal properties plants like *Picrorhiza kurrooa* [71, 72] *Aconitum* sp. [72, 73], *Polygonum bistorta* [73, 74] *Nardostachys jatamansi* [75], etc.

7. Conclusion

Unique features of the alpine habitats make them home to some of the extraordinary flora and fauna in the world. In their habitats, alpine plants experience extremely stressful conditions, which causes the production of the free radicals or ROS species in them. However, these plant species genetically or phenotypically adapted to scavenge those ROS. Enzymatic as well non-enzymatic antioxidant system efficiently protecting the alpine floras, although this protection is species-specific, as a generalized feature the antioxidant potential in alpine plants increase with altitudes. Alpine vegetation showed a range of variation in the antioxidant protection plants like *Ranunculus glacialis* has very low antioxidant protection despite this, the plant species can survive in some of the highest altitudes of the world. On the other hand, species like *Soldanella alpina* showed very high antioxidant potential with high ascorbic acid, glutathione, phenolic, and other antioxidants. Alpine plants adapted to diurnal as well as seasonal fluctuations to ROS production due to the fluctuating environmental conditions of their habitats, especially during the daily freeze–thaw cycle of the early spring and late winter as well as the seasonal cycle. However, the changing climate is interfering with this seasonal acclimation. For example, a heatwave during the winter can deacclimatized the dormant buds of woody alpine trees, and a cold wave during summer may destroy the reproductive shoots. All these disturbances interrupt the ROS-antioxidant protection dynamics in those alpine plants. Most of the alpine floras are currently facing extinction due to climate change scenarios and anthropogenic activities, and we need to protect those unique habitats and related flora and fauna.

Conflict of interest

The authors declare no conflict of interest.

Author details

Vijay Laxmi Trivedi* and Mohan Chandra Nautiyal
Hemvati Nandan Bahuguna Garhwal University, Srinagar Garhwal, Uttarakhand, India

*Address all correspondence to: vijaylaxmitrivedi@gmail.com

References

[1] Testolin R, Attorre F, Jiménez-Alfaro B. Global distribution and bioclimatic characterization of alpine biomes. Ecography. 2020; 43: 779-788. DOI: 10.1111/ecog.0501

[2] Roupioz L, Jia L, Nerry F, Menenti M. Estimation of Daily Solar Radiation Budget at Kilometer Resolution over the Tibetan Plateau by Integrating MODIS Data Products and a DEM. Remote Sensing. 2016; 8(6): 504. DOI: 10.3390/rs8060504

[3] Nievola CC, Carvalho CP, Carvalho V, Rodrigues E. Rapid responses of plants to temperature changes. Temperature (Austin). 2017; 4(4):371-405. DOI:10.1080/23328940.2017.1377812

[4] Feierabend J, Schaan C, Hertwig B. Photoinactivation of Catalase Occurs under Both High- and Low-Temperature Stress Conditions and Accompanies Photoinhibition of Photosystem II. Plant.1992; 100: 1554-1561. DOI: 0032-0889/92/100/1 554/08/$01 .00/

[5] Ball MC. The role of photoinhibition during tree seedling establishment at low temperatures. In: Baker NR, Bowyer JR, editors. Photoinhibition of photosynthesis from molecular mechanisms to the field. Oxford BIOS Scientific; 1994. p. 365-76.

[6] Germino MJ. Plants in Alpine Environments. In: Monson R, editors. Ecology and the Environment. Springer, New York, NY. DOI: 10.1007/978-1-4614-7612-2_12-4

[7] Murata N, Takahashi S, Nishiyama Y, Allakhverdiev SI. Photoinhibition of photosystem II under environmental stress. Biochimica et Biophysica Acta. 2007. 1767: 414-42. 10.1016/j.bbabio.2006.11.019.

[8] Noctor G, Foyer C H. Ascorbate and glutathione: keeping active oxygen under control. Annual Review of Plant Biology. 1998; 49: 249-279. DOI: 10.1146/annurev.arplant.49.1.249.

[9] Sharma P, Jha AB , Dubey RS, Pessarak M. Reactive Oxygen Species, Oxidative Damage, and Antioxidative Defense Mechanism in Plants under Stressful Conditions. Journal of Botany. 2012; DOI: 10.1155/2012/2170.

[10] Munné-Bosch. The role of α-tocopherol in plant stress tolerance. Journal of Plant Physiology. 2005; 162: 743-748. DOI: 10.1016/j.jplph.2005.04.022.

[11] Ort D, Baker N. A photoprotective role of O2 as an alternative electron sink in photosynthesis? Current Opinion in Plant Biology. 2002; 5:193-198. DOI: 10.1016/s1369-5266(02)00259-5

[12] Streb P, Aubert S, Gout E, Bligny R. Reversibility of cold- and light-stress tolerance and accompanying changes of metabolite and antioxidant levels in the two high mountain plant species Soldanella alpina and *Ranunculus glacialis*. Journal of Experimental Botany. 2003; 54:405-418. DOI: 10.1093/jxb/erg048

[13] Orabi S, Shaban A. Antioxidant defense mechanisms enhance oxidative stress tolerance in plants. A review. Current Science International. 2019; 8: 565-576.

[14] Zhou X, Chen S, Wu H, Yang Y, Xu H. Biochemical and proteomics analyses of antioxidant enzymes reveal the potential stress tolerance in Rhododendron chrysanthum Pall. Biology Direct. 2017;12(1):10. DOI:10.1186/s13062-017-0181-6

[15] Caverzan A, Casassola A, Brammer SP. Antioxidant responses of wheat plants under stress. Genetics and Molecular Biology. 2016;

39(1):1-6. DOI:10.1590/1678-4685-GMB-2015-0109.

[16] Bowler C, Van Montagu M, Inze D. Superoxide dismutase and stress tolerance. Annual Review of Plant Physiology and Plant Molecular Biology. 1992; 43: 83-116. DOI: 10.1146/annurev.pp.43.060192.000503.

[17] Birben E, Sahiner UM, Sackesen C, Erzurum S, Kalayci O. Oxidative stress and antioxidant defense. World Allergy Organ J. 2012; 5(1):9-19. DOI:10.1097/WOX.0b013e3182439613

[18] Streb P, Feierabend J, Bligny R. Resistance to photoinhibition of photosystem II and catalase and antioxidative protection in high mountain plants. Plant Cell Environment. 1997; 20: 1030-1040. DOI: 10.1111/j.1365-3040.1997.tb00679.x

[19] Wildi B, Lütz, C, Antioxidant composition of selected high alpine plant species from different altitudes. Plant Cell Environment. 1996; 19: 138-146. DOI: 10.1111/j.1365-3040.1996.tb00235.x

[20] Wang Y, He W, Huang H et al. Antioxidative responses to different altitudes in leaves of alpine plant *Polygonum viviparum* in summer. Acta Physiology Plantarum. 2009; 31: 839-848 DOI: 10.1007/s11738-009-0300-9.

[21] Zhou R, Zhao H. Seasonal pattern of antioxidant enzyme system in the roots of perennial forage grasses grown in alpine habitat, related to freezing tolerance. Physiologia Plantarum. 2004; 121(3): 399-408. DOI: 10.1111/j.0031-9317.2004.00313.x

[22] Guo J, Liu X, Li X, Chen S, Jin Z, Liu G. Overexpression of VTE1 from Arabidopsis resulting in high vitamin E accumulation and salt stress tolerance increase in tobacco plant Journal of Applied Environmental and Biological Sciences. 2006; 12:468-471. DOI: 10.1007/s10529-008-9672-y

[23] De Pinto MC, De Gara L. Changes in the ascorbate metabolism of apoplastic and symplastic spaces are associated with cell differentiation. Journal of Experimental Botany. 2004; 55 (408): 2559-2569. DOI: 10.1093/jxb/erh253

[24] Foyer CH, Noctor G. Redox sensing and signalling associated with reactive oxygen in chloroplasts, peroxisomes and mitochondria. Physiologia Plantarum. 2003; 119 (3): 355-364. DOI: 10.1034/j.1399-3054.2003.00223.x

[25] Foyer CH, Noctor G.] Ascorbate and Glutathione: The Heart of the Redox Hub. Plant Physiology. 2011; 155 (1) 2-18. DOI: 10.1104/pp.110.167569

[26] Laureau C, Meyer S, Baudin X, Huignard C, Streb P. In vivo epidermal UV-A absorbance is induced by sunlight and protects Soldanella alpina leaves from photoinhibition. Functional Plant Biology. 2015; 42:599-608. DOI: 10.1071/FP14240.

[27] Tausz M, Wonisch A, Peters J, Jiménez MS, Morales D, Grill D. Short-term changes in free-radical scavengers and chloroplast pigments in *Pinus canariensis* needles as affected by mild drought stress. Journal of Plant Physiology. 2001b; 158: 213-219. DOI: 10.1078/0176-1617-00178

[28] Hasanuzzaman M, Nahar K, Anee TI, Fujita M. Glutathione in plants: biosynthesis and physiological role in environmental stress tolerance. Physiology and Molecular Biology of Plants. 2017; 23(2): 249-268. DOI:10.1007/s12298-017-0422-2.

[29] Kocsy G, von Ballmoos P, Rüegsegger A, Szalai G, Galiba G, Brunold C. Increasing the glutathione content in a chilling-sensitive maize genotype using safeners increased protection against chilling-induced

injury. Plant Physiology. 2001; 127:1147-1156. DOI: 10.1104/pp.010107.

[30] Zhao S, Blumwald E. Changes in oxidation-reduction state and antioxidant enzymes in the roots of jack pine seedlings during cold acclimation. Physiologia Plantarum. 2002; 104: 134-142. DOI: 10.1034/j.1399-3054.1998.1040117.x.

[31] Foyer CH, Shigeoka S. Understanding Oxidative Stress and Antioxidant Functions to Enhance Photosynthesis. Plant Physiology. 2011; 115: 93-100. DOI: 10.1104/pp.110.166181

[32] Falk J, Munné-Bosch S. Tocochromanol functions in plants: antioxidation and beyond, Journal of Experimental Botany. 2010; 61(6) : 1549-1566. DOI: 10.1093/jxb/erq030.

[33] Fritsche S, Wang X, Jung C. Recent Advances in our Understanding of Tocopherol Biosynthesis in Plants: An Overview of Key Genes, Functions, and Breeding of Vitamin E Improved Crops. Antioxidants (Basel). 2017; 6(4):99. DOI:10.3390/antiox6040099.

[34] Sickel H, Bilger W, Ohlson M. High Levels of α-Tocopherol in Norwegian Alpine Grazing Plants. Journal of Agricultural and Food Chemistry. 2012; 60 (31) 7573-7580. DOI: 10.1021/jf301756j.

[35] Franzen J, Bausch J, Glatzle D, Wagner E. Distribution of vitamin E in spruce seedlings and mature tree organs, and within the genus. Phytochemistry. 1991; 30: 147-151.

[36] Wingsle G, Hällgren JE. Influence of SO2 and NO2 exposure on glutathione superoxide dismutase and glutathione reductase activities in Scots pine needles. Journal of Experimental Botany. 1993; 44: 463-470.

[37] Young A J. The photoprotective role of carotenoids in higher plants. Physiologia Plantarum. 1991; 83(4): 702-708. DOI:10.1111/j.1399-3054.1991.tb02490.x

[38] Merhan O. The Biochemistry and Antioxidant Properties of Carotenoids, Carotenoids, Dragan J. Cvetkovic and Goran S. Nikolic, IntechOpen, DOI: 10.5772/67592. [BOOK]

[39] Zaripheh S, Erdman Jr. JW. Factors that influence the bioavailability of xanthophylls. Journal of Nutrition. 2002; 132: 531S–534S. DOI: 10.1093/jn/132.3.531S

[40] Croce R, Weiss S, Bassi R. Carotenoid-binding sites of the major light-harvesting complex II of higher plants. Journal of Biological Chemistry. 1999b; 274: 29613-29623. DOI: 10.1074/jbc.274.42.29613

[41] Niyogi KK. Photoprotection revisited: Genetics and molecular approaches. Annual Review of Plant Physiology and Plant Molecular Biology. 1999; 50: 333-359. DOI: 10.1146/annurev.arplant.50.1.333

[42] Aro EM, Virgin I, Andersson B. Photoinhibition of PS II. Inactivation, protein damage and turnover. Biochimica et Biophysica Acta (BBA) - Bioenergetics. 1993; 1143 (2): 113-134. DOI: 10.1016/0005-2728(93)90134-2.

[43] Havaux M, Dall'Osto L, Bassi R. Zeaxanthin Has Enhanced Antioxidant Capacity with Respect to All Other Xanthophylls in Arabidopsis Leaves and Functions Independent of Binding to PSII Antennae. Plant Physiology. 2007; 145 (4) 1506-1520. DOI: 10.1104/pp.107.108480.

[44] Öncel I, Yurdakulol E, Keleş Y, Kurt L, Yıldız A. Role of antioxidant defense system and biochemical adaptation on stress tolerance of high mountain and steppe plants. Acta Oecologica. 2004; 26: 211-218. DOI: 10.1016/j.actao.2004.04.004

[45] González JA, Gallardo MG, Boero C, Cruz ML, Prado FE. Altitudinal and seasonal variation of protective and photosynthetic pigments in leaves of the world's highest elevation trees Polylepis tarapacana (Rosaceae). Acta Oecologica. 2007; 32:36-41. DOI: 10.1016/j.actao.2007.03.002

[46] Gilmore AM. Mechanistic aspects of xanthophyll cycle-dependent photoprotection in higher plant chloroplast and leaves. Physiologia Plantarum. 1997; 99:197-209.DOI: 10.1111/j.1399-3054.1997.tb03449.x.

[47] Asada K. The water-water cycle as alternative photon and electron sinks. Philosophical transactions of the Royal Society of London. Series B, Biological sciences. 2000; 355(1402): 1419-1431. DOI: 10.1098/rstb.2000.0703

[48] Grace SC (2005) Phenolics as antioxidants. In: Smirnoff N (ed) Antioxidants and reactive oxygen species in plants. Blackwell Scientific Publishers, Oxford, pp 141-168

[49] Winkel-Shirley B. Biosynthesis of flavonoids and effects of stress. Current Opinion in Plant Biology. 2002; 5:218-23. DOI: 10.1016/s1369-5266(02)00256-x.

[50] Bais HP, Park SW, Weir TL, Callaway RM, Vivanco JM. How plants communicate using the underground information superhighway. Trends in Plant Science. 2004; 9(1):26-32. DOI: 10.1016/j.tplants.2003.11.008.

[51] Robberecht R, Caldwell M, Billings W. Leaf Ultraviolet Optical Properties Along a Latitudinal Gradient in the Arctic-Alpine Life Zone. Ecology. 1980: 61(3), 612-619. DOI :10.2307/1937427.

[52] Körner, C. (2003). Alpine Plant Life: Functional Plant Ecology of High Mountain Ecosystems. Berlin: Springer.

[53] Albert A, Sareedenchai V, Heller W, Seidlitz HK, Zidorn C. Temperature is the key to altitudinal variation of phenolics in *Arnica montana* L. cv. ARBO. Oecologia. 2009 ; 160(1):1-8. DOI: 10.1007/s00442-009-1277-1.

[54] Lefebvre T, Millery-Vigues A, Gallet C. Does leaf optical absorbance reflect the polyphenol content of alpine plants along an elevational gradient? Alpine Botany. 2016; 126(2), 177-185. DOI: 10.1007/s00035-016-0167-5

[55] Jaitak V, Sharma K, Kalia K, Kumar N, et al. Antioxidant activity of Potentilla fulgens: An alpine plant of western Himalaya. Journal of Food Composition and Analysis. . 2010. 23(2): 142-147. DOI:10.1016/j.jfca.2009.02.013

[56] Bahukhandi A, PandeyA, Sekar KC, Bhatt I. Polyphenolics, Nutrients and Antioxidant Activity of Gaultheria trichophylla Royle: A High Value Wild Edible Plant of Trans Himalaya. Horticulture International Journal. 2017; 1: 1-6. DOI: 10.15406/hij.2017.01.00007.

[57] Bahukhandi A, Rawat S, Jugran AK, et al. Seasonal Variation in Phenolics and Antioxidant Activity of *Acorus calamus* Linn.: An Important Medicinal Plant of Himalaya. National Academy Science Letters. 2021; 44, 13-15. DOI: 10.1007/s40009-020-00959-3

[58] Nautiyal MC and Nautiyal BP. Agrotechniques for High Altitude Medicinal & Aromatic Plants. M/s Bishen Singh Mahendra Pal Singh; First Edition. 2004.

[59] Mayr S, Hacke U, Schmid P, Schweinbacher F, Gruber A. Frost Drought in Conifers at the Alpine Timberline: Xylem Dysfunction and Adaptations. Ecology. 2006; 87(12): 3175-3185. DOI: 10.1890/0012-9658(2006)87[3175:FDICAT]2.0.CO;2

[60] Arora R. Mechanism of freeze-thaw injury and recovery: a cool retrospective

and warming up to new ideas. Plant Science . 2018; 270: 301-313. DOI: 10.1016/j.plantsci.2018.03.002

[61] Neuner G. Frost resistance in alpine woody plants. Frontiers in plant science. 2014; 5: 654. DOI: 10.3389/fpls.2014.00654.

[62] Caldwell MM. Solar Ultraviolet Radiation as an Ecological Factor for Alpine Plants. Ecological Monographs. 1968(38)1968: 243-268. DOI: 10.2307/1942430.

[63] Sedej T T, Erznožnik T, Rovtar J. Effect of UV radiation and altitude characteristics on functional traits and leaf optical properties in Saxifraga hostii at the alpine and montane site in the Slovenian Alps. Photochemical & Photobiological Sciences. 2020; 19(2):180-192. DOI: 10.1039/c9pp00032a.

[64] Frohnmeyer H, Staiger D. Ultraviolet-B Radiation-Mediated Responses in Plants. Balancing Damage and Protection. Plant Physiology.2003; 133 (4) 1420-1428; DOI: 10.1104/pp.103.030049.

[65] Chanishvili S, Badridze G, Rapava L, Janukashvili N. Effect of altitude on the contents of antioxidants in leaves of some herbaceous plants. Russian Journal of Ecology. 2007; 38(5): 367-373. DOI:10.1134/s1067413607050128.

[66] Day T A, Vogelmann T C, Delucia E H. Are some plant life forms more effective than others in screening out ultraviolet-B radiation. Oecologia. 1992; 92(4): 513-519. DOI: 10.1007/BF00317843.

[67] Barnes PW, Ryel RJ, Flint SD. UV Screening in Native and Non-native Plant Species in the Tropical Alpine: Implications for Climate Change-Driven Migration of Species to Higher Elevations. Frontiers in Plant Science. 2017; 8:1451. DOI: 10.3389/fpls.2017.01451

[68] L€utz C, Seidlitz HK. Physiological and Ultrastructural Changes in Alpine Plants Exposed to High Levels of UV and Ozone. IN: Plants in Alpine Regions Cell Physiology of Adaption and Survival Strategies . 2012 : 29-42 . Springer-Verlag/Wien, Newyork

[69] VL Trivedi, J Sati, D Chand , Nautiyal MC. Antioxidant Potential of Herbal Tea from Rhododendron anthopogon D. Don and Hippophae salcifolia D. Don. Journal of Non-Timber Forest Products. 2017; 3: 131-135.

[70] Bhatt ID, Rawat S, Rawal RS. (2013) Antioxidants in Medicinal Plants. In: Chandra S., LATA H., Varma A. (eds) Biotechnology for Medicinal Plants. Springer, Berlin, Heidelberg. https://doi.org/10.1007/978-3-642-29974-2_13

[71] Rajkumar V, Gunjan R, Ashok R. Antioxidant and antineoplastic activities of Picrorhiza kurroa extracts. Food Chemical Toxicology. 2011; 49:363 369. DOI: 10.1016/j.fct.2010.11.009

[72] Konda VG, Eerike M, Raghuraman LP, Rajamanickam MK. Antioxidant and Nephroprotective Activities of Aconitum heterophyllum Root in Glycerol Induced Acute Renal Failure in Rats. Journal of Clinical and Diagnostic Research for doctors. 2016; 10(3):FF01-2. doi: 10.7860/JCDR/2016/10798.7388.

[73] Munir N, Ijaz W, Altaf I, Naz S. Evaluation of antifungal and antioxidant potential of two medicinal plants: Aconitum heterophyllum and *Polygonum bistorta*, Asian Pacific Journal of Tropical Biomedicine. 2014; 4 (2) : 639-S643. DOI: 10.12980/APJTB.4.201414B182.

[74] Wang ST, Gao WF , Ya-Xi , Xinguang & LKD, et al. Phenol profiles and antioxidant capacities of Bistort

Rhizoma (*Polygonum bistorta* L.) extracts. RSC Advances . 2016; 6(33)10.1039/C6RA00687F.

[75] Sharma SK, Singh AP. In vitro antioxidant and free radical scavenging activity of Nardostachys jatamansi DC. J Acupunct Meridian Stud. 2012 ;5(3):112-8. DOI: 10.1016/j.jams.2012.03.002.

Chapter 19

Use of Selected Antioxidant-Rich Spices and Herbs in Foods

Perçin Karakol and Emin Kapi

Abstract

Free radicals are chemicals that play a role in the etiopathogenesis of ischemia–reperfusion injury. To prevent or reduce this damage, many protective or therapeutic antioxidants are used effectively in alternative medicine. These antioxidants include immunological or pharmacological agents, vitamins, food and herbal products, and spices. Herbs and spices have been used for a long time as coloring or preservative agents by adding to the content of foods, and at the same time to increase the nutritional value of foods. More recently, the nutritional effects of herbs and spices have become more perceived and the area of interest for these products has increased. Concordantly, the biological contents of herbs and spices have begun to be studied in more detailed way at the cellular and molecular level. Sample plants are classified according to different chemical families, with the diet. Therefore, they have different levels of antioxidant capacity. These products also have potent anti-inflammatory, antihypertensive, glucoregulatory, antithrombotic, anticarcinogenic and so forth effects. These properties are used in the treatment of some chronic diseases. In this review, the antioxidant properties of various herbs and spices used to add flavor to foods or to extend their shelf life have been examined in the light of large-scale nutritional epidemiological studies, in vitro cellular/animal studies and clinical trials.

Keywords: antioxidant, food, herb, plant, review, spice, supplement

1. Introduction

It is known that cell or tissue damage is related to free reactive oxygen radicals (ROS; reactive oxygen species) and associated nitrogen degradation products [1–5]. These radicals are high-energy molecules that have free electrons in their outer orbits, and can easily interact with other molecules and cause DNA damage. These molecules are continuously produced in the human body secondary to some detoxification processes, phagocytosis and energy production. Although the healthy human body has the capacity to neutralize these radicals, the balances may change in the direction of increasing the ROS ratio and reducing the antioxidant capacity due to the reasons such as environmental conditions and diet, so oxidative stress develops [6]. There are many different types of ROS, and many cellular and organ system level pathologies occur in the body depending on these products [2, 7, 8]. Various antioxidant compounds are used in medicine to prevent these pathologies [1, 2, 9, 10]. These compositions include various immunological and pharmacological agents, vitamins, fruits, vegetables, food supplements, herbal products, or spices [1, 2, 4, 11].

Many types of herbs and spices have generally safe ingredients for human health and their benefits have been known for a long time [10–13]. These benefits include facilitation of digestion, anti-inflammatory, antirheumatic, antisclerotic, antimalarial, antimicrobial, antiviral, immunomodulatory, antiallergic, antiaging, antidiabetic, radioprotective, antioxidant, and antiproliferative/anticarcinogenic effects [4, 9–20]. Because of these benefits, they are used in many acute and chronic diseases (diabetes, dyslipidemia, hypertension, cancer, cardiovascular and neuro-degenerative disease, liver cirrhosis, arthritis, asthma, obesity, metabolic syndrome, etc.) [9, 10, 12–14, 19, 21, 22]. In addition, herbs and spices are used in order to increase the nutritional value, flavor and aroma of foods, have protective properties during storage and extend the shelf life of foods [3, 5, 9, 11–14, 21, 23–26]. Thanks to the spices added to foods, the lipids in the food are protected against oxidative deterioration and the formation of oxidant substances is delayed.

Antioxidant materials can be classified under two main headings, which are synthetic and natural [5, 12]. Synthetic antioxidants are widely used in the market. However, it has been determined that these synthetic products have harmful effects on human health in the long term, and cause teratogenic/carcinogenic effects. Therefore, consumers prefer foods that contain natural antioxidant agents. Concordantly, over time, herbs and spices with natural antioxidant properties were replaced by synthetic products [4]. These so-called "natural antioxidants" are claimed to be more effective than synthetic ones. The origins and uses of natural antioxidants are diverse. In this review, the main properties of herbs and spices with known antioxidant properties are studied to be presented.

2. General properties of herbs and spices with natural antioxidant effects

Many bioactive foodstuffs originate from herbs [2]. These substances are generally called as "phytochemicals" [2, 5]. Most of these phytochemicals are redox active molecules so that they have antioxidant features [2].

Many herbs and spices with antioxidant effects are from the *"labiatae (lamiaceae)"* family. Most of the herbs in this family have been used in traditional treatments to cure various diseases from ancient times until today. Besides, it has areas of use in the food, cosmetics and perfumery industries [27].

Herbs and spices contain organic sulfur, tannin, alkaloid, phenolic diterpene, diketone, polyphenol, polyphenylpropanoid, vitamin, flavonoid and anthocyanin compounds, and they have a protective effect against oxidizing agents [12–14, 27–29]. It is stated that this protective effect is mostly related to the "flavonoid" and "phenolic" content of the herbs and spices [3, 4, 9, 12, 13].

It has been suggested that being fed with a flavonoid-containing diet efficiently reduces the risk of chronic diseases [9, 10, 21]. These effects of flavonoids have been reported to be related to oxidative stress defense at the molecular level [9, 30–32]. Flavonoids scavenge and neutralize free radicals [32]. Numerous articles have been published on this subject, especially in the last two decades. In these studies, very detailed investigations have been made especially on the structures and biological activities of flavonoids [4, 9, 21, 33–35].

Phenolic compounds act with redox reactions [32]. The ratio of phenolic component is an important variable on the antioxidant activity of the product [3–5, 9, 10, 12, 26].

It has been reported that the antioxidant capacity of these products is approximately 10 times higher than that of fresh fruits and vegetables [9, 32]. Parallel to the progress made by modern medicine in the last decade, studies to determine the bioactive components in herbs have gained momentum. Although the chemical structures of most herbal components have been described in detail, tests and molecular studies on their bioactive roles are still ongoing [9, 21, 36–39].

3. Antioxidant-affected plants

In the **Figure 1**, natural herbs with potent antioxidant features and which are most commonly used are listed.

3.1 Rosemary (*Rosemarinus officinalis*)

This plant, in the "*lamiaceae/labiatae*" family, is a polyphenol-containing plant with small pointed leaves, which grows particularly in the Mediterranean region [9, 12–14, 21, 27, 40]. The plant can reach 1–2 meters in height. It has an aromatic structure and does not shed its leaves in winter. Especially in spring, white-blue flowers bloom with leaves [14, 27]. Its leaves taste bitter [27]. It is used in making salads or tea [40].

This plant is used as an antioxidant and preservative, especially in the food industry [12, 14, 27, 41–43]. In addition, it can be consumed in the form of soap, perfume and lotion [27]. Its use for food preservation is for the lipid component in food. When used as a food preservative, it has been determined that rosemary does not spoil the organoleptic contents of foods [12].

There are studies indicating that the antioxidant capacity of rosemary is closely related to the techniques in production [44]. It has been reported that the antioxidant effect of rosemary depends primarily on its type, harvest time, type of treatment, environmental and ecological characteristics of the environment it grows [27]. The way rosemary is given is also an important parameter in its effectiveness. It has been reported that the encapsulated form of rosemary essential oil exhibited more antimicrobial effects compared to the standard essential oil form [12].

Carnosol, carnosic acid, phenolic diterpene, phenolic acid, rosmanol, epirosmanol, rosmarinic acid, caffeic acid ester, tosemaridiphenol, 3- (3,4 dihydroxyphenyl) lactic acid, flavonoids (apigenin, diosmin, luteolin), tannins provide antioxidant properties to the plant [9, 11–13, 27, 40, 45]. Rosemary also contains essential oils (cineole, pinene, camphor) [13]. The dominant components in its structure are

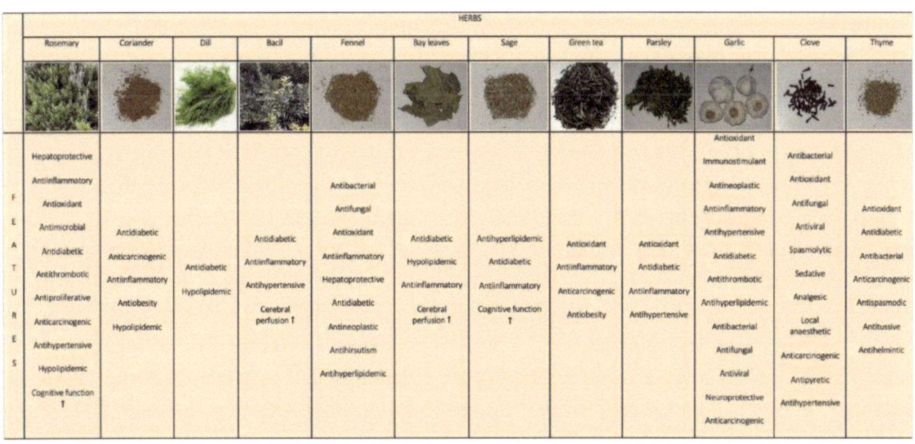

Figure 1.
Natural herbs with potent antioxidant features and which are most commonly used.

rosmarinic and carnosic acid [12, 13, 27]. Carnosic acid and carnosol are responsible for 90% of the antioxidant effect. These components reduce cell membrane damage by 40–50%. Both components also reduce DNA damage due to dietary oxidant agents [13]. The antioxidant activity of carnosic acid has been compared with synthetic antioxidants such as butylated hydroxytoluene (BHT), butylated hydroxyanisole (BHA) and tertiary butyl hydroquinone (TBHQ), and it has been proved that carnosic acid has a stronger antioxidant effect than these molecules [12].

There are many studies on rosemary in the literature. Akgül et al. determined that rosemary is among the most powerful antioxidants [46]. It has been stated that rosemary extract increases the antioxidant status and defense of aged rats [13]. Similarly, in another study, the antioxidant effect of 32 different plants and spices on lard was investigated, and rosemary was detected to be among the most important antioxidants [47]. In another study in which 15 different types of spices were tried in sausages, it was observed that one of the products with the most important antioxidant effect was rosemary [48]. In a study examining the effect of rosemary on foods prepared with some fish species, it was observed that rosemary significantly reduced the level of malondialdehyde in fish-containing foods. In a study on the oxidative stability of ground sardines, rosemary extract was determined to have an antioxidative effect over a 5-month period [27]. Rıznar et al. examined the antioxidant activity at 3 different temperatures (4, 12, 25 °C) by adding rosemary extract to chicken sausages, and observed high antioxidant effects during storage at all temperatures [49]. Lopez-Bote et al. indicated that rosemary extract is highly effective in preventing lipid peroxidation in chicken meat stored at −20 ° C for 6 days [50]. In a study of alloxan-induced diabetic rats, intraperitoneal injection of rosemary for 7 days decreased in blood glucose levels [40]. In a similar study, after administration of 100 mg/kg rosemary extract in diabetic rat models, a significant decrease in blood glucose level and an increase in serum insulin concentration were achieved [13].

The properties of rosemary include hepatoprotective, antiangiogenic, anti-inflammatory, antioxidant, antimicrobial, antidiabetic, antihypertensive, antithrombotic, antiproliferative, and anticarcinogenic effects [4, 13, 14, 40]. Its anti-inflammatory effect is thought to be because of decreased macrophage viability, inducible nitric oxide synthase (iNOS) protein expression and nitric oxide (NO) production. Rosemary can also contribute to the treatment of hypertension. Increased urinary volume and excretion of sodium, potassium, and chloride were found in healthy rats given rosemary extract daily for 7 days orally [40]. It also improves endothelial function with its antithrombotic effect [13]. Carnocic acid has an inhibitory effect on liver fibrosis [14]. Rosemary extract has been determined to have detoxifying properties on toxic chemical-related liver damage and cirrhosis in experimental animal models. In the experiments performed in mice, it was observed that fatty liver associated with obesity was decreased by giving 200 mg/kg of rosemary leaves after the diet with high fat content [13]. Another effect of rosemary is that it is hypolipidemic. In a study conducted on obese rats, it was evaluated that feeding a rosemary-rich diet for 64 days caused a decrease in body weight [40]. Rosemary extract reduces low density lipoprotein (LDL) cholesterol oxidation. In cell culture tests, it has been detected to reduce lipid peroxidation by 38–89% under oxidative stress. In a randomized clinical study conducted with rosemary inhalation in 140 subjects, it was observed that cognitive assessment and self-assessment mood scale levels and cognitive functions increased. In vivo and in vitro studies, rosemary extract has been reduced oxidative damage in fat cells on the skin surface. Rosemary is therefore a potential candidate for skin treatment. However, clinical studies with large series are needed on this subject [13]. Amoah et al. reported that this ingredient is also used in the treatment of atopic dermatitis and seasonal allergic rhinoconjunctivitis [51].

3.2 Coriander (*Coriandrum sativum*)

It is a plant with a flavonoid structure [9]. Coriander leaves and roots are used in cooking. Especially the coriander leaf type known as "*cilantro*" is frequently used for this purpose [40].

The roots of this plant contain high levels of chlorogenic acid, caffeoyl derivatives, quercetin-3-O-rutinoside and p-coumaric acid [9, 40].

Several potential benefits of chlorogenic acid have been reported [9]. These include antidiabetic, anticarcinogenic, anti-inflammatory and antiobesity effects [9, 52, 53]. In streptozotocin-induced diabetic rats, intraperitoneal injection of coriander seed extract significantly decreased serum glucose and increased insulin secretion in pancreatic β-cells. It was also observed that lipid peroxidation and protein oxidation decreased in the subjects given coriander. Coriander roots also have a hypolipidemic effect. In a study conducted in obese and hyperlipidemic rats, it was presented that total cholesterol, LDL and triglyceride levels were reduced in the group given coriander extract orally for 30 days. Additionally, serum and erythrocyte antioxidant parameters have been detected to be increased [40].

3.3 Dill (*Anethum graveolens*)

Dill has a flavonoid structure [4, 6]. It is generally consumed during feeding with seafood [40]. Fresh dill contains high levels of flavonol glucuronides, chlorogenic acid quercetin and isorhamnetin [9, 40].

It has antidiabetic potential. Dill given orally for 15 days in diabetic rats induced by dexamethasone has been determined to cause a decrease in serum glucose and insulin levels. Dill is also hypolipidemic. In rats fed a high-fat diet for 3 weeks, daily oral dill was found to cause a decrease in blood total cholesterol, triglyceride and LDL levels after 2 weeks [40].

3.4 Bacil (*Osimum basilicum*)

It is a medium density plant with flavonoid and polyphenol content [9, 40]. Bacil leaves are used in the form of a salad or cake dressing [40].

Bacil extract contains significant rosmarinic acid and catechin [40].

In studies on bacil extract, it has been determined that bacil is highly effective in preventing metabolic syndrome. Its antidiabetic and anti-inflammatory properties are known. The bacil extract also prevents the accumulation of intracellular sorbitol by providing aldose reductase inhibition. In this way, it is suggested that it reduces vascular osmotic pressure and oxidative stress, which are among diabetic complications. Due to its dense polyphenol content, it has also been closely associated with the reduction of advanced glicosylation products that occur in oxidative stress. It is also effective in the regulation of blood pressure. It increases renal function in hypertensive rats. Subjects treated with bacil had a decrease in blood urea nitrogen concentration and a decrease in creatinine and angiotensin compared to the hypertensive control group [40]. In an experimental study in which cerebral hypoperfusion and ischemia/reperfusion damage was performed in the brain in mice, it was found that it reduced the size of cerebral infarct with its antioxidant effect, but also increased short-term memory and motor coordination [21].

3.5 Fennel

This plant species belonging to the "*foenicuum vulgare*" species and often called "fennel" belongs to the "*apiaceae*" family [14]. It is consumed in salads, sauces, bread making, together with fish products and in the form of tea [40]. This product is a type of plant that is used quite often in alternative medicine. Although it often grows in the Mediterranean, it is known that it grows in different parts of the world today [14].

It contains fenchone, estragole, anise aldehyde, trans-anethole, and essential oils [14]. This ingredient gives fennel its unique smell and taste [5]. The most concentrated flavonoid in its composition is quercetin [40].

It has antibacterial, antifungal, antioxidant, hepatoprotective, antidiabetic, antineoplastic, and anti-inflammatory effects [14, 40, 54]. Anise aldehyde content of fennel is responsible for the hepatoprotective effect [14]. The reducing effect of fennel consumption on systemic complications of diabetes is through aldose and aldehyde reductase inhibition [40]. Studies have proved that *F. vulgare* accelerates the removal of harmful waste from the body by increasing body excretion. The anti-cancer potential of fennel seed methanolic extract (FSME) has been observed to be due to its reduction in oxidative stress in human MCF-7 and HepG-2 cell lines [14]. Fennel bulb has an antihyperlipidemic effect. In a study conducted on mice, it was observed that 24 hours after fennel bulb administration, a decrease was achieved in total cholesterol, triglyceride, LDL and ApoB levels [40]. In the experimental study conducted on Swiss albino mice by Mohamad et al., it was reported that oxidative stress decreased in subjects who were given 100 mg/kg FSME intraperitoneally, and they were protected from Ehrlich Ascites Carcinoma (EAC) associated with ROS [55]. In another study, it has been proved that fennel extract administered orally to mice reduces arachidonic acid-related ear edema [40].

3.6 Bay leaves (*Laurus nobilis*)

Laurus nobilis is a plant that is often grown in southern Europe and used in cooking. It contains flavonoids such as quercetin, kaempferol and sesquiterpen in particular [40].

It is especially known for its antidiabetic effect. Its hypolipidemic effect has been demonstrated in several in vivo studies. Bay leaf extract has been increased glucose uptake in rat epididymal adipocytes by acting like insulin. Besides, it causes a decrease in total plasma cholesterol level in hypercholesterolemic people. It inhibits ApoA1 glycation, oxidation of LDL particles and uptake of oxidized LDL particles from macrophages, in in vitro studies. Bay leaf additionally has an anti-inflammatory effect. Bay leaf extract reduces interleukin-6 (IL-6) production and cyclooxygenase-2 (COX-2) protein expression, particularly in stimulated macrophages [40]. It has also been detected to reduce the rate of cell death and cerebral infarction after cerebral ischemia in rats [21].

3.7 Sage (*Salvia officinalis*)

It is in the fragrant herbs class that forms the "salvia" genus from the "*lamiacea*" family. It is also known as "*Ammi majus*" and "*salvia*". It grows a lot in Asian and European countries [27]. The dried form of the leaves, which are furry and whitish, can be boiled like tea and can be used to add taste and flavor to meat dishes [27, 40].

It is dense in terms of polyphenols. It is particularly rich in phenolic and rosmarinic acid [40]. The most important phenolic components in the structure of sage, which has antioxidant effect, are carnosol, carnosic acid and rosmanol [27].

It has an antihyperlipidemic effect [40]. Fasseas et al. reported that lipid peroxidation decreased in meats treated with sage extract, but this effect may vary depending on storage temperature and time [56]. In streptozotocin-induced diabetic rats, it was observed that sage extract given intraperitoneally caused a decrease in serum glucose level after 3 hours, but it was shown that it did not cause any change in serum insulin level. However, it has been shown to contribute positively to glucose management in healthy subjects. Serum glucose levels have been decreased in healthy subjects given oral sage for 14 days. Experimental studies have been conducted on the potential anti-inflammatory effect of sage and positive results have been obtained. Inflammation at the injection site was observed to be reduced by administering sage one hour before injection of carrageenan or formalin to rats [40]. In a study conducted on people between the ages of 65 and 80 with mild or moderate Alzheimer's disease, another type of salvia called "*salvia lavandulaefolia*" was used for 4 months and significant improvement was obtained in cognitive functions. Thus, this product is thought to have the feature of increasing "speed of memory" in healthy volunteers. In a comparative study conducted between "*Salvia officinalis*" (aroma form) and "*salvia lavandulaefolia*" (oil form), it was detected that *Salvia officinalis* increased cognitive and emotional characteristics and memory quality more [21].

In a study of industrial microwave exposure of sage, it was examined that there was no change in the antioxidant properties of this plant [50].

3.8 Green tea

It is an antioxidant and anti-inflammatory product with flavonol structure [21]. It is an important component of many diets, due to its high antioxidant content [2].

Major flavonoids in green tea are monomer catechins, epigallocatechin gallate (EGCG), epigallotechin, epicatechin (EC), epicatechin-3-gallate (ECG) and epicathechin (EGC) [2, 26]. EGCG is the most active and the most concentrated component in green tea [26]. It makes up 43% of total phenol [4, 26]. Most of the stated effects of green tea are related to the EGCG component. EGCG presents its antioxidant, anti-inflammatory effect by reducing COX-2 overexpression. The polyphenol content constitutes approximately 35% of its dry weight. Compared to black tea, green tea has a higher proportion of catechins [26].

Green tea is a herb known to have positive effects on age-related chronic diseases, cardiovascular diseases, cancer, obesity, diabetes, and neurodegenerative pathologies. In many epidemiological studies, it has been suggested that green tea consumed daily reduces morbidity and mortality due to chronic diseases [26].

3.9 Parsley (*Petroselinum crispum/Petroselinum neapolitanum*)

It is an antioxidant herb with a very high flavonoid content [9, 21, 40]. It mainly contains apigenin [40].

It was observed that parsley, which was given parsley extract and administered orally to streptozotocin-induced diabetic rats for 28 days, caused a decrease in the level of glucose in the circulation. In addition, parsley also has an anti-inflammatory effect. One hour after oral administration of parsley extract in rats with paw edema induced by carrageenan, a decrease in edema was observed in the area where carrageenan injection was applied. Another benefit of parsley consumption is that it contributes to the treatment of hypertension. In a study conducted on healthy rats, it has been presented that oral administration of parsley extract leads to an increase in urinary output after 5 hours and an increase in excretion of sodium, potassium and chlorine with urine [40].

3.10 Garlic/Chive (*Allium schoenumprasum*)

It is a herb that has always had a place in traditional and modern diets [21]. Garlic, also known as "*Allium sativum*", is a plant belonging to the "*amaryllidaceae*" family that can be used prophylactically or in treatment in both the food industry and alternative medicine [14, 21].

Bioactive ingredients include organosulfide compounds such as allicin, ajoene, S-allyl-L-cysteine, dallyltrisulfide (DATS) [13]. Dallyltrisulfide (DATS), which is found in the composition of garlic, is also an important phenolic component [14].

It has various pharmacological activities accepted in the medical literature [14]. These include antioxidant, immunostimulant, antineoplastic, anti-inflammatory, antihypertensive, antithrombotic, antibacterial, antifungal and antiviral activities [13, 14, 21].

Its anti-inflammatory property is due to inhibition of nuclear factor κB (NFκB) (transcription factor regulating inflammatory response) activation, iNOS and COX-2 expression. In in vitro and in vivo animal studies, garlic has been determined to strengthen immune function, stimulate lymphocyte proliferation, increase interferon-γ (IFN-γ) release, increase macrophage phagocytosis function and natural killer (NK) cell activity [13]. Garlic has been reduced TNFα-induced ROS and NFκB activation on human umbilical vein endothelial cells. It has been proved that the anti-inflammatory effect of garlic or garlic oil derivatives is due to NO suppression in induced macrophages. However, it has reduced endotoxin-induced iNOS activity in rat intestinal mucosa and weaken monocyte chemoattractant protein-1 by IL-6 induced by macrophage-secreted factors in human preadipocytes [21].

In some studies, it has been observed that garlic has positive effects, especially in cardiovascular diseases [13, 14]. It is known that it slows down the atherosclerotic process, reduces the risk of heart attack and infarction, prevents fat accumulation in blood vessels, inhibits LDL cholesterol oxidation, reduces total cholesterol, increases HDL, and has positive effects on endothelial function [10, 13]. There are studies reporting the antioxidant effect of garlic, especially in elderly and hypertensive persons [10, 21]. It has reduced systolic blood pressure by 5.5% [10]. Garlik extracts have also reduced oxidative stress and contribute to vascular remodeling in rats given sucrose-containing water [21]. Other effects include decreasing blood glucose levels [10, 13, 21]. In a study conducted on rats fed with fructose for 8 weeks, it was demonstrated that the metabolic syndrome was attenuated, insulin sensitivity was increased, and oxidative stress was reduced by giving garlic homogenized with water. In addition, garlic has neuroprotective effects in Alzheimer's disease [21]. In rats, it reduces the infract size in rats following edema and ischemia/reperfusion injury after transient global brain ischemia [13, 21]. It has a learning and memory strengthening effect. Garlic has been detected to prevent Abeta-induced neurotoxicity and apoptosis and protect neurons [13]. In the absence of any stress environment, a significant increase in memory was observed in rats given garlic after 21 days of oral use [21]. It is known that garlic has beneficial effects on respiration and digestion. Garlic is also used in some skin diseases and parasitic infections. DATS, which is in the composition of garlic, has an effect that inhibits tumorigenesis. It achieves this effect through the Wnt/β-catenin signaling pathway. Thus, it is known to affect SW480 and DLD-1 colorectal cancer cells [14].

3.11 Clove (*Eugenia caryophyllata/Syzygium aromaticum*)

Clove (*Eugenia caryophyllata*) comes from the "*mirtaceae*" family, a medium-sized (8–12 m) tree that grows on the Maluku Islands in Eastern Indonesia.

It consists of leaves and buds. It is a widely used herb that is often combined with foods. Cloves are generally used in meat and rice dishes. In North Indian cuisine, cloves are used in almost every side dish, often mixed with curry. Previously used only as a food preservative, this herb continues to be used increasingly due to its antioxidant properties [57].

The biocomponents of this plant, which has a dominant scent, are phenolic compounds (ferulic, caffeic, ellagic, and salicylic acids) such as flavonoids (quercetin and kaempferol), β-caryophyllene, eugenol, hydroxybenzoic acids, hydroxynamic acids and hydroxyphenyl propenes [57, 58].

Its most prominent effect as a food preservative is its antibacterial and antioxidant effect. In addition, its antifungal, antiviral, spasmolytic, sedative, analgesic, local anesthetic and anticarcinogenic effects are also important. There are literature data indicating that clove increases microcirculation, lowers body temperature, provides a hypotensive effect, and may reduce cardiovascular risks and arterial sclerosis [59]. Local anesthetic effects are among the reasons that are frequently recommended by dentists. It is thought to act by depressing nociceptors, which are sensory receptors that play a role in pain perception [60]. Clove also inhibits prostaglandin biosynthesis and the release of leukotrienes in the inflammatory pathway through its potent COX-1 and 2 inhibitory activity [61].

Clove oil has antibacterial activity thanks to its β-caryophyllene and eugenol content. Bacteria with which it is effective include campylobacter jejuni, *Escherichia coli*, salmonella enteritica, *Listeria monocytogenes* and *Staphylococcus aureus*. Antifungal effects have also been reported on *Candida albicans*, trichophyton rubrum, microsporum canis, tricophyton mentagrophytes, fusarium monoliforme, microsporum gypseum, fusarium oxysporum, epidermophyton floccosum, mucor species, microsporum gypseum and aspergillus [58, 62].

3.12 Thyme/Oregano (*Thymus vulgaris/Oreganum vulgare*)

It is a member of the "*lamiaceae*" family. Although there are many species of the thymus genus, the more common one is "T*hymus vulgaris*", native to Italy and the Western Mediterranean. Oregano grows largely in temperate regions and is rare in Africa. Different studies have concluded that the use of oregano improves stability and reduces lipid oxidation throughout the shelf life of foods (meat, meat products, milk, fish or fish products). This property makes thyme an enriched functional food source [63].

Thyme includes monoterpene polyphenols such as thymol and p-cymene, with the most particular component being carvacrol, and other monoterpenes such as -pinene, 1,8-cineol, camphor, linalool and borneol [9, 21, 63]. Flavonoid content is quite high [21]. The common feature of the thyme types widely used in the industry is that they contain essential oil and the main components of these essential oils are thymol and carvacrol. These substances are phenolic compounds that give thyme its unique scent and give it antioxidant properties [27].

Thyme is a nutritional antioxidant that stands out with its antidiabetic, antibacterial and anticarcinogenic effects. The basis of its antimicrobial activity is the free hydroxyl group, its hydrophobicity and the presence of a phenol moiety [64]. Similarly, the presence of phenol is responsible for its antispasmodic and antitussive effects. There are also both animal studies and in vitro studies on its anthelmintic effects [65]. In in vitro studies, the effect of thyme oil on antibiotic-resistant enterococcus and escherichia strains, especially staphylococcus and pseudomonas strains has been presented. It is highly effective on biofilms, and its antibacterial effects are associated with direct penetration into the cell wall and matrix [66].

4. Antioxidant-affected spices

In the **Figure 2**, natural spices with potent antioxidant features and which are most commonly used are listed.

4.1 Saffron (*Crocus*)

Saffron, also known as "*Crocus sativus*", is a spice belonging to the "*iridaceae*" family. It is also called as "red gold" since it is a very precious spice in food and medicine. It is among the most valuable spices in the world [14]. It is one of the most important phytochemical carotenoids [14, 21].

Crocin/Crocetin is the most important bioactive molecule in substance of saffron. This molecule has the effect of reducing tumor growth [14].

It has potent antioxidative and anti-inflammatory effects. It has been observed that *crocetin* significantly reduces insulin resistance, corrects hyperinsulinemia, dyslipidemia and hypertension in rats that are given fructose. It reduces the oxidative damage associated with ischemia/reperfusion in the rat hippocampus. After chronic cerebral hypoperfusion in rats, it has been determined that the extracts of *crocin* and *crocetin* increase spatial cognitive abilities. A double-blind study reported significant improvement in cognitive function in individuals with Alzhemier's disease after 16 weeks of saffron use [21].

4.2 Curcumin (Turmeric/Eugenol/*Curcuma longa*)

Its use in traditional medicine, especially in dermatological diseases, in eastern societies, especially in China and India, is based on approximately 4,000 years. This product, which is accepted as a combination of plants that have a place in religious rituals in ancient times, is collected in its roots and stems and then reproduces by giving seeds again [20]. Originally, this spice, which comes from the ginger family, has been recognized to have a healing effect on many disease

	SPICES						
	Saffron	Curcumin	Cumin	Cinnamon	Ginger	Black pepper	Red chili
	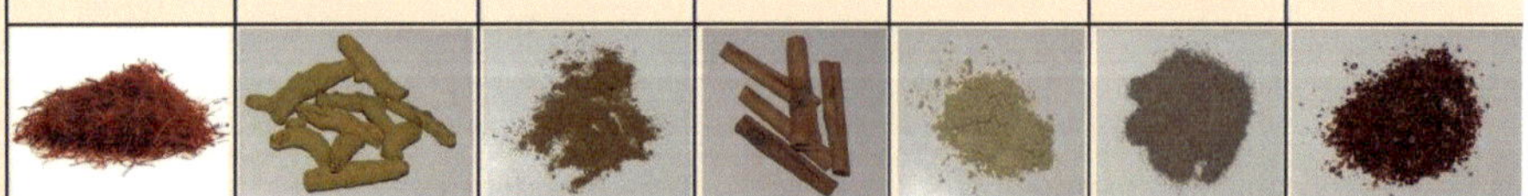						
FEATURES	Antioxidant	Antiinflammatory	Antiinflammatory	Antioxidant	Antioxidant	Antioxidant	Antioxidant
	Antiinflammatory	Antioxidant	Antioxidant	Antiinflammatory	Antiinflammatory	Antimicrobial	Antiinflammatory
	Anticarcinogenic	Antibacterial	Hypolipidemic	Sedative	Neuroprotective	Analgesic	Anticarcinogenic
	Antidiabetic	Cognitive function ↑	Antidiabetic	Antidiabetic	Antinausea	Antipiretic	Cerebral perfusion ↑
	Antilipidemic	Antidiabetic	Antibacterial	Antimicrobial	Antiobesity	Antidepressant	Antiplatelet
	Antihypertensive	Antiobesity	Antimicrobial	Antibacterial	Antilipidemic	Antifungal	Antidiabetic
	Cognitive function ↑	Anticarcinogenic	Hepatoprotective	Antifungal	Antimicrobial	Antiinflammatory	Antilipidemic
		Antilipidemic	Nefroprotective	Anticarcinogenic		Anticarcinogenic	Gastroprotective
			Neuroprotective	Antilipidemic		Antithyroid	
						Antiallergic	
						Antilipidemic	

Figure 2.
Natural spices with potent antioxidant features and which are most commonly used.

progression, although some remained only in the clinical trial phase. However, the transition from traditional medicine to modern plug was not difficult. This spice with flowers and broad leaves grows in tropical climates. Its color and taste are used by putting it in pasta, rice, vegetables, meat dishes and salads. The Food and Drug Administration (FDA) has confirmed that curcumin is a compound "generally considered safe". Curcumin has been proven to be sensitive to light, so it is recommended that biological samples containing curcumin should be protected from light [67]. Studies are underway to increase its bioavailability after oral ingestion, as its absorption from the gastrointestinal tract is poor and most of it is excreted in the feces [68].

Biologically active component of "*Curcuma longa*" is lipophilic, yellow-orange colored curcumin (diferuloylmethane). It is also referred to "Indian saffron" because of its specific color. Its antioxidant properties are due to the methoxy, phenoxy and carbon–carbon double bonds in its structure. Even though its metabolic rate and elimination are high, its bioavailability is limited. However, in the development phase of many diseases, cytokines, it plays an important role by regulating growth factors, kinases, transcription factors and enzymes. Its molecular activity on signal transduction and redox reactions has always been a curiosity. High-level methoxylation and low-level hydrogenation of curcumin content increase free radical scavenging ability [68].

Curcumin is one of the spices with the highest antioxidant and anti-inflammatory component [2, 12]. The antioxidant effect of curcumin is based on reducing TNFα and IL-1 expression and establishing balance with ROS. Curcumin, other than being beneficial for wound healing, also has an antibacterial effect by controlling the inflammatory response. Curcumin induces apoptosis of inflammatory cells and thus shortens the inflammatory phase. It accelerates healing by increasing collagen synthesis and fibroblast migration in the early phase of wound healing. However, forms suitable for topical use are not yet available. In vivo and in vitro studies on this subject continue. Therefore, it is much more effective to add oral forms of curcumin to the diet for wound healing at this stage [69]. Studies have shown that the effects of curcumin on the processes of Alzheimer's, diabetes mellitus, obesity, neurodegenerative diseases, osteoarthritis, and oncogenesis give promising results [20]. There are studies showing that curcumin reduces the proliferation and invasion of tumor cells [70]. It has been examined that curcumin is a biologically active agent that increases cancerous cell apoptosis in head–neck, pancreatic and colorectal cancer patients [70–73]. Curcumin is also a good source of ω-3 fatty acids and α-linolenic acid. It prevents atherosclerosis by reducing the level of LDL in the blood, preventing lipoperoxidation, and reducing cholesterol levels [74]. It is mostly because of this effect that it is used as a common cooking spice in developed countries where the consumption of saturated fatty acids is greatly increased. Curcumin supplementation is recommended for foods during both prevention and treatment of cardiovascular diseases in which atherosclerosis plays a major role. Curcuminoids reduced blood sugar, partly due to their effect of reducing free fatty acids, and in addition, in studies on rodent models, they prevent the reduction in antioxidant capacity caused by diabetes. As a result, it has been reported to have an antidiabetic effect in patients with insulin-resistant type-II diabetes and in in-vivo studies [75, 76].

4.3 Cumin (Cumin aldehyde/*Cuminum cyminum*)

Cumin (*Cuminum cyminum*) is a well-known culinary spice that is often used in mealtimes. It is a small herbaceous product belonging to the "*apiaceae*" family. Its oblong-shaped seeds have a strong aromatic scent and a warm bitter flavor. It is widely grown in Central Asia, Pakistan, India, Iran and China. It is traditionally used as an antiseptic agent. It is also widely used in digestive disorders such as dyspepsia and diarrhea [72].

Its bioactive components are terpenes, phenols and flavonoids. Thanks to these components, it has been proven that it has free radical scavenging and metal chelating properties [77].

It is a spice with anti-inflammatory and antioxidant properties [12]. Animal studies are available showing the hypolipidemic and antidiabetic effects of cumin [78]. Experimental studies have been conducted to support the effect of cumin on renal ischemia–reperfusion injury [79, 80]. It also has antibacterial and potent antimicrobial activity [66, 77]. Cumin seeds also have immunostimulating, gastric protective, hepatoprotective, nephroprotective, and neuroprotective activities [81].

4.4 Cinnamon (Cinnam aldehyde/*Cinnamomum zeylanicum*):

Cinnamon comes from the "*lauraceae*" family, and its leaves and shells as a spice have been in the world trade for centuries. Cinnamon is mostly obtained from the bark of the "*Cinnamomum zeylanicum*" tree originating from South and Southeast Asia. The most specific feature of cinnamon, which is an evergreen tree, is its aromatic scent. Cinnamon, which is also widely traded, is frequently consumed in Iran in the form of traditional tea. It is used to prevent lipid oxidation of bakery products such as cakes, so that it prevents the taste of foods [82].

The antioxidant activity is estimated to be due to the polysaccharide known as "daruchini" derived from cinnamon bark. Thanks to "arabinogalactan" and "glucan" in its structure, it loses protons and gives a radical scavenging effect [83].

It is a spice with a pronounced antioxidant and anti-inflammatory effect [12]. It has been observed that consuming it especially in tea form is beneficial in the treatment of diseases related to oxidative stress. It has also been presented to have a sedative effect in many human studies [83]. Cinnamon, acting like insulin, increases insulin receptor kinase activity and stimulates glycogen synthase activity. Thus, it exerts antidiabetic effect [82, 84]. Spices such as cinnamon have started to be included in prescriptions as an additional treatment, due to the toxic side effects of diabetes medications and balance problems due to long-term use. In these studies, which accelerated the development of multiple antibiotic resistances, antibacterial effects on factors such as bacillus subtilis, *Staphylococcus aureus*, *Bacillus cereus*, *Escherichia coli*, salmonella typhi, *Pseudomonas aeruginosa*, *Listeria monocytogenes*, and fungal effects such as aspergillus monocytogenes, aspergillus monocytogenes are also known [85]. In addition, NF-κB, which is known to be effective in cancer development acts an anticancer by inhibiting the production of IL-1β and TNF-α. Cinnamon is beneficial in lowering triglycerides and LDL cholesterol by affecting the blood lipid profile through the poliphenols in its structure [86]. The effect of polyphenols here is achieved by inhibiting hepatic lipid peroxidation. In this way, by cleaning hydroxy and fatty acid radicals and chelates, providing the metabolic balance of fat and carbohydrates, cinnamon has turned into a functional nutrition.

4.5 Ginger (*Zingiber officinale roscoe*):

Ginger (*Zingiber officinale roscoe*) comes from the "*zingiberaceae*" family, and especially its roots are among the most widely used functional spices in the world. With a slightly bitter but strong aroma, this root can be used in powder or ground form. It can be consumed in brine, drying, canned or fresh [20].

"Oleoresin" obtained from its roots contains various bioactive molecules. Among these are terpenes, polysaccharides, lipids, but especially gingerol, physiological effects are the most intense [20, 87]. The proportion of gingerol is higher in fresh ginger than the dried form, so consuming fresh is more important for its antioxidant effect [20]. Ginger extract is also a natural and potent antioxidant compared to synthetic antioxidants, with a high Fe^{+3}-effective chelating capacity [88].

Studies mention the effects of ginger on cardioprotective, anti-inflammatory, neuroprotective, antinausea and antiobesity. Its anti-inflammatory effects have been demonstrated in the treatment of osteomyelitis, arthritis and rheumatism [89]. Ginger, which has increased glutathione levels and suppress lipid peroxidation during its anti-inflammatory effects, is widely used as a food flavor in developed countries for colds, migraine attacks and gastrointestinal disorders. Its antimicrobial effects are related to its lipophilic property, making the fungal walls and cytoplasmic membrane permeable. Antibacterial effects on species such as *Staphylococcus aureus*, *Streptococcus pyogenes*, *Streptococcus pneumoniae* and haemophilus have been proved on various animal and human studies. The most stable metabolite, 6-gingerol derivative, has been observed to have an antinause effect by blocking 5-hydroxy tryptophan and serotonin-mediated vagal afferent neurons in patients used after chemotherapy, nephrectomy and cesarean operations [90, 91].

4.6 Black Pepper (*Piper nigrum*)

Black pepper is a product that belongs to the "*piparaceae*" family and is called as "P*iper nigrum*" [14]. It is obtained from the ripe fruits of *Piper nigrum* L [27]. Black pepper has a very common pharmaceutical use in the world [14]. It is cultivated in tropical regions, especially in India, Malaysia, Asia and Indonesia [12, 27]. It is among the best-selling spices on the market in some countries like India [14, 92].

Black pepper contains five phenolic acids (piperettine, piperanine, piperylin A, piperolein B and pipericine) amide with antioxidant effects [12, 13, 27]. Additionally, it contains alkamides, piptigrine, wisanine and dipiperamide [13]. These phenolic components have a damaging effect by preventing the growth of the bacterial membrane, and their antimicrobial activity occurs through this mechanism [12]. These compounds are non-greasy, odorless, tasteless and exhibit stronger antioxidant activity than α-tocopherol [27]. The composition in the form of essential oil has antimicrobial activity [12]. The quality of black pepper varies depending on piperine causing bitterness and the essential oils responsible for its aroma [12, 27]. Piperine is a green crystalline clear substance that was first isolated in 1819. This alkaloid is a compound that gives the pepper its bitterness. The nature of piperine, which is its active basic component, is known in detail, and its effectiveness in alternative medicine has been clearly proven [13, 14, 21]. Its content, piperine, is a bioactive component with known beneficial effects on human health [13, 14]. Piperine is absorbed by passive diffusion in the gastrointestinal tract and has a short clearance time [13]. In a study of industrial microwaving of black pepper, it was determined that no change was observed in the antioxidant properties of this herb [50].

It has antioxidant, antimicrobial and antipyretic properties [27]. Antidepressant, antifungal, anti-inflammatory, analgesic, anticarcinogenic, antithyroid activities are some of the important pharmacological effects of black pepper [13, 14, 93]. Its anti-inflammatory effect has been detected on rats in many experimental studies. Black pepper accelerates the digestion process, increases digestive enzymes, gastric acid and bile acid secretion, and shortens the food transit time. It has anti-depressant-like effect by regulating neurotransmitter metabolism, causing an increase in behavioral/cognitive effects [13]. Piperine significantly reduces cell death, brain edema, and post-reperfusion proinflammatory cytokines in rats. It has decreased hippocampal cell death after ethylcholine aziridinium ion administration in rats [21]. Piperine has reduced arthritis pain in animal models.

Piperine supplementation reduces muscle damage when given before and after exercise. Piperine reduces histamine release and eosinophil infiltration in animal models. However, it suppresses allergic airway inflammation and airway hypersensitivity. Piperine increases energy expenditure in animal experiments, activates the sympathetic nervous system, causes thermogenesis, increases catecholamine levels, and activates adrenal sympathetic nerves [13]. In a study, it was examined that lipid peroxidation was delayed in pork meat with the addition of black pepper [13, 94]. Piperine prevented lipid accumulation in mouse macrophages. Alternatively, it has been determined to transform into foamy cells in animal studies, which can reduce fat accumulation in the arterial wall [13].

4.7 Red Chili/Chili Pepper (*Capsicum annum*)

Red chili is a product belonging to the "*solanaceae*" family [14].

"Capsaicin" is the primary bioactive substance of red chili pepper [14, 21]. Capsaicin is an alkaloid. It constitutes 50–70% of total capsaicinoids. It contains 20–25% dihydrocapsaicin and 0.2–2% capsaicinoid [10]. Among its recently discovered ingredients are capsiate and dihydrocapsiate [13].

The beneficial effects of red pepper have been documented long before. In vitro and experimental studies of red pepper and capsaicin have proved potential antioxidant and anti-inflammatory effects of it against oxidative stress in various tissues and organs [13]. This spice type has the ability to induce apoptosis in major type cancers. It has been presented that capsaicin treatment in gastic cancer cells (MGC-803) and cervical cancer cells (HeLa) prevented the G1 phase in cell cycle analysis. In an experimental study performed in athymic mice, it was indicated that tumor growth in prostate cancer cells (LNCaP) was reduced in subjects given 5 mg/kg orally [14]. In another study conducted in vitro, it has been determined that it has a protective effect on rat hippocampal neurons, reduces hippocampal death after global ischemia, decreases the size of cerebral infarction after bilateral arterial occlusion in mice, and decreases the infraction volume in neonatal rats ligated in unilateral carotid arteries after hypoxia [21]. However, capsaicin regulates energy metabolism and has beneficial effects on the cardiovascular system, with its antioxidant and antiplatelet effects. In a clinical study conducted on humans, it was determined that 5 grams of red pepper (*Capsicum frutescens*) lowered blood glucose levels and maintained healthy insulin levels. In the short-term use of red pepper, it has been observed that body mass index contributes to management, decreases energy and fat intake, increases body heat production (thermogenesis), increases body metabolic rate, decreases the conversion of fat cells to mature cells (adipogenesis) and increases fat oxidation. Capsaicin has been detected to be gastroprotective in patients with peptic ulcer disease. Capsaicin reduces acid secretion, induces alkaline mucous stimulation (particularly by affecting gastric mucosal blood flow) and contributes to ulcer healing [13].

5. Comparison of natural antioxidant-affected herbs and spices

In a study comparing antioxidant effects, it was stated that the strongest antioxidant effect was in rosemary and curcumin, followed by herbs such as cinnamon, saffron, sage, and thyme [2, 27, 46].

Shahidi et al. asserted that the antioxidant activities of clove, sage, thyme and ginger in meat oil were concentration-dependent [95]. They stated that among these substances, the most effective was clove, and the least effective spices were ginger and thyme [95].

Pizzale et al. found that, on average, the antioxidant activity of sage species (*Salvia officinalis and fruticosa*) was higher than thyme species (*Origanum onites and indercedens*) in their study [96].

Another study proved that chloroform extract of dried musk sage (*Salvia sclarea*) has higher antioxidant activity than acetone extract, and both extracts have higher total antioxidant activities than α-tocopherol [27].

Nakatani et al. determined that black pepper is more effective than synthetic antioxidants such as BHT and BHA [97].

In another study, the antioxidant properties of curcuminoids were investigated, and it was determined that the antioxidant capacity of these extracts was equivalent to ascorbic acid [98].

When evaluated in terms of the density of total phenolic compounds, it has been observed that rosemary and thyme have higher phenolic content than other herbs. Also, it was presented that fresh plants have more intense phenolic content than dried plants [9].

Correspondingly, it is thought that the most potent antioxidants are fresh rosemary and curcumin, and it may be suggested to increase the consumption of these products.

6. Antioxidant combinations

Since each spice contains a wide range of phenols, many of them can provide synergistic effects with each other. The formulations of different herbs and spices were tested in vivo and in vitro, and their antimicrobial effects were compared [12].

It is predicted that the antioxidant effect increases significantly when thyme essential oil and vitamin E are mixed in half so that there is a synergistic effect between thyme essential oil and vitamin E [27].

It has been indicated that meats are effectively protected against *Listeria monocytogenes* with the combined use of curcumin and thyme [12].

In an experimental animal study, it was observed that when capsaicin (0.015%) was given alone and in combination with curcumin, it reduced triglyceride levels by 12% and 21% in animals given a high fat diet [13].

Since piperine increases the absorption of various drug and food sources, it increases their bioavailability when used with other antioxidants. It increases the absorption of compounds such as coenzyme-Q, curcumin and polyphenol. For example, bioavailability of curcumin increases by 154% when it is given with 20 mg/kg piperine in animal studies. Piperine shows its effect by decreasing the intestinal and hepatic metabolism of curcumin. In some studies, it has been presented that piperine increases the bioavailability of resveratrol in vivo by inhibiting its metabolism. In this way, it ensures that additional resveratrol doses are not required [13].

Therefore, the combined use of herbs and spices with appropriate formulations can be recommended.

7. Conclusion

Herbs and spices used in cooking, increasing the nutritional value of foods and extending the storage time are highly interesting compounds with antioxidant properties due to their bioactive content, showing beneficial effects on human health. Interest in natural antioxidants in plants around the world is increasing day by day, with the widespread use of natural additives in the food industry. Therefore, herbs and spices have become the most important focus of research for the study of natural antioxidants.

Since ancient times, herbs and spices have been used in alternative medical treatments due to their antimicrobial, anti-inflammatory and antioxidative effects. Although the use of herbs and spices in food and treatment has been available for a long time, research on this subject is limited to the recent past. In addition to the poor antioxidant features of animal origin foods, the antioxidant power of plant-based foods is much higher.

There are over 1.000 known antioxidant phytochemicals. Although they are very small in terms of weight and volume, they have a feature of increasing the value and antioxidant content of foods. Thanks to the studies conducted on this subject, the application strategies of phytochemical antioxidants in the diet can be determined, and chronic diseases related to oxidative stress such as cancer, cardiovascular diseases, hypertension, hyperlipidemia, inflammation and diabetes can be prevented or their effects can be reduced.

Various synthetic and natural products are used in the food industry to cope with dietary oxidative stress. Hence, there is a need for optimized studies of natural antioxidant products that can be used as food preservatives in the food industry. Thus, the natural storage times and nutritional values of foods can be increased.

Conflict of interest

The authors declare that there is no conflict of interest, and there have been no sources of funding.

Author details

Perçin Karakol[1]* and Emin Kapi[2]

1 Department of Plastic, Reconstructive and Aesthetic Surgery, Bagcilar Research and Training Hospital, University of Health Sciences, Istanbul, Turkey

2 Department of Plastic, Reconstructive and Aesthetic Surgery, Adana Faculty of Medicine, Health Application and Research Center, University of Health Sciences, Adana, Turkey

*Address all correspondence to: ppercin@gmail.com

References

[1] Bozkurt M, Kapi E, Kulahci Y, Gedik E, Ozekinci S, Isik FB, Celik Y, Selcuk CT, Kuvat SV. Antioxidant support in composite musculo-adipose-fasciocutaneous flap applications: an experimental study. Journal of Plastic Surgery and Hand Surgery. 2013;48:44-50. DOI: 10.3109/2000656X.2013.800527

[2] Carlsen MH, Halvorsen BL, Holte K, Bohn SV, Dragland S, Sampson L, Willey C, Senoo H, Umezono Y, Sanada C, Barikmo I, Berhe N, Willett WC, Phillips KM, Jacobs DR, Blomhoff R. The total antioxidant content of more than 3100 foods, beverages, spices, herbs and supplements used worldwide. Nutrition Journal. 2010;9:4-11.

[3] Koch CE, Ganjam GK, Steger J, Legler K, Stöhr S, Schumacher D, Hoggard N, Heldmaier G, Tups A. The dietary flavonoids naringein and quercetin acutely impair glucose metabolism in rodents possibly via inhibition of hypothalamic insülin signalling. British Journal of Nutrition. 2013;109:1040-1051. DOI: 10.1017/S0007114512003005.

[4] Leal LN, Jordan MJ, Bello JM, Otal J, Hartog L, Hendriks WH, Tereso JM. Dietary supplementation of 11 different plant extracts on the antioxidant capacity of blood and selected tissues in lightweight lambs. J Sci Food Agric. 2019;99:4296-4303. DOI: 10.1002/jsfa.9662.

[5] Dorman HJD, Bachmayer O, Kosar M, Hiltunen R. Antioxidant properties of aqueous extracts from selected lamiaceae species grown in Turkey. J Agric Food Chem. 2004;52:762-770. DOI: 10.1021/jf034908v.

[6] Schreck R, Baeuerle PA. A role for oxygen radicals as second messengers. Trends cell Biol. 1991;1:39-42.

[7] El Babili F, Bouajila J, Souchard JP, Bertrand C, Bellvert F, Fouraste I. et al. Chemical analysis and evaluation of its antimalarial, antioxidant, and cyto-toxic activities. J. Food Sci. 2011;76:C512–C518.

[8] Serafini M, Peluso I. Functional foods for health: The interrelated antioxidant and anti-inflammatory role of fruits, vegetables, herbs, spices and cocoa in humans. Curr Pharm Des. 2016;22:6701-6715.

[9] Slimestad R, Fossen T, Brede C. Flavonoids and other phenolics in herbs commonly used in Norwegian commercial kitchens. Food Chem. 2019. DOI: https://doi.org/10.1016/j.foodchem.2019.12578.

[10] Patch CS. Health benefits of herbs and spices: the past, the present, the future. The Medical Journal of Australia. 2006;185:1-24.

[11] Vallverdu-Queralt A, Reguero J, Martinez-Huelamo M, Alvarenga JFR, Leal LN, Lamuela-Raventos RM. A comprehensive study on the phenolic profile of widely used culinary herbs and spices: rosemary, oregano, cinnamon, cumin and bay. Food Chemistry. 2014. DOI: http://dx.doi.org/10.1016/j.foodchem.2013.12.106.

[12] Torres JET, Gassara F, Kouassi AP, Brar SK, Belkacemi K. Spice use in food: properties and benefits. Critical Reviews in Food Science and Nutrition. 2015; DOI: 10.1080/10408398.2013.858235.

[13] Jiang TA. Health benefits of culinary herbs and spices. Jiang: Journal of AOAC International. 2019;102:395-411. DOI: https://doi.org/10.5740/jaoacint.18-0418.

[14] Adithya JK, Bhagyalakshmi N, Sreeleksmi P, Lekshmi RN. Curry versus cancer: potential of some

selected culinary spices against cancer with in vitro, in vivo, and human trials evidences. Journal of Food Biochemistry. 2020;00:e13285.1-21. DOI: https://doi.org/10.1111/jfbc.13285.

[15] Shobana S, Akhilender Naidu K. Antioxidant activity of selected Indian spices. Prostaglandins, Leucotriens and Essential Fatty Acids. 2000;62:107-110.

[16] Velioglu YS, Mazza G, Gao L, Ooomah BD. Antioxidant activity and total phenolics in selected fruits, vegetables, and grain products. Journal of Agricultural and Food Chemistry. 1998;46:4113-4117.

[17] Zheng W, Wang SY. Antioxidant activity and phenolic compounds in selected herbs. Journal of Agricultural and Food Chemistry. 2001;49:5165-5170.

[18] Martinez-Gracia C, Gonzales-Bermudez CA, Cabelerro-Valcarcel AM, Santaella-Pascual M, Frontela-Saceta C. Use of herbs and spices for food preservation: advantages and limitations. Curr Op Sci. 2015;6:38-43.

[19] Kunnumakkara AB, Sailo BL, Banik K, Harsha C, Prasad S, Gupta SC, Aggarwal BB. Chronic diseases, inflammation, and spices: how are they linked? Journal of Translational Medicine. 2018;16(1):14. https://doi.org/10.1186/s12967-018-1381-2.

[20] Paur I, Carlsen MH, Halvorsen BL, Blomhoff R. Herbal Medicine. In: Biomolecular and Clinical Aspects. 2nd ed. Boca Raton (FL): CRC Press/Taylor&Francis; 2011. Ch 2.

[21] Kiran SP. Beneficial effects of herbs, spices and medicinal plants on the metabolic syndrome, brain and cognitive function. Central Nervous System Agents in Medicinal Chemistry. 2013;13:13-29.

[22] Surh YJ. Chemopreventive Phenolic Compounds in Common Spices; Taylor and Francis: New York, NY, USA, 2006.

[23] Kivilompolo M, Hyotylainen T. Comprehensive two-dimensional liquid chromatography in analysis of Lamiceae herbs: Characterisation and quantification of antioxidant phenolic acids. Journal of Chromatography A. 2007;1145:155-164.

[24] Park JB. Identification and quantification of a major anti-oxidant and anti-inflammatory phenolic compound found in basil, lemon thyme, mint, oregano, rosemary, sage, and thyme. International Journal of Food Sciences and Nutrition. 2011;62:577-584.

[25] Shan B, Chai YZ, Sun M, Corke H. Antioxidant capacity of 26 spice extracts and characterization of their phenolic constituents. Journal of Agricultural and Food Chemistry. 2005;53:7749-7759.

[26] Scapagnini G, Caruso C, Calabrese V. Therapeutic potentisl of dietary polyphenols against brain ageing and neurodegenerative disorders. Bio-Farms for Neutraceuticals: Functional and Safety Control by Biosensors. 2010;3:27-35.

[27] Çoban ÖE, Patır B. Use of some species and herbs antioxidant affected in foods. Electronic Journal of Food Technologies. 2010;2:7-19.

[28] Guldiken B, Ozkan G, Catalkaya G, Ceylan FD, Yalcinkaya IE, Capanoglu E. Phytochemicals of herbs and spices: health versus toxicological effects. Food and Chemical Toxicology. 2018;119:37-49. https://doi.org/10.1016/j.fct.2018.05.050.

[29] Opara EI, Chohan M. Culinary herbs and spices: their bioactive properties, the contribution of polyphenols and the challenges in deducing their true health benefits. International Journal of Molecular Sciences. 2014;15(10):19183-19202. https://doi.org/10.3390/ijms151019183.

[30] Bower A, Marquez S, Gonzalez de Mejia E. The health benefits of selected culinary herbs and spices found in the traditional mediterranean diet. Crit Rev Food Sci Nutr. 2016;56:2728-2746.

[31] Lin D, Xiao M, Zhao J, Li Z, Xing B, Li X, Kong M, Li L, Zhang Q, Liu Y, Cheng H, Qin W, Wu H, Chen S. An overview of plant phenolic compounds and their importance in human nutrition and management of thye 2 diabetes. Molecules. 2016;21:1374-1393.

[32] Yashin A, Yashin Y, Xia X, Nemzer B. Antioxidant activity of spices and their impact on human health: a review. Antioxidants. 2017;6:70-88.

[33] Xiao J. Dietary flavonoid aglycones and their glycosides: Which Show better biological significance? Crit Rev Food Sci Nutr. 2017;57:1874-1905.

[34] Raffa D, Maggio B, Raimondi MV, Plescia F, Daidone G. Recent discoveries of anticancer flavonoids. Eur J Med Chem. 2017;142:213-228.

[35] Wang T, Li Q, Bi K. Review: Bioactive flavonoids in medical plants: Structure, activity and biological fate. Asian J Pharm Sci. 2018;13:12-23.

[36] Ibrahim AHH, Herfindal L, Rathe B, Andersen HL, Almeida JRGS, Fossen T. A novel poly-oxygenated flavone glycoside from aerial parts of the Brazilian plantNeoglaziova variegate (Bromeliaceae). Heliyon. 2019;5:e051369.

[37] Rayyan S, Fossen T, Andersen QM. Flavone c-glycosides from seeds of fenugreek, trigonella foenum-graceum L. J Food Chem Agric. 2019;58:7211-7217.

[38] Slimestad R, Fossen T, Verheul M. The flavonoids of tomatoes. J Agric Food Chem. 2008;56:2436-2441.

[39] Fossen T, Slimestad R, Andersen QM. Anthocyanins from maize (zea mays) and reed canarygrass (phalaris arundinacea). J Agric Food Chem. 2001;49:2318-2321.

[40] Bower A, Marquez S, Mejia EG. The health benefits of selected culinary herbs and spices found in the traditional mediterranean diet. Critical Reviews in Food Science and Nutrition. 2016;56:2728-2746. DOI: 10.1080/10408398.2013.805713.

[41] De Oliveira JR, Camargo SEA, De Oliveira LD. Rosmarinus officinalis L. (rosemary) as the therapeutic and prophylactic agent. Journal of Biomedical Science. 2019;26(1):5.

[42] Habtemariam S. The therapeutic potential of rosemary (*Rosmarinus officinalis*) diterpenes for Alzheimer's disease. Evidence-Based Complementary and Alternative Medicine. 2016; eCAM. 2680409https://doi.org/10.1155/2016/2680409.

[43] Nieto G, Ros G, Castillo J. Antioxidant and antimicrobial properties of rosemary (*Rosmarinus officinalis*, L.): A review. Medicines. 2018;5(3):98. https://doi.org/10.3390/medicines5030098.

[44] Önenç SS, Açıkgöz Z. Antioxidant effects of aromatic herbs in animal products. Animal Production. 2005;46:50-55.

[45] Herrero M, Plaza M, Cifuentes A, Ibanez E. Green processes fort he extraction of bioactives from rosemary: chemical and functional characterization via ultra-performance liquid chromatography-tandem mass spectrometry and in-vitro assays. Journal of Chromatography A. 2010;1217:2512-2520.

[46] Akgül A, Ayar A. Antioxidant effects of local spices. Nature-TRJ of Agriculture and Foresty. 1993;17:1061-1068.

[47] Yanishlieva NV, Marinova E. Stabilisation of edible oils with natural antioxidants. Eur Journal Lipid Science Technol. 2001;103:752-767.

[48] Yanishlieva NV, Marinova E, Pokorny J. Natural antioxidants from herbs and spices. Eur Journal Lipid Science Technol. 2006;108:776-793.

[49] Rıznar K, Celan S, Knez Z, Skerget M, Bauman D, Glaser R. Antioxidant and antimicrobial activity of rosemary extract in chicken frankfurters. Journal of Food Science. 2006;71(7).

[50] Lopez-Bote CJ, Gray JI, Gomaa EA, Flegal CJ. Effect of dietary administration of oil extracts from rosemary and sage on lipid oxidation in broiler meat. British Poultry Science. 1998;39:235-240.

[51] Amoah SKS, Sandjo LP, Kratz JM, Biavatti MW. Rosmarinic acid-pharmaceutical and clinical aspects. Planta Med. 2016;82:388-406.

[52] Tajik N, Tajk M, Mack I, Enck P. The potential effects of chlorogenic acid, the main phenolic components in coffee, on health: a comprehensive review of the literature. Eur J Nutr. 2017;56:2215-2244.

[53] Jessica Elizabeth DLT, Gassara F, Kouassi AP, Brar SK, Belkacemi K. Spice use in food: properties and benefits. Critical Reviews in Food Science and Nutrition. 2017;57(6):1078-1088. https://doi.org/10.1080/10408398.2013.858235.

[54] Rather MA, Dar BA, Sofi SN, Bhat BA, Qurishi MA. Foeniculum vulgare: a comprehensive review of its traditional use, phytochemistry, parmacology, and safety. Arabian Journal of Chemistry. 2016;9:1574-1583. https://doi.org/10.1016/j.arabjc.2012.04.011.

[55] Mohamad RH, El-Bastawesy AM, Abdel-Monem MG, Noor AM, Al-Mehdar HAR, Sharawy SM, El-Merzabani MM. Antioxidant and anticarcinogenic effects of methanolic extract and volatile oil fennel seeds (foeniculum vulgare). Journal of Medicinal Food. 2011;14(9): 986-1001.

[56] Fasseas MK, Mountzouris KC, Tarantilis PA, Polissiou M, Zervas G. Antioxidant activity in meat treated with oregano and sage essential oils. Food Chemistry. 2007.

[57] Cortés-Rojas DF, de Souza CRF, Oliveira WP. Clove (Syzygium aromaticum): a precious spice. Asian Pacific Journal of Tropical Biomedicine, 2014;4(2):90-96.

[58] Park MJ, Gwak KS, Yang I, Choi WS, Jo HJ, Chang JW, Jeung EB et al. Antifungal activities of the essential oils in Syzygium aromaticum (L.) Merr. Et Perry and Leptospermum petersonii Bailey and their constituents against various dermatophytes. J Microbiol. 2007;45:460-465.

[59] Pulikottil SJ, Nath S. Potential of clove of Syzygium aromaticum in development of a therapeutic agent for periodontal disease: A review. South African Dental J. 2015;70:108-115.

[60] Kamatou GP, Vermaak I, Viljoen AM. Eugenol—From the Remote Maluku Islands to the International Market Place: A Review of a Remarkable and Versatile Molecule. Molecules. 2012;17(6):6953-6981.

[61] Kelm MA, Nair MG, Strasburg GM, DeWitt DL. Antioxidant and cyclooxygenase inhibitory phenolic compounds from Ocimum sanctum Linn. Phytomedicine 7.1 (2000):7-13.

[62] Tampieri MP, Galuppi R, Macchioni F, Carelle MS, Falcioni L, Cioni PL.et al. The inhibition of *Candida albicans* by selected essential oils and their major

components. Mycopathologia. (2005) Apr;159(3):339-45.

[63] Burt S. Essential oils: Their antibacterial properties and potential applications in foods—A review. Int. J. Food Microbiol. 2004;94:223-253.

[64] Lorenzo JM, Khaneghah AM, Gavahian M, Marszałek K, Es I, Munekata PES et al. Understanding the potential benefits of thyme and its derived products for food industry and consumer health: From extraction of value-added compounds to the evaluation of bioaccessibility, bioavailability, anti-inflammatory, and antimicrobial activities. Crit Rev Food Sci Nutr. 2019;59(18):2879-2895.

[65] Engelbertz J, Schwenk T, Kinzinger U, Schierstedt D, Verspohl EJ. Thyme extract, but not thymol, inhibits endothelin induced contractions of isolated rat trachea. Planta Med. 2008;74(12):1436-1440.

[66] Sienkiewicz M, Lysakowska M, Denys P, Kowalczyk E. The Antimicrobial Activity of Thyme Essential Oil Against Multidrug Resistant Clinical Bacterial Strains. Microbial Drug Resistance. 2012;18(2):137-148.

[67] Prasad S, Gupta S, Tyagi A, Aggarwal B. Curcumin, a component of golden spice: Frombedside to bench and back. Biotechnology Advances. 2014;32:1053-1064.

[68] Ammon HP, Wahl MA. Pharmacology of curcuma longa. Planta Med. 1991; 57:1-7.

[69] Barchitta M, Maugeri A, Favara G, Magnano San Lio R, Evola G, Agodi A et al. Nutrition andWound Healing: An Overview Focusing on the Beneficial Effects of Curcumin. Int J Mol Sci. 2019 Mar 5;20(5):1119.

[70] Devassy J, Nwachukwu I, Jones P. Curcumin and cancer: barriers to obtaining a health claim. Nutrition Reviews Vol. 2015, 73(3):155-165.

[71] Kammath AJ, Nair BPS, Nath LR. Curry versus cancer: Potential of some selected culinary spices against cancer with in vitro, in vivo, and human trials evidences. J Food Biochem. 2020;00:e13285.

[72] Patil P, Jayaprakasha GK, Chidambara Murthy KN. Vıkram A. Bioactive compounds: Historical perspectives, opportunities, and challenges. J Agric Food Chem. 2009;57:8142-8160.

[73] Sharma RA, Steward WP, Gescher AJ. Pharmacokinetics and pharmacodynamics of curcumin. In: The Molecular Targets and Therapeutic Uses of Curcumin in Health and Disease. Aggarwal BB, Surh YJ, Shisodia S, editors.; Springer; New York, 2007; pp. 453-470.

[74] Ramírez-Tortosa MC, Mesa MD, Aguilera MC, Quiles JL, Baro L, Ramírez-Tortosa CL. Oral administration of a turmeric extract inhibits LDL oxidation and has hypocholesterolemic effects in rabbits with experimental atherosclerosis. Atherosclerosis. 1999;147(2):371-378.

[75] Den Hartogh DJ, Gabriel A, Tsiani E. Antidiabetic Properties of Curcumin II: Evidence from In Vivo Studies. Nutrients. 2020 Jan;12(1):58.

[76] Das L, Vinayak M. Long Term Effect of Curcumin in Regulation of Glycolytic Pathway and Angiogenesis via Modulation of Stress Activated Genes in Prevention of Cancer. PLoS One. 2014 Jun 16;9(6):e99583.

[77] Mnif S, Aifa S. Cumin (Cuminum cyminumL.) from Traditional Uses to Potential Biomedical Applications. Chemistry&Biodiversity. 2015;12(5):733-742.

[78] Liu Q, Meng X, Li Y, Zhao CN, Tang GY, Li HB. Antibacterial and

Antifungal Activities of Spices. International Journal of Molecular Sciences. 2017;18(6):1283.

[79] Mousavi G. Study on the effect of black cumin (Nigella sativa Linn.) on experimental renal ischemia-reperfusion injury in rats. Acta Cirurgica Brasileira. 2015;30(8):542-550.

[80] Bozkurt M, Sezgic M, Karakol P, Uslu C, Balikci T. The Effect of Antioxidants on Ischemia-Reperfusion Injury in Flap Surgery. Antioxidants, Intech Open 2019.

[81] Tapsell LC, Hemphill I, Cobiac L, Sullivan DR, Fenech M, Patch CS et al. Health benefits of herbs and spices: the past, the present, the future. Medical Journal of Australia. 2006;185(S4).

[82] Ranjbar A, Ghasmeinezhad S, Zamani H, Malekirad AA, Baiaty A, Mohammadirad A et al. Antioxidative stress potential of Cinnamomum zeylanicum in humans: a comparative cross-sectional clinical study. Therapy. 2006;3(1):113-117.

[83] Ghosh T, Basu A, Adhikari D, Roy D, Pal A. K. Antioxidant activity and structural features of *Cinnamomum zeylanicum*.2015; 323 Biotech, 5(6), 939-947.

[84] Bi X, Lim J, Henry CJ. Spices in the management of diabetes mellitus. Food Chemistry. 2017;217:281-293.

[85] Jayaprakasha GK, Rao LJM. Chemistry, Biogenesis, and Biological Activities of Cinnamomum zeylanicum. Critical Reviews in Food Science and Nutrition. 2011;51(6):547-562.

[86] Muhammad DRA, Dewettinck K. Cinnamon and its derivatives as potential ingredient in functional food-A review. International Journal of Food Properties. 2017;1-27.

[87] Ho S, Chang K, Lin C. Anti-neuroinflammatory capacity of fresh ginger is attributed mainly to 10-gingerol. Food Chem. 2013;141:3183-3191.

[88] Stoilova I, Krastanov A, Stoyanova A, Denev P, Gargova S. Antioxidant activity of a ginger extract (Zingiber officinale). Food Chemistry. 2007;102(3):764-770.

[89] Mao QQ, Xu XY, Cao SY, Gan RY, Corke H, Beta T et al. Bioactive Compounds and Bioactivities of Ginger (Zingiber officinale Roscoe). Foods, 2019;8(6):185.

[90] Marx WM, Teleni L, McCarthy AL, Vitetta L, McKavanagh D, Thomson D et al. Ginger (Zingiber officinale) and chemotherapy-induced nausea and vomiting: a systematic literature review. Nutr Rev. 2013;71:245-254.

[91] Palatty PL, Haniadka R, Valder B, Arora R, Baliga MS. Ginger in the prevention of nausea and vomiting: A review. Crit Rev Food Sci. 2013;53:659-669.

[92] Do MT, Kim HG, Choi JH, Khanal T, Park BH, Tran TP, Jeong HG. Antitumor efficacy of piperine in the treatment of human HER2-overexpressing breast cancer cells. Food Chemistry. 2013;141(3):2591-2599. https://doi.org/10.1016/j.foodchem.2013.04.125.

[93] Abraham A. The trend in export, import and production performance of black pepper in India. International Journal of Pure and Applied Mathematics. 2018;118(18):4795-4802.

[94] Tipsrisukond N, Fernando LN, Clarke AD. Antioxidant effects of essential oil and oleoresin of black pepper from supercritical carbon dioxide extractions in ground pork. J Agric Food Chem. 1998;46:4329-43333.

[95] Shahidi F, Pegg RB, Saleemi ZO. Stabilization of meat lipids with ground spices. J Food Lipids. 1995;2:145-153.

[96] Pizzale L, Bortolomeazzi R, Vichi S, Überegger E, Conte LS. Antioxidant activity of sage (Salvia officinalis and S fruticosa) oregano (Origanum onites and O indercedens) extracts related their phenolic compound content. J Sci Food Agric. 2002;82:1645-1651.

[97] Nakatani N, Inatani R, Ohta H, Nishioka A. Chemical constituents of pepper and application to food preservation. Naturally occurring anti-oxidative compounds. Environ Health Perspect. 1986;67:135-147.

[98] Khanna NM. Turmeric-Nature's precious gift. Curr Sci. 1999;76:1351-1356.

Chapter 20

Cinnamomum zeylanicum: Morphology, Antioxidant Properties and Bioactive Compounds

Asel Chandula Weerasekera, Kanchana Samarasinghe, Heethaka Krishantha Sameera de Zoysa, Thushara Chathuranga Bamunuarachchige and Viduranga Yashasvi Waisundara

Abstract

Cinnamomum zeylanicum is one of the oldest spices used for culinary purposes in Asian countries. Its extracts have demonstrated a positive impact on controlling the progression of disease pathologies due to antioxidant, anti-inflammatory, antimicrobial, anticancer, anti-mutagenic, anti-tyrosinase and antidiabetic characteristics. *C. zeylanicum* also has its unique variations which makes it necessary to distinguish it from other species of cinnamon. Phenolic compounds such as cinnamaldehyde, eugenol, carvacrol, cinnamic acetate and thymol are the main compounds that can be found in essential oils of *C. zeylanicum*. However, cinnamaldehyde and eugenol act as the main bioactive antioxidant compounds found in *C. zeylanicum* because of their active functional groups in the structures. There are many examples of the use of *C. zeylanicum* extracts for medicinal purposes, specifically cinnamon metabolite proanthocyanidins which suppress inflammatory compounds and help pathways such as insulin signaling. Moreover, the bioactive compounds in essential oils of this plant are used against many pathogenic (including food-borne) and spoilage bacteria.

Keywords: Alzheimer's disease, Ayurveda, cinnamaldehyde, Ceylon cinnamon, eugenol

1. Introduction

Cinnamomum zeylanicum (family Lauraceae), known as 'Ceylon cinnamon' or 'true cinnamon', grows as an ever-green tree native to Sri Lanka (earlier Ceylon), and India including other regions of tropical Indochina and Madagascar (**Figure 1**). This is one of the oldest traditional spice species used for culinary purposes in South Asian countries [1, 2]. Additionally, according to toponymical and historical evidence, *C. zeylanicum* has been used for medicinal purposes since the establishment of Aryan settlements in the Anuradhapura kingdom [3]. Moreover, the indigenous species of Ceylon cinnamon has been used in the Ayurveda system of Sri Lanka [3, 4]. Ethnopharmacological studies show that

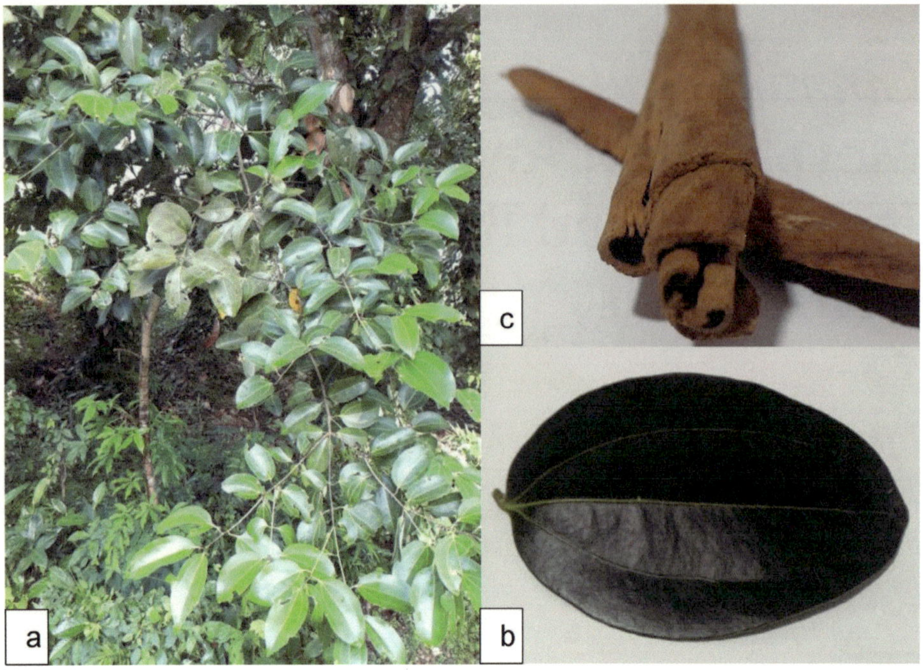

Figure 1.
Typical Cinnamomum zeylanicum *tree (a), leaf (b), and processed bark (c) in Sri Lanka.*

C. zeylanicum has gained more importance in Ayurveda and folklore medicine as it can be used in concoctions and decoctions. The inner bark of *C. zeylanicum* is used for medicine preparation in flatulence control, indigestion and in flu-prevention in the Sri Lankan Ayurveda system. *C. zeylanicum* has also been found in various other folklore treatments against inflammation of eyes, dyspnoea, leucorrhoea, rheumatism, neuralgia, wounds, toothache and diabetes [4–6].

C. zeylanicum and it extracts have demonstrated their ability to have a positive impact on controlling the progression of disease pathologies in modern times as well. This is mainly due to the functional properties of *C. zeylanicum* and its compounds behaving as antioxidant, anti-inflammatory, antimicrobial, anticancer, anti-mutagenic, anti-tyrosinase and antidiabetic agents [1, 2]. In fact, Ceylon cinnamon is considered one of the few plants in the world that have made it to the modern pharmacy in the form of pills, powders, oils and ointments.

A striking resemblance in terms of appearance exists between different Cinnamon varieties. In particular, *C. zeylanicum* is sometimes confused with other varieties resulting in incorrect information being disseminated about the functional properties and bioactive compounds. To avoid consequences of these similarities, as well as due to the lack of data about the antioxidant properties of the plant and the importance of this information to its folkloristic use and pharmacological activities, it was deemed necessary to address the morphological features and antioxidant properties of *C. zeylanicum* in detail in this chapter, as well as the culinary and traditional uses, and the phytochemical composition and pharmacological activities.

2. Morphological features of *Cinnamomum zeylanicum*

C. zeylanicum has its unique variations which are quite useful in distinguishing it from other species of cinnamon. It is generally grown in loamy, lateritic, and silver sand soil and can grow up to 12 m in height. The morphological features which enable the identification of the varieties of *C. zeylanicum* from other species of Cinnamon based on leaf traits are shown in **Table 1** [7]. While the deep vein distribution appears to be common to all Cinnamon species, the color change of the

Type	Leaf shape	Leaf color	Leaf size	Venation	References
Cinnamomum zeylanicum (Sri Wijaya)	Acute	Red leaves when young And deep green when matured.	Small to medium	Deep vein distribution pattern present.	[7, 8]
Cinnamomum zeylanicum (Sri Gemunu)	Ovate to elliptic	Red leaves when young and dark green when matured.	Medium to large	Deep vein distribution pattern present	[8]
Cinnamomum cassia	Lanceolate	Red leaves when young.	Small to medium	Deep veins	[9]
Cinnamomum burmannii	Ovate-oblong	Pale greenish brown leaves.	Small to medium	Deep veins	[10]
Cinnamomum tamala	Elliptic-oblong, ovate	Slightly pinkish when young and green when matured.	Small to medium	Deep veins. Three-nerved from close above the base almost to the apex	[11]

Table 1.
Morphological traits of leaves of varieties of cinnamon.

Type of Cinnamon	Color	Texture	Layers when rolled	Fragility	Odor	Taste	References
Cinnamomum zeylanicum	Tan brown	Thin, soft and papery	Multiple layers and curls inward from both edges.	Fragile	Exotic aroma	Mild sweet	[4, 12]
Cassia Cinnamon	Reddish dark brown	Thick and rough	Few layers and curls inward from one edge.	Harder to break	Mild aroma	Spicy	[4, 12]
Cinnamomum burmannii	Light reddish brown	Thin and soft	One layer	Fragile	Strong aroma	Marginal bitter and astringent	[12]
Cinnamomum loureiroi Nees	Reddish brown	Thin and rough	Few layers	Harder to break	Strong aroma	Slightly bitter and astringent	[4, 12]

Table 2.
Significant differences in the bark of Cinnamomum zeylanicum *and in other species of cinnamon.*

Type of Cinnamon	Flower color	Arrangement	References
Cinnamomum zeylanicum	Greenish	In panicles	[10, 13]
Cinnamomum cassia	White	In panicles	[13]
Cinnamomum burmannii	Whitish Yellow	In panicles	[14]
Cinnamomum tamala	Yellow	In panicles	[13]

Table 3.
Variations of flower and inflorescence in Cinnamomum zeylanicum *and other kinds of cinnamon.*

leaves from red to deep green and a larger size help to distinguish the *C. zeylanicum* from *C. cassia*, *C. burmannii* and *C. tamala*.

The Cinnamon bark of *C. zeylanicum* is where most of the bioactive compounds exist, and, there are certain traits which help identify the plant, based on bark characteristics which are shown in **Table 2** [4, 12]. However, it is also shown that the bark of *C. zeylanicum* in powder form is practically impossible to distinguish from other wild species of cinnamon due to its identical appearance – a character which is often misused by Cinnamon producers for adulteration. In these instances, an analytical method or a microscope is essential for the identification of Ceylon Cinnamon in its powdered form. However, the aroma from *C. zeylanicum* is more fragrant and exotic than other varieties. Owing to continued exposure to the plant, traditional Cinnamon growers would have the best sense of distinguishing *C. zeylanicum* from other varieties simply based on the aroma of the bark.

Flowers of *C. zeylanicum* are greenish in color and are arranged in panicles both from the axial or apex [10, 13, 14]. Variations in the Cinnamon flowers based on the different varieties are shown in **Table 3**. *C. zeylanicum* flowers have a noticeable green hue which would set it apart from flowers of other Cinnamon varieties.

3. Antioxidant properties and beneficial effects

Antioxidants are known as substances or compounds, that delay/stop the oxidation by ceasing the damage caused by free radicals. They are able to easily interact with free radicals by oxidation, and generally, the reaction occurs either in single or multi-step fashion. Antioxidants can also react through single electron transfer, hydrogen atom transfer or by chelating transitional metals. Moreover, antioxidants in the biological systems occur as enzymatic and non-enzymatic forms at both extracellular and intracellular environments [2, 15, 16]. The balance of free radicals and antioxidant defense mechanisms is critically important in health aspects from the perspective of mitigating oxidative stress [17–20]. Oxidative stress, which is induced by free radicals, is associated with many chronic diseases such as cancer, osteoporosis, diabetes and coronary heart disease [2, 4, 16, 21]. Reactive oxygen species (ROS) induce oxidative stress and are responsible for the cumulative damage imparted on DNA, lipids, proteins and other molecules, subsequently resulting in even permanent damage [17–19, 22]. Many spices, fruits and vegetables have already been identified as rich in antioxidant compounds such as polyphenols, vitamins, flavonoids and carotenoids [23–25]. Moreover, antioxidant-rich foodstuff are good sources to combat and prevent the incidence of many chronic diseases associated with oxidative stress [23].

C. zeylanicum is rich in phenolic compounds. These compounds and their activities are defined by their structure (reactive benzene rings), which is directly linked with quenching radicals in biological systems [17, 22, 26]. Cinnamaldehyde, eugenol, carvacrol, cinnamic acetate and thymol are the main phenolic compounds that can be found in essential oils of *C. zeylanicum* [27, 28]. Characterization of phenolic compounds in *C. zeylanicum* revealed that it can improve hyperlipidemia; possibly by lowering cholesterol production, and suppressing lipid peroxidation [1]. Among the parts used in the *C. zeylanicum* tree for various medicinal purposes, the bark demonstrated the highest antioxidant activity compared to the leaves and flowers [2]. However, essential oils appear to have the greatest antioxidant activity compared to leaves, bark and extracts from other parts of the plant [18].

Peroxynitrite (ONOO-) is a compound capable of reacting with almost every class of biomolecules due to formation of $NO2^{\bullet}$ and $OH^{\bullet}$ radicals via degradation. These radicals can promote oxidative damage to blood vessels, skin, heart, lungs, kidney, and brain. Eugenol – a component of the active oils extracted from Cinnamon was found to be effective in preventing peroxynitrite-induced damage *in vitro*. However, the concentration of eugenol present in active oil extracts differ depending on the Cinnamon variety it was extracted from, with *C. zeylanicum* activity demonstrating the highest. Therefore, from a pure peroxynitrite inhibitory standpoint, Cinnamon oil extracts with a high eugenol content can be classified as a spice to inhibit the activity of radicals $NO2^{\bullet}$ and $OH^{\bullet}$ [29].

Besides, many studies have been conducted to assess the antioxidant properties of *C. zeylanicum* with extractions from different parts of the tree, under both *in vitro* and *in vivo* conditions [2, 19]. Multiple studies have exposed the total antioxidant capacity and its beneficial results such as a decrease in blood lipid peroxide levels through the improvement of hepatic antioxidant enzyme activities [2, 19, 25], and lowered risks of male infertility, and inflammatory diseases [17]. A study done with swiss albino mice by using Cinnamon 0.25% and Cardamom 0.5%, orally administered at doses of 100 ml/mouse/day, observed that azoxymethane induced colon carcinogenesis could be significantly controlled by inhibiting lipid peroxidation and enhancing Glutathione-S-transferase (GST) activity in liver and colon [30].

In addition to the health benefits, these antioxidants have been used as a primary additive or preservative especially in food industries to prevent or delay the spoilage of food rich in fats and oils [23] and for enhancement flavor [19]. Nowadays, many food industries are concerned with producing food which is less toxic, have fewer health risks and contain a smaller number of synthetic compounds during processing. Therefore, plant-derived antioxidants, especially those coming from *C. zeylanicum*, has commanded the attention of manufacturers and consumers [2, 26, 27]. The natural compounds, which are characterized by their antioxidant properties have shown great potential in terms of their health benefits (**Table 4**) [22, 27]. Additionally, these antioxidant compounds are used as substitutes for the synthetic ones such as butylated hydroxytoluene (BHT) and butylated hydroxy anisole (BHA) [22, 27, 34]. Studies have also revealed that when *C. zeylanicum* is used as an antioxidant in food, it enhances antioxidant enzymes and remove the ROS, while decreasing malondialdehyde which is naturally present during situations of elevated oxidative stress [17]. *C. zeylanicum* compounds appear to withstand severe processing conditions as well, since a study has shown that irradiation – which is used frequently to preserve foods these days, does not affect the antioxidant properties of *C. zeylanicum* extracts [15]. This indicates its suitability as a food preservative [15, 35]. Moreover, *C. zeylanicum* is used in the pharmaceutical industry as a nutraceutical. It is also used in the essence industries due to its fragrance to produce foods, perfumes and drugs [2, 22, 23].

In terms of the bioactive antioxidant compounds present in *C. zeylanicum*, cinnamaldehyde and eugenol act as the main bioactive antioxidant compound because of their active functional groups in the structures [36]. Health benefits of antioxidant compounds present in *C. zeylanicum* are listed in **Table 5.**

C. zeylanicum plant product type or parts	Main Antioxidant compounds	Properties or benefits	Reference
Essential oils	Cinnamaldehyde, eugenol, thymol, carvacrol, safrole, menthol, 1,8-cineole, α-terpineol, p-cymene	As agro-food natural antioxidants to conserve fatty foods used in all formulations containing fats, as food additives and as a natural food preservative.	[26]
Essential oils	Cinnamaldehyde, α-pinene, eugenol, β-caryophyllene, and eucalyptol	high inhibitory effect against β-carotene discoloration, suppress lipid oxidation reaction, and as a food preservative.	[31]
Essential oils	Cinnamaldehyde, eugenol and carvacrol	As feed additives and potential alternative to antibiotics in poultry industry.	[32]
Essential oil	Cinnamaldehyde and cinnamic acetate	inhibition of 2-hexenal oxidation	[28]
Essential oil	Cinnamaldehyde and trans-cinnamaldehyde	As a drug in phytotherapy disease treatment.	[33]
Cinnamon (*C. zeylanicum*) tea	Trans-cinnamaldehyde	Decrease blood lipid peroxides, increase antioxidant capacity and total thiol molecules.	[19]

Table 4.
Antioxidant compounds of C. zeylanicum *products and their properties.*

Antioxidants compounds	Activity	Reference
Cinnacassiol, eugenol, camphene, coumarin, cinnamaldehyde, cinnamic acid and gamma-terpinene	Against high cholesterol diet toxicity	[17]
Cinnamaldehyde and other compounds of Cinnamon	Activity against the production of nitric oxide and the expression of inducible nitric oxide.	[23, 37]
Eugenol	Against peroxynitrite induced nitration and lipid peroxidation.	[23]
Essential oil rich in eugenol, (E)- cinnamaldehyde, and linalool		[37]
Cinnamaldehyde and trans-cinnamaldehyde	Anti-tyrosinase activity.	[17, 23]
Cinnamate	Improves hyperlipidemia and decrease triglyceride levels.	[1]
Cinnamaldehyde	Reduce visfatin-induced breast cancer.	[38]
Cuminaldehyde	Inhibition of proliferation and apoptosis induction.	[38]

Table 5.
Antioxidant properties of bioactive compounds present in C. zeylanicum.

There are other demonstrated beneficial properties of *C. zeylanicum*. Acetaminophen is an over-the-counter antipyretic-analgesic drug. It exhibits anti-inflammatory properties at therapeutic doses. However, it also causes hepatotoxicity and nephrotoxicity at large doses. Trials conducted by supplementing high doses of Cinnamon with acetaminophen in four rat groups discovered that pre-treatment with Cinnamon significantly ameliorated cellular alterations and apoptosis [39].

Tauopathy neurodegeneration is a subset of diseases involving a trademark neurofibrillary tangling. Hyperphosphorylation in the microtubular protein known as tau results in the protein disassociating from the microtubules and forming insoluble aggregates. These neurofibrillary tangles of tau are believed to be one of the possible central pathologies of Alzheimer's disease. Cinnamon extract was found to effectively inhibit the aggregation of human tau *in vitro*. The activity was attributed to a proanthocyanidin trimer and cinnamaldehyde. The same study observed that while the Cinnamon extract inhibited the aggregation of tau, not all polyphenols in the Cinnamon extract are active in the inhibitory process. Therefore, the inhibitory activity cannot be linked to the general antioxidant properties of the extract. However, the studies were performed *in vitro*, raising concerns about the bioavailability of compounds. Regardless, this study has set the stage and qualified Cinnamon extract for additional testing in clinical trials [40].

Cinnamon extract also exhibited significant gastroprotective effects in a study performed with Wistar albino rats. Gastric lesions were induced via an orally administered indomethacin solution. A Cinnamon suspension was administered 30 min prior to the oral indomethacin, and the animals were sacrificed 6 hours after the treatment. The results found a significant decrease in basal gastric acid secretion and ulcer protective effects across a range of models [41].

4. Bioactive compounds

C. zeylanicum antioxidant compounds are found in many of parts of the plant such as leaves, buds, flowers, fruits, bark, root bark and oils. Additionally, *C. zeylanicum* is also rich with volatile compounds, most of which act as antioxidants. *C. zeylanicum* contains cinnamyl acetate, eugenol, trans-cinnamaldehyde (the main component of Cinnamon flavor), cymene, cinnacassiol, cineol, camphene, catechins, coumarin cinnamic acid and gamma-terpinene, terpinolene, and α-thujene, α-terpineol, linalool, l-borneol, E-nerolidol, pinene, phyllandrene, proanthocyanidins, safrole, tannins constituting polymeric 5,7,3,4-tetrahydroxy-tetrahydroxy flavan-3-4-diol units, α-cubene and resins [1, 17, 23]. In addition, most of the compounds are mainly derived from cinnamyl, hydrolyzed phenol, tannins, phenylpropanoids and terpenoids compounds [42]. There are several other bioactive compounds listed in **Table 6**, according to the type of extraction using different parts of the *C. zeylanicum* tree [26]. However, eugenol, benzyl benzoate, linalool and eugenyl acetate are reported as the common antioxidants of *C. zeylanicum* species [27].

Among the bioactive constitutes of *C. zeylanicum*, cinnamaldehyde and trans-cinnamaldehyde are considered as the major compounds, especially concerning anti-tyrosinase activity [17]. The spicy and fragrance characters of *C. zeylanicum* is mainly due to cinnamaldehyde [23]. Based on the richness of bioactive compounds and its medicinal properties, *C. zeylanicum* is used traditionally to provide aroma and essence compounds. It is also used as an antioxidant, anti-inflammatory, anti-hyperglycemic, anti-lipidemic, antidiabetic, anticancer, antitumor, anthelmintic, anti-aflatoxigenic, antifungal and antimicrobial agent medicinally [1, 29, 32, 43–47]. There are many examples of its use for medicinal purposes such as Cinnamon metabolite proanthocyanidins which suppresses inflammatory compounds helping pathways such as insulin signaling. Moreover, essential oil bioactive compounds are used against many pathogenic (including food-borne) and spoilage bacteria [17, 31, 46].

Parts of *C. zeylanicum*	Antioxidant compounds	Reference
Essential oil	• Cinnamaldehyde • Trans-Cinnamaldehyde • Camphor • Cinnamyl-acetate • Caryophyllene • Carvacrol • Caryophyllene oxide • Eugenol • E-nerolidol • b-caryophyllene • Guaiol • Terpinolene • Thymol • Safrole • Menthol • 1,8-cineole • α-terpineol • p-cymene • Trans α-bergamotene • Linalool • L-borneol • L-bornyl acetate • Geraniol • Bornyl acetate • α-cubebene • α-terpineol • α-thujene • γ-elemene • α-copaene	[23, 26, 28].
Oils from the buds	• Mono and sesquiterpenes	[28]
Leaves	• Cinnamaldehyde • Eugenol	[23, 36]
Cinnamon Bark	• Cinnamaldehyde • Eugenol • Linalool • Safrole • Pinene • Phyllandrene • Cymene • Cineol • Tannins constituting polymeric 5,7,3,4-tetrahydroxy-tetrahydroxy flavan-3-4-diol units • Catechins • Proanthocyanidins • Resins	[23, 36]

Parts of *C. zeylanicum*	Antioxidant compounds	Reference
Root Bark	• Camper	[23, 36]
Flowers and fruits and in lower amounts in buds	• Trans-Cinnamaldehyde • Terpene hydrocarbons • *alpha*-Bergamotene • *alpha*-Copaene • Oxygenated terpenoids • (E)-Cinnamyl acetate • *trans-alpha*-Bergamotene • Caryophyllene oxide	[23, 28, 36]

Table 6.
Bioactive compounds find in the C. zeylanicum *species.*

5. Conclusion

Based on the evidence presented above, it is only pertinent to identify *C. zeylanicum* as a potent disease-preventing herb due to its superior antioxidant power. While most of the bioactive compounds responsible for this functional property have been isolated and identified, it is evident that the compounds vary with the variety of the plant, environmental conditions as well as the analytical method used for the characterization process. Thus, it is inevitable that more potent antioxidant compounds can be discovered in *C. zeylanicum*. Even though currently considered as a spice and a traditional medicinal herb, *C. zeylanicum* has the potential to serve as the source for generating compounds for clinical trials for further evaluation of efficacy and ability to prevent specific diseases.

Author details

Asel Chandula Weerasekera[1], Kanchana Samarasinghe[2],
Heethaka Krishantha Sameera de Zoysa[3,4],
Thushara Chathuranga Bamunuarachchige[3] and Viduranga Yashasvi Waisundara[2*]

1 Western Sydney University, Sydney, Australia

2 Australian College of Business and Technology – Kandy Campus, Kandy, Sri Lanka

3 Department of Bioprocess Technology, Faculty of Technology, Rajarata University of Sri Lanka, Mihintale, Sri Lanka

4 Department of Biology, University of Naples Federico II, Naples, Italy

*Address all correspondence to: viduranga@gmail.com

References

[1] Abdelgadir AA, Hassan HM, Abdelgadir AA, Hassan HM, Eltaher AM, Mohammed KG, et al. Hypolipidemic Effect of Cinnamon (*Cinnamomum zeylanicum*) Bark Ethanolic Extract on Triton X-100 induced Hyperlipidemia in Albino Rats. Med Aromat Plants [Internet]. 2020 [cited 2021 Jan 9];9(3):1-6. Available from: https://www.researchgate.net/publication/342096168

[2] Abeysekera WPKM, Premakumara GAS, Ratnasooriya WD. In Vitro Antioxidant Properties of Leaf and Bark Extracts of Ceylon Cinnamon (*Cinnamomum zeylanicum* Blume). Trop Agric Res. 2013;24(2):128-38.

[3] Patel A, Tiwari S, Pandey N, Gupta D. Role of Spices Beyond a Flavouring Agent: The Antioxidant and Medicinal Properties. In: Mishra N, editor. Ethnopharmacological Investigation of Indian Spices [Internet]. 2020 [cited 2021 Jan 9]. p. 5-35. Available from: https://orcid.org/0000-0002-1335-0267

[4] Ranasinghe P, Galappaththy P. Health benefits of Ceylon cinnamon (Cinnamomum zeylanicum): a summary of the current evidence Clinical trials View project Acute Coronary Syndrome Sri Lanka Audit Project View project THE CEYLON MEDICAL JOURNAL Health benefits of Ceylon cinnamon (Cinnamom. Off Publ Sri Lanka Med Assoc [Internet]. 2016 [cited 2021 Jan 9];61(1):1-5. Available from: http://doi.org/10.4038/cmj.v61i1.8251

[5] Das M, Mandal S, Mallick B, Hazra J. Ethnobotany, phytochemical and pharmacological aspects of *Cinnamomum zeylanicum* blume. Int Res J Pharm. 2016 Nov 21;4(4):58-63.

[6] Kumar V, MarkoviĆ T, Emerald M, Dey A. Herbs: Composition and Dietary Importance. In: Caballero B, Finglas PM, Toldrá F, editors. Encyclopedia of Food and Health. Elsevier Inc.; 2015. p. 332-7.

[7] Azad R, Ranawaka RAAK, Senanayake G, Kumara KLW, Pushpakumara DKNG, Wijesinghe KGG, et al. Morphological variation of cinnamon (*Cinnamomum verum* Persl) germplasm in Matara district of Sri Lanka. Int J Minor Fruits, Med Aromat Plants. 2016;2(1):6-14.

[8] Ariyarathne HBMA, Weerasuriya SN, Senarath WTPSK. Comparison of morphological and chemical characteristics of two selected accessions and six wild species of genus *Cinnamomum* Schaeff. Sri Lankan J Biol. 2018 Jan 30;3(1):23.

[9] Wilson L. Spices and Flavoring Crops: Leaf and Floral Structures. In: Caballero B, Finglas PM, Toldrá F, editors. Encyclopedia of Food and Health. Elsevier Inc.; 2015. p. 84-92.

[10] Chen P, Sun J, Ford P. Differentiation of the four major species of cinnamons (*C. burmannii*, *C. verum*, *C. cassia*, and *C. loureiroi*) using a flow injection mass spectrometric (FIMS) fingerprinting method. J Agric Food Chem [Internet]. 2014 Mar 26 [cited 2021 Jan 9];62(12):2516-21. Available from: https://pubs.acs.org/sharingguidelines

[11] Lamichhane D, Karna N. Harvesting methods of Cinnamomum tamala leaves in private land: a case study from Udayapur district, Nepal. Banko Janakari [Internet]. 1970 Jan 1 [cited 2021 Jan 9];19(2):20-4. Available from: https://www.nepjol.info/index.php/BANKO/article/view/2981

[12] Bandusekara BS, Pushpakumara DKNG, Bandaranayake PCG, Wijesinghe KGG, Jayasinghe GG. Field Level

Identification of <em>Cinnamomum</em> Species in Sri Lanka Using a Morphological Index. Trop Agric Res. 2020 Oct 6;31(4):53.

[13] Azad R, Kumara KLW, Senanayake G, Ranawaka RAAK, Pushpakumara DKNG, Geekiyanage S. Flower morphological diversity of cinnamon (*Cinnamomum verum* Presl) in Matara District, Sri Lanka. Open Agric [Internet]. 2018 Jan 1 [cited 2021 Jan 9];3(1):236-44. Available from: https://doi.org/10.1515/opag-2018-0025

[14] Sharma G, Nautiyal AR. *Cinnamomum tamala*: A valuable tree of Himalayas. J Med Aromat Plants [Internet]. 2011 [cited 2021 Jan 9]; 1(1):1-4. Available from: https://www.researchgate.net/publication/267692908

[15] Kitazuru ER, Moreira AVB, Mancini-Filho J, Delincée H, Villavicencio ALCH. Effects of irradiation on natural antioxidants of cinnamon (*Cinnamomum zeylanicum* N.). Radiat Phys Chem. 2004 Sep 1;71(1-2):39-41.

[16] Nimse SB, Pal D. Free radicals, natural antioxidants, and their reaction mechanisms. RSC Adv [Internet]. 2015 Mar 20 [cited 2021 Jan 24];5(35):27986-8006. Available from: www.rsc.org/advances

[17] Arisha SM, Sakr SA, Abd-Elhaseeb FR. *Cinnamomum zeylanicum* alleviate testicular damage induced by high fat diet in albino rats; histological and ultrastructural studies. Heliyon. 2020 Nov 1;6(11):1-14.

[18] Castro JC, Pante GC, Centenaro BM, Almeida RTR De, Pilau EJ, Dias Filho BP, et al. Antifungal and antimycotoxigenic effects of *Zingiber officinale, Cinnamomum zeylanicum* and *Cymbopogon martinii* essential oils against *Fusarium verticillioides*. Food Addit Contam Part A [Internet]. 2020 Sep 1 [cited 2021 Jan 11];37(9):1531-41. Available from: https://www.tandfonline.com/doi/full/10.1080/19440049.2020.1778183

[19] Ranjbar A, Ghasmeinezhad S, Zamani H, Malekirad AA, Baiaty A, Mohammadirad A, et al. Antioxidative stress potential of *Cinnamomum zeylanicum* in humans: a comparative cross-sectional clinical study. Therapy [Internet]. 2006 [cited 2021 Jan 21];3(1):113-7. Available from: www.future-drugs.com

[20] Ghosh T, Basu A, Adhikari D, Roy D, Pal AK. Antioxidant activity and structural features of *Cinnamomum zeylanicum*. 3 Biotech. 2015 Dec 1;5(6):939-47.

[21] El-Baroty GS, Abd El-Baky HH, Farag RS, Saleh MA. Characterization of antioxidant and antimicrobial compounds of cinnamon and ginger essential oils. African J Biochem Res [Internet]. 2010 Jun 30 [cited 2021 Jan 16];4(6):167-74. Available from: http://www.academicjournals.org/AJBR

[22] Dudonné S, Vitrac X, Coutiére P, Woillez M, Mérillon JM. Comparative study of antioxidant properties and total phenolic content of 30 plant extracts of industrial interest using DPPH, ABTS, FRAP, SOD, and ORAC assays. J Agric Food Chem [Internet]. 2009 Mar 11 [cited 2021 Jan 14];57(5):1768-74. Available from: https://pubs.acs.org/sharingguidelines

[23] Rao PV, Gan SH. Cinnamon: A multifaceted medicinal plant. Evidence-based Complement Altern Med. 2014;2014:1-13.

[24] Singh R, Lawrence R, Lawrence K, Agarwal B, Gupta RK, Dar S. Antioxidant and Antibacterial Activity of *Syzigium aromaticum*, *Zingiber officinale* and *Cinnamomum zeylanicum* Essential Oils. Chem Sci Trans [Internet]. 2015 [cited 2021 Jan 23];

4(1):239-45. Available from: http://www.e-journals.in

[25] Borzoei A, Rafraf M, Niromanesh S, Farzadi L, Narimani F, Doostan F. Effects of cinnamon supplementation on antioxidant status and serum lipids in women with polycystic ovary syndrome. J Tradit Complement Med. 2018 Jan 1;8(1):128-33.

[26] Wilson AA, Pierre MDJ, Leopold NT, Priya P, Nisha P. Stabilisation potentials of the essential oils of *Thymus vulgaris* L., *Cinnamomum zeylanicum* B. and *Mentha piperita* L. on palm olein at accelerated storage. African J Biotechnol [Internet]. 2020 Jul 31 [cited 2021 Jan 10];19(7):464-77. Available from: http://www.academicjournals.org/AJB

[27] Schmidt E, Jirovetz L, Buchbauer G, Eller GA, Stoilova I, Krastanov A, et al. Composition and antioxidant activities of the essential oil of cinnamon (*Cinnamomum zeylanicum* blume) leaves from Sri Lanka. J Essent Oil-Bearing Plants [Internet]. 2006 [cited 2021 Jan 22];9(2):170-82. Available from: https://www.tandfonline.com/action/journalInformation?journalCode=teop20

[28] Cardoso-Ugarte GA, López-Malo A, Sosa-Morales ME. Cinnamon (*Cinnamomum zeylanicum*) essential oils. In: Preedy VR, editor. Essential Oils in Food Preservation, Flavor and Safety. Elsevier Inc.; 2016. p. 339-47.

[29] Chericoni S, Prieto JM, Iacopini P, Cioni P, Morelli I. In vitro activity of the essential oil of *Cinnamomum zeylanicum* and eugenol in peroxynitrite-induced oxidative processes. J Agric Food Chem [Internet]. 2005 Jun 15 [cited 2021 Jan 9];53(12):4762-5. Available from: https://pubs.acs.org/sharingguidelines

[30] Bhattacharjee S, Rana T, Sengupta A. Inhibition of Lipid Peroxidation and Enhancement of GST Activity by Cardamom and Cinnamon During Chemically Induced Colon Carcinogenesis in Swiss Albino Mice. Asian Pacific J Cancer Prev [Internet]. 2007 [cited 2021 Jan 9];8:578-82. Available from: https://www.researchgate.net/publication/5590955

[31] Behbahani AB, Falah F, Lavi Arab F, Vasiee M, Tabatabaee Yazdi F. Chemical Composition and Antioxidant, Antimicrobial, and Antiproliferative Activities of Cinnamomum zeylanicum Bark Essential Oil. Evidence-based Complement Altern Med. 2020;2020:1-8.

[32] El-Hack MEA, Alagawany M, Abdel-Moneim A-ME, Mohammed NG, Khafaga AF, Bin-Jumah M, et al. Cinnamon (*Cinnamomum zeylanicum*) Oil as a Potential Alternative to Antibiotics in Poultry. Antibiotics [Internet]. 2020 Apr 26 [cited 2021 Jan 16];9(5):1-12. Available from: https://www.mdpi.com/2079-6382/9/5/210

[33] Khaki A. Effect of *Cinnamomum zeylanicumon* on spermatogenesis. Iran Red Crescent Med J [Internet]. 2015 Dec 1 [cited 2021 Jan 18];17(2):1-5. Available from: /pmc/articles/PMC4376985/?report=abstract

[34] Hamidpour R, Hamidpour M, Hamidpour S, Shahlari M. Cinnamon from the selection of traditional applications to its novel effects on the inhibition of angiogenesis in cancer cells and prevention of Alzheimer's disease, and a series of functions such as antioxidant, anticholesterol, antidiabetes, antibacterial, antifungal, nematicidal, acaracidal, and repellent activities. J Tradit Complement Med. 2015 Apr 1;5(2):66-70.

[35] Bhatia S, Saraswat S. CINNAMON: ALL ROUND MEDICINAL SPICE. Plant Arch [Internet]. 2020 [cited 2021 Jan 10];20(Special Issue

(AIAAS-2020)):95-9. Available from: http://plantarchives.org/SPL ISSUE AIAAS 2020/95-99.pdf

[36] Adarsh A, Chettiyar B, Kanthesh B, Raghu N. Phytochemical Screening and Antimicrobial Activity of "*Cinnamon zeylanicum*." Int J Pharm Res Innov. 2020;13:22-33.

[37] Jayaprakasha GK, Rao LJM. Chemistry, Biogenesis, and Biological Activities of *Cinnamomum zeylanicum*. Crit Rev Food Sci Nutr [Internet]. 2011 Jul [cited 2021 Jan 18];51(6):547-62. Available from: http://www.tandfonline.com/doi/abs/10.1080/10408391003699550

[38] Kubatka P, Kello M, Kajo K, Samec M, Jasek K, Vybohova D, et al. Chemopreventive and Therapeutic Efficacy of *Cinnamomum zeylanicum* L. Bark in Experimental Breast Carcinoma: Mechanistic In Vivo and In Vitro Analyses. Molecules [Internet]. 2020 Mar 19 [cited 2021 Jan 20];25(6):1-32. Available from: https://www.mdpi.com/1420-3049/25/6/1399

[39] Abdeen A, Abdelkader A, Abdo M, Wareth G, Aboubakr M, Aleya L, et al. Protective effect of cinnamon against acetaminophen-mediated cellular damage and apoptosis in renal tissue. 2019 [cited 2021 Jan 9];26:240-9. Available from: https://doi.org/10.1007/s11356-018-3553-2

[40] Peterson DW, George RC, Scaramozzino F, Lapointe NE, Anderson RA, Graves DJ, et al. Cinnamon extract inhibits tau aggregation associated with alzheimer's disease in vitro. J Alzheimer's Dis. 2009 Jan 1;17(3):585-97.

[41] Alqasoumi S. Anti-secretagogue and antiulcer effects of "cinnamon" *Cinnamomum zeylanicum* in rats. J Pharmacogn Phyther [Internet]. 2012 Jul 31 [cited 2021 Jan 9];4(4):53-61. Available from: http://www.academicjournals.org/JPP

[42] Tang PL, Chen YT, Qin J, Hou X, Deng J. Effect of cinnamon bark and twig extracts on the chemical, physicochemical and antioxidant properties of fermented milk. J Food Meas Charact [Internet]. 2020 Aug 1 [cited 2021 Jan 20];14(4):2271-81. Available from: https://doi.org/10.1007/s11694-020-00474-5

[43] Fabbri J, Maggiore MA, Pensel PE, Denegri GM, Elissondo MC. In vitro efficacy study of *Cinnamomum zeylanicum* essential oil and cinnamaldehyde against the larval stage of *Echinococcus granulosus*. Exp Parasitol. 2020 Jul 1;214:107904.

[44] Beji RS, Khemir S, Wannes WA, Ayari K, Ksouri R. Antidiabetic, antihyperlipidemic and antioxidant influences of the spice cinnamon (*Cinnamomum zeylanicumon*) in experimental rats. Brazilian J Pharm Sci [Internet]. 2018 [cited 2021 Jan 10];54(2):17576. Available from: http://dx.doi.org/10.1590/s2175-97902018000217576

[45] Dorri M, Hashemitabar S, Hosseinzadeh H. Cinnamon (*Cinnamomum zeylanicum*) as an antidote or a protective agent against natural or chemical toxicities: a review. Drug Chem Toxicol [Internet]. 2018 Jul 3 [cited 2021 Jan 12];41(3):338-51. Available from: https://www.tandfonline.com/doi/abs/10.1080/01480545.2017.1417995

[46] Elgammal E, El Gendy AEN, Elgamal AE-B. Mechanism of action and bioactivities of *Cinnamomum zeylanicum* essential oil against some pathogenic microbes. Egypt Pharm J [Internet]. 2020 [cited 2021 Jan 16];19(2):171. Available from: http://www.epj.eg.net/text.asp?2020/19/2/162/288661

[47] Diniz do Nascimento L, Moraes AAB de, Costa KS da, Pereira Galúcio JM, Taube PS, Costa CML, et al. Bioactive Natural Compounds and Antioxidant Activity of Essential Oils from Spice Plants: New Findings and Potential Applications. Biomolecules [Internet]. 2020 Jul 1 [cited 2021 Jan 21];10(7):1-35. Available from: https://www.mdpi.com/2218-273X/10/7/988

Chapter 21

Dietary Phytochemicals: As a Natural Source of Antioxidants

Manju Singh Makhaik, Arvind K. Shakya and Raosaheb Kale

Abstract

Since time immemorial, plants are used as the source of food and medicine. It can be traced back to the start of humanity. Bringing plant-based food, such as fruits, vegetables, and whole grains, rich in phytochemicals, with beneficial nutrients, opens the door for healthy living. The health benefits are partly attributed to the compounds which possess antioxidants. Several epidemiological observations have shown an opposite relationship between consumption of plant-based foods, rich in phytochemicals, and many diseases including cancer. The majority of the ailments are related to oxidative stress induced by free radicals. Free radicals are extremely unstable with a very short half-life, highly reactive molecule which leads to oxidative damage to macromolecules such as proteins, DNA, and lipids. Free radical induced cellular inflammation appears to be a major contributing factor to cause aging, and degenerative diseases such as cancer, cardiovascular diseases, diabetes, hepatic diseases, renal ailments, and brain dysfunction. Free radicals have been caught up in the pathogenesis of several diseases. Providentially, free radical formation is controlled naturally by phytochemicals, through their antioxidant potential which plays a key role in preventing many diseases including cancer by suppressing oxidative stress-induced DNA damage. Keeping these facts in mind, an attempt has been made to highlight the oxidative stress, enzymatic and non-enzymatic antioxidant, dietary phytochemicals and their role of in disease prevention and cure.

Keywords: Oxidative stress, antioxidants, reactive oxygen species, antioxidant enzymes, phytochemicals

1. Introduction

Life threatening diseases such as cardiovascular diseases, neurodisorders, diabetes, and cancers are world health problems and account for morbidity and mortality to millions of people. These diseases/disorders are mainly linked to oxidative stress due to free radical induced toxicity. The free radicals (oxidants) are unstable species with a very short half-life, but they are highly reactive metabolites which are harmful to normal functions of the cells and body. They produce oxidative damage toward macromolecules like proteins, DNA, and lipids. In general, the reactive oxygen species circulating in the body tend to react with the electron of other molecules in the body and these also affect various enzyme systems and cause DNA damage which may further contribute to oxidative damage and inflammatory diseases and conditions such as cancer, ischemia, aging, adult respiratory distress syndromes, rheumatoid arthritis, etc. Oxidative stress occurs as result of an imbalance between free radicals and antioxidant defense system. A plant-based diet protects against chronic oxidative stress-related diseases. Many researchers reported that dietary fruits, vegetables, and grains apply a protective effect against the development of these chronic diseases [1–4]. This protective role can be predominantly credited to the phytochemicals in them, which are defined as bioactive non-nutrient compounds in fruits, vegetables, grains, and other parts [5]. Antioxidants or inhibitors of oxidation are compounds that retard or prevent the oxidation in general, and prolong the life of the oxidizable matter.

Plants kingdom contains variable chemical families and amounts of antioxidants. It has been hypothesized that antioxidants from dietary plants may contribute to the beneficial health effects. Among these, routine dietary sources are also easily available and more suitable for dietary interventions.

The need is to identify and generate awareness about these sources, which can be rated from top to down regarding antioxidant potential. The people who are habitual of consuming these vegetables and fruits in their routine diet are proved to be less suffered by various chronic diseases [6], and studies have also endorsed the long-term health impact of consuming these plant based diets. This chapter presents certain information about oxidative stress, antioxidant categories, phytochemicals, and their role in prevention and cure of several diseases.

2. Free radicals and oxidative stress

Free radicals are highly reactive species because they have unpaired electrons which seek an electron to stabilize the molecule. Free radicals can be generated by a variety of sources which can be classified as endogenous (within the body) and exogenous sources (outside the body). They are essential intermediates in natural processes and readily react with other molecules result in oxidative stress. **Figure 1** represents the generation of free radicals. Reactive oxygen species (ROS) is a collective term which include hydroxyl radical (OH•), perhydroxyl radical (HO_2•), hypochlorous acid (HOCl), superoxide anion radical ($O_2•^-$), hydrogen peroxide (H_2O_2), singlet oxygen ($^1O_2$), nitric oxide radical (NO•), hypochlorite radical (OCl•), peroxynitrite (ONOO),

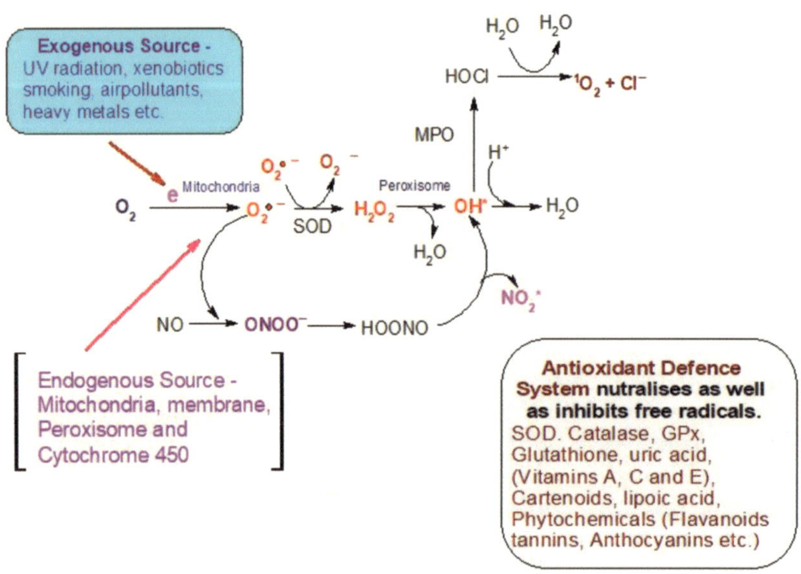

Figure 1.
Overview of generation of reactive oxygen species (free radicals).

and different lipid peroxides. Reactive nitrogen species (RNS) such as $ONOO^-$ and NO• are formed by the reaction of nitric oxide with $O_2\bullet^-$ while RSS are easily produced from thiols through a reaction with ROS [7, 8]. Though, the free radicals are produced naturally by normal process of metabolism and lifestyle also influences their production in the body such as smoking, exposure of toxic chemicals, alcohols and fried foods. Although, cells have antioxidant defense system (antioxidant enzymes) to encounter harmful effects of free radicals. These free radicals are linked to the diseases such as cardiovascular, neurodisorders, diabetes, liver diseases, cancer and aging.

An imbalance between antioxidant defense system and reactive oxygen species result in oxidative stress which further leads to necrosis and cell damage. Cells experience oxidative stress when they are exposed with excess level of free radicals (ROS) as result of depletion of antioxidant level within cells. Free radicals contain uneven number of electrons which can harm biomolecules by producing lipid peroxides, protein carbonyls and various degenerative changes that can cause DNA damage and apoptotic events which lead to damage cell's survival capacity and finally cause cell death. Cells use endogenous and exogenous antioxidants defense mechanism to detoxify these reactive products.

2.1 Oxidative stress and cellular damage

Reactive oxygen species (ROS) are typical by-products of cellular metabolism, playing a role as secondary messengers and influencing different normal physiological functions of the body. In some cases, oxidative stress is also useful for intracellular signaling which is necessary for physiological adaptation of the body.

Furthermore, there is growing evidence supporting the role of ROS in numerous pathological conditions, that is, diseases (**Figure 2**). The paired character of ROS with their beneficial and detrimental characteristics indicates the sophistication of their specific roles at a biological compartment and the difficulties in attaining applicable procedures to treat ROS-related diseases. From basic science research to clinical trials, the biomedical scientific society has promptly progressed toward an improved interpretation of ROS-metabolizing systems and their impact on specific

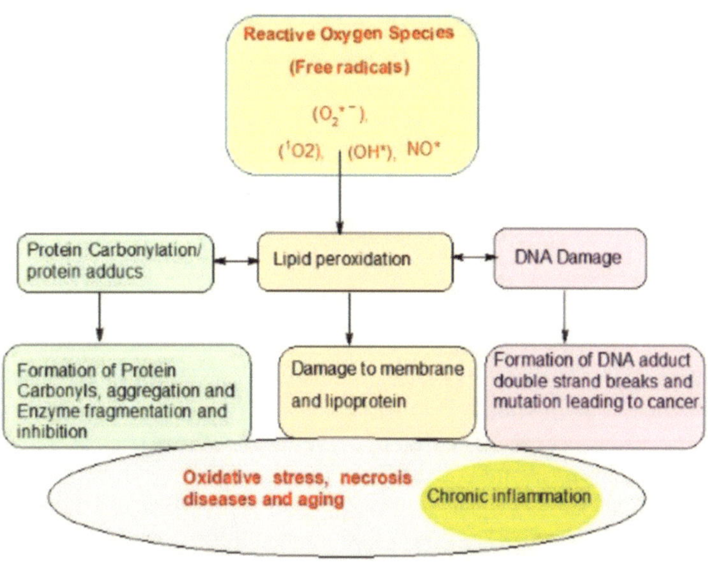

Figure 2.
Impact of free radicals on cellular system.

conditions. The free radicals often involve in cell–cell communication, apoptosis, ion transportation, and gene expression [8].

Oxidation is a normal and necessary process that takes place in the body. Whereas, oxidative stress, on the other hand, takes place when there's an imbalance between oxidants and antioxidants within the body due to lack of antioxidants or increased production of free radicals (ROS) [9, 10]. Free radicals due to unpaired electrons can start oxidation to biomolecules i.e. carbohydrates, proteins, lipids, and nucleic acids. These consequences can lead to heart disease, inflammatory disease, cancer, diabetes mellitus, Alzheimer's disease, autism, and to the aging process [7, 11].

2.2 Antioxidant defense system

Antioxidants are molecule that reduce and prevent the harmful effect of free radicals. Humans have a complex antioxidant protection system, which functions interactively and synergistically to neutralize free radicals. There are several antioxidant enzymes that can neutralize free radicals and ROS. These enzymes form the body's endogenous defense mechanisms from free radicals to protect the cell. Enzymatic defense system mainly includes enzymes such as glutathione peroxidases, superoxide dismutase and catalase, which decrease the concentration of the most harmful ROS whereas non-enzymatic antioxidants are vitamins C and E, β-carotene, uric acid and glutathione.

Antioxidant enzymes are important protein components that offer protection against ROS via removing potential oxidants/transferring ROS/RNS into relatively stable compounds [11]. For optimum catalytic activity, these enzymes require micronutrient cofactors such as Se, Fe, Cu, Zn, and Mn [12]. The following three antioxidant enzymes play significant roles in protecting cells from oxidative stress:

2.2.1 Superoxide dismutases (SOD)

Mc Cord and Fridovich first discovered this enzyme in 1969. Superoxide Dismutase (SOD), is the best known and perhaps most important of the antioxidant enzymes. It converts the harmful free radicals superoxide to the less active peroxide, which then can be further converted by other antioxidant enzyme (catalase) into water. The enzyme dismutase converts two molecules of superoxide radical to form H_2O_2 and O_2. The SOD family consists of four metallo forms which require copper, zinc, one manganese and one iron Cu for their free radical detoxifying activity. ZnSOD is found in the cytosol of most eukaryotic cells [13]. A different form of Cu, ZnSOD is found in extracellular fluids (EC), where it is called EC-SOD [14, 15]. The two superoxide radicals converted into hydrogen peroxide and oxygen during the catalytic reaction of SOD.

$$O_2^{\bullet -} + O_2^{\bullet -} \xrightarrow{\text{SOD}} O_2 + \mathbf{H_2O_2}$$

This is important, because free radicals are highly active and unstable, and will attack any molecule in the body. Organ or tissue damage can occur whenever production of free radicals exceeds to that of scavenger enzymes such as SOD, which are the first-line defense system of the body's tissues.

2.2.2 Catalase (CAT)

Catalase is localized exclusively in peroxisomes and deals with the large amount of H_2O_2 present in them. It requires iron as a cofactor to degrade hydrogen peroxide to water and oxygen. Human CAT composes four identical subunits of 62 kDa [16]. It's optimum pH lies in the alkaline range. At the subcellular level, CAT is found mostly in perxoisomes (80%) and cytosol (20%), and deals with a large amount of hydrogen peroxides (H_2O_2) present in them.

$$2H_2O_2 \xrightarrow{\text{CAT}} 2H_2O + O_2$$

2.2.3 Glutathione peroxidase (GPx)

Gutathione peroxidase (GPx) is a group of cytosolic enzymes which contains a single selenocysteine residue, in which selenium is covalently bound in its active site. This selenium dependent enzyme which converts hydroperoxides to H_2O where GSH represent reduced state and GSSH represent the glutathione disulfie (oxidized state) [17].

$$H_2O_2 + 2GSH \xrightarrow{\text{GPx}} GSSH + O_2$$

2.2.4 Non-enzymatic antioxidants

The non-enzymatic antioxidants also play important role to neutralize intracellular free radicals which are discussed as follows:

2.2.4.1 Glutathione

Glutathione (GSH) is present in all plant and animal cells and is a tripeptide (glutamyl-cysteinyl-glycine). The cysteine provides an exposed free sulphydryl group (SH) that is highly reactive, providing an abundant target for radical attack. It is mainly synthesized in the liver [18] and exists in several redox forms, among which the most predominant is the reduced glutathione. GSH is a hydrosoluble antioxidant present in high cellular concentrations (1–10 mM) in the nucleus, mitochondria, and cytoplasm. GSH is involved in several lines of defense against ROS. First, the thiol group confers GSH with the ability to protect other thiol functions in proteins against oxidative damage [19]. Thiol groups (-SH) are widespread and highly reactive chemical entities in cells. They make complex with metal ions, participate in oxidation reactions by getting oxidized themselves to sulfonic acids, and form thiol radicals and disulfides [20].

2.2.4.2 Uric acid

Uric acid (UA) is a strong reducing agent (donates electrons) which acts as a powerful antioxidant and scavenge the singlet oxygen and radicals. Normally in humans, one of the main antioxidants in plasma is uric acid.UA is a hydrophilic antioxidant generated during the metabolism of purine nucleotides and accounts nearly for 66% of the total oxygen scavenging activity in the blood serum. Mammals and humans are capable of producing UA, making it the most predominant aqueous antioxidant present in humans [21, 22] with an approximate blood level of 3.5–7.5 mg/dL. UA is an effective metabolite that can stop free radicals produced by xanthine oxidase (XO) in catalysis reaction of xanthine and hypoxanthine [23]. UA gives cellular protection from oxidants, which related to a variety of physiological situation [24, 25].

In addition, there are diverse dietary foods and medicinal plants which are rich sources of vitamins and phytochemicals, provide additional protection to the body against oxidative stress. The major among those antioxidants are vitamin E, Vitamin A, vitamin C and flavonoids, carotenoids, lipoic acids and tannins etc.

2.2.4.3 Vitamin E

Vitamin E is exogenous (lipid-soluble antioxidant) and must be obtained through diet in small amounts since the organism cannot synthesize it. Its biosynthesis is restricted to plants, photosynthetic algae, and certain cyanobacteria. It plays a vital role in protecting membranes from oxidative damage and thus its primary activity is to trap peroxy radicals in cellular membranes. It inhibits the lipid peroxidation induced by free radicals [26]. α-Tocopherol is the most active form of vitamin E that has antioxidant activity and immune functions. It has been revealed to be a more effective free radical scavenging vitamins that prevent peroxynitrite-induced lipid peroxidation and inflammatory reactions [27].

2.2.4.4 Vitamin C

Vitamin C (L-ascorbic acid) is an optically-active hydrosoluble antioxidant which scavenges free radicals from a variety of sources. It bears a highly acidic hydroxyl group (pKa = 4.2) known to be completely ionized at neutral pH [28, 29]. It acts as an antioxidant and reducing agent by donating electrons to various enzymatic and nonenzymatic reactions. It reduces the transition metal ions of several biosynthetic enzymes, thus preventing biological oxidation of macromolecules. Interestingly, it also functions as an enzyme cofactor [23].

2.2.4.5 Vitamin A

Vitamin A, a lipid soluble vitamin, is localization within the lipophilic compartment of membranes and lipoproteins. It has free radicals scavenging feature and thus play important role in human health. It has been shown to be essential for many physiological processes, such as cell metabolism, reproduction, embryonic development, immunity and bone metabolism, in all vertebrates [30–32]. It is essential for vision. The retinal and retinoic acid are the dietary components of vitamin A [33].

2.2.4.6 Carotenoids

Carotenoids are important antioxidants for plants and animals which are present in fruits and vegetables. Carotenoids are known to be very efficient physical and chemical quenchers of singlet oxygen ($^1O_2$), as well as potent scavengers of other reactive oxygen species (ROS) [34–36]. This is of special significance, because the uncontrolled generation and concomitant increase of ROS level in the body results in "oxidative stress", an essential contributor to the pathogenic processes of many diseases. Carotenoids have a protective role against ROS-mediated disorders, such as cardiovascular diseases, cancer as well as photosensitive or eye-related disorders.

2.2.4.7 Lipoic acid

Lipoic acid is one of the most versatile antioxidants known. Aside from its ability to function in both aqueous and lipid media, lipoic acid is capable of neutralizing a wide variety of free radicals: singlet oxygen, superoxides, peroxyl and hydroxyl radicals, hypochlorite, and peroxynitrite [37]. These radicals are believed to play a significant role in disease processes such as hardening of the arteries (atherosclerosis), cancer, cataract formation and diabetes.

2.2.4.8 Flavonoids

Flavonoids are rich source of antioxidants, which are low-molecular-weight phenolic compounds. They are broadly present in fruits, vegetables and certain beverages. They belong to a class of plant secondary metabolites. Flavonoids are, in particular, important antioxidants that can act as reducing agents, free radical scavenger, hydrogen donors, and singlet oxygen quenchers. In addition, they have also metal chelating potential [38]. Their structures and impact on human health is discussed in details in subsequent sections.

2.2.4.9 Tannins

Tannins are naturally found in a variety of edible and inedible plants, including tree bark, leaves, spices, nuts, seeds, fruits, and legumes. They are potentially very important antioxidants. Plants produce them as a natural defense against pests. Tannins also give color and flavor to plant foods. Tannins are phenolics such as flavan-3-ols: (−)-epicatechin and (+)-catechin. Hydrolysable tannins are heterogeneous polymers compound for example phenolic acids and gallic acid (3,4,5trihydroxyl benzoic acid) [23, 39].

3. Phytochemicals: classification and dietary sources

The basic skeleton of polyphenols is made up of 15 carbon chain that arranged in two aromatic rings A and B connected by a unit of carbon–carbon bridge and it can also form ring C. They have conjugated double bonds and functional groups (hydroxyl or other substituents). Flavonoid can occur as a form in aglycones, glycosides and methylated derivatives in plants. They are present in all parts of plant such as stem, root, flower and leaf and seed. The structure of phytochemicals possesses functional groups such as hydroxyl groups (OH), aromatic compounds (CH), Carbonyl and carboxylic groups (CO) and organosulfur groups (SO). The major class of phytochemicals are polyphenols and caratenoids. Based on heterocyclic ring structure, flavonoids are divided into six chemical structures: flavones, flavonols, flavanones, catechins, or flavanols, anthocyanidins and isoflavones (**Figure 3**) [40].

The dietary sources of different phytochemicals are given in **Table 1**. Polyphenols are known for their unique property of activation at multiple levels, through the modulation of A mitogen-activated protein kinase (MAPK), protein kinase B (PKB), and NF-κB signaling pathways, inhibiting the production of inflammatory cytokines and chemokines, suppressing the activity of cyclooxygenase (COX) and Inducible nitric oxide synthase (iNOS) and thus decreasing the production of free radicals. Several phytochemicals including genistein, curcuminoids, and catechins are known to suppress the activation of Akt, thus, inhibiting cancer cell growth. Some phenols like resveratrol, curcumin, and green tea catechins have been shown to suppress COX-2 giving the benefit of decreasing the production of reactive oxygen species (ROS) [41]. The health benefits of functional foods and nutraceuticals fortified with natural polyphenols. Flavonoids exert many biological and pharmacological properties

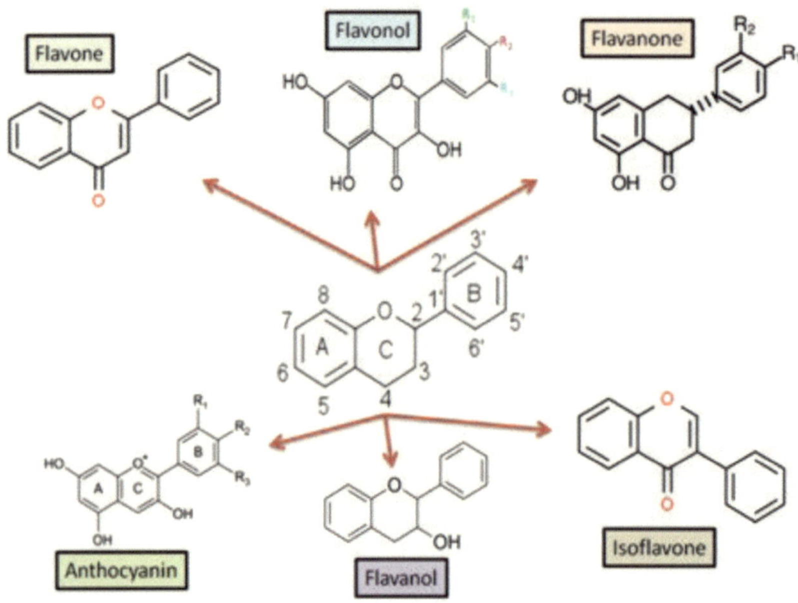

Figure 3.
Basic flavonoid structure.

Phytochemical Class	Phytochemical constituents	Major dietary food sources
Flavones	Luteolin and Apigenine	Celery, chill paper and green vegetables
Flavonols	Quercetin, kaempferol	Garlic, onion, Raw Broccoli, onion, chill paper, Parsely, Blueberries
Flavanones	HesperetinTangeretin	Carrot, Grapefruit juice, citrus fruit,
Isoflavones	Genistein, Daidzein	Soybean, tofu soymilk and black bean
Flavanols	Epicatechinecatechin and epigallocatechin	Tea, fruits and cocoa Chocolate
Anthocyanins	Cyanidin, delphinidin, malvidin, peonidin, petunidin, and pelargonidin	Strawberries Green vegetable and fruits

Table 1.
Dietary phytochemicals and their sources.

for instance, cardioprotective inflammatory, antiviral, anti-cancer, anti-diabetic and cytoprotective etc.

4. Biological role of phytochemical antioxidants in prevention and cure of several chronic diseases

Oxidative stress is accountable for pathogenesis of several human diseases, including CVD, certain types of cancers, and aging [42, 43]. Antioxidant phytochemicals play a therapeutic role against chronic diseases caused by oxidative stress [44]. The schematic overview of the therapeutic properties of flavonoid-rich foods is given in **Figure 4**. The phytochemicals are the recent area of drug research to find the promising herbal drug for the treatment of various human diseases such as diabetes, cancer, tuberculosis, malaria and viral diseases etc.

Edible fruits and vegetable have medicinal properties with antioxidant potential. They contain various types of phytochemicals which are proven to reduce the impact of various diseases. The dietary fruits such as strawberries, citrus fruits or green vegetables, cereals are rich source of vitamins and phytochemicals [45]. The medicinal plant rich in flavonoids have been reported to have antioxidant potential [46]. α-tocopherol is good free radicals scavenging vitamins that reduced the oxidative stress in the body and prevents the aging process. Consumption of dietary plants lessens the development of life style related diseases because they are rich in polyphenols an show synergistic effect on metabolic pathway of diseases cells [47]. In addition, polyphenols may enhance the antioxidant defense system against free radical induced toxicity [48]. Many medicinal plant are known to provide defensive role against microbial and viral infections [49, 50]. Pathogens and oxidative stress can cause chronic inflammation that assist in the pathogenesis ofmany chronic diseases including CVD, cancers, neurodegenerative diseases, diabetes [51–53]. Most antioxidant phytochemicals have been scientifically investigated for their anti-inflammatory action, hepatoprotective, cardioprotective, neuro-protective and anticancer and antidiabetes and antimalerial and antiaging effects. Phytochemicals including resveratrol, anthocyanins, and curcumin etc. are known to have medicine like properties that mediate protection via inhibition of lipid peroxidation, lower the prostaglandin production and modulate the nuclear factor-κB activity, enzyme inhibition, as well as improve the immunity [54]. Usually, the phytochemicals have strong antioxidant abilities as well as anti-inflammatory action, which account for other bioactivities with health benefits [55].

Though, the phytochemicals have been reported to exert wide range of biological activities. These include:

4.1 Cardioprotective activity

Cardiovascular disease (CVD) is common health problem in modern society and is the leading cause of morbidity and mortality worldwide. Rising blood pressure

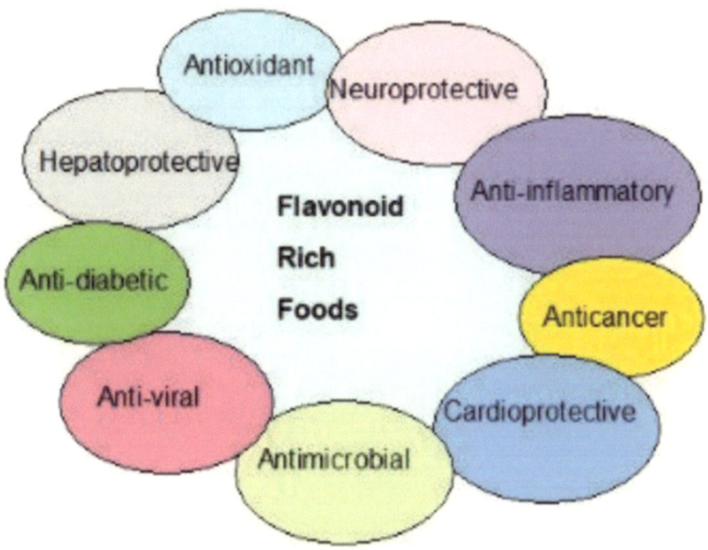

Figure 4.
The schematic overview of the therapeutic properties of flavonoids.

and atherosclerosis diseases are common heart problem in all age group of people. The modern medicine and treatment can reduce the symptoms of the CVD but allopathic treatment sometime produce adverse side effect on the body. The adequate intake of phytochemical rich food can reduce the impact of CVD [56]. The phytochemicals constituents such as Epicatechin, catechin, garlic, Apigenin, luteolin are known to possess cardioprotective properties. Dietary foods containing flavonoids can suppress the cholesterol and lipoproteins to protect the heart.

Catechin is a known flavonoid found in green tea, *Camellia sinensis*. Many experimental and clinical studies have recently reported that catechin has multiple cardiovascular health benefits such as prevention of atherosclerosis, hypertension, endothelial dysfunction, ischemic heart diseases, and cardiomyopathy. It protects normal heart function by decreasing oxidative stress and reducing the inflammatory events [57].

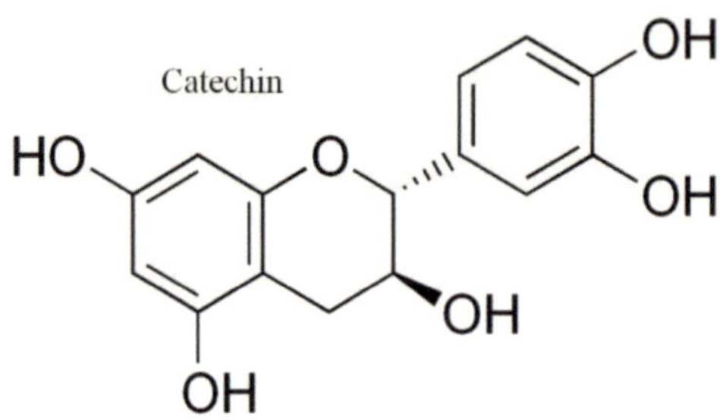

Lutein is a bioactive flavonoid possesses good efficacy as an anti-oxidative, antitumor, and anti-inflammatory properties [58]. Recent scientific studies have reported the lutein has cardiac protective effects *in vitro* and *in vivo*. Epicatechin and procyanidins have been reported to have good cardioprotective health benefits [59].

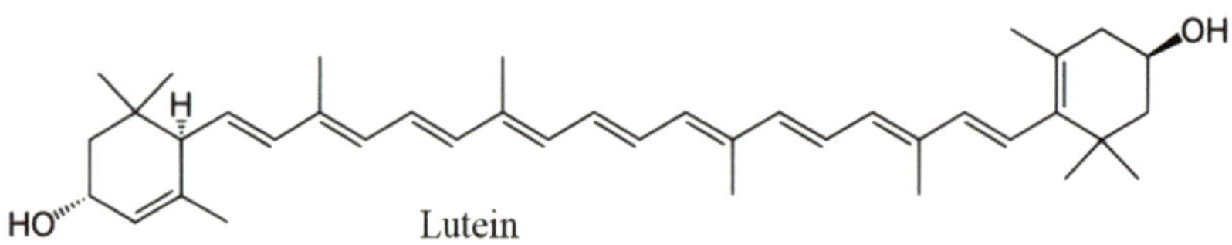

Allicin is one of the key ingredients of *Allium sativum* (Garlic) said to be good regulator of blood pressure and hypertension. It is an organosulfure phytochemical and possesses many medicinal properties such as anticancer, antidiabetic, hepatoprotective and cardioprotective. Many research reports suggested that allicin has shown positive effects on the heart and it can lower high cholesterol levels against atherosclerosis. People use raw garlic to get some relief from blood pressure [60].

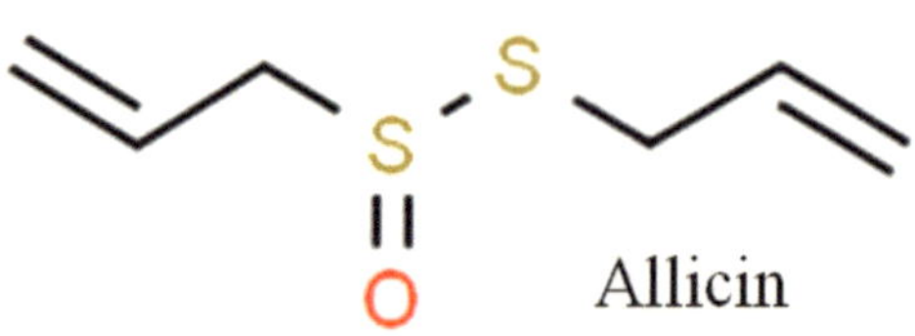

Allicin

4.2 Hepatoprotective activity

Nowadays, hepatic diseases are common concern in modern societies due to the unhealthy eating habits and over consumption of synthetic medicines, pathogen infection and environmental pollutants. Jaundice and cirrhosis are the most common liver diseases. There are many edible plant and fruits which keep liver healthy against drug induced liver toxicity. The plants contain many hepatoprotective phytochemicals such as resveratrol; saponin, Gallic acid, emodin, and tannin provide protection to liver against free radical induced damage.

Gallic acid well known flavonoid is found in fruits like pomegranates, gooseberry and strawberries and other plant foods, is one of the well-studied phytochemical. It shows antioxidant, anti-inflammatory, hepatoprotective, antimutagenic, and anticancer properties. It has been investigated for its hepatoprotective activity against ethanol, Carbon tetrachloride (CCL_4) and paracetamol-induced hepatotoxicity [61]. Both have shown protection of liver against drug induced hepatotoxicity. Consumption of dietary fruits contain ellagicangallic can cure the liver problems. These flavonoids have restored the normal level of hepatic markers i.e. bilirubin, aminotransferases, lipid peroxides, and improve the antioxidant defense system.

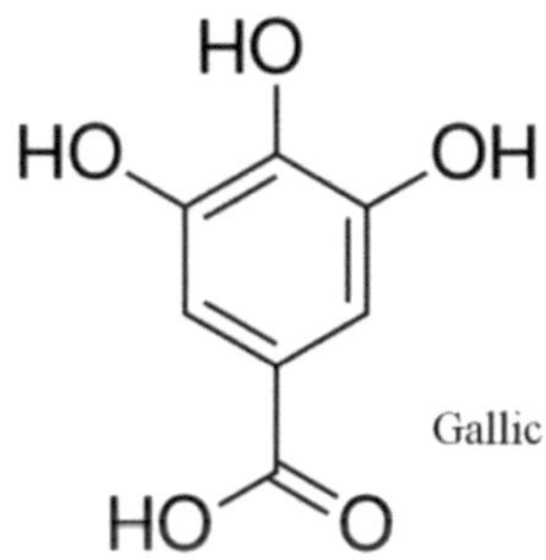

Gallic acid

Silymarin is a well-known Hepatoprotective plant having many flavonolignan. Experimental studies reported that silymarin has improved the level of hepatic enzymes and reversed the normal cellular structure of liver against drug induced hepatotoxicity. It is used for treatment of alcoholic fatty liver, jaundice, viral hepatitis and drug-induced liver diseases. Many researchers across the world reported Hepatoprotective activity of silymarin against the carbon tetrachloride, alcohol, paracetamol, galactosamine and thioacetamide toxicity [62, 63]. Several scientific evidences and clinical studies suggested that Silibinin, is a main bioactive flavonoid which has antioxidant, hepatoprotective and anti-inflammatory properties [64].

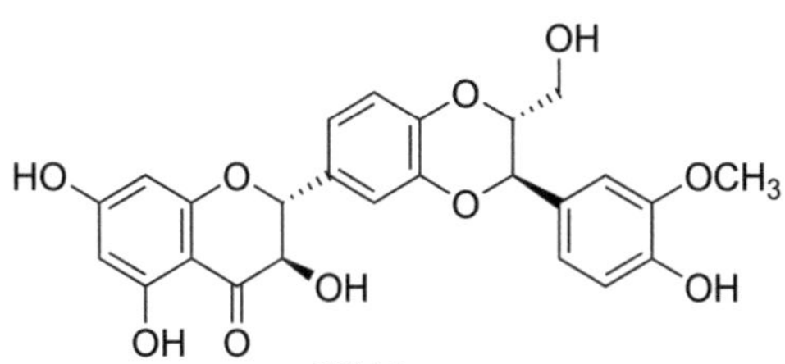

Silibinin

4.3 Neuroprotective activity

Alzheimer's disease (AD) is a chronic brain disorder generally seen in the elderly people. Oxidative stress and neuroinflammation can account for neurodegenerative diseases like Alzheimer's and Dementia (memory loss). A dietary food such as walnut is a rich source of many antioxidants (vitamin E and folate), minerals (selenium) and phytochemicals including flavonoids, phenolic acid (ellagic acid), and proanthocyanidins etc. Experimental evidence suggested that walnuts have anti-inflammatory effect which may show the synergistic effect to reduce the risk of neurogenerative disorders and enhance the activeness of neurotransmitter in brain cells. Withaferin A is the main active ingredient of Ayurvedic medicinal plant *Withania somnifera*. It is an oldest medicine used to treat various neurodegenrative diseases [65, 66]. The root extracts of *W. somnifera* has been reported to possess free radical scavenging properties [67] and is associated to induce the Neurons & Glial Cells [68, 69]. The root extract of *W. somnifera* is reported to induce outgrowth in SK-N-SH cells [70].

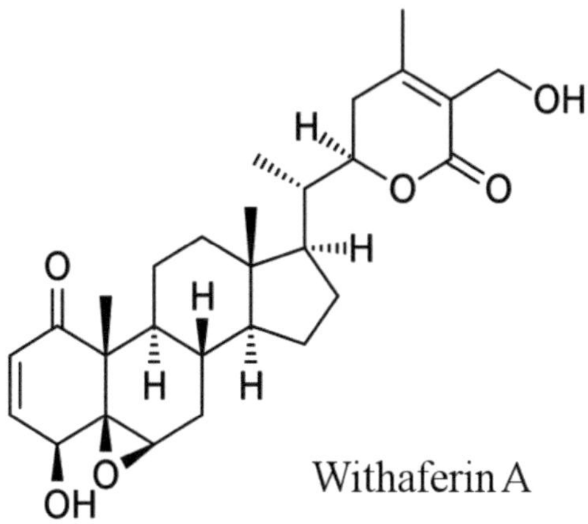

Withaferin A

Bacopamonnieri is known as Brahmi an herbal nutraceutical herb which is popular for brain tonic or nootropic agent which is described for use of memory improvement, epilepsy, insomnia, and anxiolytic in Ayurveda. It is rich source of various phytochemicals such as bacoside A, bacoside B, bacopasaponins, D-mannitol, apigenin, luteonin, brahmine, herpestine, hydrocotyline. In addition, sapogeninjujubacogenin, pseudojuju, bacogenin are the major ingredient of B. moneieri. Latest research reports indicated that *B. monnieri* has neuroprotective effect against brain inflammation and Alzheimer's disease [71].

4.4 Anti-inflammatory activity

Inflammation is a normal phenomenon of the body upon pathogen infection. The inflammation is characterized by physical appearance like swelling, redness, heat, pain, and loss of function. It is the series of transformation of infection site as a result of immunological response [72]. Flavonoids intake can inhibit the cyclooxygenase pathway involved in the inflammatory process.

Curcuma longa (turmeric) is popular spice used in making home food. It is the oldest traditional medicine for the treatment of various health problem, joint pain, inflammatory conditions and cancer and diabetes and liver ailments. Its consumption provides healing effect to cure infection and inflammation in the body. The curcumin is main active component of *Curcuma longa* which has various medicinal properties such as hepatoprotecctive, anticancer and antidiabetic and anti-inflammatory. It is the efficient antioxidant that reduces the level of oxidative stress caused by toxic elements [73].

Ginger is a popular edible root of *Zingiberofficinale* plant. It is widely used for treatment of cough and cold due to its anti-inflammatory property. Gingerols is the main bioactive compounds of ginger. It has reduced the level of inflammation markers cytokines and tumor necrosis factors.

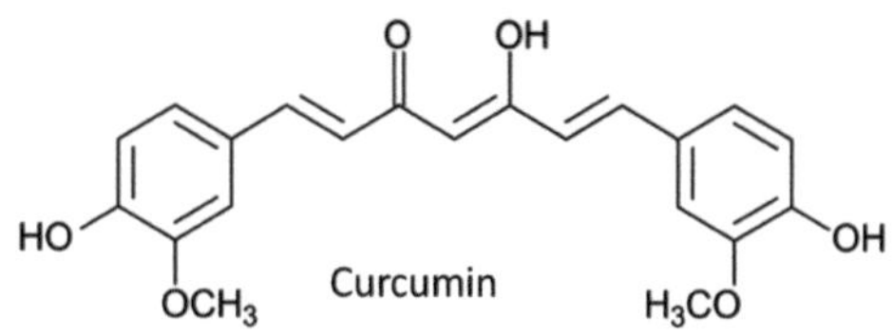

Curcumin

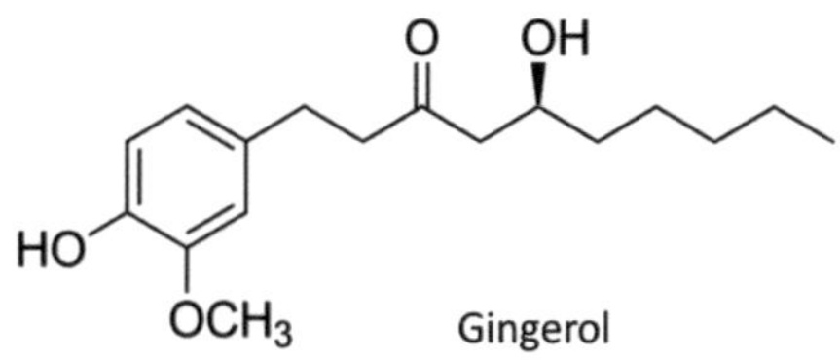

Gingerol

4.5 Anticancer activity

Cancer, a disease is characterized by uncontrolled cell division [74, 75]. Many flavonoids have shown to possess the anticancer properties. There are many dietary flavonoids such as apigenin, karmpferol, quercetin and resveratrol showed the anticancer effect against various cancers such as breast, lung, liver, skin, blood, colon, prostate, pancreatic, cervical, oral, and stomach by modulating the signal pathway of apoptosis. The experimental results showed the protective efficacy of flavonoids on cancer cells by modulating the pathway of cell cycles. The molecular mechanism of flavonoid is due their antiproliferation activity, cell cycle arrest, inhibition of P53 protein and down regulation of tyrosin kinases. Flavonoids are evidenced to be effective chemopreventive agents.

Apigenin is plant derived flavonoid belonging to the flavone structural class. It is found in several edible vegetables and fruits. It has been reported as anticancer molecule *in vitro* and *invivo* experiments. It showed promising antioxidative and antiproliferation effect against cancer disease [76, 77].

Kaempferol is very effective herbal medicine and present in grapes and onion. It has antioxidant and anticarcinogenic activity. It acts as a chemopreventive agent against metastasis and angiogenesis. *In vitro* studies reported that Kaempferol was found to have good cytotoxic effect on cancer cells. It is reported to reduce proliferation of cancer cells by arrest cell cycle events of various cell lines such as glioblastoma leukemia, lung cancer, and breast adenocarcinoma [78].

Quercetin is one of the dietary flavonoids, which suppresses tumor growth by inhibiting protein tyrosine kinase (PTK). Fruits and vegetables are having an enormous amount of quercetin, which have been used as cancer chemopreventive agents. The mechanism of action of flavonoids is dues their interphase arrest, heat-shock protein inhibition, tyrosine kinase inhibition, down regulation of p53 protein, inhibition of Ras protein, and expression of Ras protein [79].

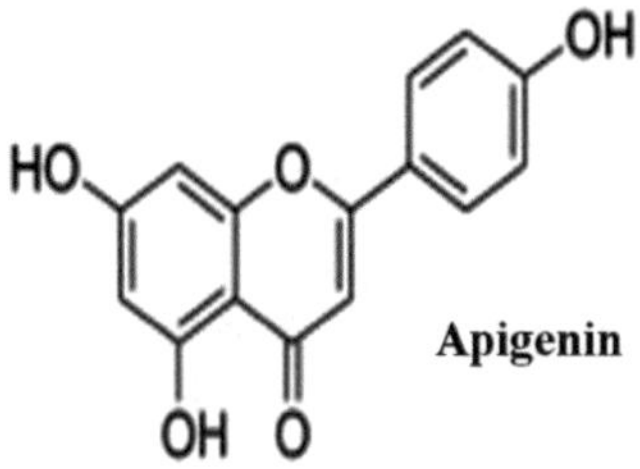

Apigenin

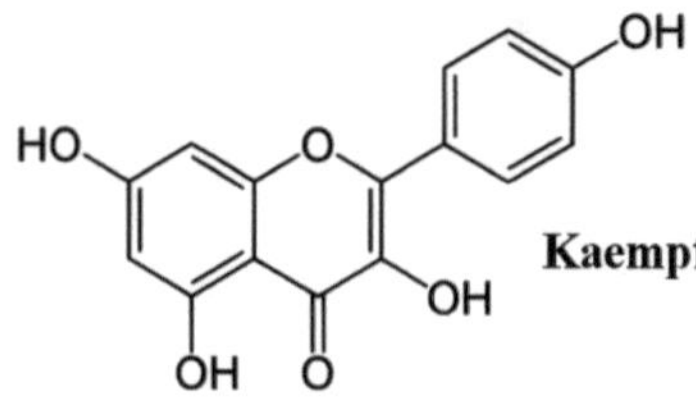

Kaempferol

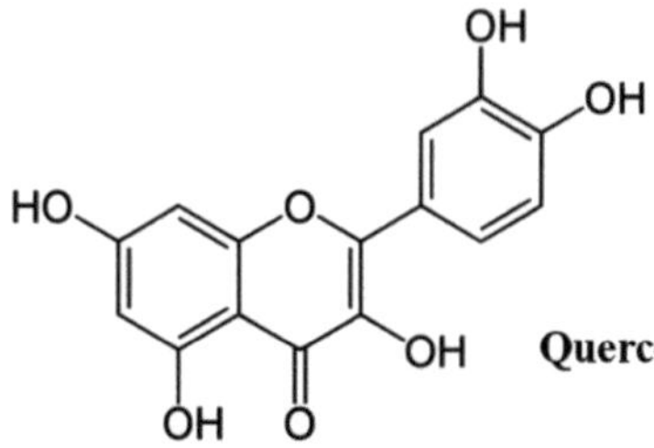

Quercetin

4.6 Antidiabetic activity

Diabetes is one of the emerging health disease caused by metabolic abnormalities of carbohydrate. The presence of higher blood sugar level in blood and urine is the main the sign of the diabetes. There are many dietary flavonoids such as bitter guard, *fenugreek* leaves and *seeds and* Curry Leaves or KadiPatta that exert anti-diabetic effects by targeting various cellular signaling pathways in pancreas, liver, skeletal muscle, and white adipose tissue sources, that can reduce the higher blood sugar level in diabetic patient. These dietary foods are rich source of phytochemicals that can reverse the abnormal sugar level into normal level.

Morin, a natural flavonoid, is found in the edible plant *Moringaoleifera*. Its oral consumption for 30 days significantly improved the blood sugar level, glucose intolerance, and promotes the pancreas to release sufficient insulin in the body. It also inhibits the insulin resistance [80].

Rutin is a glycosylated flavonoid found in the citrus fruits. The anti-diabetic effects of rutin have been experimentally evaluated and suggested the rutin has good antidiabetic efficacy. It enhances the glucose uptake by the suppression of tissue gluconeogenesis resulting in lowering glucose level in blood. It can activate insulin secretion from β-cells. It also decreases the free radical formation produced due to higher glucose level [81].

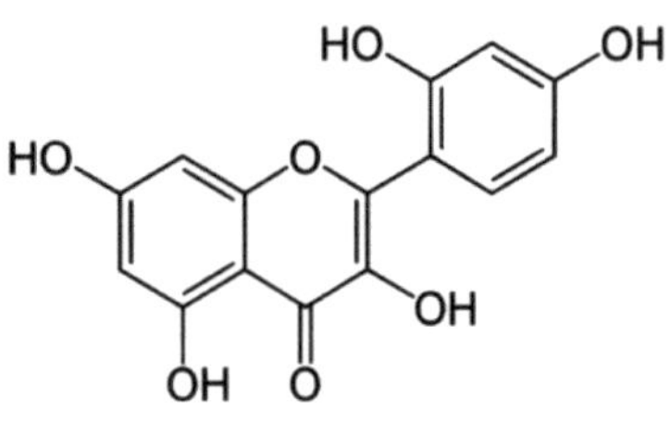

Morin

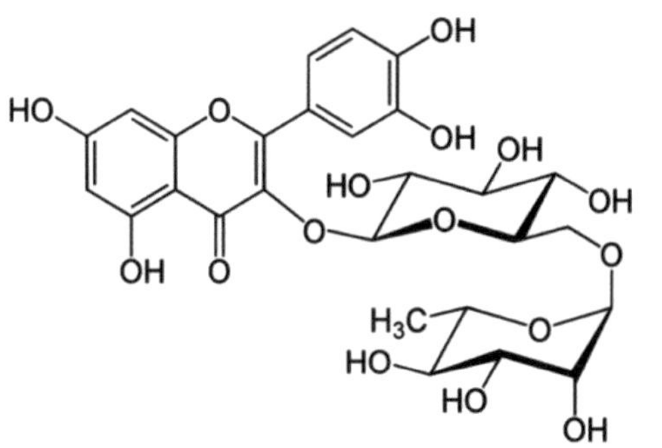

Rutin

4.7 Antiviral activity

G. glabra or **Licorice** is a traditional remedy for the treatment of liver diseases like jaundice. **Glycyrrhizin** is an active biocompound in the licorice root, that has antioxidant, anti-inflammatory and hepatoprotective and antiviral activity. It also prevents oxidative damage produced by oxidative stress. Scientific studies reported that Glycyrrhizin can inhibit the growth of hepatitis A and hepatitis C virus and effectively control the viral replication [82].

Naringin is a citrus dietary favonoid found in tomatoes, grapefruit and orange and known to have positive biological effect on human health as antioxidant, anti-inflammatory, and antiviral. It was found that **Naringin** can reduce the viral growth in the cell culture. It also investigated to have antiviral effect against HSV-1 and HSV-2 [83].

Quercetin, a naturally occurring dietary flavonoid, is well known to ameliorate chronic diseases and aging processes in humans, and its antiviral properties have been investigated in numerous studies. In silico and in vitro studies demonstrated that quercetin can interfere with various growth stages of the coronavirus replication cycle [84].

Epigallocatechin-3-gallate (EGCG), is a principal tea derived catechin which know have many pharmacological properties like cardioprotective, haptoprotective and antiviral. Many research studied confirmed that EGCG has antiviral protective effect against influenza virus [85–87]. It has experimentally shown the protection against DNA and RNA viruses [88].

Silymarin has also shown the promising antiviral effect against hepatitis C and B virus [89].

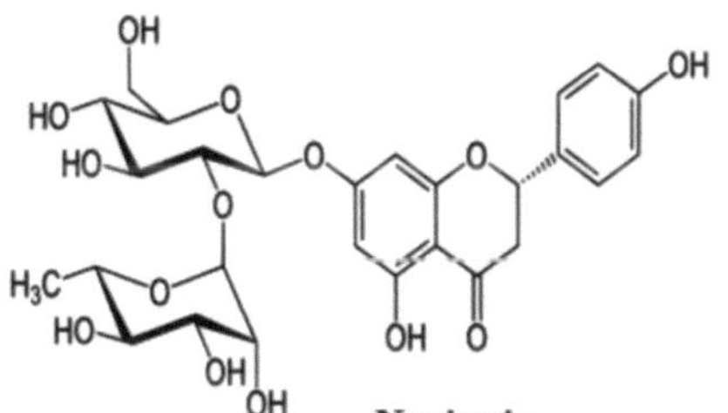

Naringin

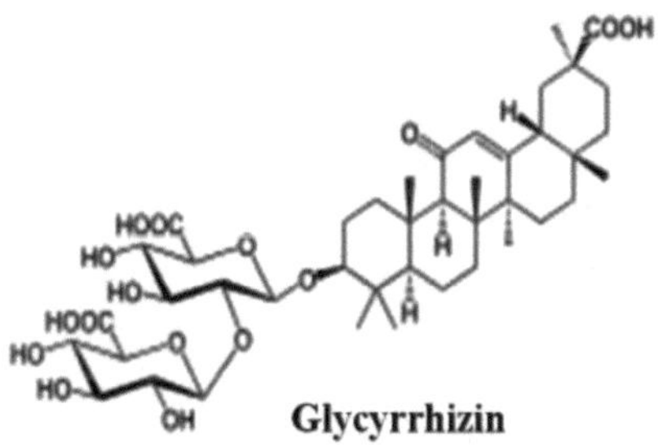

Glycyrrhizin

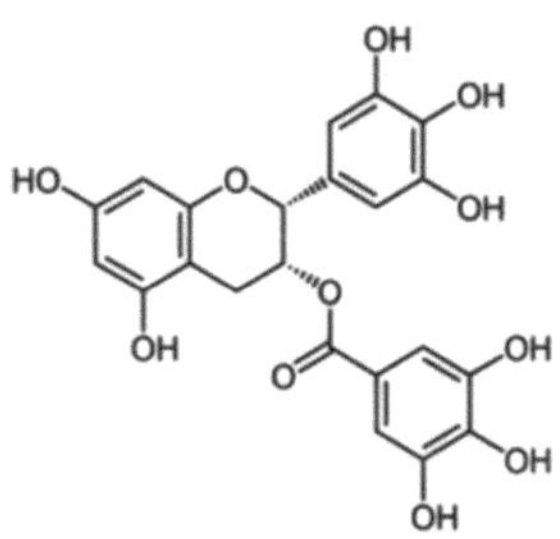

Epigallocatechin-3-gallate

4.8 Antiparasitic activity

Parasites are organism that live in the another organism called host. They use other organism to survive and get food from them. The common parasite that live on or in human body are scabies (skin mites), threadworm (stomach), and hookworm (gut worms). Parasites are microscopic organisms such asprotozoa, helminths, and ectoparasites that cause diseases such as malaria and leishmaniasisin human [90, 91].

Many plant derived phytochemicals have been tested for their antiparasite activity. Quinine is an alkaloid isolated from the Cinchona species is well known effective herbal medicine for its antimalarial properties. It is used to treat malaria disease. Another popular alkaloid, **artemisinin** is a quite useful for the treatment of maleria diseases. Artemisinin is an active component of *Artemisia annua has* been investigated for it antimalarial activity [92].

Quinine

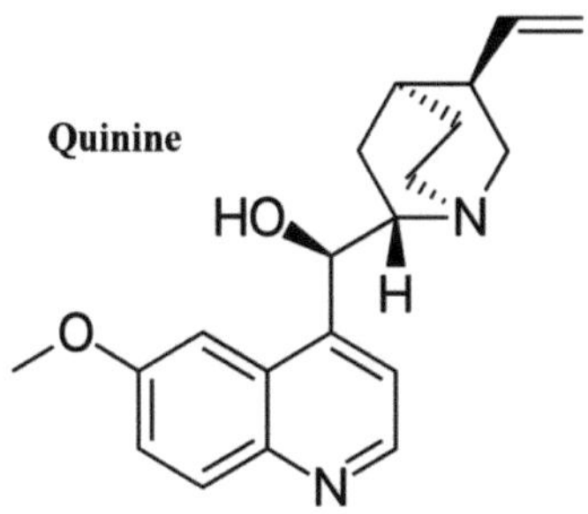

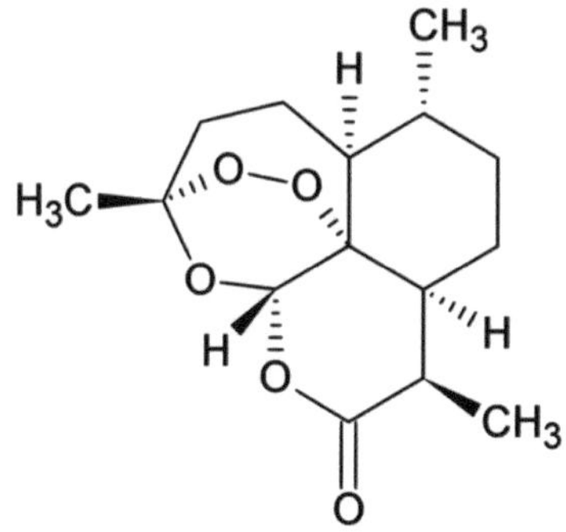

Artemisinin

4.9 Antiaging activity

Aging is a well-established risk factor for a wide range of diseases such as neurodegenerative diseases, and presently, there is no effective treatment for age-related neurodegenerative diseases [93].

Grapes and citrus fruits have a high content of polyphenols which showed free radical scavenging activity [94]. Curcumin and vitamin E are promising antiaging compounds that may delay the symptoms of aging. Vitamin E is lipid soluble antioxidants that scavenges the peroxide radical and stop the chain reaction of free radicals which are involved in aging process [95]. Being a efficient antioxidant and anti-inflammatory molecules, curcumin is modulated cellular senescence involved in aging [96, 97].

4.10 Renoprotective activity

Chronic kidney disorders are common world health problem including India. People with chronic diabetes are at risk of diabetonephropathy. Nephrotoxicity can occur by chemotherapy treatment with cisplatin medicine which causes the oxidative stress and inflammation in kidney [98].

Medicinal plants are used traditionally in ethnomedicine for the treatment of kidney disease. *Bryophyllumpinnatum*, is commonly known as Pattharcaṭṭa, is popular medicine for kidney stone and urinary insufficiency. Some plant derived flavonoids are used in combination as a herbal formulation to cure the kidney diseases [99]. Some antioxidants like kaemferol [100], catechin [101], and quercitrin [102] have been reported to have renoprotective effect.

5. How do phytochemicals work?

Medicinal plants are natural source of phytochemical antioxidants that are known to prevent different diseased states. The medicinal plants contain phytochemical ingredients as source of antioxidants. Phytochemicals are antioxidants compounds that inhibit or delay onset of biological oxidation. They are nitrogenous cyclinphytols compounds which possess functional groups such as hydroxyl groups, ketone groups and aldehyde. Phytochemicals work at different level to provide protection and boost the body defense mechanism against oxidative stress.

5.1 Antioxidant

Antioxidants are such anti molecules which work against oxidation reaction. It means they prevent oxidation of biomolecules caused by free radicals. Many phytochemicals work as antioxidant helping to scavenge free radicals. They donate electron to stabilize the free radicals in order to maintain the imbalance between antioxidant defense system and free radicals. The phytochemicals are subtle molecules or compounds that work like as an antioxidant.

5.2 Hormonal action

Some phytochemical can influence the hormonal activity in the body. Genistein a soy isoflavones, it works like estrogen hormone which inhibit the menopausal hot flushes in some women [103].

5.3 Biological action

Different phytochemicals play different role in the biological system. There are many different groups of phytochemicals which all have different chemical structures which may induce different health benefits. Caroteniods may inhibit the cancer cell growth and reduce the risk of cardiovascular disease and boost immunity. Dietary anthocyanins may help lower the high blood pressure. Phytochemicals as an antioxidant scavenge the free radicals and reduce the oxidative damage.

6. Summary

Oxidative stress has been linked to the various chronic diseases including cardiovascular diseases (CVD), cancer, neurological disorders, hepatic diseases, diabetes and aging. Free radicals (reactive oxygen species and reactive nitrogen species) are accountable for the pathogenesis of such diseases. Free radicals that naturally produced by the normal process of metabolism are generally neutralized by antioxidant enzymes (SOD, catalase and GPx) and non-antioxidants molecules *i.e.* GSH, uric acid and phytochemicals. Sedentary life style factors may accelerate the free radical formation that create imbalance between the antioxidant defense system and oxidative stress which leads to inflammation, necrosis and eventually cell death. Vitamins A, E and C are the primary major antioxidant vitamins which play a significant role in physiological functions of the body. Scientific reports suggested that medicinal plants contain thousands of phytochemicals (alkaloids, flavonoid, carotenoids and tannins, isoflavones and glycosides etc.) that possess antioxidant properties as well as biological activities. Dietary fruits and vegetables provide such vital molecules to our body. Many research studies reported that adequate intake of vegetables and fruits may prevent or reduce the symptoms of chronic diseases caused by oxidative stress or pathogens. Antioxidant phytochemicals are considered to be responsible for these health benefits. They often possess efficient antioxidant properties that neutralize the free radicals as well as anti-inflammatory action. Phytochemicals possess drug like effect and they are considered as therapeutic medicine which are the basis of other bioactivities and health benefits. Flavonoids, alkaloid, carotenoids and anthocyanins are the major groups of phytochemicals that possess many pharmacological properties such as anticancer, anti-aging, anti-diabetic, hepato-protective, anti-microbial, antiviral and neuroprotective. Due to variety of pharmacological properties, phytochemicals are considered as neutraceuticals. Medicinal plants are rich sources of antioxidants that are known to prevent different diseased states. Phytochemicals are nitrogenous cyclinphytols compound that are rich mostly in functional groups such as hydroxyl groups (OH), aromatic compounds (CH), Carbonyl and carboxylic groups (CO) and organosulfur groups (SO). Their functional group can donate electron to stabilize the free radicals in order to maintain the imbalance between antioxidant defense system and oxidative stress.

There are many different subclasses of phytochemicals which all have different chemical structures responsible for different positive health effects. Scientific communities across the world focusing on the alternative medicinal system in exploring the natural ingredients to be used in the food and food products for the prevention of human diseases. Herbal based medicine can be more safe, convenient and efficient as dietary components for the prevention or treatment of human diseases.

Acknowledgements

Authors are thankful to Jawaharlal Nehru University, New Delhi, India and Indira Gandhi National Open University, New Delhi India for providing necessary facilities.

Conflicts of interest

The authors declare no conflict of interest.

Author details

Manju Singh Makhaik[1]*, Arvind K. Shakya[2] and Raosaheb Kale[1]

1 School of Life Sciences, Jawaharlal Nehru University, New Delhi, India

2 Biochemistry Discipline, School of Sciences, Indira Gandhi National Open University, New Delhi, India

*Address all correspondence to: ommanjusingh@gmail.com

References

[1] Yamada T, Hayasaka S, Shibata Y, Ojima T, Saegusa T, Gotoh T, Ishikawa S, Nakamura Y, Kayaba K. Frequency of citrus fruit intake is associated with the incidence of cardiovascular disease: TheJichi Medical School cohort study. Journal epidemiology. 2011;21:169-175.

[2] Mursu J, Virtanen JK, Tuomainen TP, Nurmi T, Voutilainen S. Intake of fruit, berries, and vegetablesand risk of type 2 diabetes in Finnish men: The kuopioischaemicheart disease risk factor study. American Journal Clinical Nutrition. 2014; 9: 328-333.

[3] KrukJ. Association between vegetable, fruit and carbohydrate intake and breast cancer risk in relation tophysical activity. Asian Pacific Journal Cancer Prevention.2014;15 4429-4436.

[4] KyroC,Skeie G, Loft S, Landberg R, Christensen J, Lund E, Nilsson LM, Palmqvist R, TJonnel, A,OlsenA. Intake of whole grains from different cereal and food sources and incidence ofcolorectal cancer in the Scandinavian HELGA cohort. Cancer Causes Control.2013;24:1363-1374.

[5] Wang LF, Chen JY, Xie HH, Ju XR, Liu RH.Phytochemical profiles and antioxidant activity of adlayvarieties. JournalAgriculture Food Chemistry.2013; 61:5103-5113.

[6] Dembinska-Kiec A,Otto Mykkänen, BeataKiec-Wilk, HannuMykkänen. Antioxidant phytochemicals against type 2 diabetes.British Journal of Nutrition. 2008;99(E-S1):ES109-ES117.

[7] Krishnamurthy P, Wadhwani A. Antioxidant enzymes and human health. In: El-Missiry MA, editor. Antioxidant Enzyme. Croatia: In Tech; 2012. pp. 3-18. DOI: 10.3109/0886022X.2015.1103654.

[8] Lü JM, Lin PH, Yao Q, Chen C. Chemical and molecular mechanisms of antioxidants: Experimental approaches and model systems. Journal of Cellular and Molecular Medicine. 2009;14(4):840-860.

[9] Law BMH, Waye MMY, So WKW, Chair SY. Hypotheses on the potential of rice bran intake to prevent gastrointestinal cancer through the modulation of oxidative stress. International Journal of Molecular Sciences. 2017;18:1-20.

[10] Aziz MA, Ghanim HM, Diab KS, Al-Tamimi RJ. The association of oxidant-antioxidant status in patients with chronic renal failure.Renal Failure. 2016;38(1):20-26.

[11] Pandey KB, Rizvi SI. Markers of oxidative stress in erythrocytes and plasma during aging in humans. Oxidative Medicine and Cellular Longevity. 2010;3(1):2-12.

[12] Butnariu M, Grozea I. Antioxidant (antiradical) compounds.Journal of Bioequivalence and Bioavailability. 2012;4(6):4-6.

[13] McCord J, Fridovich M.Superoxide dismutase. An enzymic function for erythrocuprein(hemocuprein).Journal of Biological Chemistry. 1969; 244(22):6049-55.

[14] Marklund, S.L. Human copper-containing superoxide dismutase of high molecular weight. Proc. Natl. Acad. Sci. USA. 1982; 79; 7634-7638.

[15] Marklund S. Properties of extracellular superoxide dismutase from human lung. Biochemical Journal.1984; 220:269-272.

[16] Buschfort C, MullerMR, SeeberS, RajewskyMF, ThomaleJ. DNA excision repair profiles of normal and leukemic

human lymphocytes: Functional analysis at the single cell level. Cancer Research. 1997;57:65-658.

[17] Esworthy RS, Ho YS, Chu FF. The GPx1 gene encodes mitochondrial glutathione peroxidase in the mouse liver. Archives Biochemistry Biophysics. 1997;340:59-63.

[18] Lu SC. Glutathione synthesis. BiochimicaetBiophysicaActa. 2013;1830:3143-3153

[19] Samuelsson M, Vainikka L, Öllinger K. Glutathione in the blood and cerebrospinal fluid: A study in healthy male volunteers. Neuropeptides. 2011;45:287-292

[20] Lushchak VI. Glutathione homeostasis and functions: Potential targets for medical interventions. Journal of Amino Acids. 2012;2012:1-26.

[21] Stinefelt B, Leonard SS, Blemings KP, Shi X, Klandorf H. Free radical scavenging, DNA protection, and inhibition of lipid peroxidation mediated by uric acid. Annals of Clinicaland Laboratory Science. 2005;35:37-45.

[22] Warning WS. Uric acid: An important antioxidant in acute Ischaemic stroke. QJM: An International Journal of Medicine. 2002;95:691-693.

[23] Skowyra M. Antioxidant properties of extracts from selected plant materials (*Caesalpiniaspinosa*, Perillafrutescens, *Artemisia annua* and *Viola wittrockiana*) *in vitro* and in model food systems [thesis]. Department of Chemical Engineering, UniversitatPolitècnica de Catalunya; 2014.

[24] Ames BN, Cathcart R, Schwiers E, Hochstein P. Uric acid provides an antioxidant defense in humans against oxidant-and radical-caused aging and cancer: A hypothesis. Proceedings of the National Academy Sciences of the United States of America.1981;78: 6858-6862.

[25] Johnson RJ. Essential hypertension, progressive renal disease, and uric acid: A pathogenetic link? Journal of American Nephrology. 2005;16:1909-1919.

[26] Herrera E, Barbas C. Vitamin E: Action, metabolism and perspective. Journal of Physiology and Biochemistry. 2001;57:43-56.

[27] McCormick CC, Parker RS. The cytotoxicity of vitamin E is both vitamer and cell specific and involves a selectable trait. Journal of Nutrition. 2004;134:3335.

[28] Morales-Gonzalez JA, editor. Oxidative stress and chronic degenerative diseases: A role for antioxidants. In: The Exogenous Antioxidants. London, United Kingdom: IntechOpen; 2013. pp. 33-57.

[29] Pehlivan FE. Vitamin C: An Antioxidant Agent. IntechOpen; 2017.

[30] Mora JR, Iwata M, Von Andrian UH. 2008. Vitamin effects on the immune system: vitamins A and D take center stage. Nat Rev Immunol.8:685-698.

[31] Gutierrez-Mazariegos J, Theodosiou M, Campo-Paysaa F, Schubert M. Vitamin A: a multifunctional tool for development. Semin Cell Dev Biol. 2011; 22:603-610.

[32] Lind T, Lind PM, Jacobson A, Hu L, Sundqvist A, Risteli J, YebraRodriguezd A, Rodrig uez-Navarroe A, Anderssonf G, Melhus H. High dietary intake of retinol leads to bone marrow hypoxia and diaphysealendosteal mineralization in rats. Bone.2011;48:496-506.

[33] Arredondo ML. Relationship between vitamin intake and total antioxidant capacity in elderly adults.

UniversitasScientiarum. 2016;21(2): 167-177.

[34] Fiedor J, Fiedor L, Haessner R, Scheer H. Cyclic ednoperoxides of β-carotene, potential pro-oxidants, as products of chemical quenching of singlet oxygen. Biochemical Biophysics Acta. 2005;1709:1-4.

[35] Edge R, Truscott TG. Properties of Carotenoid Radicals and Excited States and Their Potential Role in Biological Systems. In: Landrum J.T., editor. *Carotenoids: Physical, Chemical, and Biological Functions and Properties.* CRC Press; Boca Raton, FL, USA: 2010. pp. 283-308.

[36] Cvetkovic D, Fiedor L, Fiedor J, Wiśniewska-Becker A, Markovic D. Molecular Base for Carotenoids Antioxidant Activity in Model and Biological Systems: The Health-Related Effects. In: Yamaguchi M., editor. Carotenoids: Food Sources, Production and Health Benefits. Nova Science Publishers; Hauppauge, NY, USA: 2013. pp. 93-126.

[37] Biewanga G, G R Haenen, ABast. The pharmacology of the antioxidant lipoic acid.Gen Pharmacology The Vascular System.1997;29(3):315-31

[38] Fai-Chu W, Ann-Li Y, EvonPeir-Shan T, Sim-Chyi K, Hean-Chooi O, and Tsun-Thai C. Antioxidant, Metal Chelating, Anti-glucosidase Activities and Phytochemical Analysis of Selected Tropical Medicinal Plants.Iranian JournalPharmacuetical Research. 2014;13(4):1409-1415.

[39] Walter M, Marchesan E. Phenolic compounds and antioxidant activity of rice. Brazilizn Archives of Biology and Technology. 2011;54(1):371-377.

[40] Chia-Jui W, Gow-Chin Y. Flavonoids, a ubiquitous dietary phenolic subclass, exert extensive *in vitro* anti-invasive and *in vivo* anti-metastatic activities. Cancer Metastasis Review. 2012;31(1-2):323-51.

[41] NourY,,NawalA, MajedJ,and Chantal M. The Immunomodulatory and Anti-Inflammatory Role of Polyphenols.Nutrients. 2018;10(11):1618

[42] Poulose SM, Miller MG, Shukitt-Hale B. Role of walnuts in maintaining brain health with age. Journal Nutrition. 2014;144:561S-566S.

[43] Singh M, Suman S, ShuklaY. New enlightenment of skin cancer chemoprevention through phytochemicals: In vitro and in vivo studies and the underlying mechanisms. Biomed Research International. 2014;243452.

[44] Soobrattee MA, Neergheen VS, Luximon-Ramma A, AruomaOI, Bahorun T. Phenolics as potential antioxidant therapeutic agents: Mechanism and actions. Mutation Research. 2005;579: 200-213.

[45] Cao G, Russell RM, Lischner N, Prior RL. Serum antioxidant capacity is increased by consumption of strawberries, spinach, red wine or vitamin C in elderly women. Journal Nutrition.1998; 128:2383-2390.

[46] Cao G, Booth SL, Sadowski JA, Prior RL. Increases in human plasma antioxidant capacity after consumption of controlled diets high in fruit and vegetables.American Journal Clinical Nutrition.1998; 68: 1081-1087.

[47] Mazza G, Kay CD, Cottrell T, Holub BJ.Absorption of anthocyanins from blueberries and serum antioxidant status in human subjects.Journal Agriculture Food Chemisttry.2002; 50:7731-7737.

[48] Koren E, Kohen R, Ginsburg I. Polyphenols enhance total oxidant-scavenging capacities of human blood

by binding to red blood cells. Experimental Biology Medicine. 2010; 235: 689-699.

[49] Liu RH. Health benefits of fruit and vegetables are from additive and synergistic combinations of phytochemicals. American Journal Clinical Nutrition.2003;78:517S-520S.

[50] Liu RH. Potential synergy of phytochemicals in cancer prevention: Mechanism of action. Journal Nutrition 2004; 134 (Suppl. S12), 3479-3485.

[51] Dahlen EM, Tengblad A, Lanne T, Clinchy B, Ernerudh J, Nystrom FH, Ostgren CJ. Abdominal obesity and low-grade systemic inflammation as markers of subclinical organ damage in type 2 diabetes. Diabetes Metabolism. 2014;40:76-81.

[52] Qiao L, Li X. Role of chronic inflammation in cancers of the gastrointestinal system and the liver: Where we are now. Cancer Letters. 2014;345:150-152.

[53] Steinberg GR, Schertzer JD. AMPK promotes macrophage fatty acid oxidative metabolism to mitigate inflammation: Implications for diabetes and cardiovascular disease. Immunologyand Cell Biology 2014;92:340-345.

[54] Hutchins-Wolfbrandt A, Mistry AM. Dietary turmeric potentially reduces the risk of cancer. Asian Pacific Journal Cancer Prevention. 2011;12:3169-3173.

[55] Robert E, Joshua AB, and David BM. bioactivities of resveratrol. Comprehensive Review in Food Sciences and Food Safety.2006;5:65-70

[56] Yu-Jie Zhang,Ren-You Gan,, Sha Li, Yue Zhou,, An-Na Li,, Dong-Ping Xu and Hua-Bin Li.Antioxidant Phytochemicals for the Prevention andTreatment of Chronic Diseases. Molecules 2015;20:211382-1156.

[57] PoojaB, DeepaK. Green tea catechins: defensive role in cardiovascular disorders. Chinese Journal Natural Medicine. 2013;11(4):345-53.

[58] YuanyuanLuo, Pingping S, and Dongye L. Luteolin: A Flavonoid that Has Multiple Cardio-Protective Effects and Its Molecular Mechanisms. Front Pharmacol. 2017: 6;8:692.

[59] Babu PV, Liu D. Green tea catechins and cardiovascular health: an update. Current Medicinal Chemistry 2008;15:1840-50.

[60] Leyla B,PeirHK, Ali G. Garlic: a review of potential therapeutic effects. Avicenna Jounral of Phytomedicine. 2014;4(1):1-14.

[61] KazimK, AyşegülO, HakanŞ, GökhanB, MedihaC, GüngörK. Investigation of the possible protective role of gallic acid on paraoxanase and arylesterase activities in livers of rats with acute alcohol intoxication. CellBiochemistry Function. 2013;31(3):208-13.

[62] Haddad Y, Diane V, Antoine B, Haddad PS. Antioxidant and Hepatoprotective Effects of Silibinin in a Rat Model of NonalcoholicSteatohepatitis. Evidence Based Complementantry and Alternative Medicine. 2011;1-10.

[63] Dixit N, Baboota S, Kohli K, Ahmad S, Ali J. Silymarin: A review of pharmacological aspects and bioavailability enhancement approaches. Indian Journal of Pharmacology. 2007;39(4):172-9.

[64] Papackova Z, Heczkova M, Dankova H, Sticova E, Lodererova A, Bartonova L, *et al*. Silymarin prevents acetaminophen-induced hepatotoxicity in mice. PLoS One. 2018;13(1):e0191353.

[65] Senthil K, Thirugnana SP, Oh TJ, Kim SH, Choi HK. Free radical

scavenging activity and comparative metabolic profiling of in vitro cultured and field grown *Withania somnifera* roots.PLoS One 2015;10:e0123360.

[66] RajaS, Manivasagam T, Sankar V, Prakash S, Muthusamy R, Krishnamurti A, *et al.* *Withaniasomnifera* root extract improves catecholamines and physiological abnormalities seen in a parkinson's disease model mouse. JournalEthnopharmacology 2009;125:369-73.

[67] Sumathi S, Padma PR, Gathampari S, Vidhya S. Free radical scavenging activity of different parts of Withaniasomnifera. Ancient Scienceof Life. 2007;26:30-4

[68] Kesava RVK, Venkata SA, Thangavel S, Madhavan PN. Ashwagandha (*Withania somnifera*) Reverses β-Amyloid1-42 Induced Toxicity in Human Neuronal Cells: Implications in HIV-Associated Neurocognitive Disorders (HAND). PLoS One. 2013; 8(10): e77624.

[69] Francesca M, Giulia G, Liliana B, and Daniela R. Withaferin AInhibits Nuclear Factor- κB-Dependent Pro-Inflammatory and Stress Response Pathways in the Astrocytes. Neural Plasticity. 2015; 2015: 381964.

[70] Mohammad RB, MuhammedIK, Prabu SR. Neuroprotective efficacy of withaferina on aging mediated oxidative stress in striatum and Substantianigra of wistar albino rat. Drug Invention Today 2019: 12:(3) 425-431.

[71] Kaustubh S. Chaudhari, Nishant R. Tiwari,cRakesh R. Tiwari, and Rohan S. Neurocognitive Effect of Nootropic Drug Brahmi (Bacopamonnieri) in Alzheimer's Disease. Annals of Neuroscience.2017;24(2): 111-122

[72] Linlin C, Huidan D,Hengmin C, Jing F, Zhicai Z, Junliang D, Yinglun L, Xun W, and Ling Z. Inflammatory responses and inflammation-associated diseases in organs. Oncotarget. 2018;23; 9(6): 7204-7218.

[73] Julie SJ. Anti-inflammatory properties of curcumin, a major constituent of *Curcuma longa*: a review of preclinical and clinical research. Alternative Medicine Review. 2009;14(2):141-53.

[74] Tobias O, Piotr S. Cell cycle proteins as promising targets in cancer therapy. Nature Review: Cancer. 2017;17(2): 93-115.

[75] Rustelle JV, Michelle H. Visagie, Anne E. Theron, Annie MJ. Antimitotic drugs in the treatment of cancer.Cancer Chemotherapy and Pharmacology.2015;76; 1101-1112.

[76] Shankar E, Goel A, Gupta K, Gupta S. Plant flavone Apigenin: An emerging anticancer agent. Current Pharmacology Reports. 2017: 3(6): 423-446.

[77] Imran M, Salehi B, Sharifi-Rad J, AslamGondal T, Saeed F, Imran A, Shahbaz M, TsouhFokou PV,UmairArshad M, Khan H, Guerreiro SG, Martins N,Estevinho LM. Kaempferol: A Key Emphasis to Its Anticancer Potential. Molecules.2019; 24:2277.https://doi.org/10.3390/molecules24122277

[78] Seung-Hee K, Kyung-Chul. Anti-cancer Effect and Underlying Mechanism(s) of Kaempferol, a Phytoestrogen, on the Regulation of Apoptosis in Diverse Cancer Cell Models.Toxicology Research. 2013;29(4):229-234.

[79] Rauf A, Imran M, Khan IA, Ur-Rehman M, Gilani SA, Mehmood Z, Mubarak MS. Anticancer potential of quercetin: A comprehensive review.

Phytotherapy Research. 2018;32(11): 2109-2130.

[80] Abuohashish HM, Al-Rejaie SS, Al-Hosaini KA, Parmar MY, Ahmed MM. Alleviating effects of morin against experimentally-induced diabetic osteopenia. Diabetology and Metabolic Syndrome. 2013;5:5.

[81] Stanley Mainzen P, Kamalakkannan N. Rutin improves glucose homeostasis in streptozotocin diabetic tissues by altering glycolytic and gluconeogenic enzymes. Journal of Biochemical and Molecular Toxicology. 2006;20:96-102.

[82] Ashfaq UA, Masoud MS, Nawaz Z, Riazuddin S. Glycyrrhizin as antiviral agent against Hepatitis C Virus.Journal of Translational Medicine.2011; 9:112. doi: 10.1186/1479-5876-9-112.

[83] TutunchiH, NaeiniFA. Ostadrahimi MJ. Hosseinzadeh-Attar. Naringenin, a flavanone with antiviral and anti-inflammatory effects: A promising treatment strategy against COVID-19. PhytotherapyResearch. 2020;34(12):3137-3147.

[84] AgrawalKP,Chandan A, Gerald B. Quercetin: Antiviral Significance and Possible COVID-19 Integrative Considerations. Natural Product Communications. 2020;15(12): 1-10.

[85] Steinmann J, Buer J, Pietschmann T, Steinmann E.Anti-infective properties of epigallocatechin-3-gallate (EGCG), a component of green tea.BritishJournal Pharmacology.2013;168(5):1059-73.

[86] Xu J, Xu Z, Zheng W.A Review of the Antiviral Role of Green Tea Catechins. Molecules. 2017;12; 22(8):1337.

[87] Kim M, Kim SY, Lee HW, Shin JS, Kim P, Jung YS, Jeong HS, Hyun JK, Lee CK .Inhibition of influenza virus internalization by (-)-epigallocatechin-3-gallate.Antiviral Res. 2013;100(2):460-72.

[88] KunihiroK Miyuki Y, YasuhitoE. Antiviral Mechanism of Action of Epigallocatechin-3- O-gallate and Its Fatty Acid Esters. Molecules. 2018; 27;23(10):2475.

[89] Liu CH, Jassey A, Hsu HY, Lin LT. Antiviral Activities of Silymarin and Derivatives. Molecules. 2019;24(8):1552. doi: 10.3390/molecules24081552.

[90] Nuria T, Maria RG, Maria TF, Maria DO, Africa G, David N, Mercedes C, Jose LR, Concepcion G. Immunity to Parasites. Journal Name: Current Immunology Reviews. 2011;7(1):25-43.

[91] Bin Mohanna MA. Leishmaniasis, malaria, and schistosomiasis concurrently in an 8- year-old boy.Saudi Medical Journal. 2015; 36(4): 494-496.

[92] Wright CW. Antiprotozoal Natural Products. In: Evans EC, editor. Trease and Evans Pharmacognosy. 16th ed. Edinburgh: Saunders; pp. 428-434. 2009.

[93] Sikora E., Bielak-Zmijewska A., Mosieniak G, Piwocka K. The Promise of Slow Down Ageing May Come from Curcumin. Current Pharmaceutical Design. 2010;16:884-892.

[94] Lisa M. Health foods in anti-aging therapy: reducers of physiological decline and degenerative diseases Advances in Phytomedicine. 2002;15(1):173-180.

[95] Sadowska-Bartosz I, Bartosz G. Effect of Antioxidants Supplementation on Aging and Longevity.BioMed Research International. 2014;404680. doi: 10.1155/2014/404680

[96] Bielak-Zmijewska A, Grabowska W, Ciolko A, Bojko A, Mosieniak G, Bijoch Ł, SikoraE. The Role of Curcumin

in the Modulation of Ageing. International Journal of Molecular Science.2019; 20(5): 1239.doi: 10.3390/ijms20051239.

[97] Sikora E, Scapagnini G, Barbagallo M.Curcumin, inflammation, ageing and age-related diseases. Immunity and Aging. 2010;17;7(1):1.

[98] Miller RP, Tadagavadi RK, Ramesh G, Reeves WB.Mechanisms of Cisplatin Nephrotoxicity.Toxins (Basel). 2010;2(11): 2490-2518.

[99] Vargas F, Romecín P, García-Guillén AI, Wangesteen R, Vargas-Tendero P, Paredes MD, Atucha NM, García-EstañJ.Flavonoids in Kidney Health and Disease. Frontier in Physiology. 2018;9:394.doi: 10.3389/fphys.2018.00394

[100] Zhu W,Wansen S, Xi S, Ye W,Meilan Z. Kaempferol ameliorates Cisplatin induced nephrotoxicity by modulating oxidative stress, inflammation and apoptosis via ERK and NF-κB pathways.AMB Express. 2020;10:58. doi: 10.1186/s13568-020-00993-w

[101] Orawan W, Wachirasek P, Anongporn K. Catechin supplementation prevents kidney damage in rats repeatedly exposed to cadmium through mitochondrial protection. Naunyn-Schmiedeberg's Archives of Pharmacology. 2018;391(4):385-394.

[102] Yang H, Yan S,Ya-nan L, Rong Li. Quercetin Treatment Improves Renal Function and Protects the Kidney in a Rat Model of Adenine-Induced Chronic Kidney Disease. MedicalScience Monitor. 2018;24:4760-4766.

[103] Chen LR, Ko NY, Chen KH. Isoflavone Supplements for Menopausal Women: A Systematic Review. Nutrients. 2019;11(11):2649.doi: 10.3390/nu11112649.

Chapter 22

Biosynthesis and Regulation of Antioxidant Flavonolignans in Milk Thistle

Samantha Drouet and Christophe Hano

Abstract

Mature fruits (achenes) of milk thistle (*Silybum marianum* (L.) Gaertner, Asteraceae) accumulate high amounts of silymarin, a complex mixture of bioactive antioxidant flavonolignans deriving from taxifolin. Their biological activities in relation with human health promotion and disease prevention have been well described. The conditions of their biosynthesis *in planta*, however, have long been elusive and thus tend to be a limiting factor for their future applications. Significant advances in understanding their biosynthesis and regulation have been made over the last decade and are outlined in the current chapter.

Keywords: *Silybum marianum*, flavonolignans, silymarin, biosynthesis, regulation

1. Introduction

Plant products, as food or as an "herbal medicine" preparation have been used by humans throughout history with varying success to prevent and/or cure various diseases [1]. Neanderthals had already understood the importance of plants in their diet but also their medicinal capacity [2]. For centuries, medicine has relied heavily on the use of plants. In many countries, traditional medicines, based on medicinal plants, are an essential part of their health system [3]. Some of these medicinal plants are still today, either collected from the wild or cultivated to ensure their availability for industry or traditional medicine. Nowadays, the badly named "weeds" such as thistles, nettle or burdock, represent a significant part of agricultural production [4]. These weeds are considered as pests, yet they are medicinal plants traditionally used for their beneficial properties. There is indeed a strong potential for the use of these plants as sources of pharmaceutical or cosmetic antioxidants [4]. In particular, the craze for silymarin from milk thistle is directly linked to the biological properties of this mixture. Silymarin is a complex mixture of bioactive flavonolignans accumulated in mature fruits (achenes) of milk thistle. Numerous biological activities, in particular hepatoprotective, anti-proliferative, immunomodulatory, anti-inflammatory and antioxidant, have demonstrated the high potential of these compounds [5, 6].

Free radicals, including superoxide radical ($O_2^{-\bullet}$), hydroxyl radical ($OH^{-\bullet}$), hydrogen peroxide (H_2O_2) and peroxide radical ($ROO^{-\bullet}$), are implicated in liver disease [7, 8]. These reactive oxygen species (ROS) are produced through biochemical processes (cell metabolism) or induced by inflammatory diseases, cancers, or treatments such as radiotherapy or chemotherapy [9]. ROS play an important role in many signaling pathways (proliferation, cell activation, migration, etc.). However, when they are produced in large quantities in certain cellular compartments, they can become harmful to the body. This phenomenon is called "oxidative stress". To protect themselves, cells respond by regulating the production of cellular antioxidants such as glutathione (GSH) and/or the activity of antioxidant enzymes such as superoxide dismutase (SOD) and catalase (CAT), glutathione peroxidase (GPx) [9, 10].

The abilities of silibinin (mixture of silybin A and B), which are among the main flavonolignans accumulated in *S. marianum* fruits, to fight certain oxidative stresses or oxidants such as superoxide anion radicals, hydrogen peroxide, hydroxyl radical and hypochlorous acid (HOCl) was studied [11–13]. The mixture of silybins does not seem to be a good $O_2^{-\bullet}$ scavenger and no reaction with hydrogen peroxide has been shown. On the other hand, these flavonolignans react rapidly in free solution with $OH^{-\bullet}$ radicals [11]. Besides, in lymphocytes of patients with cirrhosis, *in vitro* incubation with silymarin markedly increases the expression of superoxide dismutase (SOD) [10]. Silymarin also helps increase the glutathione content in the cell leading to inhibition of lipid peroxidation, which enhances membrane stability [14].

The silymarin mixture also reduces oxidative stress induced by UV in epidermal and dermal cells. In certain skin conditions, it therefore exerts on humans a chemo-preventive effect on oxidative stress induced by solar UV rays (photo-aging and photo-carcinogenesis) [15–17]. Systemic and local administration of silymarin to burns is effective against oxidative damage (and morphological alterations) induced by sunburns to rat skin [18]. The study of the individual effect of some silymarin compounds has shown some differences. Other flavonolignans from milk thistle, isosilybin and silydianin, protect against glutathione depletion, ROS generation and activation of caspase-3 which plays a central role in the activation of apoptotic cell death. Both silychristin and silydianin only seem to reduce the levels of caspase-3 [19].

Hemisynthetic derivatives of silybins were found to be the effective radical scavengers and lipid peroxidation inhibitors [20–23].

The biological activities in relation with human health promotion and disease prevention of the antioxidant milk thistle flavonolignans are well described. However, the conditions of their biosynthesis in plants are still unclear and have been a limiting factor for their potential developments. During the last decade, studies have paved the way toward a better understanding of the biosynthetic regulation of these flavonolignans during the maturation of *S. marianum* fruit. Providing important insights to better control the production of these medicinally important antioxidant compounds. This chapter summarizes these major outcomes.

2. Botanical description of *Silybum marianum*

Milk Thistle, *S. marianum* (L. Gaertner) is one of the oldest known medicinal plants belonging to the Asteraceae family. It was described and named by Carl von Linné, then replaced in the current classification by Joseph Gaertner in 1791. The term *Silybum* designates, in Greek and Latin, an edible thistle, as for the qualifier *marianum*, it would be linked to the Virgin Mary. Legend has it that during her journey from Judea to Herod's escape, the Virgin Mary sheltered herself under a grove of thistles with the infant Jesus, where she breastfed him. Her breast milk would then have fallen on the leaves of thistles, hence the characteristic white mottling of this species. This legend could be the origin of the use of milk thistle to promote lactation, although its effectiveness in this area has never been demonstrated. Within the plant kingdom, *S. marianum* is an angiosperm (Magnoliophytes) commonly a flowering, fruit-bearing plant or Magnoliopsida (formerly dicotyledonous). The biological aspects of milk thistle (phenotype, life cycle) will be discussed in this section, followed by its worldwide distribution and its characteristics. Although this Asteraceae is considered a weed, it is valuable because of its interesting biological properties and antioxidant activities, in particular for applications in medicine, cosmetics, or even in the food industry.

Milk thistle is an annual or biennial herbaceous plant native to the Mediterranean basin. Due to its ecological abundance, this plant is considered as a common, even invasive species, it is nevertheless valuable. *S. marianum* can grow over a meter in height and diameter (at its base). Its stem is grooved, with a slightly cottony internal pith and branched at its top. This plant can be identified by its green leaves, marbled with white stripes, with an elliptical, toothed and thorny blade (**Figure 1**).

There is a plethora of thistles in the world, possessing similar morphological characteristics (**Figure 2**). Depending on the stage of development, it will be more or less easy to determine precisely the plant species. Indeed, many specific traits are unique to the flower or inflorescence, such as color or size. It is important to respect the "keys" of morphological identification. These taxonomic keys, based on aspects of fruits, flowers, stems, are often used as the main elements for the identification of most genera of plants [25]. The number, size, hairiness and shape of the organs often distinguish closely related species. In order not to confuse milk thistle with other species, flavonolignans could be used as taxonomic markers. It is important to have a critical look at different botanical, molecular and chemical techniques for the authentication of plant material for cosmetic applications. Molecular or phytochemical criteria are sometimes necessary, particularly when plants arrive crushed, as is customary in the industry. Identification, as well as the authentication of species, requires a wide range of technical knowledge and skills. It is easy to confuse one species with another, if only certain morphological characters, assumed to be specific to a species, are observed [25].

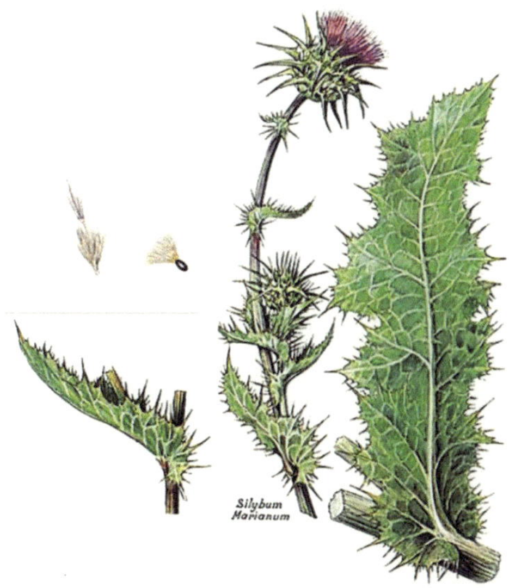

Figure 1.
Silybum marianum, *redrawn from Bonnier and Douin, 1990 [24].*

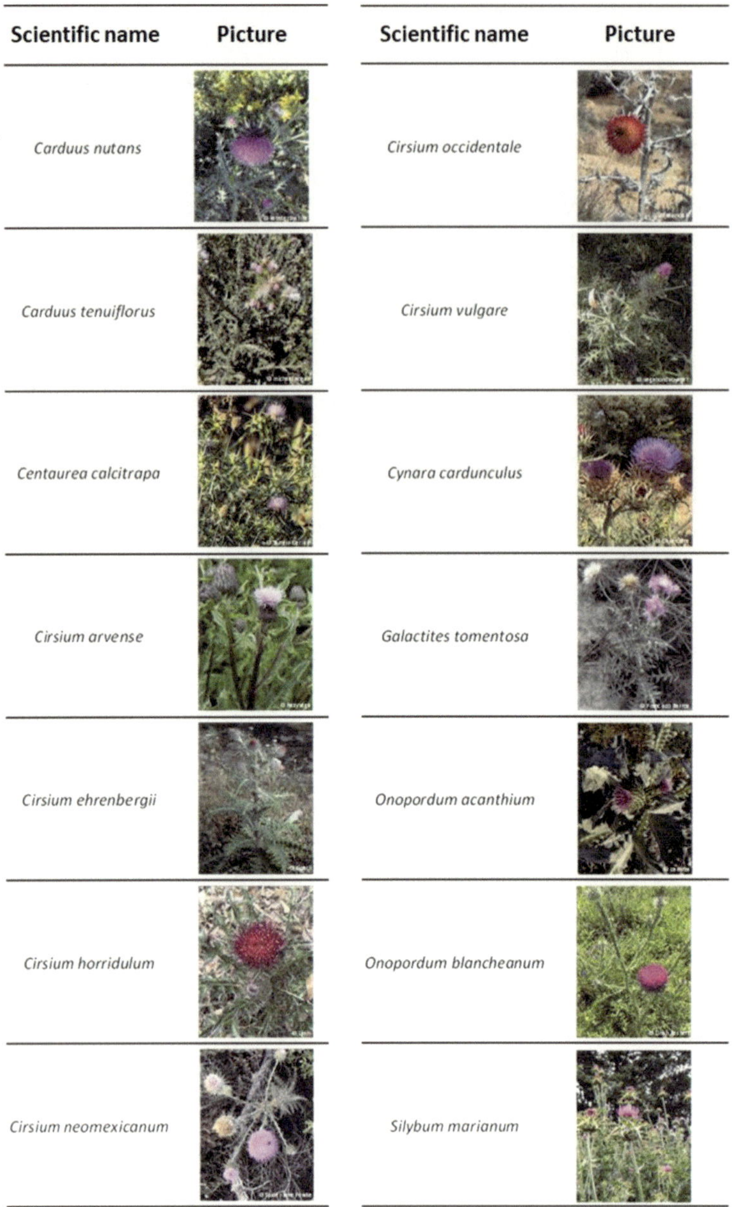
Scientific name
Picture
Scientific name
Picture
Carduus nutans
Cirsium occidentale
Carduus tenuiflorus
Cirsium vulgare
Centaurea calcitrapa
Cynara cardunculus
Cirsium arvense
Galactites tomentosa
Cirsium ehrenbergii
Onopordum acanthium
Cirsium horridulum
Onopordum blancheanum
Cirsium neomexicanum
Silybum marianum

Figure 2.
Example of plant species that can be confused with S. marianum, *all from the Asteraceae family.*

S. marianum is native to southern Europe, specifically the mountains of the Mediterranean region, western Asia, and Russia, from where it has spread to most temperate regions of the world (**Figure 3**). This plant has also been introduced widely outside its natural range, such as North America, Japan, Iran, Australia, and New Zealand, and is now found all over the world. In some parts of the world, it is considered an invasive species, notably in Israel, Australia, Tasmania and Kansas in the USA [26]. *S. marianum* was introduced to the United States as an ornamental/medicinal plant and is also believed to have been introduced to the Pacific Northwest through the importation of contaminated hay. It is probably this species that Darwin calls the "giant pampas thistle" in his journal of the Voyage of the Beagle, 1831–1836 [27].

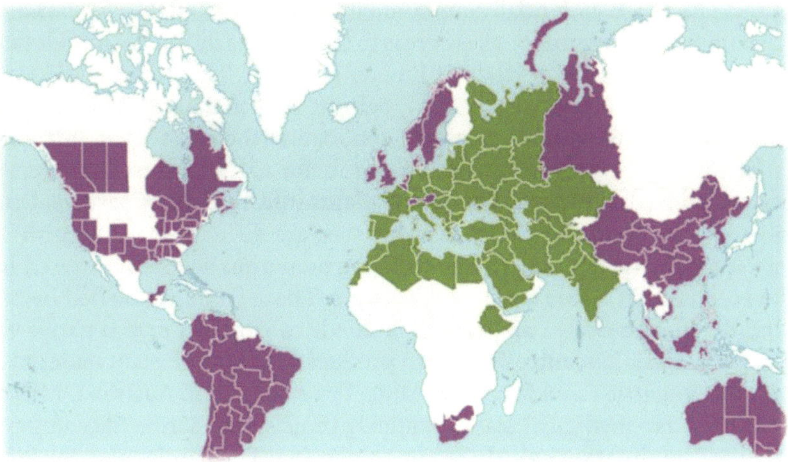

Figure 3.
Distribution of S. marianum, *in green the native species and in purple the introduced species.*

Speaking of the abundance of these species and their invasiveness, Darwin says, "There were immense beds of the thistle, as well as of the cardoon [i.e., *Cynaria cardunculus*]; the whole country, indeed, may be called one great bed. The two sorts [i.e., *S. marianum* and *Cynaria cardunculus* (artichoke and cardoon, edible and cultivated)] grow separate, each plant in company with its own kind. The cardoon is as high as a horse's back, but the Pampas thistle is often higher than the crown of the rider's head. To leave the road for a yard is out of the question; and the road itself is partly, and in some cases entirely closed" reported in Bulletin of the Torrey Botanical Club [27]. Milk thistle is also cultivated for industry and the production of large-scale pharmaceutical raw materials, in Austria (Waldviertel region), Germany, Hungary, Poland, China and Argentina, but also in France in the Loire Valley region.

Most medicinal plants can be harvested from the wild, but their cultivation ensures their availability for industry. Both traditional and biotechnological breeding techniques can be applied to improve yield and uniformity [4]. Conventional methods of plant breeding can improve both agronomic and medicinal characteristics [28] and in particular increase the content of active compounds. The time of harvest depends on the maturity stage of the considered crop. Flowering in flower heads is spread over time, maturation is not simultaneous throughout the plan [4], which is the general case with non-domesticated plants. In Poland, Andrzejewska and Sadowska [29] reported that the harvest of *S. marianum* should take place around the last days of July or early August when 40–50% of the inflorescences were in flower. After harvesting, the achene pappus should be removed with a knife and the harvested achenes should be dried at 50 °C at 8% humidity [30]. Carrier et al., [31] found that the highest silymarin content came from the late stages of development when the achenes are dark brown or even black [4]. Harvesting should be done just before the flower heads start to tear, for this an ordinary combine can be used. The large thorns present on the stems, leaves and inflorescences of milk thistle make manual harvesting of flower heads an extremely unpleasant task. However, in terms of efficiency, it is much better to harvest thistle flower heads manually rather than by machine, otherwise the yield and quality of the seeds could be compromised.

Milk thistle has been called an invasive plant because of its rapid growth and low requirement in terms of nutrients or the environment. This plant tends to grow outside its range, potentially contaminating other crop fields. *S. marianum* grows in compact groups and makes access to some paths or roads difficult due to its thorns. This plant can reach over 1 meter in height. This creates shadows for nearby plants (especially fodder species), helps to reduce their development, causes native vegetation to move or, in the worst case, causes them to wither. Introduced non-native thistles can invade an area, substitute for native plants, reduce crop yield or create problems for animals, when these plants infest a field or pasture. One of the problems with controlling thistles is that they are difficult to distinguish and to eradicate. Milk thistle reproduces thanks to the numerous achenes scattered in the soil. They can remain viable for up to nine years. These fruits are carried by rain, water and the movements of animals. Milk thistle can quickly invade native vegetation in natural areas. Uncontrolled, it can produce four tons of plant material every 4,000m^2, leaving little room for other plants. For example, in Australia, Milk thistle was introduced as a medicinal plant. It quickly proliferated across the country, as far as Tasmania. The situation quickly became worrying. The species was quickly recognized as an invasive plant, leading to its inclusion as noxious grass in Australian and English legislation of 1851 and 1856 [32].

3. Phytochemical considerations on *Silybum marianum*

Milk thistle fruit extract contains 65–80% silymarin and 20–35% fatty acids, including linoleic and palmitic acid [33], but also many flavonoids (quercetin, kaempferol, apigenin, taxifolin) and phenolic compounds. Besides, around 38% of carbohydrates (mainly starch) and up to 23% of protein can be found, as well as some amines (tyramine, histamine). Silymarin is a mixture of polyphenolic molecules comprising seven closely related flavonolignans (silybin A, silybin B, isosilybin A, isosilybin B, silychristin, isosilychristin, silydianin) and a flavonoid (taxifolin).

Pelter and Haensel were the first, in 1968, to propose the generic term "flavonolignan" to designate these hybrid molecules of natural origin [34]. According to the definition recommended by the "International Union of Pure and Applied Chemistry" (IUPAC), the structure of flavonolignans is defined by the condensation of a $C_6C_3C_6$ flavonoid unit with one or more C_6C_3 lignan precursors [35]. The precursors of lignans can be found under the general name of the unit phenylpropane (also called monolignols) which are generally in the form of hydroxycinnamic alcohol (**Figure 4**).

Silibinin, a semi-purified fraction of silymarin, is mainly a mixture of 2 diastereomers, silybin A and silybin B, in an almost equimolar ratio (close to 1:1) [36].

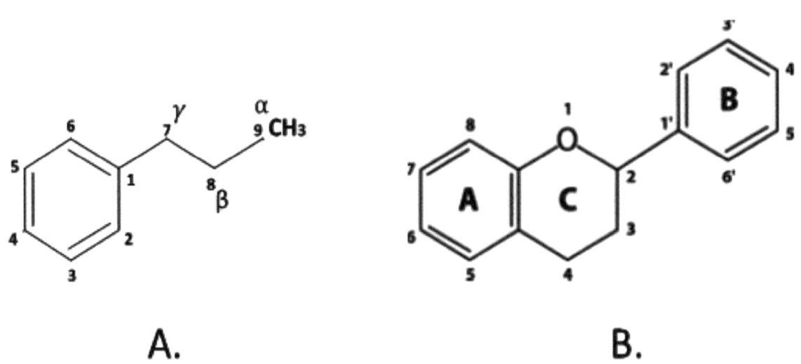

Figure 4.
Structure of a phenylpropane unit (A) and a flavonoid (B).

The silymarin content in fruits strongly depends on the selected ecotype. The geographical location of the crop (physical properties of the soil, weather conditions), as well as the agronomic conditions (sowing period, fertilization, irrigation, harvest period, seed maturity), greatly influence the composition of the flavonolignans constituting silymarin [37–39]. It is thanks to its compounds that this plant has been used for over 2,000 years in the European Pharmacopeia, making it one of the oldest medicinal plants in the Pharmacopeia.

Milk thistle is the model plant for the study of flavonolignans. The silymarin contained in the extract of milk thistle fruit, is used in diverse pharmaceutical and nutraceutical preparations. For example, Legalon® is used in the treatment of acute and chronic liver conditions. This mixture of several flavonolignans and a flavonoid account for 65–80% of the extract from the fruit of *S. marianum*. The constituents of silymarin are silybin, isosilybin, silychristin and silydianin [34, 40–43]. These are the best known and most studied flavonolignans in the literature. These compounds are produced by the condensation of taxifolin and coniferyl alcohol.

In 1968, when the German phytochemist Hildebert Wagner and his colleagues described the mixture of flavonolignans extracted from milk thistle, only silybins, isosilybins, silydianin and silychristin had been characterized [44]. The different isomers were described later. What was initially described as a "simple" mixture of 4 molecules, actually turned out to be much more complex. In this mixture, most of the silymarin compounds are (regio)isomers and therefore contain the same number of atoms, but linked in different ways. Silybins and isosilybins are stereoisomers. These isomeric molecules differ in the three-dimensional orientations of their atoms, they are therefore diastereomers [45]. To date, by taking into account the various isomeric forms, nearly 23 flavonolignans have been identified in the genus *Silybum* [46]. Their structural similarity made the identification of these isomers difficult, especially by NMR, where their ^{1}H and ^{13}C spectra are similar, and no characteristic signal makes it possible to distinguish the three-dimensional orientations [47]. The different diastereomers were not isolated and fully characterized until 2003. These compounds were separated by column chromatography on silica gel, reverse phase HPLC, followed by recrystallization [48]. After the improvement of the various techniques and equipment, the study of silybins and isosilybins was facilitated, in particular by approaches based on chemistry, the generation of analogues, X-ray crystallography (to verify the structures of the four main isomers) and the development of tools making it possible to discern and quantify flavonolignans by ^{1}H NMR spectroscopy, despite almost identical spectra [49, 50] (**Figure 5**).

Isosilybin C and isosilybin D also exist (**Figure 6**). The regiochemistry of these two compounds is similar to that of isosilybin A and isosilybin B. The major structural difference between these compounds and the other flavonolignans lies in their 1,3,5 substitution profile in the aromatic ring derived from the lignan precursor [47]. These two compounds are present in small quantities in the mixture of flavonolignans of milk thistle. They are therefore more rarely studied or analyzed in extracts from this plant.

The other three silymarin flavonolignans are silychristin, isosilychristin, and silydianin. These are the structural isomers of the compounds mentioned above. Among these 3 compounds, only silychristin was characterized as two diastereoisomers (silychristin A and silychristin B) (**Figure 7**).

The coupling, considered as non-stereo-selective, of taxifolin and coniferyl alcohol gives the two pairs of diastereomers (silybins and isosilybins). It is therefore not surprising to observe the existence of two diastereomers of silychristin in silymarin [51]. However, unlike silibinin (silybin A + silybin B) and isosilibinin (isosilybin A + isosilybin B) whose ratio between diastereomers varies according to the considered ecotype [52, 53], the silychristin A/silychristin B diastereomeric ratio

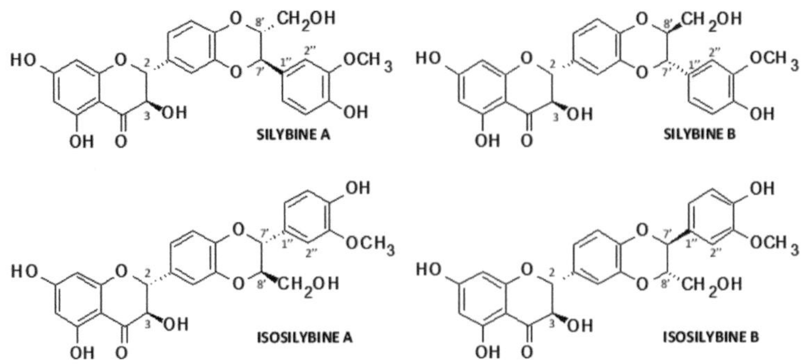

Figure 5.
Chemical structure of the diastereomers of silybin and isosilybin. Complete structural assignments in C-2, C-3, C-7 'and C-8' of these flavonolignans have thus been possible. The stereochemistry of these diastereomers was determined in the form of silybin A: 2R, 3R 7'R, 8'R; silybin B: 2R, 3R, 7'S, 8'S; isosilybin A: 2R, 3R, 7'R, 8'R; and isosilybin B: 2R, 3R, 7'S, 8'S [48].

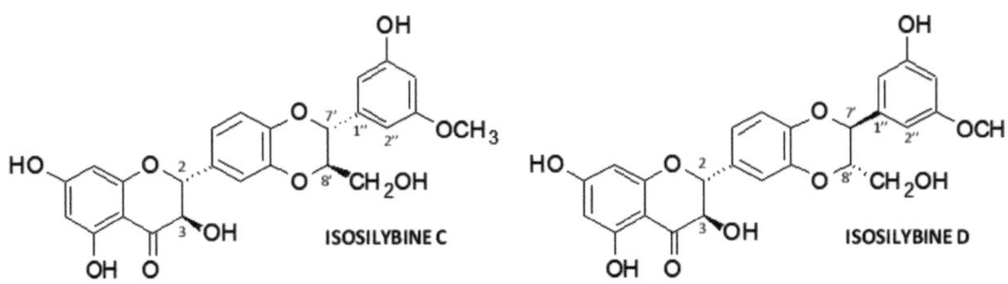

Figure 6.
Chemical structure of other isosilybins present in minor amounts in milk thistle extract.

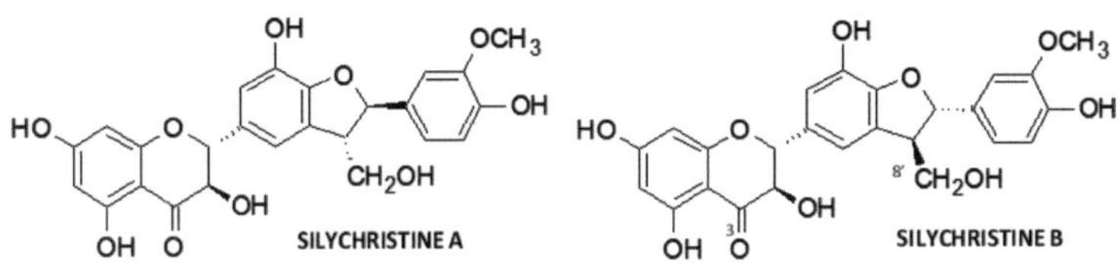

Figure 7.
Chemical structure of silychristin diastereomers.

is largely unbalanced, about 95: 5 in favor of silychristin A [51]. To date, no diastereoisomers of silydianin or isosilychristin have been reported. However, due to the low content of silychristin B, it is highly likely that a diastereomer of isosilychristin is also present but at a trace level. The presence of silydianin diastereomers cannot be excluded. However, the cyclic and compact structure of this molecule places these stereocenters close to the pre-existing stereocenters of taxifolin, which could explain the high stereoselectivity of this compound [51].

4. Flavonolignans biosynthesis in *Silybum marianum*

Most of the studies on flavonolignans focus on their pharmacological use and the chemistry of silymarin. In comparison, their biosynthesis remains less. Two different branches of the phenylpropanoids biosynthetic pathway are involved in the biosynthesis of their precursors, those of monolignols and flavonoids. In the case of the flavonolignans of purple milk thistle, the oxidative coupling allowing these molecules to be obtained occurs via the condensation of taxifolin and coniferyl alcohol. The reaction would take place via a radical coupling mechanism by oxidizing enzymes forming radicals, such as peroxidases or laccases, in a similar way to the formation of monolignol radicals and polymerization, during lignification [38, 45]. The synthesis would therefore involve three pathways: that of monolignols, that of flavonoids, and finally that specific to flavonolignans, which begins with the coupling of a flavonoid and a monolignol, possibly followed by intramolecular rearrangements.

Flavonolignans are produced mainly by oxidative coupling between a monolignol (generally coniferyl alcohol and a flavonoid). Their biosynthetic pathway includes a common element, *p*-coumaroyl-CoA, a key metabolite and precursor of multiple compounds, such as stilbenes, lignans, but also many phenolic compounds. The shikimate pathway generates the main metabolic flow of the flavonoid pathway. It provides the systemic phenylpropanoids pathway with a link with the primary metabolism in the form of L-phenylalanine [54]. The first enzyme acting on L -phenylalanine is L-phenylalanine ammonia lyase (PAL), followed by cinnamate 4-hydroxylase (C4H) and then *p*-coumarate-CoA ligase (4CL). These enzymes represent the first steps in the phenylpropanoid pathway and convert L-phenylalanine into a variety of secondary metabolites: lignin, lignans, coumarins, stilbenes and flavonoids [54–56].

The monolignols pathway allows the formation of various precursors, necessary for the formation of multiple phenylpropanoid compounds, such as lignin, lignans, neolignans, coumarins, flavonoids, stilbenes, etc. [57–61]. This pathway plays a central role in the secondary metabolism of plants [62]. Monolignols are synthesized from L-phenylalanine by the general route of phenylpropanoids. Several enzymatic steps are involved to obtain coniferyl alcohol, used in the biosynthesis of flavonolignans from purple milk thistle. Coniferyl alcohol is derived from the reduction of cinnamic acid by a NADPH-dependent reaction with coenzyme A, followed by aromatic hydroxylation and methylation (OMT). Then, the feruloyl-CoA is reduced by the enzyme cinnamoyl-CoA reductase to coniferyl aldehyde. The final step in the synthesis of coniferyl alcohol is catalyzed by cinnamyl alcohol dehydrogenase (CAD). This enzyme also catalyzes the final step in monomer biosynthesis, also synthesizing *p*-coumaryl alcohol and sinapyl alcohol. Monolignols are mainly known to be the precursors of lignin. The main components of lignin are derived from hydroxycinnamyl alcohols (or monolignols), such as coniferyl alcohol, sinapyl alcohol and *p*-coumaryl alcohol (usually present in minor amounts). The existence of these three monolignols is responsible for the significant structural variety of lignin within plant species [63]. The units resulting from these monolignols, when incorporated into the lignin polymer, are called guaiacyl (G), syringyl (S) and p-hydroxyphenyl (H) units and play a crucial role in the process of lignification. Lignin is one of the most common biopolymers along with cellulose [45, 64]. These three alcohols are also involved in the synthesis of certain flavonolignans, at present, the contribution of *p*-coumaryl alcohol and sinapyl alcohol remains largely less widespread than that of coniferyl alcohol. However, interest in flavonolignans continues to increase and there is no indication that other flavonolignans, derived from these two alcohols, will not be discovered.

Flavonoids include more than 9,000 known structures [54] and are found in almost all plant tissue [65]. The flavonoid pathway is a major branch of the phenylpropanoid pathway and therefore has the same enzymes, PAL, C4H and 4CL, involved in the early stages of the phenylpropanoid pathway, to obtain monolignols. Generally, in plants, chalcones are not the end products. These compounds go through several enzymatic steps before giving rise to other classes of flavonoids, such as dihydroflavonols, flavanols or anthocyanins, the main water-soluble pigments of flowers and fruits [66]. Certain classes of flavonoids, (namely isoflavones,

flavones, pro-anthocyanidins and flavonols) represent secondary branches of the flavonoid pathway and are derived from intermediates that allow the formation of anthocyanins [66]. Flavonoids play a large number of roles and perform certain functions [67–70]: 1) pigmentation of flowers, fruits and seeds, 2) protection against ultraviolet rays, 3) defense of plants against pathogens, microorganisms, 4) plant fertility and pollen germination.

In *S. marianum*, the precursor of silymarin, the flavanonol taxifolin, belongs to the flavonoids. After being formed through the phenylpropanoid, *p*-coumaroyl-CoA serves as a starting precursor for the biosynthesis of flavonoids. The *p*-coumaroyl-CoA molecule is associated with 3 units of malonyl-CoA, thanks to chalcone synthase (CHS) which catalyzes the reaction to give the naringenin chalcone [45]. The latter is a chalcone containing two aromatic rings. Subsequent cyclization results in other flavonoids [71].

In the next step, chalcone isomerase (CHI) converts chalcones into flavanones (naringenin, eriodictyol and dihydrotricin) and vice versa. For the rest of the biosynthesis leading to the flavanonols, the naringenin obtained can be hydroxylated twice, (once in the C3 position and a second time in the C3' position) to obtain taxifolin (2,3-dihydroquercetin). The synthesis of taxifolin involves two enzymes flavanones-3-hydroxylases (F3H and F3'H) which allow the two successive hydroxylation steps from naringerin. The F3H enzyme belongs to the family of 2-oxoglutarate-dependent dioxygenases. It is highly conserved in plant species [72, 73]. Hydroxylation at the C3 position of flavanones to dihydroflavonols has been demonstrated in a wide variety of plant species, including *Petunia hybrida*, *Antirrhinum majus* or *Zea mays* [74, 75].

Silymarin flavonolignans are supposed derived from taxifolin and coniferyl alcohol by one of the two proposed mechanisms: 1) the traditional Freudenburg hypothesis or 2) Althagafy's proposal.

The Freudenburg hypothesis suggests an oxidative coupling reaction between taxifolin and coniferyl alcohol, induced by the formation of free radicals, and probably catalyzed by an enzyme of the peroxidase or laccase type, known to generate radicals [52]. Mechanically, the reaction assumes the formation of two distinct radicals, one at the phenoxyl group of taxifolin, and the other at the side chain of coniferyl alcohol, leading to a very reactive quinone methide intermediate [45]. The free radical of taxifolin therefore couples with the quinone methide radical, generated from coniferyl alcohol, to produce a molecule via a mechanism which is neither regio- nor enantioselective [76, 77]. The last step in biosynthesis is therefore a thermodynamically controlled nucleophilic attack, of a free intramolecular hydroxyl group, on the quinone methide nucleus of the monolignol part. Some rearrangement and cyclization are necessary to lead to the two molecules of diastereomeric flavonolignans, called silybins A and B. The *O-β* coupling step is neither regio- nor enantioselective [42, 45, 78]. Similar radical coupling could also result in the formation of regioisomers, isosilybin A and isosilybin B isolated from *S. marianum* [71].

Besides the regioisomer of silybin, two other isomers, silychristin and silydianin, having different binding modes between dihydroflavonol and coniferyl alcohol, have been described. In both cases, these two molecules are derived from a mesomer of the free radical derived from taxifolin [52].

Silychristin illustrates another structural variant of flavonolignans, with the formation of a furan nucleus [71]. This structure would be obtained via a mesomerism of the taxifolin radical which differs from that allowing the synthesis of silybins and isosilybins. There is a resonance form of taxifolin where the unpaired electron is located on the carbon of the B ring at position 4′ depending on the original 4-hydroxyl [76]. It is this difference in the resonance shape of taxifolin that allows the formation of the furan ring. In the case of silydianin, the mesomerism of taxifolin is analogous to that allowing the production of silybins and isosilybins, with the unpaired electron located on the carbon of the B ring at position 3′ [76]. But its unique and more complex structure suggests a more complicated mechanism [76]. Indeed, the only significant difference here lies in the formation of two new C-C bonds during the radical coupling during which the product cyclizes again, thus creating a bi-cyclo structure [79]. Subsequently, an intramolecular attack of an enolate on quinone methide (hemiacetalization) occurs, thus forming the original ketone-hemiketal structure of silydianin [76, 79].

However, Althagafy suggests, based on a biomimetic synthesis of the 4 major flavonolignans of silymarin (silybins and isosilybins), that the latter would be produced by a different mechanism, via the coupling of coniferyl alcohol and taxifolin [80]. There would be the formation of an intermediate quinone methide, via an oxidation causing the loss of an electron on the coniferyl alcohol. This intermediate would then add to taxifolin, via one of its hydroxyl groups, at the level of its catechol part. A second oxidation would allow the synthesis of silybins and isosilybins constituting silymarin. This is contrary to the mechanism proposed by Freudenburg for this process. Althagafy et al. [80], exclusively studied oxidative couplings carried out using silver (I) oxide (Ag_2O) instead of enzyme, to form flavonolignans. It is postulated that a similar reaction mechanism could occur in the biosynthesis of flavonolignans *in vivo*.

Although the Althagafy hypothesis is shown to be functional *in vitro*, it does not offer any hypothesis on the mechanism of silydianin or silychristin biosynthesis. This second hypothesis focuses exclusively on silybins and isosilybins, which are the major components of silymarin.

The protein(s) responsible for the formation of flavonolignans, during the oxidative coupling step between taxifolin and coniferyl alcohol, remains to be identified. As stated above, the reaction could take place via a radical coupling mechanism by the intervention of oxidative radical-forming enzymes, such as peroxidases or laccases [38]. These enzymes are associated with the formation of monolignol radicals, with polymerization during lignification and lignan synthesis [38]. These two types of enzymes cause electron loss by catalyzing the oxidation of phenolic substrates [61], especially monolignols such as coniferyl alcohol, *p*-coumaryl alcohol and alcohol. Sinapylic thus leading to the formation of radicals with a view to their polymerization [81]. Peroxidases are among the most common and widespread enzymes. Many peroxidases incorporate an iron-porphyrin (heme) derivative at the heart of their active site. They can catalyze the oxidation of a wide variety of organic compounds using hydrogen peroxide (H_2O_2) [82]. The most studied function of peroxidases is their role in the polymerization of lignin (polymer constituent of the plant cell wall). Peroxidases have been shown to catalyze the polymerization of lignin monomers (*p*-coumaryl alcohol, coniferyl alcohol, and sinapyl alcohol) *in vitro* to form a lignin-like polymer [83]. Peroxidases are very widespread, especially in Arabidopsis where around 73 different peroxidase genes have been identified [84, 85]. So far, the expression of 23 peroxidases has been studied in different organs of this plant [85]. Numerous examples of functional characterization *in vivo* confirm this role in planta [86]. A peroxidase potentially involved in the formation of flavonolignans could be structured in the same way as class III peroxidases [45, 87]. Extracellular peroxidases are believed to be also responsible for the oxidation of taxifolin [88, 89]. Laccases are widely distributed oxidases, harboring a multi-copper center, among plants, insects and fungi [90]. They are mainly monomeric, dimeric or tetrameric glycoproteins [91]. These enzymes catalyze oxidations on a wide variety of organic and inorganic substrates, in particular mono-, di- and polyphenols, with simultaneous reduction of oxygen to water by 4 electrons from their multi-copper center [92]. These oxidases play a role in the degradation, but also in the formation of polymers of lignin, by promoting the oxidative coupling of monolignol units [45]. In comparison with peroxidases, besides the different structural aspects, laccases are generally considered to have a lower oxidative power than that of peroxidases [93].

The proposed biosynthetic sequence leading to flavonolignans accumulation in *S. marianum* fruit is summarized in **Figure 8**.

A recent study on the spatial organization of silybin biosynthesis in *S. marianum* demonstrated, through biomimetic synthesis, that peroxidase and laccase can both

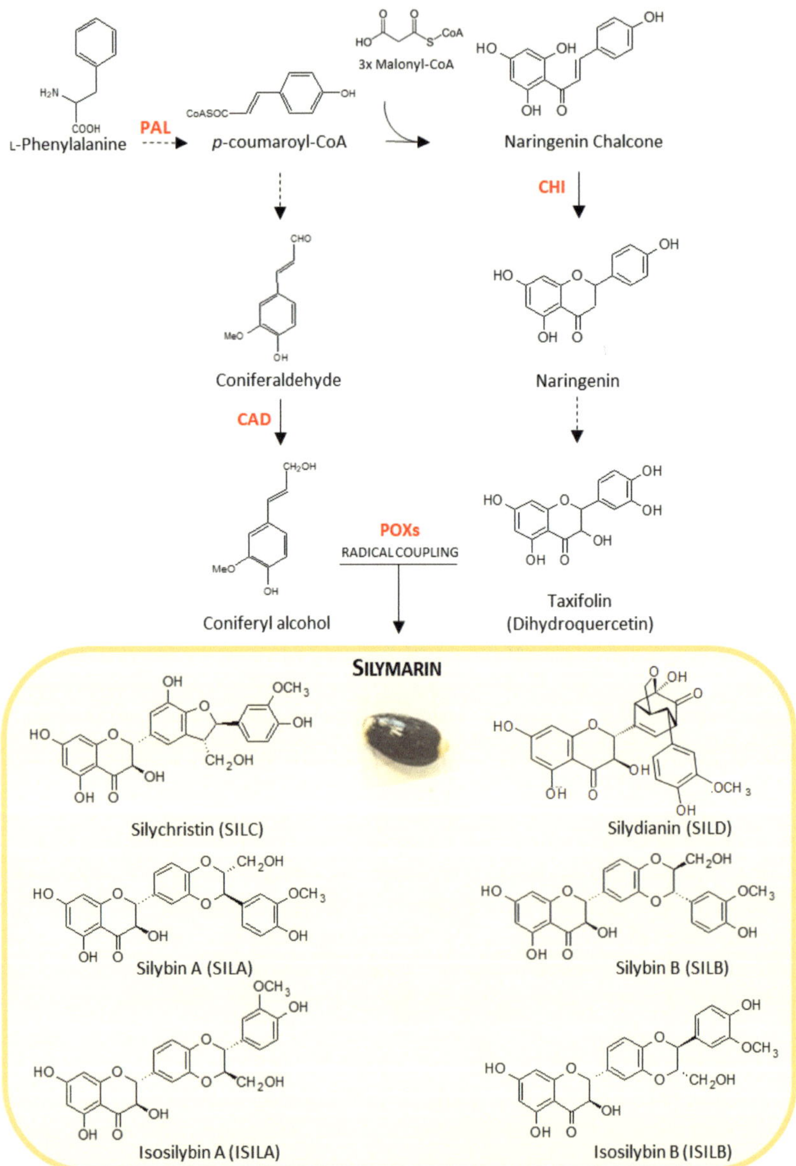

Figure 8.
Partial scheme of the silymarin (SILM) flavonolignans biosynthesis pathway in S. marianum. *Flavonolignans are mainly accumulated in mature achenes (yellow box). In red are presented genes potentially involved in this pathway: PAL (L-phenylalanine ammonia-lyase), CAD (cinnamyl alcohol dehydrogenase), CHS (chalcone synthase), flavanone 3-dioxygenase (F3H), flavone 3′-hydroxylase (F3′H), LAC (laccases) and POX (peroxidases). The dotted arrows indicate a single step, while dashed arrows indicate several steps in the metabolic pathway while the full arrows indicate direct synthesis of the compound through an enzyme.*

catalyze silybin synthesis [94]. This study was further developed by identifying, through an RNAseq sequencing study, five peroxidase candidates involved in the production of silybins and isolybins. Among these, APX1 (ascorbate peroxidase 1) exhibits distinct peroxidase activity and the ability to synthesize silybins [94]. This first step provides a better understanding of the biosynthesis of silybin and other flavonolignans. Despite these encouraging results, it is still unknown, at this time, whether peroxidases are the only enzymes involved in the final stage of flavonolignan biosynthesis [88, 89]. Based on these results, two different coupling modes can be suggested, depending on the type of flavonolignan obtained. One would involve a classic, simple coupling, while the other would be a more complex coupling, with complementary proteins depending on the flavonolignans synthesized, suggesting the possible intervention of dirigent proteins (DIRs).

The two mechanisms proposed above are radical types. They are therefore, a priori, non-stereospecific and non-regioselective, which implies a wide variety of possibilities at the coupling level, and therefore of the isomers formed. Based on this information, the diastereomers of silybin and isosilybin are described as equimolar mixtures reflecting the lack of stereospecificity of the initial radical couplings [76, 95]. Among the available experimental data, none confirms the 1: 1 ratio between these diastereoisomeric couples [31, 37, 88, 96, 97]. Also, the theory of random radical coupling cannot explain the proportions obtained in the mixture of silymarin, since in certain genotypes, silydianin is practically non-existent [37, 88, 97]. An important question then arises on the biosynthetic pathway of flavonolignans [45] is how to explain the strong disparities observed during the quantification of the constituents of silymarin in the fruits of various origins of milk thistle since 3 distinct chemotypes have already been described in *S. marianum* based on their phytochemical diversity in silymarin [37–39, 52].

The in-depth study of these chemotypes could provide important information on the biosynthetic pathways leading to the different flavonolignans of silymarin. This could allow relational models to be established, based on the levels of metabolites in chemotypes, to infer the presence of steps in a metabolic pathway [88]. To study flavonolignans from a scientific point of view, it would be interesting to understand the underlying mechanism allowing to obtain the different chemotypes and positional isomers in *S. marianum*, and more generally. Despite the hypotheses made and studied about the biosynthesis of flavonolignans, little investigation has been carried out on how the proportional differences of isomers arise, and how the plant differentiates them [45]. In 1995, the discovery of DIRs by Davin and Lewis opened up new perspectives on how free radical coupling of plant phenols is controlled in the production of lignans and lignin [98]. DIRs, by their abundance, would be the first essential elements of phenoxy-radical couplings. The first action hypotheses of these proteins concerned the stereoselective biosynthesis of (+)-pinoresinol from coniferyl alcohol monomers. Coniferyl alcohol (or the resulting radical) was oriented and directed by a DIR and allowed specific synthesis of (+)-pinoresinol during bimolecular coupling [99]. Until recently, DIRs were not considered as enzymes, due to their lack of oxidative activity. The proper binding and orientation of the substrate radicals appeared sufficient for DIR activity. In 2016, the structure of the AtDIR6 from *Arabidopsis thaliana* confirms that DIRs are actively involved and that they have a catalytic function in the cyclization step of the quinone methide intermediate [45, 100, 101]. This has been attributed to the active donation of protons by the formation of hydrogen bonds or by acid catalysis [100]. Other DIRs have been identified, notably in *Arabidopsis thaliana*, with DIR responsible for the enantioselective synthesis of (−)-pinoresinol [102]. Other DIRs have been described in other plant species including flax [103], *Schisandra* [102, 104] or *Isatis indigotica* [105]. In *Gossypium hirsutum* (cotton), a leader protein has been characterized. It is involved in the stereoselective coupling of hemigossypol in the formation of the terpene (+)-gossypol [106, 107]. In 2018, the study of the leader proteins of *Linum usitatissimum* made it possible to highlight around forty DIRs in the flax genome [103] and to identify new conserved motifs linked to functions specific biochemicals. The mechanism of reactions by oxidative coupling leading to the accumulation of different steroisomers in the synthesis of flavonolignans and lignans, in *S. marianum*, makes possible the hypothesis of the involvement of DIRs [53, 108].

5. Regulation of flavonolignans biosynthesis in *Silybum marianum*

The genes, the expression of which has been studied in milk thistle, are the genes involved in the formation of precursors to taxifolin and coniferyl alcohol. The mixture of flavonolignans from Milk Thistle mainly accumulates in the pericarp of the fruit of milk thistle. It is therefore necessary to wait several months for the plant to produce its fruits and the molecules of interest. Experiments have shown that the accumulation of silymarin in the fruits of *S. marianum* is associated with the ripening process. The study of gene expression in milk thistle fruit is very recent. So far, it has only concerned 5 genes, involved in the pathway of flavonoids biosynthesis, *CHS* [109, 110], *CHI*, *F3H*, *F3'H* and *CAD* [108, 111]. The objective was to verify their roles in the biosynthesis of flavonolignans. These first functional studies showed the potential association of these genes in the synthesis of silymarin, because their expression coincides with the accumulation of taxifolin in fruits. In addition, induction of the *CAD* gene appears to be necessary for the accumulation of silymarin in ripe fruits [108, 111].

Recently, Drouet et al. [108] precisely described development stages of fruit to study the kinetics of accumulation of silymarin constituents during fruit ripening (**Figure 9**). During fruit maturation, the accumulation profiles of the silymarin components were evaluated by LC–MS analysis at each of the development stages identified [108]. Reference genes have been identified, selected and validated to allow accurate gene expression profiling of candidate biosynthetic genes [108]. Enzyme activity and biosynthetic gene expression indicated a possible in situ biosynthesis of silymarin from L-Phenylalanine during fruit ripening [108]. The gene expression profiles were well correlated with silymarin kinetic accumulation and preferential location in pericarp during *S. marianum* fruit maturation, reaching maximum biosynthesis when desiccation occurs [108]. This observation led us to consider the possible involvement of abscisic acid (ABA), a key phytohormone in fruit ripening control, for which accumulation timing and location during fruit ripening were consistent with the potential regulation of the silymarin accumulation. This possible transcriptional regulation of silymarin biosynthesis by ABA was further supported by the presence of ABA-responsive *cis*-acting elements in the silymarin biosynthetic gene promoter regions studied [108].

Biotechnological approaches have been used to increase the production of these molecules *in vitro*. The *in vitro* culture of a plant is a possible source of secondary metabolites. The use of in vitro models makes it possible to overcome the constraints of plant growth and makes it possible to have a biomass containing the molecules of interest more quickly. The cell models used aim to increase the yields of flavonolignans, by optimizing their biosynthesis. The main objective is therefore to modify the expression of one or more genes, or/and to elicit cultures, to overcome the steps limiting the accumulation of these compounds in the biosynthetic pathway [111]. However, one of the major constraints is the limited information available on the coupling of flavonolignans, for the genes and proteins involved.

A.

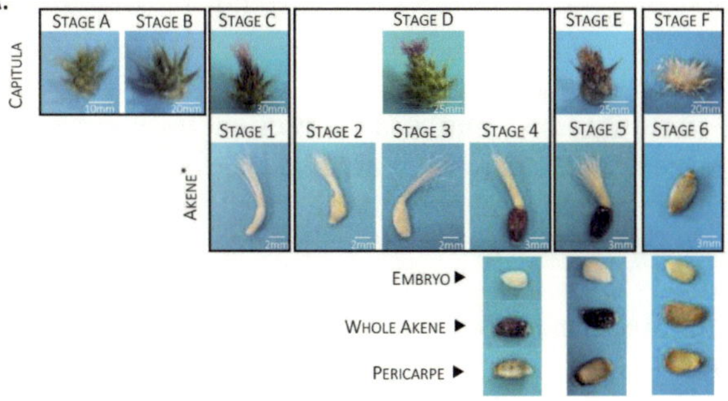

B.

DEVELOPMENT STAGES	DAY AFTER FLOWERING	WHOLE AKENE FW (mg)	PERICARPE FW (mg)	EMBRYO FW (mg)	LENGHT (mm)	MORPHOLOGICAL FEATURES
WA1	7	4.83±0.20	4.83±0.20	-	3.8	White akene without visible embryo
WA2	10	7.70±0.36	7.70±0.36	-	5	White akene without visible embryo
WA3	15	9.53±0.09	9.53±0.09	-	6	White akene without visible embryo
WA4	24	38.10±1.68	30.17±1.79	7.93±0.27	6	Akene color purple/brown
WA5	32	45.50±0.47	23.83±1.97	21.67±1.65	6	Color of akene darker
WA6	50	29.13±1.28	13.33±0.84	15.80±1.40	6.3	Dry mature akene

Figure 9.
Development stages of the S. marianum *achene defined according to their morphological characteristic. (A) Six achene developmental stages were defined. For the developmental stages 4, 5 and 6 achenes were manually dissected to allow the visualization of both seed and pericarp. The capitula morphology corresponding to each defined achene developmental stage is presented. Note that the capitula morphology is not predictive of the fruit developmental stage. (B) Morphological features of achene maturation during time such as achene, seed, and pericarp length, dry weight (DW) and day of flowering (DAF). Each value represents means ± SD of n = 10 independent sampling.*

S. marianum in vitro cultures can constitute an alternative and renewable source of this natural product. However, the concentration of silymarin in this type of crop is often lower than that found naturally in fruit [111, 112]. A higher accumulation was observed in cell suspensions obtained from calli [113]. To obtain silymarin in sufficiently high concentrations for commercial purposes, techniques have been proposed to stimulate its production in calli and cultured cells of *S. marianum*, via the use of elicitors or by the addition of precursors. The elicited systems are a starting point in improving the production of silymarin for industrial purposes. Elicitation is one of the most effective approaches to increase the yield of secondary metabolites in *in vitro* cultures [114]. It modulates the rates of biosynthesis and accumulation [112, 115]. The use of stress mediators such as methyl jasmonate, exposure to certain lights [116, 117], auxin, [118], yeast extracts, chitosan [119], cyclodextrin, strongly induce the extracellular accumulation of coniferyl alcohol and Silymarin [111, 120]. The "feeding" experiments consisting in providing the initial substrates to increase the content of flavonolignans are less conclusive. Coniferyl alcohol added to cultures allows for a significant and more surprisingly increase in silydianin, but no other component of silymarin has been detected [121].

Hairy root cultures have multiple advantages, in particular their genetic/biochemical stability and the ability to rapidly produce large biomasses [112].

Hairy roots are roots of plant tissue obtained by genetic transformation using a bacteria naturally present in the soil, *Agrobacterium rhizogenes*. Hairy root cultures of *S. marianum* have been established [122–124]. Elicitation experiments have been undertaken on this model. Salicylic acid is effective in increasing the content of flavonolignans, the content of linoleic acid and the activity of lipoxygenase (an important enzyme in jasmonate biosynthesis) in hairy root crops [125]. It is therefore likely that elicitation by salicylic acid regulates the jasmonate pathway which in turn mediates the accumulation of silymarin [125].

A recent and comprehensive review summarized these different biotechnological strategies [126].

6. Conclusions

Many experiments have provided a deeper understanding of the biosynthesis and control of silymarin flavonolignans from *S. marianum* over the last decade. However, to completely take advantage of their multiple biological activities, including antioxidant activity, for pharmaceutical and/or cosmeceutical uses, this view is still partial and further study is needed. To allow a better understanding of the biosynthetic steps leading to these flavonolignans, more detailed enzymatic and genetic studies are therefore needed. Only a thorough and comprehensive understanding of the metabolic regulation of these pathways in *S. marianum* can make it possible to identify andpromote their accumulations, the limiting steps and key points toward their regulation on which it will be possible to act.

Acknowledgements

S.D. acknowledges research fellowships of Loire Valley Region. This research was part of the MariLine project (grant number ICO16029) focusing on the cosmetic application of the milk thistle flavonolignans, supported by Cosmetosciences, a global training and research program dedicated to the cosmetic industry. Located in the heart of the cosmetic valley, this program led by University of Orléans is funded by the Region Centre-Val de Loire.

Conflict of interest

The authors declare no conflict of interest.

Author details

Samantha Drouet and Christophe Hano*
LBLGC, INRAE USC1328, University of Orleans, Chartres, France

*Address all correspondence to: hano@univ-orleans.fr

References

[1] Raskin I, Ribnicky DM, Komarnytsky S, Ilic N, Poulev A, Borisjuk N, et al. Plants and human health in the 21st century. Trends Biotechnol [Internet]. 2002;20(12):522-531. Available from: http://tibtech.trends.com

[2] Shipley GP, Kindscher K. Evidence for the Paleoethnobotany of the Neanderthal: A Review of the Literature. Scientifica (Cairo). 2016;2016:1-12.

[3] Ma JKC, Chikwamba R, Sparrow P, Fischer R, Mahoney R, Twyman RM. Plant-derived pharmaceuticals - The road forward. Trends Plant Sci. 2005;10(12):580-585.

[4] Karkanis A, Bilalis D, Efthimiadou A. Cultivation of milk thistle (*Silybum marianum* L. Gaertn.), a medicinal weed. Ind Crops Prod [Internet]. 2011;34(1):825-30. Available from: http://dx.doi.org/10.1016/j.indcrop.2011.03.027

[5] Shaker E, Mahmoud H, Mnaa S. Silymarin, the antioxidant component and Silybum marianum extracts prevent liver damage. Food Chem Toxicol [Internet]. 2010;48(3):803-806. Available from: http://dx.doi.org/10.1016/j.fct.2009.12.011

[6] Bijak M. Silybin, a Major Bioactive Component of Milk Thistle (Silybum marianum L. Gaernt.)—Chemistry, Bioavailability, and Metabolism. Molecules. 2017;22(11):1942.

[7] Abenavoli L, Capasso R, Milic N, Capasso F. Milk Thistle in Liver Diseases: Past, Present, Future. Phyther Res. 2010;24(June):1423-1432.

[8] Urtasun R, Rosa LC de la, Nieto N. Oxidative and Nitrosative Stress and Fibrogenic Response. Clin Livers Dis. 2008;12(4).

[9] Wu D, Yotnda P. Production and Detection of Reactive Oxygen Species (ROS) in Cancers. J Vis Exp. 2011;(57):2-5.

[10] Pradhan S, Girish C. Hepatoprotective herbal drug, silymarin from experimental pharmacology to clinical medicine. Indian J Med Res. 2006;124:491-504.

[11] Detaille D, Sanchez C, Sanz N, Lopez-Novoa JM, Leverve X, El-Mir MY. Interrelation between the inhibition of glycolytic flux by silibinin and the lowering of mitochondrial ROS production in perifused rat hepatocytes. Life Sci. 2008;82(21-22):1070-1076.

[12] Polyak SJ, Morishima C, Lohmann V, Pal S, Lee DYW, Liu Y, et al. Identi fi cation of hepatoprotective fl avonolignans from silymarin. 2010;107(13).

[13] Drouet S, Leclerc EA, Garros L, Tungmunnithum D, Kabra A, Abbasi BH, et al. A Green Ultrasound-Assisted Extraction Optimization of the Natural Antioxidant and Anti-Aging Flavonolignans from Milk Thistle Silybum marianum (L .) Gaertn . Fruits for Cosmetic Applications. Antioxidants. 2019;8(304):1-19.

[14] Karimi G, Vahabzadeh M, Lari P, Rashedinia M, Moshiri M. Silymarin, a promising pharmacological agent for treatment of diseases. Iran J Basic Med Sci. 2011;14(4):308-317.

[15] Katiyar SK. Silymarin and skin cancer prevention: Anti-inflammatory, antioxidant and immunomodulatory effects (Review). Int J Oncol. 2005;26:169-176.

[16] Katiyar SK, Meleth S, Sharma SD. Silymarin, a flavonoid from milk thistle (Silybum marianum L.), inhibits UV-induced oxidative stress through

targeting infiltrating CD11b+cells in mouse skin. Photochem Photobiol. 2008;84(2):266-271.

[17] Meeran SM, Katiyar S, Elmets C a, Katiyar SK. Silymarin inhibits UV radiation-induced immunosuppression through augmentation of interleukin-12 in mice. Mol Cancer Ther. 2006;5(7):1660-1668.

[18] Toklu HZ, Tunali-Akbay T, Erkanli G, Yüksel M, Ercan F, Şener G. Silymarin, the antioxidant component of Silybum marianum, protects against burn-induced oxidative skin injury. Burns. 2007;33(7):908-916.

[19] Rajnochová A, Eva S, Jitka G, Bohumil U, David Z. A pilot study of the UVA - photoprotective potential of dehydrosilybin , isosilybin , silychristin , and silydianin on human dermal fibroblasts. Arch Dermatol Res [Internet]. 2019; Available from: https://doi.org/10.1007/s00403-019-01928-7

[20] Gažák R, Purchartová K, Marhol P, Živná L, Petr Sedmera, Valentová K, et al. Antioxidant and antiviral activities of silybin fatty acid conjugates. Eur J Med Chem. 2010;45:1059-1067.

[21] Zarrelli A, Romanucci V, Greca M Della, De Napoli L, Previtera L, Di Fabio G. New silybin scaffold for chemical diversification: Synthesis of novel 23-phosphodiester silybin conjugates. SYNLETT. 2013;24(1):45-48.

[22] Zarrelli A, Romanucci V, Tuccillo C, Federico A, Loguercio C, Gravante R, et al. New silibinin glyco-conjugates: Synthesis and evaluation of antioxidant properties. Bioorganic Med Chem Lett [Internet]. 2014;24(22):5147-5149. Available from: http://dx.doi.org/10.1016/j.bmcl.2014.10.023

[23] Drouet S, Doussot J, Garros L, Mathiron D, Bassard S, Favre-Réguillon A, et al. Selective Synthesis of 3-O-Palmitoyl-Silybin, a New-to-Nature Flavonolignan with Increased Protective Action against Oxidative Damages in Lipophilic Media. Molecules. 2018;23(10):2594.

[24] Bonnier G, Douin R. La grande flore. Belin, editor. 1990.

[25] Drouet S, Garros L, Hano C, Lainé É. A Critical View of Different Botanical , Molecular , and Chemical Techniques Used in Authentication of Plant Materials for Cosmetic Applications. 2018;

[26] International C. CABI, 2018. Invasive species compendium [Internet]. 2018. Available from: http://www.cabi.org/isc/

[27] W.E Safford. The Flora of Banda Oriental. In: Bulletin of the Torrey Botanical Club [Internet]. New York : Torrey Botanical Club,; 1887 [cited 2019 Apr 12]. p. 159-64. Available from: https://www.biodiversitylibrary.org/item/7990

[28] Canter PH, Thomas H, Ernst E. Bringing medicinal plants into cultivation: Opportunities and challenges for biotechnology. Trends Biotechnol. 2005;23(4):180-185.

[29] Andrzejewska J, Sadowska K. Effect of cultivation conditions on the variability and interrelation of yield and raw material quality in Milk thistle (Silybum marianum (L.) GAERTN.). Acta Sci Pol Agric. 2008;7(3):3-11.

[30] Andrzejewska J, Sadowska K, Mielcarek S. Effect of sowing date and rate on the yield and flavonolignan content of the fruits of milk thistle (Silybum marianum L. Gaertn.) grown on light soil in a moderate climate. Ind Crops Prod [Internet]. 2011;33(2):462-468. Available from: http://dx.doi.org/10.1016/j.indcrop.2010.10.027

[31] Carrier DJ, Crowe T, Sokhansanj S, Wahab J, Branka B. Milk Thistle,

Silybum marianum (L.) Gaertn., flower head development and associated marker compound profile. J Herbs, Spices Med Plants. 2003;10(1):65-74.

[32] Parsons WT, Cuthbertson EG. Noxious Weeds of Australia. Inkata Pre. 1992.

[33] Greenlee H, Abascal K, Yarnell E, Ladas E. Clinical applications of Silybum marianum in oncology. Integr Cancer Ther. 2007;6(2): 158-165.

[34] Pelter A, Hansel R. The structure of silybin (Silybum substance E6), the first flavonolignan. Tetrahedron Lett. 1968;1(25):2911-2916.

[35] Rauter AP, Ennis M, Hellwich K-H, Herold BJ, Horton D, Moss GP, et al. Nomenclature of flavonoids (IUPAC Recommendations 2017). Vol. 90, Pure and Applied Chemistry. 2018. 1429-1486 p.

[36] Kroll DJ, Shaw HS, Oberlies NH, Kroll BDJ, Shaw HS, Oberlies NH. Milk thistle nomenclature: why it matters in cancer research and pharmacokinetic studies. Integr Cancer Ther. 2007;6(2):110-119.

[37] Martin RJ, Lauren DR, Smith WA, Jensen DJ, Deo B, Douglas JA, et al. Factors influencing silymarin content and composition in variegated thistle (Silybum marianum). New Zeal J Crop Hortic Sci. 2006;34(3):239-245.

[38] Poppe L, Petersen M. Variation in the flavonolignan composition of fruits from different *Silybum marianum* chemotypes and suspension cultures derived therefrom. Phytochemistry [Internet]. 2016;131:68-75. Available from: http://dx.doi.org/10.1016/j.phytochem.2016.09.003

[39] Radjabian T, Rezazadeh SH, Huseini HF. Analysis of silymarin components in the seed extracts of some milk thistle ecotypes from Iran by HPLc. Iran J Sci Technol. 2008;32:6-8.

[40] Delfini M, Cocco MED, Gaggelli E, Lepri A, Valensin G. H-1 delineation of conformational parameters of constituents of silybum marianum in solution. Spectrosc Lett. 1990;23(8):1007-1025.

[41] Hansel R, Janiak VB. Phytochemisch-pharmakognostische untersuchungen über fructus Cardui mariae. Planta Med. 1960;8:71-84.

[42] Nam-Cheol K, Graf TN, Sparacino CM, Wani MC, Wall ME. Complete isolation and structure identification of hepatoprotective flavonolignans silybins and isosilybins from the medicinal herb milk thistle (Silybum marianum). Org Biomol Chem. 2003;1:1684-1689.

[43] Wagner H, Diesel P, Seitz M. The chemistry and analysis of silymarin from *Silybum marianum* Gaertn. Arzneimittelforschung [Internet]. 1974;24(4):466—471. Available from: http://europepmc.org/abstract/MED/4408125

[44] Wagner H, Hörhammer L, Münster R. On the chemistry of silymarin (silybin), the active principle of the fruits from Silybum marianum (L.) Gaertn. (Carduus marianus L.). Naturwissenschaften [Internet]. 1965;18(6):688—696. Available from: http://europepmc.org/abstract/MED/5755805

[45] Poppe L. Thesis: Flavonolignan Biosynthesis in *Silybum marianum* – Potential Regulatory Mechanisms and Candidate Genes. 2017.

[46] Csupor D, Csorba A, Hohmann J, Cuspor DD, Csorba A, Hohmann J. Recent advances in the analysis of flavonolignans of Silybum marianum. J Pharm Biomed Anal. 2016;130:301-317.

[47] Abouzid S, Ahmed OM. Silymarin flavonolignans: Structure-activity relationship and biosynthesis. 1st ed. Vol. 40, Studies in Natural Products Chemistry. © 2013 Elsevier B.V. All rights reserved.; 2013. 469-484 p.

[48] Lee DY, Liu Y. Molecular structure and stereochemistry of Silybin A, Silybin B , Isosilybin , and Isosilybin B, isolated from Silybum marianum (Milk Thistle). J Nat Prod. 2003;66:1171-1174.

[49] Althagafy HS, Meza-Aviña ME, Oberlies NH, Croatt MP. Mechanistic study of the biomimetic synthesis of flavonolignan diastereoisomers in milk thistle. J Org Chem. 2013;78(15):7594-7600.

[50] Napolitano JG, Lankin DC, Graf TN, Brent Friesen J, Chen SN, McAlpine JB, et al. HiFSA fingerprinting applied to isomers with near-identical NMR Spectra: The silybin/isosilybin case. J Org Chem. 2013;78(7):2827-2839.

[51] Smith WA, Lauren DR, Burgess EJ, Perry NB, Martin RJ. A silychristin isomer and variation of flavonolignan levels in milk thistle (Silybum marianum) fruits. Planta Med. 2005;71(9):877-880.

[52] Chambers CS, Hole V, Petrásková L, Biedermann D, Buchta M, Vladimír K. The silymarin composition ... and why does it matter??? Food Res Int. 2017;100(July):339-353.

[53] Drouet S, Abbasi BH, Falguières A, Ahmad W, Sumaira, Ferroud C, et al. Single Laboratory Validation of a Quantitative Core Shell-Based LC Separation for the Evaluation of Silymarin Variability and Associated Antioxidant Activity of Pakistani Ecotypes of Milk Thistle (*Silybum marianum* L.). Molecules. 2018;23(904).

[54] Bashandy H. Flavonoid metabolomics in Gerbera hybrida and elucidation of complexity in the flavonoid biosynthetic pathway. 2016.

[55] Tohge T, Watanabe M, Hoefgen R, Fernie AR. The evolution of phenylpropanoid metabolism in the green lineage. Crit Rev Biochem Mol Biol. 2013;48(2):123-152.

[56] Winkel-shirley B. Flavonoid Biosynthesis. A Colorful Model for Genetics, Biochemistry, Cell Biology, and Biotechnology. Plant Physiol. 2001;126(June):485-493.

[57] Attoumbre J, Hano C, Mesnard F, Lamblin F, Bensaddek L, Raynaud-Le Grandic S, et al. Identification by NMR and accumulation of a neolignan, the dehydrodiconiferyl alcohol-4-$β$-D-glucoside, in *Linum usitatissimum* cell cultures. Comptes Rendus Chim. 2006;9(3-4).

[58] Hano C, Addi M, Bensaddek L, Crônier D, Baltora-Rosset S, Doussot J, et al. Differential accumulation of monolignol-derived compounds in elicited flax (Linum usitatissimum) cell suspension cultures. Planta. 2006 Apr;223(5):975-989.

[59] Martins V, Garcia A, Costa C, Sottomayor M, Gerós H. Calcium- and hormone-driven regulation of secondary metabolism and cell wall enzymes in grape berry cells. J Plant Physiol [Internet]. 2018;231(August):57-67. Available from: https://doi.org/10.1016/j.jplph.2018.08.011

[60] Umezawa T. Diversity in lignan biosynthesis. Phytochem Rev. 2003;2(3):371-390.

[61] Vanholme R, Demedts B, Morreel K, Ralph J, Boerjan W. Lignin Biosynthesis and Structure. Plant Physiol. 2010;153(3):895-905.

[62] Umezawa T. The cinnamate/monolignol pathway. Phytochem Rev. 2010;9(1):1-17.

[63] Rodrigo CP, James WH, Zwier TS. Single-Conformation ultraviolet and infrared spectra of jet-cooled monolignols: P-coumaryl alcohol, coniferyl alcohol, and sinapyl alcohol. J Am Chem Soc. 2011;133(8):2632-2641.

[64] Freudenberg K, Neish AC. Constitution and biosynthesis of lignin. Springer. Science. Berlin; 1968.

[65] Martens S, Mithöfer A. Flavones and flavone synthases. Phytochemistry. 2005;66(20):2399-2407.

[66] Schijlen EGWM, Ric de Vos C, Tunen AJ Van, Bovy AG. Modification of flavonoid biosynthesis in crop plants. Phytochemistry. 2004;65:2631-2648.

[67] Dooner HK, Robbins TP, Jorgensen RA. Genetic and Developmental Control of Anthocy an in. Most. 1991;

[68] Spangenberg G. Flavonoids : a metabolic network mediating plants adaptation to their real estate. Front Plant Sci. 2014;5(November):1-16.

[69] Vasilev N, Schmitz C, Dong L, Ritala A, Imseng N, Häkkinen S, et al. Comparison of plant-based expression platforms for the heterologous production of geraniol. Plant Cell, Tissue Organ Cult [Internet]. 2014;117(3):373-80. Available from: http://dx.doi.org/10.1007/s11240-014-0446-z

[70] Winkel-shirley B. Biosynthesis of flavonoids and effects of stress. 2002;218-23.

[71] Begum S., Sahai M, Ray A. Non-conventional Lignans: Coumarinolignans, Flavonolignans, and Stilbenolignans. Kinghorn A., Falk H, Kobayashi J, editors. SpringerWienNewYork; 2010. 28-49 p.

[72] Britsch L, Dedio J, Saedler H, Forkmann G. Molecular characterization of flayanone 3β-hydroxylases: Consensus sequence, comparison with related enzymes and the role of conserved histidine residues. Eur J Biochem. 1993;217(2):745-754.

[73] Hall J, Ananga A, Georgiev V, Ochieng J, Cebert E, Tsolova V. Molecular Cloning, Characterization, and Expression Analysis of Flavanone 3-Hydroxylase (F3H) Gene during Muscadine Grape Berry Development. J Biotechnol Biomater [Internet]. 2015;05(02). Available from: http://www.omicsonline.org/open-access/molecular-cloning-characterization-and-expression-analysis-of-flavanone-3hydroxylase-f3h-gene-during-muscadine-grape-berry-development-2155-952X-1000180.php?aid=54383%0Ahttps://www.omicsonline.org/open-access/molecul

[74] Weiss D, van der Luit AH, Kroon JTM, Mol JNM, Kooter JM. The petunia homologue of the Antirrhinum majus candi and Zea mays A2 flavonoid genes; homology to flavanone 3-hydroxylase and ethylene-forming enzyme. Plant Mol Biol. 1993;22(5):893-897.

[75] Deboo GB, Albertsen MC, P.Taylor L. Flavanone 3-hydroxylase transcripts and flavonol accumulation are temporally coordinate in maize anthers. plant J. 1995;7(5):703-713.

[76] Dewick PM. The shikimate pathway: aromatic amino acids and phenylpropanoids. In: Medicinal Natural Products: A Biosynthetic Approach. John Wiley. 2007. p. 137-184.

[77] Merlini L, Zanarotti A, Pelter A, Rochefort MP, Hänsel R. Benzodioxans by oxidative phenol coupling. Synthesis of silybin. J Chem Soc, Perkin Trans 1. 1980;(0):775-778.

[78] Mascher H, Kikuta C, Weyhenmeyer R. Diastereomeric separation of free and conjugated

silibinin in plasma by reversed phase hplc after specific extraction. J Liq Chromatogr. 1993;16(13):2777-2789.

[79] Biedermann D, Moravcová V, Valentová K, Kuzma M, Petrásková L, Císařová I, et al. Oxidation of flavonolignan silydianin to unexpected lactone-acid derivative. Phytochem Lett [Internet]. 2019;30(October 2018):14-20. Available from: https://doi.org/10.1016/j.phytol.2019.01.006

[80] Althagafy HS, Meza-Aviña ME, Oberlies NH, Croatt MP. Mechanistic study of the biomimetic synthesis of flavonolignan diastereoisomers in milk thistle. J Org Chem. 2013;78(15):7594-7600.

[81] Kersten PJ, Kalyanaraman B, Hammel KE, Reinhammar B, Kirk TK. Comparison of lignin peroxidase, horseradish peroxidase and laccase in the oxidation of methoxybenzenes. Biochem J. 1990;268(2):475-480.

[82] Watanabe Y, Nakajima H. Creation of a Thermally Tolerant Peroxidase [Internet]. 1st ed. Vol. 580, Methods in Enzymology. Elsevier Inc.; 2016. 455-470 p. Available from: http://dx.doi.org/10.1016/bs.mie.2016.05.038

[83] Christensen JH, Montagu M Van, Bauw G, Boerjan W. Xylem peroxidases: Purification and altered expression. Prog Biotechnol. 2001;18(C):171-176.

[84] Tognolli M, Overney S, Penel C, Greppin H, Simon P. A genetic and enzymatic survey of *Arabidopsis thaliana* peroxidases. Plant Perox. 2000;

[85] Tognolli M, Penel C, Greppin H, Simon P. Analysis and expression of the class III peroxidase large gene family in Arabidopsis thaliana. Gene. 2002;288(1-2):129-138.

[86] Boerjan W, Ralph J, Baucher M. Lignin biosynthesis. Annu Rev Plant Biol [Internet]. 2003;54(1):519-546. Available from: http://www.annualreviews.org/doi/10.1146/annurev.arplant.54.031902.134938

[87] Veitch NC. Horseradish peroxidase: a modern view of a classic enzyme. Phytochemistry [Internet]. 2004;65(3):249-59. Available from: http://www.ncbi.nlm.nih.gov/pubmed/14751298

[88] Martinelli T, Whittaker A, Benedettelli S, Carboni A. The study of flavonolignan association patterns in fruits of diverging *Silybum marianum* (L.) Gaertn. chemotypes provides new insights into the silymarin biosynthetic pathway. Phytochemistry [Internet]. 2017;144:9-18. Available from: http://dx.doi.org/10.1016/j.phytochem.2017.08.013

[89] Sánchez-Sampedro A, Kim HK, Choi YH, Verpoorte R, Corchete P. Metabolomic alterations in elicitor treated Silybum marianum suspension cultures monitored by nuclear magnetic resonance spectroscopy. J Biotechnol. 2007;130(2):133-142.

[90] Yaropolov AI, Skorobogat'ko O V., Vartanov SS, Varfolomeyev S. Laccase: Properties, Catalytic Mechanism, and Applicability. Appl Biochem Biotechnol. 1994;49:257-280.

[91] Shraddha, Shekher R, Sehgal S, Kamthania M, Kumar A. Laccase: microbial sources, production, purification, and potential biotechnological applications. Enzyme Res [Internet]. 2011;2011:217861. Available from: http://www.ncbi.nlm.nih.gov/pubmed/21755038%0Ahttp://www.pubmedcentral.nih.gov/articlerender.fcgi?artid=PMC3132468

[92] Madhavi V, Lele SS. Laccase: Properties and applications. BioResources. 2009;4(4):1694-1717.

[93] Heinzkill M, Bech L, Halkier T, Schneider P, Anke T. Characterization

of laccases and peroxidases from wood-rotting fungi (family Coprinaceae). Appl Environ Microbiol. 1998;64(5):1601-1606.

[94] Lv Y, Gao S, Xu S, Du G, Zhou J, Chen J, et al. Spatial organization of silybin biosynthesis in milk thistle (Silybum marianum (L.) Gaertn.). Plant J. 2017;92:995-1004.

[95] Nyiredy S, Szücs Z, Antus S, Samu Z. New Components from Silybum marianum L.Fruits: A Theory Comes True. Chromatographia. 2008;68:5-11.

[96] Abouzid SF, Ahmed HS, Moawad AS, Owis AI, Chen S, Nachtergael A, et al. Chemotaxonomic and biosynthetic relationships between flavonolignans produced by Silybum marianum populations. Fitoterapia [Internet]. 2017;119(April):175-184. Available from: http://dx.doi.org/10.1016/j.fitote.2017.04.002

[97] Martinelli T, Potenza E, Moschella A, Zaccheria F, Benedettelli S, Andrzejewska J. Phenotypic Evaluation of a Milk Thistle Phenotypic Evaluation of a Milk Thistle Germplasm Collection: Fruit Morphology and Chemical Composition. Crop Sci. 2016;56(September).

[98] Davin LB, Lewis NG. Dirigent Proteins and Dirigent Sites Explain the Mystery of Specificity of Radical Precursor Coupling in Lignan and Lignin Biosynthesis. Plant Physiol. 2000;123:453-461.

[99] Davin LB, Wang H, Crowell AL, Bedgar DL, Martin DM, Sarkanen S, et al. Stereoselective Bimolecular Phenoxy Radical Coupling by Auxialiary (Dirigent) Protein Without an Active Center. Reports. 1997;275(16).

[100] Gasper R, Effenberger I, Kolesinski P, Terlecka B, Hofmann E, Schaller A. Dirigent Protein Mode of Action Revealed by the Crystal Structure of AtDIR6. Plant Physiol. 2016;172(4):2165-2175.

[101] Kim KW, Smith CA, Daily MD, Cort JR, Davin LB, Lewis NG. Trimeric structure of (+)-pinoresinol-forming dirigent protein at 1.95 A° resolution with three isolated active sites. J Biol Chem. 2015;290(3):1308-1318.

[102] Pickel B, Constantin MA, Pfannstiel J, Conrad J, Beifuss U, Schaller A. An enantiocomplementary dirigent protein for the enantioselective lacease-catalyzed oxidative coupling of phenols. Angew Chemie - Int Ed. 2010;49(1):202-204.

[103] Corbin C, Drouet S, Markulin L, Auguin D, Lainé É, Davin LB, et al. A genome-wide analysis of the flax (*Linum usitatissimum* L .) dirigent protein family: from gene identification and evolution to differential regulation. Plant Mol Biol [Internet]. 2018;97(1-2):73-101. Available from: http://dx.doi.org/10.1007/s11103-018-0725-x

[104] Kim K-W, Moinuddin SGA, Atwell KM, Costa MA, Davin LB, Lewis NG. Opposite Stereoselectivities of Dirigent Proteins in Arabidopsis and Schizandra Species. J Biol Chem [Internet]. 2012 Oct 5;287(41):33957-33972. Available from: http://www.jbc.org/lookup/doi/10.1074/jbc.M112.387423

[105] Li Q, Chen J, Xiao Y, Di P, Zhang L, Chen W. The dirigent multigene family in Isatis indigotica: Gene discovery and differential transcript abundance. BMC Genomics. 2014;15(1):1-13.

[106] Benedict CR, Liu J, Stipanovic RD, Ho O, C H, Oh HO, et al. The peroxidative coupling of hemigossypol to (+)- and (–_)-gossypol in cottonseed extracts. Contents / Phytochem. 2006;67(4):323-326.

[107] Liu J, Stipanovic RD, Bell AA, Puckhaber LS, Magill CW. Stereoselective coupling of hemigossypol to form (+)-gossypol in moco cotton is mediated by a dirigent protein. Phytochemistry. 2008;69(18):3038-3042.

[108] Drouet S, Tungmunnithum D, Lainé É, Hano C. Gene Expression Analysis and Metabolite Profiling of Silymarin Biosynthesis during Milk Thistle (Silybum marianum (L.) Gaertn.) Fruit Ripening. Int J Mol Sci. 2020;21(13):4730.

[109] El-garhy HAS, Khattab S, Moustafa MMA, Abou R, Abdel AZ, Elhalwagi A, et al. Silybin content and overexpression of chalcone synthase genes in *Silybum marianum* L. plants under abiotic elicitation. Plant Physiol Biochem [Internet]. 2016;108:191-202. Available from: http://dx.doi.org/10.1016/j.plaphy.2016.07.011

[110] Sepideh S, Shobbar ZS, Ebrahimi M, Hasanloo T, Sadat-Noori S-A, Tirnaz S. Chalcone synthase genes from milk thistle (Silybum marianum): isolation and expression. J Genet. 2015;94(4):611-617.

[111] Torres M, Corchete P. Gene expression and flavonolignan production in fruits and cell cultures of Silybum marianum. J Plant Physiol [Internet]. 2016;192:111-117. Available from: http://dx.doi.org/10.1016/j.jplph.2016.02.004

[112] Abouzid S. Silymarin , Natural Flavonolignans from Milk Thistle. Rao DV, editor. A Global Perspective of Their Role in Nutrition and Health. 2012. 255-272 p.

[113] Cacho M, Mora M, Ferna J. Influence of medium composition on the accumulation of flavonolignans in cultured cells of Silybum marianum (L.) Gaertn. Plant Sci. 1999;144:63-68.

[114] Namdeo A. Plant Cell Elicitation for Production of Secondary Metabolites: A Review. Pharmacogn Rev. 2007;1(1):69-79.

[115] Barz W, Beimen A, Drager B, Jaques U. Turnover and storage of secondary products in cell cultures. Second Prod from Plant Tissue Cult [Internet]. 1990 [cited 2019 May 15];79-102. Available from: http://ci.nii.ac.jp/naid/10006440628/en/

[116] Shah M, Ullah MA, Drouet S, Younas M, Tungmunnithum D, Giglioli-Guivarc'h N, et al. Interactive effects of light and melatonin on biosynthesis of silymarin and anti-inflammatory potential in callus cultures of *Silybum marianum* (L.) gaertn. Molecules. 2019;24(7).

[117] Younas M, Drouet S, Nadeem M, Giglioli-Guivarc'h N, Hano C, Abbasi BH. Differential accumulation of silymarin induced by exposure of Silybum marianum L. callus cultures to several spectres of monochromatic lights. J Photochem Photobiol B Biol [Internet]. 2018;184(February):61-70. Available from: https://doi.org/10.1016/j.jphotobiol.2018.05.018

[118] Hasanloo T, Majidi E, Ardakani MRS. Flavonolignan Production in Cell Suspension Culture of *Silybum marianum*. 2008;46(12):876-882.

[119] Shah M, Jan H, Drouet S, Tungmunnithum D, Shirazi JH, Hano C, et al. Chitosan Elicitation Impacts Flavonolignan Biosynthesis in *Silybum marianum* (L.) Gaertn Cell Suspension and Enhances Antioxidant and Anti-Inflammatory Activities of Cell Extracts. Molecules [Internet]. 2021;26(4). Available from: https://www.mdpi.com/1420-3049/26/4/791

[120] Sánchez-Sampedro MA, Fernández-Tárrago J, Corchete P. Yeast

extract and methyl jasmonate-induced silymarin production in cell cultures of Silybum marianum (L.) Gaertn. J Biotechnol. 2005;119(1):60-69.

[121] Tůmová L, Řimáková J, Tůma J, Dušek J. *Silybum marianum* in vitro-flavonolignan production. 2006;2006(10):454-458.

[122] Alikaridis FU, Papadakis D, Pantelia K, Kephalas T. Flavonolignan production from Silybum marianum transfored and untransfromed root cultures. Fitoterapia. 2000;71:379-384.

[123] Hasanloo T, Rahnama H, Sepehrifar R, Shams M. Silymarin production in hairy root cultures of Silybum marianum L. Gaertn. Planta Med. 2008;74(09):109-114.

[124] Rahnama H, Hasanloo T, Shams MR, Sepehrifar R. Silymarin production by hairy root culture of Silybum marianum (L.) Gaertn. Iran J Biotechnol. 2008;6(2):113-118.

[125] Khalili M, Hasanloo T, Tabar KSK, Rahnama H. Influence of exogenous salicylic acid on flavonolignans and lipoxygenase activity in the hairy root cultures of Silybum marianum. Cell Biol Int. 2009;33(9):988-994.

[126] Elateeq AA, Sun Y, Nxumalo W, Gabr AMM. Biotechnological production of silymarin in *Silybum marianum* L.: A review. Biocatal Agric Biotechnol [Internet]. 2020;29:101775. Available from: https://www.sciencedirect.com/science/article/pii/S1878818119317967

Chapter 23

Reappraisal of Dietary Phytochemicals for Coronavirus Infection: Focus on Hesperidin and Quercetin

Paolo Bellavite

Abstract

Food polyphenols constitute a large family of substances with beneficial properties in a large group of communicable and non-communicable diseases. These compounds support and improve the body's defences against oxidative stress and are helpful in the prevention of pathologies related to metabolic syndrome. Furthermore, they exhibit anti-inflammatory, antiviral, and antimicrobial properties. This chapter draws attention to certain nutritional components such as hesperidin and quercetin, which are emerging as good candidates for a complementary beneficial effect in the case of diseases caused by viruses, including COVID-19. These nutraceuticals have a complex mechanism of action, which involves both cellular defence against oxidative stress and the modulation of inflammation, which although normally is a defence, repair and activation mechanism of the immune system, it can elude its controls and become a systemic and destructive pathology (cytokine storm, respiratory distress syndrome). Furthermore, recent in silico simulation tests suggest that both hesperidin and quercetin may interfere with SARS-CoV-2 by binding to cell receptors and the proteolytic enzymes involved in its replication. In addition to the inhibitory effects on the virus at cellular level, the two flavonoids can have indirect effects in respiratory infectious diseases as they prevent or improve metabolic and vascular comorbidities that can complicate the clinical course. This brief review focuses on biochemical and pharmacological mechanisms of action of polyphenols in the context of the revaluation of dietary approaches to the prevention and treatment of infectious diseases caused by viruses, with a special application to COVID-19.

Keywords: hesperidin, quercetin, citrus flavanones, functional food, nutraceuticals, respiratory virus, oxidative stress, SARS-CoV-2, COVID-19, metabolic syndrome, Nrf2

1. Introduction

In modern medicine and chiefly in the approach infectious diseases, nutrition seems to be a neglected or at least underestimated aspect, although it is recognised that it often plays an important role in the prevention of various diseases, including infectious ones [1, 2]. Flavonoids are abundant functional substances in plants with potential health benefits and are used as valuable food components or as supplements. Some of these substances may have an antiviral action or in any case be important in modulating the immune system and defending cells from the oxidative stress associated with infection.

Flavonoids are hydroxylated polyphenolic compounds based on the structure of the 15-carbon backbone of the parent flavone (2-phenyl-1,4-benzopyrone), which consists of two phenyl rings (A and B) and a heterocyclic ring (C) (**Figure 1A**). They can be divided into various classes based on their molecular structure and according to the C-ring replacements scheme: flavones, flavonols, isoflavones, anthocyanins, flavanols and flavanones. More than 4,000 varieties of flavonoids have been identified.

In the human diet, flavonols are widespread with quercetin standing out among them (**Figure 1B**). The most represented flavanone is hesperetin (**Figure 1C**) which is found in citrus fruits in glycosylated form as hesperidin (**Figure 1D**). Flavanones lack a double bond between C2 and C3 and this makes them chiral in the C2 position. Chirality implies that the B ring is not planar like in flavonols and is twisted with respect to the A-C rings. Such a difference in molecular orientation is relevant because it can affect the way the different flavonoids interact with their biological targets and therefore their bioactive properties.

Quercetin [International Union of Pure and Applied Chemistry (IUPAC) name: 2-(3,4-dihydroxyphenyl)-3,5,7-trihydroxychromen-4-one, with a molecular weight of 302.23 g/Mol] contains five hydroxyl groups linked in position 3,5,7,3′ and 4′ to the basic flavonol skeleton. In plants and as a consequence of biotransformation by the intestinal bacterial flora, some of these hydroxyl groups are glycosylated and constitute the main derivatives of quercetin. Hesperidin (with a molecular weight 610.6 g/Mol) is a glycosylated derivative of hesperetin [IUPAC name: (2S)-5,7-dihydroxy-2-(3-hydroxy-4-methoxyphenyl)-2,3-dihydrochromen-4-one, with a molecular weight of 302.28 g/Mol], with a 6-O-(alpha-L-rhamnopyranosyl) -beta-D-glucopyranosyl disaccharide in position 7 via a glycosidic bond.

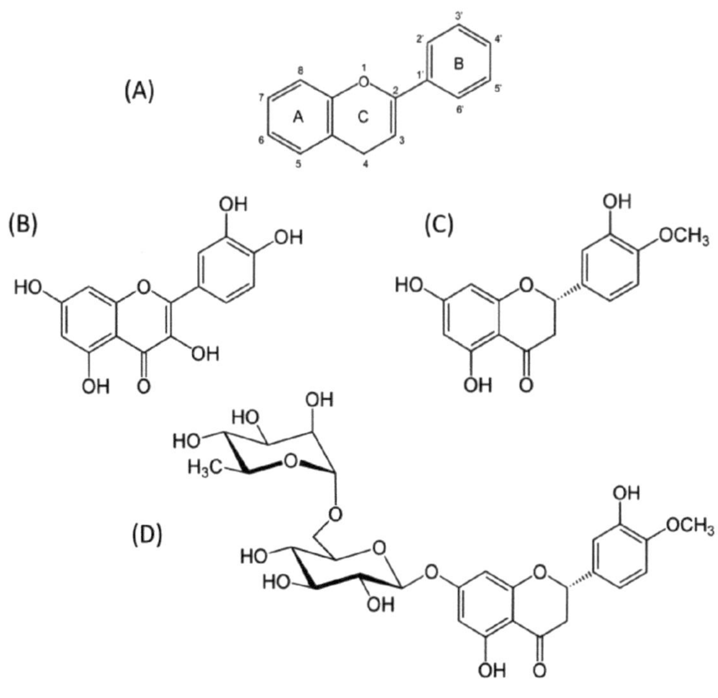

Figure 1.
Molecular structure of flavone (A), quercetin (B), hesperetin (C) and hesperidin (D).

The structure–activity studies show that the antioxidant and anti-free radical properties of flavonoids are due to the ketone group, the double bond between the 2 and 3 carbons, the 3′, 4′-catechol and the 3-hydroxyl moiety in the flavonoid skeleton (the latter two are present in quercetin but not in hesperidin) [3]. The C2-C3 double bond extends the π conjugation to the carbonyl group in the C ring, so the radical elimination capacity of unsaturated flavonoids is greater than saturated structures, such as flavanones [4]. The antiradical capacity of flavonols in aqueous solvents is mainly exerted by the mechanism of electron transfer with sequential proton loss, associated with the C3 hydroxyl group, or of electron-proton transfer in the catechol component. Therefore, the type of substitution of the B ring is also considered as a determinant of the antiradical potency of flavonoids [4].

Many of the biological effects of flavonoids appear to be related to their ability to modulate receptors, enzymes, cell signalling cascades, rather than to a direct antioxidant effect. In fact, the maximum concentrations of flavonoids that can be reached in the blood with very high intakes (~ 2 μmol/L) are much lower than the concentrations of other antioxidants, such as ascorbic acid (~50 μmol/L) uric acid (200–400 μmol/L) and glutathione (700–1500 μmol/L). The functional interaction between flavonoids and enzymes or receptors occurs through hydrogen bonds and hydrophobic interactions with key amino acids of targeted proteins. For example, an inhibition of the activity of the enzyme xanthine oxidase by quercetin is exerted thanks to hydroxyl groups of C5 and C4 [5], and the anti-inflammatory activity depends not only on the number of free hydroxyl groups, but also on the methyl group [6]. Here the binding capacity of quercetin and hesperidin to some important proteins of the SARS-CoV-2 virus will be described in more detail.

In fresh orange juice the hesperidin content represents about 30 mg per 100 ml [7], but it is found in greater quantities in the white part of the peel [8]. Quercetin is widely present in the plant kingdom [9, 10] with an average daily consumption of 25–50 milligrams [11], up to about 250 mg per day in "high-consumers" of fruit and vegetables [12].

Both hesperidin and quercetin have long been known for their antioxidant, anti-inflammatory and anti-lipemic properties. This review will focus on their effects in viral infections, with special prominence on the recently exploded COVID-19 pandemic and its SARS-CoV-2 responsible virus. With the outbreak of COVID-19 and the scientific world's focus on the search for preventive, antiviral and immunomodulatory substances, other particularly interesting characteristics of dietary phytochemicals have emerged. Many studies have highlighted the importance of the intracellular redox state as a new target for natural or synthetic drugs aimed at blocking both viral replication and excess inflammation [13, 14]. It has therefore been suggested that early flavonoid treatment may be a way to restore redox balance, prevent cell damage and the resulting inflammatory storm that causes lung damage with respiratory dysfunction [15–18].

Although there is still no clinical evidence of efficacy for COVID-19, the two flavonoids are emerging as some of the most capable substances of specifically inhibiting binding to cellular receptors of the SARS-CoV-2 virus and its replication [8, 14, 19–21]. A recent randomised study, which appeared in as a preprint version, suggests that quercetin, administered together with vitamin C, could help health care workers in the prevention of SARS-CoV-2 infection [22].

Here we will examine the known mechanisms of action of hesperidin and quercetin, taking SARS-CoV-2 as a paradigm, and without neglecting to mention the important properties of these natural substances for health care in general. Following a logical order, the various passages of the disease will be dealt with starting from cellular infection to clinical consequences, specifying the points where these flavonoids could act.

2. Effects at cellular level

Tests on laboratory animals have shown the ability of flavonoids to inhibit infection by various viruses such as herpes simplex-1, parainfluenza and respiratory syncytial virus [23, 24], poliomyelitis-1 [25], rhinovirus [26, 27], hepatitis C [28], rotavirus [29], influenza [30–36], SARS-coronavirus-1 [37]. Here we will examine recent evidence regarding the SARS-CoV-2 virus in more detail.

Coronaviruses are a group of single-stranded RNA viruses with a corona-like morphology, mainly causing enteric and respiratory diseases of varying extents. Once the first mucosal barriers and possible intervention of the immune system have been overcome, the viruses enter the cell via specific receptors, the nucleic acid is then expressed causing various intracellular changes, including replication into multiple copies and various types of damage to the host cell. In each of these steps it is possible to imagine the action of compounds that tend to block entry or slow down replication and its pathological consequences (**Figure 2**).

2.1 Receptor binding and entry

The internalisation of SARS-CoV-2 in human cells is mediated by the binding of the virus' spike glycoprotein (S) to its receptor on cell membranes, which is the angiotensin converting enzyme 2 (ACE2) [38, 39]. ACE2 is expressed in many tissues including the lung, liver, heart, colon, oesophagus, intestine, kidney, and even the brain, which is consistent with the variety of cell types that can be infected, and the variety of symptoms reported in COVID-19 patients [40–45]. The S protein has two subunits, the first of which contains a receptor binding domain (RBD), which is responsible for binding to ACE2. Binding and entry are also favoured by the presence of a polybasic cleavage site between the two subunits of the spike and by proteolytic enzymes attached to the receptor, of which trans membrane serine protease-2 (TMPRSS2) is particularly important.

The discovery that the hesperidin molecule has a chemical–physical structure suitable for binding to the spike of the SARS-CoV-2 virus (* 1 in **Figure 2**) has recently aroused scientific interest [14, 46–51]. Wu et al. [46] used in silico

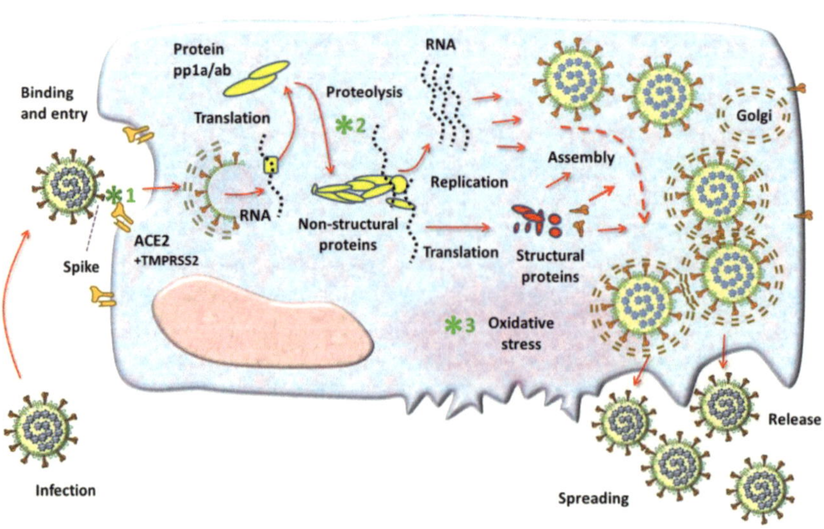

Figure 2.
Intracellular cycle of the SARS-CoV-2 virus. Green asterisks and numbers indicate the points of the flavonoid actions described in the text.

simulation techniques to screen 1066 natural substances with a potential antiviral effect, plus 78 antiviral drugs already known in the literature. Of all of them, hesperidin was the most suitable for binding to the SARS-CoV-2 spike, wedging into the shallow middle sulcus of the RBD, where some hydrophobic amino acids, including Tyr436, Try440, Leu442, Phe443, Phe476, Try475, Try481 and Tyr49 form a hydrophobic pocket to contain the compound.

Various authors have confirmed the affinity of hesperidin for the RBD fragment of the spike protein and its ability to hinder the binding with ACE2 or to make the interaction unstable (**Figure 3**) [52, 53]. The anchoring of hesperidin is stabilised by two hydrogen bonds (shown with green lines in **Figure 3**) with the amino acids Phe457 and Glu455 on the spike protein. According to other in silico screening studies, hesperidin also has an affinity for TMPRSS2 protease, which is involved in the functioning of the receptor when the vesicle is internalised with the virus [54, 55].

Molecular dynamics simulations and energy landscape studies revealed that other flavonoids such as fisetin, quercetin and kaempferol bind to the ACE2-spike complex with favourable free energy [56]. Another group reported studies showing that quercetin has a high affinity for viral spikes, blocking the sites of interaction with cellular receptors [19]. According to other authors who followed a gene expression approach [57], quercetin is identifiable as one of the highest scoring natural substances, altering the expression of numerous human genes that encode SARS-CoV-2 protein targets, including ACE2.

2.2 Proteolysis and assembly

A second theoretical site of flavonoid action is the main protease that allows the processing of the first proteins transferred from the viral genome (point *2 in **Figure 1**).

After interacting with membrane receptors and their associated proteases, the viral particle is internalised by means of a vesicle formed by the same membrane, the shell of which is then removed, allowing the release of the genomic RNA into the cytoplasm. The coding sequences of the genomic RNA are translated into pp1a

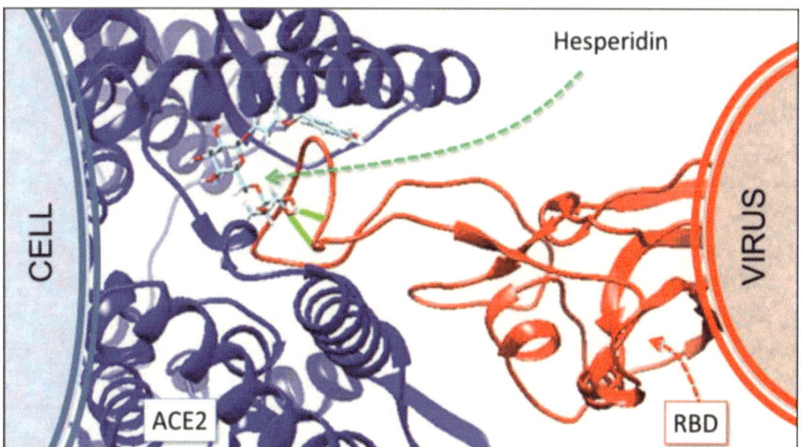

Figure 3.
Binding of the ACE2 protein with the spike in the presence of hesperidin. The RBD fragment of the spike protein (331–524) is shown in red, and the hesperidin molecule in the stick model and human ACE2 is shown in blue. Figure created using a diagram component from the cited work [52] with authorisation from Creative Commons.

and pp1ab proteins, which are then broken down by a proteolytic process for a total of 16 non-structural proteins. The main enzyme that carries out this transformation is called 3-chymotrypsin-like protease (3Clpro) or major protease (Mpro) by various authors and is in fact the target of many chemical antiviral drugs.

Some non-structural proteins then form a replication complex that uses genomic (+) RNA as a template. Eventually, the subgenomic RNAs produced through transcription are translated into structural proteins that will form new viral particles. For this purpose, structural proteins are incorporated into the membrane and the nucleocapsid N protein combines with the RNA produced through the replication process to become a nucleoprotein complex. The various components fuse into the complete viral particle in the Golgi endoplasmic reticulum apparatus, which is finally excreted in the extracellular region.

A strong affinity of hesperidin to Mpro has been discovered by various authors [46, 47, 50] in the screening of thousands of potential molecules using molecular docking techniques. Hesperidin binds with hydrogen bonds to various amino acids, mainly Thr24, Thr25, Thr45, His4, Ser46, Cys145 [50]. An important precedent exists when the authors investigated natural compounds capable of inhibiting Mpro of the SARS virus [37], using cell-based proteolytic cleavage assays. Out of seven phenolic compounds tested, hesperetin inhibited proteolytic activity efficiently with an IC50 of 8.3 μmol/L. Since the coronavirus main protease structure and active site conformation are preserved despite sequence variations [51], it is conceivable that the inhibitory effect of hesperidin, previously observed in the SARS virus, could also be exploited in SARS-CoV-2. Furthermore, hesperidin binds to structural protein 16 (nsp16) of the coronavirus, which is a methyltransferase dependent on S-adenosyl methionine [58]. This protein plays an important role in viral replication and prevents recognition by the innate immune system.

Quercetin has also been shown to inhibit the Mpro of the SARS-CoV [59], MERS-CoV [60] and SARS-CoV-2 [61] coronaviruses. The binding points of quercetin and hesperetin on SARS-CoV-2 Mpro are partially different [19]: the first in fact binds to Glu288, Asp289 and Glu290, while the second to Glu290, Asp289, Lys5. Furthermore, hesperetin, naringenin and kaempferol bind to the regulatory site Leu286, which quercetin does not do. All this suggests that the different molecules do not overlap as a pharmacological activity on the Mpro, but can synergise.

An even more recent study [62] confirms the affinity of quercetin to Mpro using the measurement of the enzymatic activity. Evidence of its inhibitory effect was obtained with a fairly low dose of quercetin (7.7 μmol/L). **Figure 4** shows the molecular complex formed by quercetin bound in the cavity that constitutes the active site of Mpro (in blue), in the most favourable position to inhibit the protein enzymatic activity in order to block the replication of the coronavirus.

Da Silva et al. [63] have expanded the search for molecules interacting with Mpro to a series of flavonoid glycosides using a molecular docking approach. The interactions and binding affinity with the protease by quercetin and even more by its glycosidic derivatives quercetin-3-O-rutinoside (rutin), quercetin-3-O-glucuronide, quercetin-3′- O-sulphate, quercetin-7-O-glucuronide, quercetin-7-O-sulfate were thus predicted. It should be noted that the absorbed flavonoids normally undergo extensive metabolism in the epithelial cells of the small intestine and in the liver. Metabolites conjugated with the methyl, glucuronate and sulphate groups are the predominant forms present in plasma [64–66]. Quercetin has also been indicated as one of the substances capable of binding and thus inhibiting RNA-dependent RNA polymerase, an essential enzyme in the replication of viral RNA in the host cell [63].

Russo et al. [20] further confirmed the ability of known flavonoids (e.g. quercetin, baicalin, luteolin, hesperetin, gallocatechin gallate, epigallocatechin gallate)

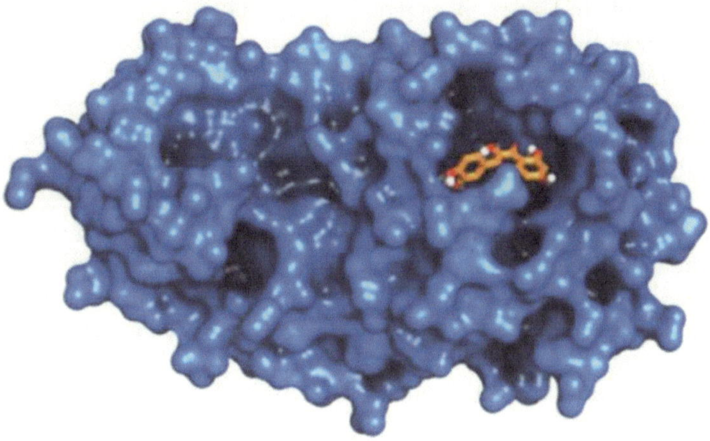

Figure 4.
Representation of the quercetin molecule (in orange) within the active site of the Mpro of the SARS-CoV-2 virus. Developed by Bruno Rizzuti on the basis of the study of which he is co-author [62]. Reproduction authorised by the author.

to inhibit the key proteins involved in the infectious cycle of SARS-CoV-2. They suggested that flavonoids and their derivatives, due to their pleiotropic activities and lack of systemic toxicity, may represent target compounds to be tested in future clinical trials to enrich the arsenal of drugs against coronavirus infections.

2.3 Oxidative stress

Oxidative stress is an important cell pathology mechanism which is involved in many diseases, including those caused by viruses. Viral respiratory infections are generally associated with the production of cytokines, inflammation, cell death and other pathophysiological processes, which could be linked to increased production of reactive oxygen species (ROS), redox imbalance and oxidative stress.

Many lines of evidence suggest that viral infections are accompanied by signs of increased production of ROS, presence of oxidation products in blood plasma and urine, and reduced antioxidant capacity [67]. This pathological and pathogenic phenomenon has been observed in the infection of viruses such as hepatitis B [68], hepatitis C [69], influenza [70] and SARS-CoV-2 [71]. In the latter, ROS could also determine an unfavourable evolution in elderly subjects with low antioxidant capacity [72, 73], perhaps because the intracellular redox environment alters the presentation of antigens [74] and the expression of ACE2 [75, 76]. In fact, the severity and mortality risk of SARS-CoV-2 or COVID-19 have been associated with age [73].

Studies have shown that the ability of viral envelope glycoproteins to fuse to the surface of a cell membrane depends on the disulphide-thiol balance of the cell, even if the binding of coronaviruses to cell receptors seems rather insensitive to these parameters [77]. It seems possible that the oxidation of thiols to disulphides, under an oxidative stress mechanism, increases the affinity of spike proteins for the ACE2 receptor and, therefore, increases the severity of COVID-19 [75]. In this regard, reduced glutathione (GSH) may also have direct anti-SARS-CoV-2 potential: in fact, a computational study indicates that the binding of the spike protein to ACE2 is at its highest when the ACE2-sulfur groups are in the form of disulphides and are altered when they are fully reduced to thiols: therefore a pro-oxidant environment with low levels of GSH would favour the cellular entry of viruses [75, 78].

In the course of viral diseases, analgesic and antipyretic drugs are widely used, and of these one of the most common is paracetamol (acetaminophen). However, the fact that this drug depletes glutathione reserves and can worsen oxidative stress is not always taken into account [78, 79]. This type of biochemical modifications can decrease the antiviral defences [80] or complicate the course especially in patients with abnormal liver tests or liver failure [81, 82].

As described in the Introduction, flavonoids have a molecular structure capable of participating in redox reactions and free radical scavenging, which are involved in the biochemical phenomena described here and in the cellular pathology resulting from viral infection (point * 3 in **Figure 2**). Hesperidin contributes significantly to antioxidant defence systems and has been reported to act as an effective agent against superoxide and hydroxyl radicals [83], while hesperetin inhibits the production of nitric oxide by lipopolysaccharide (LPS)-stimulated microglial cells [84].

Quercetin also acts as a free radical scavenger, donating two electrons to oxidised species which are reduced. When this occurs with the transfer of one electron at a time, a semiquinonic intermediate molecule is formed. This antioxidant activity of quercetin is exploited in synergy with vitamin C, thanks to the ability of ascorbate to recycle the flavonol molecule, protecting it from oxidation and recycling its oxidised quinonic form after the scavenger action on free radicals [85]. In addition to ascorbic acid, glutathione is also important for maintaining quercetin in its reduced and therefore functional form and preventing the risk that quercetin quinone, in turn, may oxidise the thiol groups of proteins [86, 87].

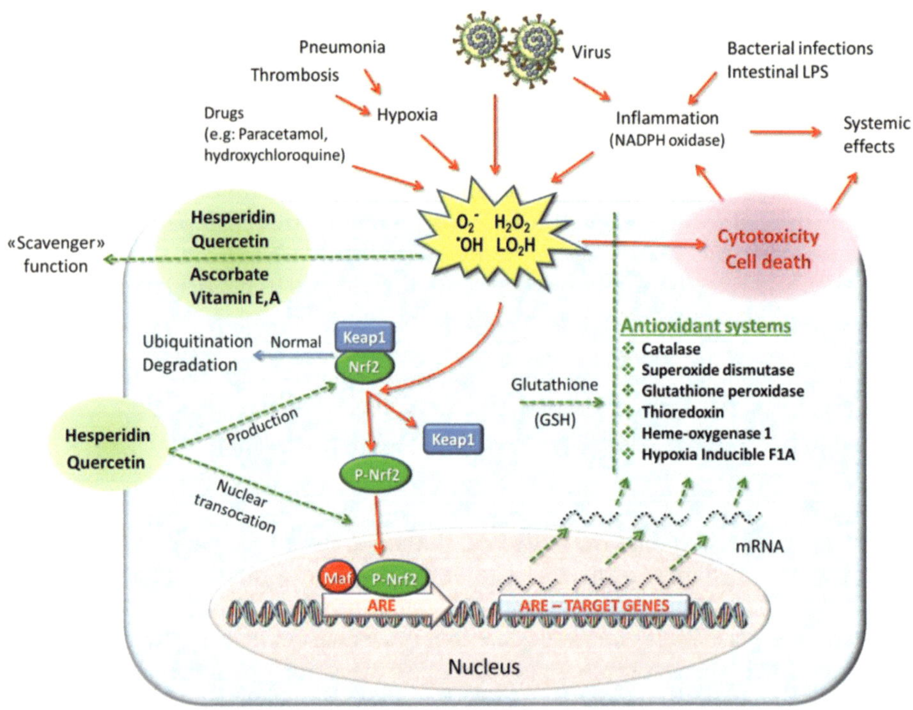

Figure 5.
Oxidative stress induced by several pathogenic factors (top part) and cellular defensive effects of flavonoids, functioning as direct free radicals scavengers in synergy with ascorbate and other liposoluble vitamins (A, E) and as stimulants of the Nrf2/ARE pathway. O2-: Superoxide anion; H2O2: hydrogen peroxide; °OH: hydroxyl radical; LO2H: Lipid hydroperoxide; LPS: lipopolysaccharide; Keap1: Kelch-like ECH-associated protein 1; Nrf2: nuclear factor erythroid 2–related factor 2; Maf: musculoaponeurotic fibrosarcoma element; ARE: antioxidant response element.

Various in vitro and in vivo studies have shown that the antioxidant activity of hesperidin and quercetin is not limited to their scavenger activity, but actually increases cellular defences against oxidative stress through the signalling path Nrf2/ARE [88–95] (**Figure 5**).

The nuclear factor erythroid 2–related factor 2 (Nrf2) is of primary importance because it regulates gene expression through a promoter sequence known as the antioxidant response element (ARE). Normally Nrf2 is attached to another protein called Kelch-like ECH-associated protein 1 (Keap1) and is rapidly degraded through the ubiquitination and proteasome system, without performing any functions. On the other hand, in the presence of ROS, Nrf2 detaches from Keap1, is phosphorylated and translocates to the nucleus, where it combines with a small musculoaponeurotic fibrosarcoma (Maf) protein to form a dimer and binds to the antioxidant response element upstream of the promoter. This ARE + Nrf2 dimer then initiates the messenger RNA transcription of a series of target genes such as those encoding antioxidant enzymes ("Antioxidant systems" in **Figure 5**).

The ability of hesperidin to fight damage from toxic oxygen radicals and stimulate the expression of Nrf2 has been reported by various authors in other experimental models namely in hepatocarcinogenesis [96], hepatotoxicity [97], neuroinflammation and neurodegeneration [91, 98–102]. The protective effects of quercetin in neurodegenerative disorders and cerebrovascular diseases, demonstrated both in in vitro and in vivo studies are also largely linked to its ability to stimulate the defences against oxidative stress [103].

3. Organ failure and systemic pathology

Once they have reproduced in the cells of the entry tissues and overcome the first barriers of innate defences, the viruses spread to target organs and cause various types of clinical consequences in different individuals. It is known that the severity of COVID-19 as well as other viral respiratory infections is related to many different parameters (age, gender, nutritional status, comorbidities, etc.) and that people with pre-existing conditions such as diabetes, hypertension, and lung, heart and kidney diseases (all diseases in which ROS play a pathogenetic role) are at increased risk of developing severe effects. In serious cases, endothelial dysfunction, coagulopathy and pulmonary thrombosis cause hypoxia, mitochondrial chain abnormalities, mitochondrial dysfunction, oxidative stress, DNA damage [104, 105]. Another mechanism that links systemic inflammation syndrome and oxidative stress is hyperferritinemia, which often characterises COVID-19 [106, 107].

These mechanisms are involved in the extensive systemic lesions observed during severe complications associated with influenza. It has therefore been suggested that agents with antioxidant properties could be drugs of choice for the treatment of patients with such severe complications [108]. N-acetylcysteine, which supports glutathione and thus the main antioxidant defence systems [109], was used with good results in influenza syndromes [110] and acute respiratory distress syndrome (ARDS) [111], and it was suggested as a potential therapeutic agent for COVID-19 [112–114].

Figure 6 summarises the main critical points of the SARS-CoV-2 virus in the whole body and the possible interventions of the two flavonoids considered here, based on the knowledge acquired so far in other types of systemic and metabolic disorders.

Experimental evidence showed that treatment with hesperidin safeguards the aged rat's heart by increasing the levels of the Nrf2 factor and the activity of enzymatic antioxidants [115]. The same group showed a protective effect of hesperetin

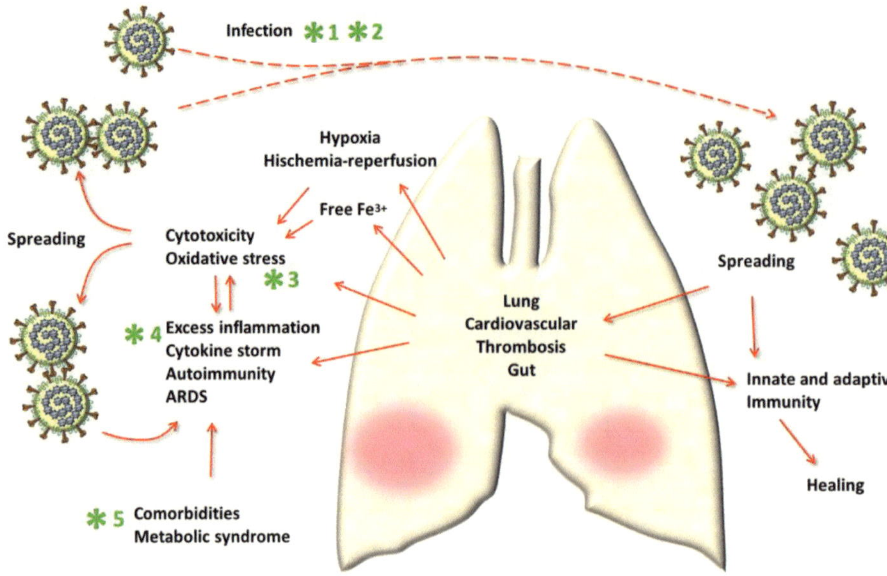

Figure 6.
*Diagram of the major systemic effects of COVID-19. The asterisks show the possible operation points of the flavonoids, as discussed in chapter 2 (*1, *2, *3) and in this chapter (*3, *4 and *5).*

on experimental heart failure in the rat [116]. The authors conclude that it is conceivable that hesperetin could be a potential therapeutic candidate that enhances Nrf2 signalling and thereby improves cardiac remodelling. Results from another study show the beneficial effects of citrus flavanones in the liver of aged rats, where nirangerin and hesperidin prevented the age-related decrease in catalase, superoxide dismutase and glutathione reductase [117].

The mechanism of ischemia–reperfusion liver injury was studied in a murine model by measuring oxidative stress indicators, serum enzymes and inflammation indices [118]. Hesperidin (100–400 mg/kg) significantly improved liver ischemia–reperfusion injury measured by serum alanine aminotransferase levels, reduced malondialdehyde content, but it increased superoxide dismutase, catalase, glutathione peroxidase levels. Furthermore, hesperidin significantly alleviated the expression levels of TNF-α, IL 6 and IL-1β. Hesperidin (100 mg/kg) protects rats from liver damage and dyslipidaemia caused by cadmium chloride [119].

The antioxidant effect of quercetin was studied in a two-week, randomised, crossover-controlled intervention trial [120]. Fourteen individuals ingested 2 capsules (total 1 g/d) of quercetin or a placebo. Blood samples were collected before, after 2 weeks of supplementation and after a period of strenuous exercise. Quercetin significantly reduced erythrocyte lipid peroxidation levels and susceptibility to haemolysis induced by free radicals, while no differences were found in antioxidant enzyme activities and glutathione homeostasis between the two groups. After a single period of intense exercise, quercetin supplementation improved redox status as assessed by the reduced glutathione/oxidised glutathione ratio and by thiobarbituric acid reactive substances levels in both erythrocytes and plasma.

3.1 Excess inflammation

During the spread of the virus in the tissues (first of all in the lung) and systemically (lymph, blood, immune system, coagulation, kidney, liver), an inflammatory reaction develops which can be clinically very serious, especially in patients with comorbidities. Excessive and "vicious" inflammation can be mediated by a distorted activation of the cytokine network, by coagulation disorders, even by a paradoxical excess of the immune reaction (autoimmunity, cytotoxic lymphocytes) [121]. Oxidative stress and excess inflammation are linked, as shown in **Figure 6** (points *3 e *4). Autoimmune phenomena are also likely to be involved in the attack on the cell infected with SARS-CoV-2, which could have implications both in the clinical course of the disease [122, 123] and in the safety of vaccines [124].

The two flavonoids which are reviewed here have a remarkable ability to modulate local and systemic inflammatory responses, through various mechanisms. Hesperidin showed antioxidant activity in rats after an intense training programme and, at the same time, alleviated cytokine secretion by stimulated macrophages [125, 126]. Furthermore, the administration of hesperetin has been shown to significantly reduce the levels of myeloperoxidase, malondialdehyde (a marker of lipid peroxidation) and inflammation in experimental models of colitis [127] and hepatic trauma [128]. A study on macrophage cells in culture induced by bacterial endotoxin (LPS) clearly highlighted the main molecular effects of hesperetin capable of modulating inflammation [129].

One of the most frequently used experimental models is LPS-induced pneumonia in mice, which somewhat mimics ARDS. Three separate studies have shown that hesperidin (in doses between 10 and 200 mg/kg) significantly reduces the accumulation of fluid in the lung and proinflammatory cytokines [130–132]. The protective and anti-inflammatory effect of hesperidin or hesperetin was also demonstrated in rats with acute lung injury induced by mechanical ventilation [133] and lung infection with the H1N1 influenza virus [36]. Finally, hesperidin has anti-inflammatory and antioxidant effects in chronic obstructive pulmonary disease (COPD) caused by smoking, reducing the levels of IL-6, IL-8 and malondialdehyde [134].

Quercetin is a powerful antioxidant but also acts as an enzymatic inhibitor in a series of mechanisms involved with inflammation [135]. In LPS-stimulated macrophages, quercetin treatment inhibited NF-kB activation and proinflammatory cytokines [136]. A randomised, parallel-group, controlled polycentric study showed the efficacy of a dietary supplement based on quercetin (150 mg), perilla dry extract (80 mg) and vitamin D3 (5 μg) in preventing allergic rhinitis flare-ups in children [137, 138].

The antiallergic property of quercetin has been explored in the laboratory setting by studying the secretory response of activated mast cells in both human and animal models [139–143], and by evaluating the release of histamine from human basophils [144, 145]. This flavonol inhibits several protein tyrosine and serine/threonine kinases involved in signal transduction in inflammatory cells [26, 103, 139, 146–148]. These inhibitory properties on the release of histamine could also be interesting for COVID-19, given that the pulmonary mast cells are involved in the phenomenon of worsening the pulmonary picture in the event of a "cytokine storm" [149].

A meta-analysis of seven randomised trials sought to quantify the effect of quercetin on inflammatory mechanisms in vivo by measuring plasma C-reactive protein (CRP) concentrations. Meta-analysis showed a significant reduction in circulating CRP levels following supplementation with quercetin, especially at doses of 500 mg /day or more and in patients with CRP <3 mg/l [150].

3.2 Comorbidities

Since COVID-19 is a multi-organ disease and has more serious clinical consequences in patients with pulmonary, intestinal, hepatic and cardiovascular comorbidities, it is conceivable that its clinical course may profit from the multiple beneficial effects of hesperidin and quercetin in systemic pathologies of this type (point * 5 in **Figure 6**). Epidemiological studies have reported an inverse relationship between citrus flavonoid intake and the risk of cardiovascular disease [151, 152]. From a careful review of the literature [153], the use of natural antioxidant polyphenols seems to be an excellent approach as they have strong antioxidant and anti-inflammatory properties.

A constellation of risk factors for cardiovascular disease is called metabolic syndrome (MetS), whose determining factors are, in order of importance: weight, genetics, ageing and lifestyle [154]. The criteria for defining MetS are based on the presence of 3 out of 5 factors, including obesity, elevated triglycerides, reduced HDL-C, elevated blood pressure and elevated fasting glucose [155]. It has been shown that individuals with these characteristics are also commonly prone to a chronic, low-grade inflammatory states. Oxidative stress phenomena are also involved in MetS, probably due to the disturbance of the nutrient metabolism at the mitochondrial level [154].

In this context, it is interesting to note that good results have been obtained in clinical studies with the integration of orange juice, polyphenols and particularly with both hesperidin and quercetin, with antioxidant and antihypertensive effects, and by regulating glucose metabolism and lipid profiles. A recent experimental study showed that hesperidin (15 or 30 mg/kg) improved biochemical alterations and cardiac dysfunction in a high-fat diet-induced MetS model in rats [156].

Soy isoflavones, citrus products, hesperidin and quercetin improved lipid metabolism [157]. Rizza et al. [158] performed a randomised, placebo-controlled study to investigate whether oral administration of hesperidin (500 mg once daily for 3 weeks) improves endothelial function in individuals with MetS. As a measure of efficacy, they measured the difference in flow-mediated dilation of the brachial artery between subjects receiving placebo or hesperidin. In the clinical study, hesperidin treatment increased flow-mediated dilation and decreased the circulating inflammatory biomarkers (highly sensitive C-reactive protein, serum amyloid A protein, soluble E-selectin). The authors concluded that hesperidin recovers endothelial dysfunction and reduces circulating markers of inflammation. Such vasculoprotective actions may explain the beneficial cardiovascular effects of citrus fruit consumption.

A double-blind study documented the beneficial effects of hesperidin supplementation (500 mg/day) on blood pressure and inflammatory markers in type 2 diabetes [159]. The mechanisms by which hesperidin could contribute to blood pressure control are associated with improvements in endothelial function, oxidative stress and inflammation [160]. In a study with a parallel group design, 49 patients with MetS received either 500 mg of hesperidin or a placebo, twice daily for 12 weeks [155]. Hesperidin led to a significant decrease in serum levels of glucose, insulin, triglycerides, total cholesterol, low density lipoprotein cholesterol, TNF-α and high sensitive-CRP. The data on the antihypertensive effect of hesperidin is more uncertain but recently Valls et al. published a study on healthy volunteers in which they actually showed an antihypertensive effect of orange juice enriched with hesperidin [152].

A systematic review has highlighted the potential antidiabetic action of citrus flavonoids and their molecular mechanisms based on in vitro and in vivo studies [161]. The research identified 38 articles, mostly on experimental animals, which reported that citrus flavonoids regulate glycaemic control biomarkers, lipid profiles, kidney function, liver enzymes and antioxidant enzymes, and modulated signalling pathways related to glucose uptake and insulin sensitivity that are involved in the pathogenesis of diabetes and its related complications. Citrus flavonoids, therefore, are promising antidiabetic candidates, while their antidiabetic effects have yet to be verified in upcoming human studies.

Quercetin supplementation also may have positive effects among patients with MetS and related disorders [162]. A meta-analysis identified 9 studies on this topic, which showed overall that quercetin supplementation did not affect fasting plasma glucose or insulin resistance. However, in the subgroup analysis, quercetin supplementation slightly but significantly reduced fasting glucose in studies lasting 8 weeks and using quercetin in doses equal to or > 500 mg/day. Better effects were found in individuals <45 years of age. Regarding lipid levels, a meta-analysis of 9 clinical studies [163] found a significant reduction in LDL in overweight and obese human subjects who took doses ≥250 mg/day of quercetin for rather extended periods, reaching a total dose of ≥14,000 mg; however, HDL cholesterol, triglyceride and total cholesterol levels remained unchanged ($p > 0.05$).

The supplementation of nutrition with quercetin on blood pressure and endothelial function among patients with MetS was investigated with a meta-analysis [164]. The authors found a significant reduction in systolic blood pressure but not diastolic pressure.

Finally, the health of the intestine cannot be neglected, which is an organ where viral infections tend to be found, and it is also fundamental because the release of endotoxins (LPS) due to an increased mucosa permeability or intestinal dysmicrobism could enhance systemic inflammatory reactions. It has been argued that the interaction between the lung and gut could lead to a vicious cycle of lung and intestinal inflammation which may be a potential factor leading to the death of patients with COVID-19 [165]. Citrus flavanones may have an impact on the intestinal microbiome, exerting beneficial effects on the intestinal barrier function and gastrointestinal inflammation [166]. In intervention studies on volunteers, orange juice positively modulated the composition and metabolic activity of the microbiota, increasing the population of Bifidobacterium spp. and Lactobacillus spp. [167] or of Lactobacillus spp., Akkermansia spp. and Ruminococcus spp. according to other authors [168], suggesting that orange juice showed a prebiotic effect, modulating the intestinal microbiota by improving blood sugar and the lipid profile. In a recent review [169], it was highlighted how the beneficial effects of hesperidin on cardiovascular risk factors can be partly attributed to the modulation of the intestinal microbiota. Based on the current evidence, some of the contradictory effects of hesperidin in human studies are in part due to the interindividual variability of hesperidin in its bioavailability. Quercetin also has a profound influence on the intestinal microbiome, which in turn modulates its bioavailability [170].

In conclusion, the results indicate that supplementation with hesperidin or quercetin may have mild antihypertensive effects, improve metabolic lipid abnormalities and inflammatory status in patients with MetS. All these beneficial effects can only be reflected in a more favourable clinical course when viral infectious diseases cause systemic disorders involving oxidative stress and inflammation.

4. Conclusions

The scientific literature is filled with works that support the beneficial effects of citrus flavonoids and quercetin on viral respiratory diseases, including COVID-19, and there are several possible mechanisms by which this effect is carried out (**Figure** 7).

Inhibition of cellular infection can occur through the intercalation of these molecules between viruses and receptors and by inhibition of intracellular replication. This phenomenon could have a protective role especially in the oral cavity and in the gastrointestinal system, where the concentrations of the active ingredients are undoubtedly higher than in the blood after intestinal absorption and diffusion

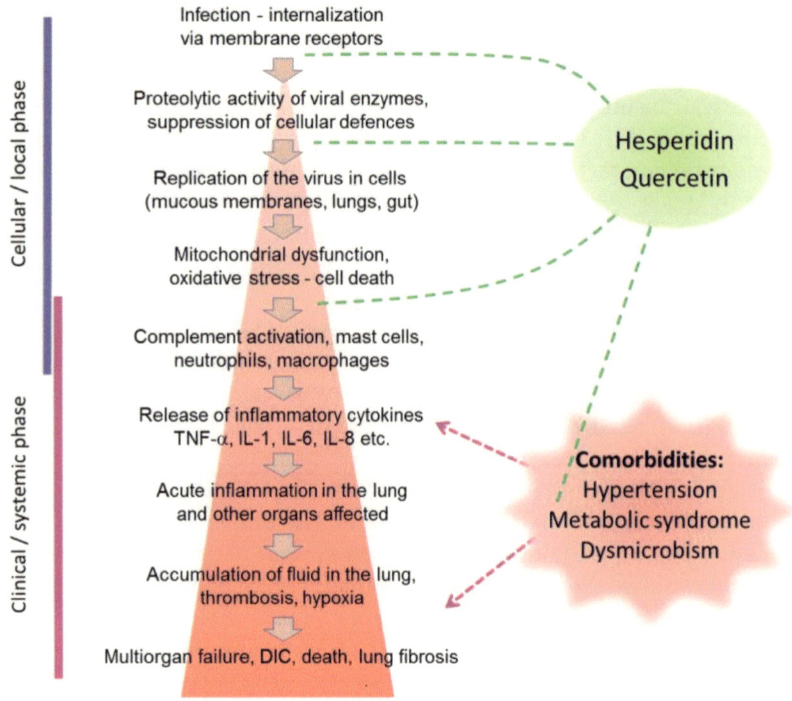

Figure 7.
Summary of the possible actions of flavonoids hesperidin and quercetin to prevent the progression of SARS-CoV-2 virus infection and its major clinical consequences.

in the body. Furthermore, the two flavonoids are able to prevent cell damage due to the virus by enhancing the antioxidant defences through the Nrf2 system and by the direct scavenger action.

The close relationship between cell damage/death and inflammation means that a positive effect can be expected in mitigating the systemic consequences of an inflammation that has eluded controls. Finally, hesperidin and quercetin can exert an indirect beneficial effect, favouring carbohydrate and lipid metabolism, improving general health conditions and thus preventing comorbidities that are contributory causes of the most serious complications. All the experimental models cited here would make it plausible for an increase in the consumption of flavonoid-rich foods, or flavonoid supplementation during periods of increased commitment of the body defences, to help the immune system in the fight against virus infections. It is therefore desirable that further suitable clinical studies are conducted to investigate the potential of these natural substances and to define effective dosages.

Acknowledgements

The article processing charges were borne by Vanda Omeopatici s.r.l. (Frascati, Roma). The sponsor had no role in the conception, writing or revision of the manuscript.

Conflict of interest

The author is scientific consultant from Vanda Omeopatici s.r.l. (Frascati, Roma), a company that produces food supplements.

Author details

Paolo Bellavite
Department of Medicine, Section of General Pathology, University of Verona, Verona, Italy

*Address all correspondence to: paolo.bellavite@univr.it

References

[1] Aune D, Keum N, Giovannucci E, Fadnes LT, Boffetta P, Greenwood DC, et al. Dietary intake and blood concentrations of antioxidants and the risk of cardiovascular disease, total cancer, and all-cause mortality: a systematic review and dose-response meta-analysis of prospective studies. Am J Clin Nutr. 2018;108(5):1069-1091.

[2] Wallace TC, Bailey RL, Blumberg JB, Burton-Freeman B, Chen CO, Crowe-White KM, et al. Fruits, vegetables, and health: A comprehensive narrative, umbrella review of the science and recommendations for enhanced public policy to improve intake. Crit Rev Food Sci Nutr. 2019;1-38.

[3] Zhang Q, Yang W, Liu J, Liu H, Lv Z, Zhang C, et al. Identification of Six Flavonoids as Novel Cellular Antioxidants and Their Structure-Activity Relationship. Oxid Med Cell Longev. 2020;2020:4150897.

[4] Spiegel M, Andruniów T, Sroka Z. Flavones' and Flavonols' Antiradical Structure-Activity Relationship-A Quantum Chemical Study. Antioxidants (Basel). 2020;9(6).

[5] Zhao J, Huang L, Sun C, Zhao D, Tang H. Studies on the structure-activity relationship and interaction mechanism of flavonoids and xanthine oxidase through enzyme kinetics, spectroscopy methods and molecular simulations. Food Chem. 2020;323:126807.

[6] Magar RT, Sohng JK. A Review on Structure, Modifications and Structure-Activity Relation of Quercetin and Its Derivatives. J Microbiol Biotechnol. 2020;30(1):11-20.

[7] Gattuso G, Barreca D, Gargiulli C, Leuzzi U, Caristi C. Flavonoid composition of Citrus juices. Molecules. 2007;12(8):1641-1673.

[8] Meneguzzo F, Ciriminna R, Zabini F, Pagliaro M. Review of Evidence Available on Hesperidin-Rich Products as Potential Tools against COVID-19 and Hydrodynamic Cavitation-Based Extraction as a Method of Increasing Their Production. Processes. 2020; 8: 549.

[9] Kawai M, Hirano T, Higa S, Arimitsu J, Maruta M, Kuwahara Y, et al. Flavonoids and related compounds as anti-allergic substances. Allergol Int. 2007;56(2):113-123.

[10] Boots AW, Wilms LC, Swennen EL, Kleinjans JC, Bast A, Haenen GR. In vitro and ex vivo anti-inflammatory activity of quercetin in healthy volunteers. Nutrition. 2008;24(7-8):703-710.

[11] Formica JV, Regelson W. Review of the biology of Quercetin and related bioflavonoids. Food Chem Toxicol. 1995;33(12):1061-1080.

[12] Andres S, Pevny S, Ziegenhagen R, Bakhiya N, Schäfer B, Hirsch-Ernst KI, et al. Safety Aspects of the Use of Quercetin as a Dietary Supplement. Mol Nutr Food Res. 2018;62(1).

[13] Checconi P, De AM, Marcocci ME, Fraternale A, Magnani M, Palamara AT, et al. Redox-Modulating Agents in the Treatment of Viral Infections. Int J Mol Sci. 2020;21(11).

[14] Bellavite P, Donzelli A. Hesperidin and SARS-CoV-2: New Light on the Healthy Function of Citrus Fruits. Antioxidants (Basel). 2020;9(8): 9080742

[15] Iddir M, Brito A, Dingeo G, Fernandez Del Campo SS, Samouda H, La Frano MR, et al. Strengthening the Immune System and Reducing Inflammation and Oxidative Stress through Diet and Nutrition:

Considerations during the COVID-19 Crisis. Nutrients. 2020;12(6).

[16] Filardo S, Di PM, Mastromarino P, Sessa R. Therapeutic potential of resveratrol against emerging respiratory viral infections. Pharmacol Ther. 2020;107613.

[17] Marinella MA. Indomethacin and resveratrol as potential treatment adjuncts for SARS-CoV-2/COVID-19. Int J Clin Pract. 2020;e13535.

[18] Mrityunjaya M, Pavithra V, Neelam R, Janhavi P, Halami PM, Ravindra PV. Immune-Boosting, Antioxidant and Anti-inflammatory Food Supplements Targeting Pathogenesis of COVID-19. Front Immunol. 2020;11:570122.

[19] Vijayakumar BG, Ramesh D, Joji A, Jayachandra PJ, Kannan T. In silico pharmacokinetic and molecular docking studies of natural flavonoids and synthetic indole chalcones against essential proteins of SARS-CoV-2. Eur J Pharmacol. 2020;886:173448.

[20] Russo M, Moccia S, Spagnuolo C, Tedesco I, Russo GL. Roles of flavonoids against coronavirus infection. Chem Biol Interact. 2020;328:109211.

[21] Mani JS, Johnson JB, Steel JC, Broszczak DA, Neilsen PM, Walsh KB, et al. Natural product-derived phytochemicals as potential agents against coronaviruses: A review. Virus Res. 2020;284:197989.

[22] Arslan B, Ergun NU, Topuz S, Semerci SY, Suner N, Kocatas A, et al. Synergistic effect of quercetin and vitamin C against COVID-19: Is a possible guard for front liners. Lancet (Preprints). 2020. https://papers.ssrn.com/sol3/papers.cfm?abstract_id=3682517.

[23] Kaul TN, Middleton E Jr, Ogra PL. Antiviral effect of flavonoids on human viruses. J Med Virol. 1985;15(1):71-79.

[24] Piva HMR, Sa JM, Miranda AS, Tasic L, Fossey MA, Souza FP, et al. Insights into Interactions of Flavanones with Target Human Respiratory Syncytial Virus M2-1 Protein from STD-NMR, Fluorescence Spectroscopy, and Computational Simulations. Int J Mol Sci. 2020;21(6).

[25] Neznanov N, Kondratova A, Chumakov KM, Neznanova L, Kondratov R, Banerjee AK, et al. Quercetinase pirin makes poliovirus replication resistant to flavonoid quercetin. DNA Cell Biol. 2008;27(4):191-198.

[26] Ganesan S, Faris AN, Comstock AT, Wang Q, Nanua S, Hershenson MB, et al. Quercetin inhibits rhinovirus replication in vitro and in vivo. Antiviral Res. 2012;94(3):258-271.

[27] Farazuddin M, Mishra R, Jing Y, Srivastava V, Comstock AT, Sajjan US. Quercetin prevents rhinovirus-induced progression of lung disease in mice with COPD phenotype. PLoS ONE. 2018;13(7):e0199612.

[28] Gonzalez O, Fontanes V, Raychaudhuri S, Loo R, Loo J, Arumugaswami V, et al. The heat shock protein inhibitor Quercetin attenuates hepatitis C virus production. Hepatology. 2009;50(6):1756-1764.

[29] Lipson SM, Ozen FS, Louis S, Karthikeyan L. Comparison of Î±-glucosyl hesperidin of citrus fruits and epigallocatechin gallate of green tea on the Loss of Rotavirus Infectivity in Cell Culture. Front Microbiol. 2015;6:359.

[30] Davis JM, Murphy EA, McClellan JL, Carmichael MD, Gangemi JD. Quercetin reduces susceptibility to influenza infection following stressful exercise. Am J Physiol Regul Integr Comp Physiol. 2008;295(2):R505-R509.

[31] Saha RK, Takahashi T, Suzuki T. Glucosyl hesperidin prevents influenza a virus replication in vitro by inhibition of viral sialidase. Biol Pharm Bull. 2009;32(7):1188-1192.

[32] Choi HJ, Song JH, Park KS, Kwon DH. Inhibitory effects of quercetin 3-rhamnoside on influenza A virus replication. Eur J Pharm Sci. 2009;37(3-4):329-333.

[33] Kim Y, Narayanan S, Chang KO. Inhibition of influenza virus replication by plant-derived isoquercetin. Antiviral Res. 2010;88(2):227-235.

[34] Dong W, Wei X, Zhang F, Hao J, Huang F, Zhang C, et al. A dual character of flavonoids in influenza A virus replication and spread through modulating cell-autonomous immunity by MAPK signaling pathways. Sci Rep. 2014;4.

[35] Wu W, Li R, Li X, He J, Jiang S, Liu S, et al. Quercetin as an Antiviral Agent Inhibits Influenza A Virus (IAV) Entry. Viruses. 2015;8(1).

[36] Ding Z, Sun G, Zhu Z. Hesperidin attenuates influenza A virus (H1N1) induced lung injury in rats through its anti-inflammatory effect. Antivir Ther. 2018;23(7):611-615.

[37] Lin CW, Tsai FJ, Tsai CH, Lai CC, Wan L, Ho TY, et al. Anti-SARS coronavirus 3C-like protease effects of Isatis indigotica root and plant-derived phenolic compounds. Antiviral Res. 2005;68(1):36-42.

[38] Wang Q, Zhang Y, Wu L, Niu S, Song C, Zhang Z, et al. Structural and Functional Basis of SARS-CoV-2 Entry by Using Human ACE2. Cell. 2020;181(4):894-904.

[39] Lan J, Ge J, Yu J, Shan S, Zhou H, Fan S, et al. Structure of the SARS-CoV-2 spike receptor-binding domain bound to the ACE2 receptor. Nature. 2020;581(7807):215-220.

[40] Ni W, Yang X, Yang D, Bao J, Li R, Xiao Y, et al. Role of angiotensin-converting enzyme 2 (ACE2) in COVID-19. Crit Care. 2020;24(1):422.

[41] Gupta A, Madhavan MV, Sehgal K, Nair N, Mahajan S, Sehrawat TS, et al. Extrapulmonary manifestations of COVID-19. Nat Med. 2020;26(7):1017-1032.

[42] Xu H, Zhong L, Deng J, Peng J, Dan H, Zeng X, et al. High expression of ACE2 receptor of 2019-nCoV on the epithelial cells of oral mucosa. Int J Oral Sci. 2020;12(1):8.

[43] Nuzzo D, Picone P. Potential neurological effects of severe COVID-19 infection. Neurosci Res. 2020;158:1-5.

[44] Watzky M, de DM, Letessier A, Saint-Ruf C, Miotto B. Assessing the consequences of environmental exposures on the expression of the human receptor and proteases involved in SARS-CoV-2 cell-entry. Environ Res. 2020;110317.

[45] Lamers MM, Beumer J, van d, V, Knoops K, Puschhof J, Breugem TI, et al. SARS-CoV-2 productively infects human gut enterocytes. Science. 2020;369(6499):50-54.

[46] Wu C, Liu Y, Yang Y, Zhang P, Zhong W, et al. Analysis of therapeutic targets for SARS-CoV-2 and discovery of potential drugs by computational methods. Acta Pharm. Sin. B. 2020; 5:766-788.

[47] Chen YW, Yiu CB, Wong KY. Prediction of the SARS-CoV-2 (2019-nCoV) 3C-like protease (3CL (pro)) structure: virtual screening reveals velpatasvir, ledipasvir, and other drug repurposing candidates. F1000Res. 2020;9:129.

[48] Adem S, Eyupoglu V, Sarfraz I, Rasul A, Ali M. Identification of Potent COVID-19 Main Protease (Mpro) Inhibitors from Natural Polyphenols: An in Silico Strategy Unveils a Hope against CORONA. Preprints. 2020; 2020030333.

[49] Utomo RY, Ikawati M, Meyianto E. Revealing the potency of citrus and galangal constituents to halt SARS-CoV-2 infection. Preprints. 2020. doi:10.20944/preprints202003.0214.v1

[50] Das S, Sarmah S, Lyndem S, Singha RA. An investigation into the identification of potential inhibitors of SARS-CoV-2 main protease using molecular docking study. J Biomol Struct Dyn. 2020;1-11.

[51] Joshi RS, Jagdale SS, Bansode SB, Shankar SS, Tellis MB, Pandya VK, et al. Discovery of potential multi-target-directed ligands by targeting host-specific SARS-CoV-2 structurally conserved main protease. J Biomol Struct Dyn. 2020;1-16.

[52] Basu A, Sarkar A, Maulik U. Molecular docking study of potential phytochemicals and their effects on the complex of SARS-CoV2 spike protein and human ACE2. Sci Rep. 2020;10(1):17699.

[53] Behloul N, Baha S, Guo Y, Yang Z, Shi R, Meng J. In silico identification of strong binders of the SARS-CoV-2 receptor-binding domain. Eur J Pharmacol. 2020;173701.

[54] Mahdian S, Ebrahim-Habibi A, Zarrabi M. Drug repurposing using computational methods to identify therapeutic options for COVID-19. J Diabetes Metab Disord. 2020;1-9.

[55] Balmeh N, Mahmoudi S, Mohammadi N, Karabedianhajiabadi A. Predicted therapeutic targets for COVID-19 disease by inhibiting SARS-CoV-2 and its related receptors. Inform Med Unlocked. 2020;20:100407.

[56] Pandey P, Rane JS, Chatterjee A, Kumar A, Khan R, Prakash A, et al. Targeting SARS-CoV-2 spike protein of COVID-19 with naturally occurring phytochemicals: an in silico study for drug development. J Biomol Struct Dyn. 2020;1-11.

[57] Glinsky GV. Tripartite Combination of Candidate Pandemic Mitigation Agents: Vitamin D, Quercetin, and Estradiol Manifest Properties of Medicinal Agents for Targeted Mitigation of the COVID-19 Pandemic Defined by Genomics-Guided Tracing of SARS-CoV-2 Targets in Human Cells. Biomedicines. 2020;8(5).

[58] Jiang Y, Liu L, Manning M, Bonahoom M, Lotvola A, Yang Z, et al. Structural analysis, virtual screening and molecular simulation to identify potential inhibitors targeting 2'-O-ribose methyltransferase of SARS-CoV-2 coronavirus. J Biomol Struct Dyn. 2020;1-16.

[59] Nguyen TT, Woo HJ, Kang HK, Nguyen VD, Kim YM, Kim DW, et al. Flavonoid-mediated inhibition of SARS coronavirus 3C-like protease expressed in Pichia pastoris. Biotechnol Lett. 2012;34(5):831-838.

[60] Park JY, Yuk HJ, Ryu HW, Lim SH, Kim KS, Park KH, et al. Evaluation of polyphenols from Broussonetia papyrifera as coronavirus protease inhibitors. J Enzyme Inhib Med Chem. 2017;32(1):504-515.

[61] Khaerunnisa S, Kurniawan H, Awaluddin R, Suhartati S, Soetjipto S. Potential Inhibitor of COVID-19 Main Protease (Mpro) From Several Medicinal Plant Compounds by Molecular Docking Study. Preprints. 2020;202003.0226.v1.

[62] Abian O, Ortega-Alarcon D, Jimenez-Alesanco A, Ceballos-Laita L, Vega S, Reyburn HT, et al. Structural stability of SARS-CoV-2 3CLpro

and identification of quercetin as an inhibitor by experimental screening. Int J Biol Macromol. 2020;164:1693-1703.

[63] da Silva FMA, da Silva KPA, de Oliveira LPM, Costa EV, Koolen HH, Pinheiro MLB, et al. Flavonoid glycosides and their putative human metabolites as potential inhibitors of the SARS-CoV-2 main protease (Mpro) and RNA-dependent RNA polymerase (RdRp). Mem Inst Oswaldo Cruz. 2020;115:e200207.

[64] Erlund I, Kosonen T, Alfthan G, Mäenpää J, Perttunen K, Kenraali J, et al. Pharmacokinetics of quercetin from quercetin aglycone and rutin in healthy volunteers. Eur J Clin Pharmacol. 2000;56(8):545-553.

[65] Manach C, Donovan JL. Pharmacokinetics and metabolism of dietary flavonoids in humans. Free Radic Res. 2004;38(8):771-785.

[66] Manach C, Williamson G, Morand C, Scalbert A, Rémésy C C. Bioavailability and bioefficacy of polyphenols in humans. I. Review of 97 bioavailability studies. Am J Clin Nutr. 2005;81(1 Suppl):230S–242S.

[67] Khomich OA, Kochetkov SN, Bartosch B, Ivanov AV. Redox Biology of Respiratory Viral Infections. Viruses. 2018;10(8).

[68] Zhang X, Wu X, Hu Q, Wu J, Wang G, Hong Z, et al. Mitochondrial DNA in liver inflammation and oxidative stress. Life Sci. 2019;236:116464.

[69] Bhargava A, Raghuram GV, Pathak N, Varshney S, Jatawa SK, Jain D, et al. Occult hepatitis C virus elicits mitochondrial oxidative stress in lymphocytes and triggers PI3-kinase-mediated DNA damage response. Free Radic Biol Med. 2011;51(9):1806-1814.

[70] Kido H, Indalao IL, Kim H, Kimoto T, Sakai S, Takahashi E. Energy metabolic disorder is a major risk factor in severe influenza virus infection: Proposals for new therapeutic options based on animal model experiments. Respir Investig. 2016;54(5):312-319.

[71] Saleh J, Peyssonnaux C, Singh KK, Edeas M. Mitochondria and microbiota dysfunction in COVID-19 pathogenesis. Mitochondrion. 2020;54:1-7.

[72] Keles ES. Mild SARS-CoV-2 infections in children might be based on evolutionary biology and linked with host reactive oxidative stress and antioxidant capabilities. New Microbes New Infect. 2020;36:100723.

[73] Delgado-Roche L, Mesta F. Oxidative Stress as Key Player in Severe Acute Respiratory Syndrome Coronavirus (SARS-CoV) Infection. Arch Med Res. 2020;51(5):384-387.

[74] Trujillo JA, Croft NP, Dudek NL, Channappanavar R, Theodossis A, Webb AI, et al. The cellular redox environment alters antigen presentation. J Biol Chem. 2014;289(40):27979-27991.

[75] Hati S, Bhattacharyya S. Impact of Thiol-Disulfide Balance on the Binding of Covid-19 Spike Protein with Angiotensin-Converting Enzyme 2 Receptor. ACS Omega. 2020;5(26):16292-16298.

[76] Dalan R, Bornstein SR, El-Armouche A, Rodionov RN, Markov A, Wielockx B, et al. The ACE-2 in COVID-19: Foe or Friend? Horm Metab Res. 2020;52(5):257-263.

[77] Lavillette D, Barbouche R, Yao Y, Boson B, Cosset FL, Jones IM, et al. Significant redox insensitivity of the functions of the SARS-CoV spike glycoprotein: comparison with HIV envelope. J Biol Chem. 2006;281(14):9200-9204.

[78] Sestili P, Fimognari C. Paracetamol-Induced Glutathione Consumption:

Is There a Link With Severe COVID-19 Illness? Front Pharmacol. 2020;11:579944.

[79] Silvagno F, Vernone A, Pescarmona GP. The Role of Glutathione in Protecting against the Severe Inflammatory Response Triggered by COVID-19. Antioxidants (Basel). 2020;9(7).

[80] Dattilo M. The role of host defences in Covid 19 and treatments thereof. Mol Med. 2020;26(1):90.

[81] Bertolini A, van de Peppel IP, Bodewes FAJA, Moshage H, Fantin A, Farinati F, et al. Abnormal Liver Function Tests in Patients With COVID-19: Relevance and Potential Pathogenesis. Hepatology. 2020 ;72(5):1864-1872.

[82] Piano S, Dalbeni A, Vettore E, Benfaremo D, Mattioli M, Gambino CG, et al. Abnormal liver function tests predict transfer to intensive care unit and death in COVID-19. Liver Int. 2020;40(10):2394-2406.

[83] Park HK, Kang SW, Park MS. Hesperidin Ameliorates Hepatic Ischemia-Reperfusion Injury in Sprague-Dawley Rats. Transplant Proc. 2019;51(8):2828-2832.

[84] Jo SH, Kim ME, Cho JH, Lee Y, Lee J, Park YD, et al. Hesperetin inhibits neuroinflammation on microglia by suppressing inflammatory cytokines and MAPK pathways. Arch Pharm Res. 2019;42(8):695-703.

[85] Colunga Biancatelli RML, Berrill M, Catravas JD, Marik PE. Quercetin and Vitamin C: An Experimental, Synergistic Therapy for the Prevention and Treatment of SARS-CoV-2 Related Disease (COVID-19). Front Immunol. 2020;11:1451.

[86] Boots AW, Kubben N, Haenen GR, Bast A. Oxidized quercetin reacts with thiols rather than with ascorbate: implication for quercetin supplementation. Biochem Biophys Res Commun. 2003;308(3):560-565.

[87] Kerimi A, Williamson G. Differential Impact of Flavonoids on Redox Modulation, Bioenergetics, and Cell Signaling in Normal and Tumor Cells: A Comprehensive Review. Antioxid Redox Signal. 2018;29(16):1633-1659.

[88] Chen M, Gu H, Ye Y, Lin B, Sun L, Deng W, et al. Protective effects of hesperidin against oxidative stress of tert-butyl hydroperoxide in human hepatocytes. Food Chem Toxicol. 2010;48(10):2980-2987.

[89] Roohbakhsh A, Parhiz H, Soltani F, Rezaee R, Iranshahi M. Molecular mechanisms behind the biological effects of hesperidin and hesperetin for the prevention of cancer and cardiovascular diseases. Life Sci. 2015;124:64-74.

[90] Oh YS, Jun HS. Effects of Glucagon-Like Peptide-1 on Oxidative Stress and Nrf2 Signaling. Int J Mol Sci. 2017;19(1).

[91] Ikram M, Muhammad T, Rehman SU, Khan A, Jo MG, Ali T, et al. Hesperetin Confers Neuroprotection by Regulating Nrf2/TLR4/NF-Î°B Signaling in an AÎ² Mouse Model. Mol Neurobiol. 2019;56(9):6293-6309.

[92] Wu J, Huang G, Li Y, Li X. Flavonoids from Aurantii Fructus Immaturus and Aurantii Fructus: promising phytomedicines for the treatment of liver diseases. Chin Med. 2020;15:89.

[93] Kwatra M, Ahmed S, Gawali B, Panda SR, Naidu VGM. Hesperidin alleviates chronic restraint stress and lipopolysaccharide-induced Hippocampus and Frontal cortex damage in mice: Role of TLR4/NF-Î°B,

p38 MAPK/JNK, Nrf2/ARE signaling. Neurochem Int. 2020;104835.

[94] Sun GY, Chen Z, Jasmer KJ, Chuang DY, Gu Z, Hannink M, et al. Quercetin Attenuates Inflammatory Responses in BV-2 Microglial Cells: Role of MAPKs on the Nrf2 Pathway and Induction of Heme Oxygenase-1. PLoS ONE. 2015;10(10):e0141509.

[95] Costa LG, Garrick JM, RoquÃ¨ PJ, Pellacani C. Mechanisms of Neuroprotection by Quercetin: Counteracting Oxidative Stress and More. Oxid Med Cell Longev. 2016;2016:2986796.

[96] Mahmoud AM, Mohammed HM, Khadrawy SM, Galaly SR. Hesperidin protects against chemically induced hepatocarcinogenesis via modulation of Nrf2/ARE/HO-1, PPARγ and TGF-β1/ Smad$_3$ signaling, and amelioration of oxidative stress and inflammation. Chem Biol Interact. 2017;277:146-158.

[97] Tabeshpour J, Hosseinzadeh H, Hashemzaei M, Karimi G. A review of the hepatoprotective effects of hesperidin, a flavanon glycoside in citrus fruits, against natural and chemical toxicities. Daru. 2020;28(1):305-317.

[98] Hong Y, An Z. Hesperidin attenuates learning and memory deficits in APP/PS1 mice through activation of Akt/Nrf2 signaling and inhibition of RAGE/NF-kB signaling. Arch Pharm Res. 2018;41(6):655-663.

[99] Hannan MA, Dash R, Sohag AAM, Haque MN, Moon IS. Neuroprotection Against Oxidative Stress: Phytochemicals Targeting TrkB Signaling and the Nrf2-ARE Antioxidant System. Front Mol Neurosci. 2020;13:116.

[100] Elyasi L, Jahanshahi M, Jameie SB, Hamid Abadi HG, Nikmahzar E, Khalili M, et al. 6-OHDA mediated neurotoxicity in SH-SY5Y cellular model of Parkinson disease suppressed by pretreatment with hesperidin through activating L-type calcium channels. J Basic Clin Physiol Pharmacol. 2020. DOI: 10.1515/jbcpp-2019-0270

[101] Kesh S, Kannan RR, Sivaji K, Balakrishnan A. Hesperidin downregulates kinases lrrk2 and Gsk3β in a 6-OHDA induced Parkinson's disease model. Neurosci Lett. 2020;740:135426.

[102] Antunes MS, Cattelan SL, Ladd FVL, Ladd AABL, Moreira AL, Bortolotto VC, et al. Hesperidin Ameliorates Anxiety-Depressive-Like Behavior in 6-OHDA Model of Parkinson's Disease by Regulating Striatal Cytokine and Neurotrophic Factors Levels and Dopaminergic Innervation Loss in the Striatum of Mice. Mol Neurobiol. 2020;57(7):3027-3041.

[103] Suganthy N, Devi KP, Nabavi SF, Braidy N, Nabavi SM. Bioactive effects of quercetin in the central nervous system: Focusing on the mechanisms of actions. Biomed Pharmacother. 2016;84:892-908.

[104] Erlich JR, To EE, Liong S, Brooks R, Vlahos R, O'Leary JJ, et al. Targeting Evolutionary Conserved Oxidative Stress and Immunometabolic Pathways for the Treatment of Respiratory Infectious Diseases. Antioxid Redox Signal. 2020;32(13):993-1013.

[105] Potus F, Mai V, Lebret M, Malenfant S, Breton-Gagnon E, Lajoie AC, et al. Novel insights on the pulmonary vascular consequences of COVID-19. Am J Physiol Lung Cell Mol Physiol. 2020;319(2):L277-L288.

[106] Perricone C, Bartoloni E, Bursi R, Cafaro G, Guidelli GM, Shoenfeld Y, et al. COVID-19 as part of the hyperferritinemic syndromes: the role

of iron depletion therapy. Immunol Res. 2020;1-12.

[107] Ruscitti P, Berardicurti O, Di BP, Cipriani P, Iagnocco A, Shoenfeld Y, et al. Severe COVID-19, Another Piece in the Puzzle of the Hyperferritinemic Syndrome. An Immunomodulatory Perspective to Alleviate the Storm. Front Immunol. 2020;11.

[108] Uchide N, Toyoda H. Antioxidant therapy as a potential approach to severe influenza-associated complications. Molecules. 2011;16(3):2032-2052.

[109] Santus P, Corsico A, Solidoro P, Braido F, Di MF, Scichilone N. Oxidative stress and respiratory system: pharmacological and clinical reappraisal of N-acetylcysteine. COPD. 2014;11(6):705-717.

[110] De FS, Grassi C, Carati L. Attenuation of influenza-like symptomatology and improvement of cell-mediated immunity with long-term N-acetylcysteine treatment. Eur Respir J. 1997;10(7):1535-1541.

[111] Soltan-Sharifi MS, Mojtahedzadeh M, Najafi A, Reza KM, Reza RM, Moradi M, et al. Improvement by N-acetylcysteine of acute respiratory distress syndrome through increasing intracellular glutathione, and extracellular thiol molecules and anti-oxidant power: evidence for underlying toxicological mechanisms. Hum Exp Toxicol. 2007;26(9):697-703.

[112] Poe FL, Corn J. N-Acetylcysteine: A potential therapeutic agent for SARS-CoV-2. Med Hypotheses. 2020;143:109862.

[113] Wu J. Tackle the free radicals damage in COVID-19. Nitric Oxide. 2020;102:39-41.

[114] De Flora S, Balansky R, La Maestra S. Rationale for the use of N-acetylcysteine in both prevention and adjuvant therapy of COVID-19. FASEB J. 2020;34(10):13185-13193.

[115] Elavarasan J, Velusamy P, Ganesan T, Ramakrishnan SK, Rajasekaran D, Periandavan K. Hesperidin-mediated expression of Nrf2 and upregulation of antioxidant status in senescent rat heart. J Pharm Pharmacol. 2012;64(10):1472-1482.

[116] Velusamy P, Mohan T, Ravi DB, Kishore Kumar SN, Srinivasan A, Chakrapani LN, et al. Targeting the Nrf2/ARE Signalling Pathway to Mitigate Isoproterenol-Induced Cardiac Hypertrophy: Plausible Role of Hesperetin in Redox Homeostasis. Oxid Med Cell Longev. 2020;2020:9568278.

[117] Miler M, Zivanovic J, Ajdzanovic V, Orescanin-Dusic Z, Milenkovic D, Konic-Ristic A, et al. Citrus flavanones naringenin and hesperetin improve antioxidant status and membrane lipid compositions in the liver of old-aged Wistar rats. Exp Gerontol. 2016;84:49-60.

[118] Li S, Qin Q, Luo D, Pan W, Wei Y, Xu Y, et al. Hesperidin ameliorates liver ischemia/reperfusion injury via activation of the Akt pathway. Mol Med Rep. 2020;22(6):4519-4530.

[119] Aja PM, Ekpono EU, Awoke JN, Famurewa AC, Izekwe FI, Okoro EJ, et al. Hesperidin ameliorates hepatic dysfunction and dyslipidemia in male Wistar rats exposed to cadmium chloride. Toxicol Rep. 2020;7:1331-1338.

[120] Duranti G, Ceci R, Patrizio F, Sgrò P, Di LL, Sabatini S, et al. Chronic consumption of quercetin reduces erythrocytes oxidative damage: Evaluation at resting and after eccentric exercise in humans. Nutr Res. 2018;50:73-81.

[121] Cavalli E, Bramanti A, Ciurleo R, Tchorbanov AI, Giordano A, Fagone P, et al. Entangling COVID-19

associated thrombosis into a secondary antiphospholipid antibody syndrome: Diagnostic and therapeutic perspectives (Review). Int J Mol Med. 2020;46(3):903-912.

[122] Lyons-Weiler J. Pathogenic Priming Likely Contributes to Serious and Critical Illness and Mortality in COVID-19 via Autoimmunity. J Transl Autoimmun. 2020;100051.

[123] Ehrenfeld M, Tincani A, Andreoli L, Cattalini M, Greenbaum A, Kanduc D, et al. Covid-19 and autoimmunity. Autoimmun Rev. 2020;19(8):102597.

[124] Shoenfeld Y. Corona (COVID-19) time musings: Our involvement in COVID-19 pathogenesis, diagnosis, treatment and vaccine planning. Autoimmun Rev. 2020;19(6):102538.

[125] Ruiz-Iglesias P, Estruel-Amades S, Camps-Bossacoma M, Massot-Cladera M, Franch Ã, Pérez-Cano FJ, et al. Influence of Hesperidin on Systemic Immunity of Rats Following an Intensive Training and Exhausting Exercise. Nutrients. 2020;12(5).

[126] Estruel-Amades S, Massot-Cladera M, Garcia-CerdÃ P, Pérez-Cano FJ, Franch Ã, Castell M, et al. Protective Effect of Hesperidin on the Oxidative Stress Induced by an Exhausting Exercise in Intensively Trained Rats. Nutrients. 2019;11(4).

[127] Polat FR, Karaboga I, Polat MS, Erboga Z, Yilmaz A, Guzel S. Effect of hesperetin on inflammatory and oxidative status in trinitrobenzene sulfonic acid-induced experimental colitis model. Cell Mol Biol (Noisy -le-grand). 2018;64(11):58-65.

[128] Duran Y, Karaboga I. Effect of hesperetin on systemic inflammation and hepatic injury after blunt chest trauma in rats. Biotech Histochem. 2020;95(4):297-304.

[129] Ren H, Hao J, Liu T, Zhang D, Lv H, Song E, et al. Hesperetin Suppresses Inflammatory Responses in Lipopolysaccharide-Induced RAW 264.7 Cells via the Inhibition of NF-Î°B and Activation of Nrf2/HO-1 Pathways. Inflammation. 2016;39(3):964-973.

[130] Yeh CC, Kao SJ, Lin CC, Wang SD, Liu CJ, Kao ST. The immunomodulation of endotoxin-induced acute lung injury by hesperidin in vivo and in vitro. Life Sci. 2007;80(20):1821-1831.

[131] Wang N, Geng C, Sun H, Wang X, Li F, Liu X. Hesperetin ameliorates lipopolysaccharide-induced acute lung injury in mice through regulating the TLR4-MyD88-NF-kappaB signaling pathway. Arch Pharm Res. 2019;42(12):1063-1070.

[132] Dong J, Zhou H, Zhao H, Zhao Y, Chang C. Hesperetin ameliorates lipopolysaccharide-induced acute lung injury via the miR-410/SOX18 axis. J Biochem Mol Toxicol. 2020;e22588.

[133] Ma H, Feng X, Ding S. Hesperetin attenuates ventilator-induced acute lung injury through inhibition of NF-kB-mediated inflammation. Eur J Pharmacol. 2015;769:333-341.

[134] Wang S, He N, Xing H, Sun Y, Ding J, Liu L. Function of hesperidin alleviating inflammation and oxidative stress responses in COPD mice might be related to SIRT1/PGC-1α/NF-kB signaling axis. J Recept Signal Transduct Res. 2020 Aug;40(4):388-394.

[135] Shaik YB, Castellani ML, Perrella A, Conti F, Salini V, Tete S, et al. Role of quercetin (a natural herbal compound) in allergy and inflammation. J Biol Regul Homeost Agents. 2006;20(3-4):47-52.

[136] Cho SY, Park SJ, Kwon MJ, Jeong TS, Bok SH, Choi WY, et al. Quercetin suppresses proinflammatory cytokines production through MAP

kinases andNF-kappaB pathway in lipopolysaccharide-stimulated macrophage. Mol Cell Biochem. 2003;243(1-2):153-160.

[137] Marseglia GL, Licari A, Ciprandi G. A polycentric, randomized, double blind, parallel-group, placebo-controlled study on Lertal®, a multicomponent nutraceutical, as add-on treatment in children with allergic rhinoconjunctivitis: phase I during active treatment. J Biol Regul Homeost Agents. 2019;33(2):617-622.

[138] Marseglia G, Licari A, Leonardi S, Papale M, Zicari AM, Schiavi L, et al. A polycentric, randomized, parallel-group, study on Lertal®, a multicomponent nutraceutical, as preventive treatment in children with allergic rhinoconjunctivitis: phase II. Ital J Pediatr. 2019;45(1):84.

[139] Kimata M, Shichijo M, Miura T, Serizawa I, Inagaki N, Nagai H. Effects of luteolin, quercetin and baicalein on immunoglobulin E-mediated mediator release from human cultured mast cells. Clin Exp Allergy. 2000;30(4):501-508.

[140] Min YD, Choi CH, Bark H, Son HY, Park HH, Lee S, et al. Quercetin inhibits expression of inflammatory cytokines through attenuation of NF-kappaB and p38 MAPK in HMC-1 human mast cell line. Inflamm Res. 2007;56(5):210-215.

[141] Kalogeromitros D, Makris M, Chliva C, Aggelides X, Kempuraj D, Theoharides TC. A quercetin containing supplement reduces niacin-induced flush in humans. Int J Immunopathol Pharmacol. 2008;21(3):509-514.

[142] Park SJ, Chung HY, Lee JH. Rapid in vivo screening system for anti-oxidant activity using bacterial redox sensor strains. J Appl Microbiol. 2010;108(4):1217-1225..

[143] Lee EJ, Ji GE, Sung MK. Quercetin and kaempferol suppress immunoglobulin E-mediated allergic inflammation in RBL-2H3 and Caco-2 cells. Inflamm Res. 2010; 59(10):847-854.

[144] Middleton E Jr, Drzewiecki G. Flavonoid inhibition of human basophil histamine release stimulated by various agents. Biochem Pharmacol. 1984;33(21):3333-3338.

[145] Chirumbolo S, Conforti A, Ortolani R, Vella A, Marzotto M, Bellavite P. Stimulus-specific regulation of CD63 and CD203c membrane expression in human basophils by the flavonoid quercetin. Int Immunopharmacol. 2010;10(2):183-192.

[146] Ying B, Yang T, Song X, Hu X, Fan H, Lu X, et al. Quercetin inhibits IL-1 beta-induced ICAM-1 expression in pulmonary epithelial cell line A549 through the MAPK pathways. Mol Biol Rep. 2009;36(7):1825-1832.

[147] Chirumbolo S, Marzotto M, Conforti A, Vella A, Ortolani R, Bellavite P. Bimodal action of the flavonoid quercetin on basophil function: an investigation of the putative biochemical targets. Clin Mol Allergy. 2010;8:13.

[148] Zaplatic E, Bule M, Shah SZA, Uddin MS, Niaz K. Molecular mechanisms underlying protective role of quercetin in attenuating Alzheimer's disease. Life Sci. 2019;224:109-119.

[149] Theoharides TC. COVID-19, pulmonary mast cells, cytokine storms, and beneficial actions of luteolin. Biofactors. 2020;46(3):306-308.

[150] Mohammadi-Sartang M, Mazloom Z, Sherafatmanesh S, Ghorbani M, Firoozi D. Effects of supplementation with quercetin on plasma C-reactive protein concentrations: a systematic review and meta-analysis of randomized

controlled trials. Eur J Clin Nutr. 2017;71(9):1033-1039.

[151] Chanet A, Milenkovic D, Manach C, Mazur A, Morand C. Citrus flavanones: what is their role in cardiovascular protection? J Agric Food Chem. 2012;60(36):8809-8822.

[152] Valls RM, Pedret A, Calderon-Perez L, Llaurado E, Pla-Paga L, Companys J, et al. Effects of hesperidin in orange juice on blood and pulse pressures in mildly hypertensive individuals: a randomized controlled trial (Citrus study). Eur J Nutr. 2020 Jul 13. DOI: 10.1007/s00394-020-02279-0.

[153] Pittala V, Vanella L, Salerno L, Romeo G, Marrazzo A, Di GC, et al. Effects of Polyphenolic Derivatives on Heme Oxygenase-System in Metabolic Dysfunctions. Curr Med Chem. 2018;25(13):1577-1595.

[154] Garcia-Garcia FJ, Monistrol-Mula A, Cardellach F, Garrabou G. Nutrition, Bioenergetics, and Metabolic Syndrome. Nutrients. 2020;12(9).

[155] Yari Z, Movahedian M, Imani H, Alavian SM, Hedayati M, Hekmatdoost A. The effect of hesperidin supplementation on metabolic profiles in patients with metabolic syndrome: a randomized, double-blind, placebo-controlled clinical trial. Eur J Nutr. 2020;59(6):2569-2577.

[156] Prasatthong P, Meephat S, Rattanakanokchai S, Bunbupha S, Prachaney P, Maneesai P, et al. Hesperidin ameliorates signs of the metabolic syndrome and cardiac dysfunction via IRS/Akt/GLUT4 signaling pathway in a rat model of diet-induced metabolic syndrome. Eur J Nutr. 2020 May 27. doi: 10.1007/s00394-020-02291-4.

[157] Amiot MJ, Riva C, Vinet A. Effects of dietary polyphenols on metabolic syndrome features in humans: a systematic review. Obes Rev. 2016 ;17(7):573-586.

[158] Rizza S, Muniyappa R, Iantorno M, Kim JA, Chen H, Pullikotil P, et al. Citrus polyphenol hesperidin stimulates production of nitric oxide in endothelial cells while improving endothelial function and reducing inflammatory markers in patients with metabolic syndrome. J Clin Endocrinol Metab. 2011;96(5):E782-E792.

[159] Homayouni F, Haidari F, Hedayati M, Zakerkish M, Ahmadi K. Blood pressure lowering and anti-inflammatory effects of hesperidin in type 2 diabetes; a randomized double-blind controlled clinical trial. Phytother Res. 2018;32(6):1073-1079.

[160] Cassidy A, Bertoia M, Chiuve S, Flint A, Forman J, Rimm EB. Habitual intake of anthocyanins and flavanones and risk of cardiovascular disease in men. Am J Clin Nutr. 2016;104(3):587-594.

[161] Gandhi GR, Vasconcelos ABS, Wu DT, Li HB, Antony PJ, Li H, et al. Citrus Flavonoids as Promising Phytochemicals Targeting Diabetes and Related Complications: A Systematic Review of In Vitro and In Vivo Studies. Nutrients. 2020;12(10).

[162] Ostadmohammadi V, Milajerdi A, Ayati E, Kolahdooz F, Asemi Z. Effects of quercetin supplementation on glycemic control among patients with metabolic syndrome and related disorders: A systematic review and meta-analysis of randomized controlled trials. Phytother Res. 2019;33(5):1330-1340.

[163] Guo W, Gong X, Li M. Quercetin Actions on Lipid Profiles in Overweight and Obese Individuals: A Systematic Review and Meta-Analysis. Curr Pharm Des. 2019;25(28):3087-3095.

[164] Tamtaji OR, Milajerdi A, Dadgostar E, Kolahdooz F, Chamani M,

Amirani E, et al. The Effects of Quercetin Supplementation on Blood Pressures and Endothelial Function Among Patients with Metabolic Syndrome and Related Disorders: A Systematic Review and Meta-analysis of Randomized Controlled Trials. Curr Pharm Des. 2019;25(12):1372-1384.

[165] Zhang M, Zhou Y, Li H, Peng Y, Qiu P, Shi X, et al. COVID-19: gastrointestinal symptoms from the view of gut-lung axis. Eur J Gastroenterol Hepatol. 2020 Oct 29. doi: 10.1097/MEG.0000000000001984

[166] Stevens Y, Rymenant EV, Grootaert C, Camp JV, Possemiers S, Masclee A, et al. The Intestinal Fate of Citrus Flavanones and Their Effects on Gastrointestinal Health. Nutrients. 2019; 11(7).

[167] Lima ACD, Cecatti C, Fidélix MP, Adorno MAT, Sakamoto IK, Cesar TB, et al. Effect of Daily Consumption of Orange Juice on the Levels of Blood Glucose, Lipids, and Gut Microbiota Metabolites: Controlled Clinical Trials. J Med Food. 2019;22(2):202-210.

[168] Fidelix M, Milenkovic D, Sivieri K, Cesar T. Microbiota modulation and effects on metabolic biomarkers by orange juice: a controlled clinical trial. Food Funct. 2020;11(2):1599-1610.

[169] Mas-Capdevila A, Teichenne J, Domenech-Coca C, Caimari A, Del Bas JM, Escotà X, et al. Effect of Hesperidin on Cardiovascular Disease Risk Factors: The Role of Intestinal Microbiota on Hesperidin Bioavailability. Nutrients. 2020;12(5).

[170] Murota K, Nakamura Y, Uehara M. Flavonoid metabolism: the interaction of metabolites and gut microbiota. Biosci Biotechnol Biochem. 2018;82(4):600-610.

Section 4

Recent Topics in Antioxidant Research

Chapter 24

Evolutionary Strategies of Highly Functional Catalases for Adaptation to High H_2O_2 Environments

Isao Yumoto, Yoshiko Hanaoka and Isao Hara

Abstract

Enzymatic evolutionary strategies for adaptation to a high H_2O_2 environment have been evaluated using catalases with high catalytic efficiency isolated from two H_2O_2-tolerant bacteria, *Exiguobacterium oxidotolerans* and *Psychrobacter piscatori*. The entrance size of the narrow main channel in catalase has been estimated by determining the formation rate of the intermediate state of peracetic acid (b), which is a larger substrate than H_2O_2 versus that of catalase activity with H_2O_2 (a) (calculated as b/a). The ratio of b/a in *E. oxidotolerans* catalase (EKTA) is much higher than that of *P. piscatori* catalase (PKTA). To elucidate the structural differences between the catalases, the amino acids present in the main channel have been compared between the two catalases and other catalases in the database. The combination of amino acid residues, which contribute high catalytic efficiency in the narrow main channel of EKTA were different from those in PKTA. In this review, we discuss strategic differences in the elimination of high concentration of H_2O_2 owing to differences in the phylogenetic positions of catalases. In addition, we describe the relationships between the environmental distributions of genera involved in H_2O_2-resistant bacteria and their catalase functions based on the main channel structure of catalase.

Keywords: H_2O_2-tolerant bacteria, *Exiguobacterium*, *Psychrobacter*, *Vibrio*, catalase, narrow main channel, bottleneck size

1. Introduction

Oxygen is important for metabolism, acting as a terminal electron acceptor in aerobic bacteria, and these bacteria produce intracellular reactive oxygen species (ROS), such as hydrogen peroxide (H_2O_2), superoxide ($O^{2\bullet-}$), and hydroxyl radical ($OH^{\bullet}$) as by-products of oxygen metabolism [1–4]. H_2O_2 is not a strongly harmful substance; however, the presence of H_2O_2 in bacterial cells may lead to the generation of harmful ROS, such as $OH^{\bullet}$, via the Fenton reaction. Therefore, the presence of catalase is critical for the protection of cellular components, such as DNA, RNA, proteins, and lipids, from strongly harmful $OH^{\bullet}$ [5–7]. Moreover, the production of intracellular catalases is important for the metabolism of aerobic microorganisms to conduct their metabolisms.

 IntechOpen

Bacteria possess catalases for the elimination of toxic by-products of oxygen metabolism produced inside the cells and for preserving their niches by eliminating the H_2O_2 produced by host organisms [8–10]. This function is important, particularly for pathogenic and symbiotic microorganisms or microorganisms needing to maintain their niches in the host. In such cases, bacterial catalases may have evolved during interactions with the host (to degrade active oxygen species generated by the host for parasites elimination) or parasitic/symbiotic microorganisms (to eliminate active oxygen species generated by the parasites/symbionts). For example, *Aliivibrio fischeri* (formerly *Vibrio fischeri*) exhibits a symbiotic relationship with the host squid by colonising the light-emitting organs of the squid. The host squid possesses a protective mechanism associated with the production of H_2O_2 to prevent the colonization of unfavourable pathogenic bacteria. In contrast, *A. fischeri* produces highly efficient catalase in the periplasmic space to eliminate H_2O_2 produced by the host squid. Thus, production of catalase in the vicinity of the cell surface is important for helping microorganisms to establish their niche.

The oral biofilm community consists of various microorganisms, including foe and companion bacteria and functions to maintain the ecological balance among constituents [11]. Among these community members, *Streptococcus gordonii* is known to produce H_2O_2 to expel its competitors. Additionally, *Veillonella atypica* is able to support the growth of the obligate anaerobe, *Fusobacterium nucleatum* under microaerophilic conditions and can also protect the microorganism from *S. gordonii* via production of catalase. Thus, extracellular catalase production is important for protection not only of the niche of the producer but also of other companion microorganisms to facilitate the formation of microbial communities within biofilm.

Catalase is commonly observed in various aerobic bacteria. Bacteria that do not possess catalase cannot grow on the agar plates owing to the presence of H_2O_2 on agar plates [12]. However, many bacterial strains have been isolated from agar plates, suggesting that these bacteria likely express catalase and these bacteria are likely to encounter H_2O_2. Moreover, these data suggest that H_2O_2 may be ubiquitously present in various environments in which many microorganisms live. Accordingly, investigation of the molecular strategies through which catalase eliminates H_2O_2 in various physiological, ecological, and taxonomic background is essential.

In this review, we evaluate the relationships between catalase evolution and structural changes in the main channel structure of catalases, based on various catalases including those isolated from H_2O_2- tolerant bacteria. In addition, considering the taxonomic backgrounds of H_2O_2-tolerant bacteria, we compared the main channel structures of catalases derived from the same genera of H_2O_2-tolerant bacteria and discussed the reasons for the distribution of these H_2O_2-tolerant bacteria. This systematic approach will bring deeper understanding in strategic evolutionary changes in bacterial catalases and strategic bacterial distributions in the environment.

2. Phylogeny of catalases

The dismutation of H_2O_2 in microorganisms occurs mainly via three phylogenetically unrelated catalases: monofunctional catalase, catalase-peroxidase, and Mn-catalase [2, 13]. Here, we focus on monofunctional catalases.

Bacterial monofunctional catalases are classified into clades 1–3 according to phylogenetic analysis based on their amino acid sequences [14, 15]. Clade 1 catalases contain approximately 500 amino acid residues per subunit and are mainly of plant origin, except a subgroup that is of bacterial origin, including Firmicutes group A and Proteobacterial minor group (*Sinorhizobium* clade). Clade 2 catalases, which exhibit larger molecular masses than catalases from other clades, consist of approximately 750 amino acid residues. The catalases in this clade originated from fungi, bacteria including Actionbacteria, Bacteroides, and Proteobacteria (*Polaromonas, Burkholderia* and *Akkermansia*) and archaea. Clade 3 catalases, with nearly 500 residues per subunit, occur in fungi, bacteria including Chloroflexi, Firmicutes group B and Proteobacteria, fungi, and some eukaryotes. Reports have shown that pathogenic or symbiotic bacteria possess only one clade 3 catalase (e.g., *Haemophilus influenzae*, *Neiseria gonorrhoeae*, and *A. fischeri* [described above]). These catalases evolved through interactions between the host and parasite. Moreover, many prokaryotic clade 3 catalases exhibit distinct NADP(H) binding compared with clade 1 catalases, discrimination of catalases between the two clades based on apparent molecular features and enzymatic characteristics is difficult.

3. Reaction mechanisms of catalases

Catalase consists of four identical subunits and each subunit, each of which possesses heme *b* or *d* at the reaction centre. The catalytic reaction cycle consists of the following two steps. The first step involves the formation of compound I, which is produced by oxidation of Fe^{3+} (Fe^{3+} Pro) in the heme moiety to an oxoiron (IV) porphyrin π-cation radical species, $Fe^{4+} = O\ Pro^{+\bullet}$, by the first reacted H_2O_2 molecule [16]. During this reaction, the oxygen–oxygen bond in the peroxide (R–O–O–H) bound to the heme, that is the first H_2O_2 molecule, is cleaved heterolytically. As a result, one oxygen binds to the ion with the by-product of a water molecule. This reaction intermediate, compound I, is subsequently reduced by second reaction of H_2O_2 to the resting state (Fe^{3+} Pro). This reaction leads to the production of molecular oxygen (O_2) and water molecules (H_2O) [17, 18]. Compound I can also be observed if organic peroxides are used as substrates instead of H_2O_2. The compound I formation rate decreases as the molecular size of the substrates increases (i.e., $H_2O_2 > CH_3COO_2H$). Therefore, estimation of the compound I formation rate may be an indicator of the size of the bottleneck structure of the narrow main channel, which is directly accessible to the reaction centre, heme.

4. Characteristics of H_2O_2-resistant bacteria

Catalase is important for cellular protection intra- and extracellular elimination of H_2O_2. Because H_2O_2-tolerant microorganisms may evolve in artificially high H_2O_2 environments, we have studied H_2O_2-tolerant microorganisms and their catalases. First, strain S-1^T can survive downstream of drain pools (sedimentation tank [8°C, 1.5–6 mM]) from herring egg processing factory, which uses H_2O_2 as a breaching agent [19, 20]. This strain was identified as a new species, *Vibrio rumoiensis* S-1^T. The growth temperature range of strain S-1^T is 2–34°C. The catalase activity of cell extracts of strain S-1^T was found to be 4000–8000 U/mg protein, which was one or two orders of magnitude higher than those of *Alcaligenes faecalis*, *Corynebacterium glutamicum*, and *Pseudomonas fluorescens*. Strain S-1^T possesses only one type of clade 3 catalase, which accounts for 1.8% of the protein in cell extracts. The isolate produces catalase not only inside the cell but also in the periplasmic space and on the cell surface [21–24]. Therefore, *V. rumoiensis* S-1^T cells exhibit catalase activity, and expression of catalase on the surface of *V. rumoiensis* cells may help to protect the cell in high H_2O_2 environments. According to several reports on symbiotic or pathogenic strains involving the genus *Vibrio* and its related genus *Aliivibrio*, strain S-1^T was predicted to be derived from marine environments or organisms.

Strain T-2-2^T, an H_2O_2-tolerant microorganism, was isolated from the upstream region of a water treatment system (pretreatment tank to decrease H_2O_2 concentration [8°C, 6–38 mM]) of a herring egg processing factory [25]. The isolate was identified as a new species, *E. oxidotolerans* T-2-2^T. The growth temperature range of this strain was 4–40°C (optimum 34°C). The cell extract of strain T-2-2^T exhibited catalase activity of 28,000 U/mg protein and catalase accounted for 6.5% of protein in the cell extract. The bacterium produced catalase (*E. oxidotolerans* [EKTA]) both intercellularly and extracellularly [26–29]. The immunolocalization of catalase suggests that the enzyme is present on the inner surface of the cells [28]. Catalase that bind to the cell surface and localise to the inner surface are also important for defence against extracellular H_2O_2 in *E. oxidotolerans* T-2-2^T. The localisation of catalase changes from inside of the cells to the cell surface as the culture period is extended. The catalase is induced by H_2O_2 stimulation prior to initiation of growth and low aeration growth condition [27, 29]. Thus, catalase activity is required inside the cells and is essential for extracellular defence as the cell age increases. *Exiguobacterium* spp. are distributed in various environments, including marine environments [30, 31]. Therefore, strain T-2-2^T may have originated from marine environments or organisms. Additionally, although strain T-2-2^T possesses a catalase gene sequence belonging to clade 2, only clade 1 catalase can be purified [32].

Strain T-3-2^T, an H_2O_2-tolerant microorganism, was isolated from the upstream of the water treatment system (pretreatment tank to decrease H_2O_2 concentration [8°C, 6–38 mM]) of a herring egg processing factory [33]. The growth temperature range of strain T-3-2^T is 0–30°C, and the localisation of catalase has not yet been clarified. However, strain T-3-2^T exhibits high resistance against H_2O_2. The isolate was identified as a new species, *P. piscatorii* T-3-2^T and cell extracts of strain T-3-2^T exhibit much higher catalase activity (12,000 U/mg protein) than those of other stains belonging to the same genus, including *Psychrobacter nivimaris* (15 U/ mg protein), *Psychrobacter proteolyticus* (29 U/mg protein) and *Psychrobacter aquamaris* (1800 U/mg protein). Strain T-3 belongs to *P. piscatorii* as well [34, 35] and exhibits higher catalase activity (19,700 U/mg), with catalase accounting for 10% of all proteins in the cell extract. Several reports have described *Psychrobacter* spp. were isolated from marine origins [36]; therefore, it is possible that strains T-3-2^T and T-3 originated from marine environments or organisms. Although the strain T-3 possesses catalase gene sequences belonging to clade 2, only clade 3 catalase can be purified [32].

5. Characteristics of catalases from H_2O_2-resistant bacteria

Catalases derived from H_2O_2-tolerant microorganisms in clade 3 and clade 1 have been purified from *V. rumoiensis* S-1^T, *P. piscatorii* T-3, and from *E. oxidotolerans* T-2-2^T. The kinetic parameters (k_{cat}/K_m) of these catalases were higher or equivalent to the highest values comparing with those of catalases reported by Switala and Loewen (2002) [37]. In addition, these catalase activities exhibited distinctive temperature dependencies comparing with ordinary catalase such as *Micrococcus luteus* catalase (MLC) and bovine liver catalase (BLC) [32]. These characteristics reflect the environmental conditions in which these bacteria were isolated (8°C, 1.5–38 mM H_2O_2). Thus, multiple environmental factors (including low temperature and high H_2O_2) have affected the characteristics of enzymes via evolutionary and/or environmental selection processes.

The catalase from *V. rumoiensis* S-1^T (VKTA) can be purified by two steps of anion-chromatography and one step of gel filtration chromatography [25]. The purified VKTA exhibits 395,000 U/mg protein under standard reaction conditions (30 mM H_2O_2, pH 7), with a V_{max} and K_m of 8.0 × 10^5 μmol H_2O_2/μmol heme/s and 35 mM for H_2O_2, respectively, as determined spectrophotometrically. The catalytic efficiency k_{cat}/K_m of VKTA is 2.3 × 10^7/s/M, which is the highest among reported clade 3 catalases owing to the low K_m value [31]. Additionally, because of the fragility of *V. rumoiensis* S-1^T cells, high affinity to H_2O_2 and high catalytic efficiency are required for protection of the cells. It is known that catalase activity is not as dependent on temperature as the activity of ordinary enzymes. Moreover, VKTA exhibits an obvious temperature dependence between 10°C and 70°C with an optimum temperature at 40°C. The amino acid sequence of VKTA contains active sites (H^{61}, T^{100} and N^{134}), proximal sites of heme (Y^{344} and R^{351}), and binding sites for the distal region of heme (V^{102}, T^{124} and F^{139}). VKTA possesses NADPH- binding sites (H^{180}, R^{189}, V^{288} and K^{291}). The active site containing "T^{100}" is unique compared with that of the other catalases listed in **Figure 1**. Indeed, other catalases contain an "S residue at this position", making the site less hydrophobic. However, the effect of this amino acid substitution on the function is unknown.

EKTA can be purified by two steps of anion-chromatography and one step of gel filtration chromatography. The purified EKTA exhibits an activity of 430,000 U/mg protein under standard reaction condition [26] with a V_{max} and K_m of 1.5 × 10^6 μmol H_2O_2/μmol heme/s and 40 mM for H_2O_2, respectively, as determined by spectrophotometry [28]. The catalytic efficiency k_{cat}/K_m of EKTA is 3.8 × 10^7/s/M, which is the highest among reported clade 1 catalases owing to the high k_{cat} and low K_m values. EKTA exhibits a temperature dependency between 10°C and 70°C with an optimum temperature of 45°C. Catalase activity decreases from 100–60% as the temperature increases from 45–50°C and then is further decreased to approximately 10% at 70°C. Moreover, this catalase exhibits the highest temperature sensitivity among the three catalases purified from the three H_2O_2- tolerant bacteria. The amino acid sequence of EKTA contains active sites (H^{56}, S^{104} and N^{138}), proximal sites of heme (Y^{339} and R^{346}) and binding sites for the distal region of heme (V^{97}, T^{119} and F^{142}), as shown in **Figure 1**. There is no NADPH-binding site in the amino acid sequence of this catalase. These important residues for catalase activity are well conserved in EKTA.

The catalase from *P. piscatorii* T-3 (PKTA) can be purified by one step of anion-chromatography and one step of hydrophobic chromatography [35]. The purified PKTA exhibits an activity of 222,000 U/mg protein under standard reaction conditions, with V_{max} and K_m of 2.4 × 10^5 μmol H_2O_2/μmol heme/s and 75 mM for H_2O_2, respectively. The catalytic efficiency k_{cat}/K_m of PKTA is 3.2 × 10^6/s/M as determined with O_2 electrode [34]. PKTA exhibits a temperature dependency between 10°C and 80°C with an optimum temperature of 45°C. The activity decreases at temperature over 50°C, showing approximately 10% at 70°C and complete deactivation at 85°C. The amino acid sequence of PKTA contains active sites (H^{65}, S^{104} and N^{138}), proximal sites of heme (Y^{348} and R^{355}), and binding sites for the distal region of heme (V^{106}, T^{128} and F^{143}). This PKTA also contains NADPH-binding sites (H^{184}, R^{193}, V^{292} and K^{295}), as shown in **Figure 1**. These important residues for catalase activity are well conserved in PKTA.

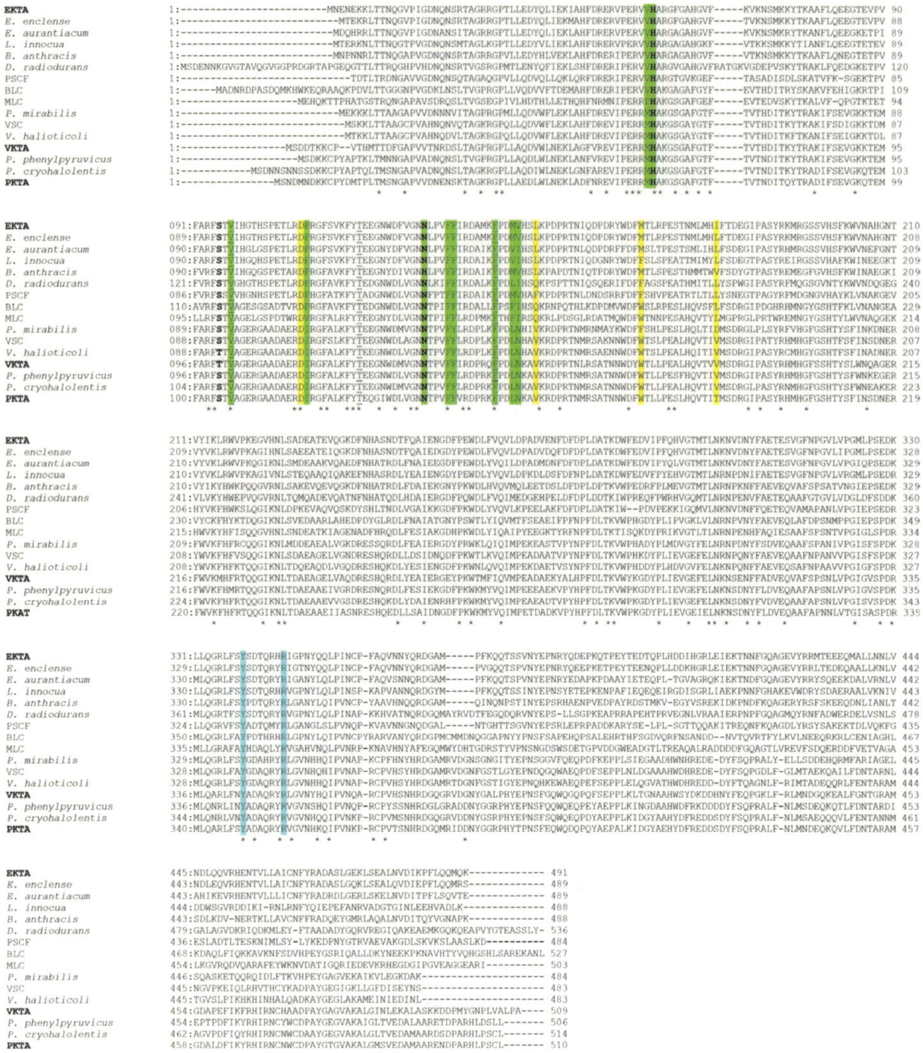

Figure 1.
Amino acid sequence alignment of EKTA, Exiguobacterium enclense *catalase,* Exiguobacterium aurantiacum *catalase,* Listeria innocua *catalase,* Deinococcus radiodurans *KatA, PSCF, MLC,* Proteus mirabilis *catalase,* Aliivibrio salmonicida *(VSC) catalase,* Vibrio halioticoli *catalase, VKTA,* Psychrobacter phenylpyruvicus *catalase and* Psychrobacter cryohalolentis *catalase. The amino acid residues involved in the narrow main channel are highlighted by green or yellow (bottleneck residues). The active sites are indicated in bold font, the proximal sites of heme are marked in blue and the binding sites of distal region of heme are marked by underlined text.*

6. Relationship between the compound formation rate with peracetic acid and the bottle neck amino acid residue in the narrow main channel

Catalase is known to have high activity owing to its superior substrate selectivity for H_2O_2. The interactions of substrate molecules larger than H_2O_2 are strongly inhibited due to selection of the substrate by the narrow main channel, which reaches the active site. The formation rate of the reactive intermediate (compound I) in the reaction of EKTA with peracetic acid is 77 times higher than that of BLC and 1200 times higher than that of MLC [26]. A comparison of the structural and functional data on EKTA (a clade 1 catalase) with the data for two clade 3 catalases (BLC and MLC) revealed that the size of the bottleneck defines the compound I formation rate, which corresponds to the size of the substrate molecule. The atom-to-atom distance for combinations of amino acid residues showed that, the L^{149} (BN [bottleneck] 2) to I^{180} (BN4) and D^{109} (BN1) to M^{167} (BN3) combinations at the bottleneck of EKTA resulted in larger bottleneck sizes than the combinations in BLC and MLC [26]. The sizes of the amino acids and the probability of occurrence of the corresponding amino acids (based on a comparison of catalase sequences in the database) indicated that M^{167} may play a key role in determining the size of the bottleneck of EKTA. Clade 3 catalases, i.e., BLC and MLC contain W (Phe) in the corresponding position of M^{167} in EKTA. The volume of W (Phe) is 231.7 Å^3, whereas that of M (Met) is 167.7 Å^3 [38, 39]. Therefore, the size of the key residue M^{167} in EKTA is the major reason for the high the compound I formation rate with peracetic acid.

7. Comparison of amino acid residues in the narrow main channel of catalase

The main channel of catalase consists upper and lower narrow parts. The narrow part, which is nearer to the reaction centre, heme consists of 14 amino acid residues [26] (**Figures 1** and **2**). The seven residues forming the channel (H^{56}, V^{97}, D^{109}, N^{129}, F^{134}, F^{135} and F^{142} in EKTA) are well conserved (≥95% homology). V^{55} is relatively highly conserved (≥ 80%) followed by P^{110} (54%). The other amino acid residues, including M^{145} (approximately 20%), V^{146} (approximately 30%) and L^{149} (approximately 20%) are relatively rarely conserved. Both M^{167} and I^{180} are very rarely conserved (≤ 3%) among catalases. Among the 14 amino acid residues described above, D^{109} (BN1), L^{149} (BN2), M^{167} (BN3) and I^{180} (BN4) are located in the bottleneck structure in between the upper and lower parts of the main channel of catalase. Among these four amino acid residues only D^{109} is well conserved. Therefore,

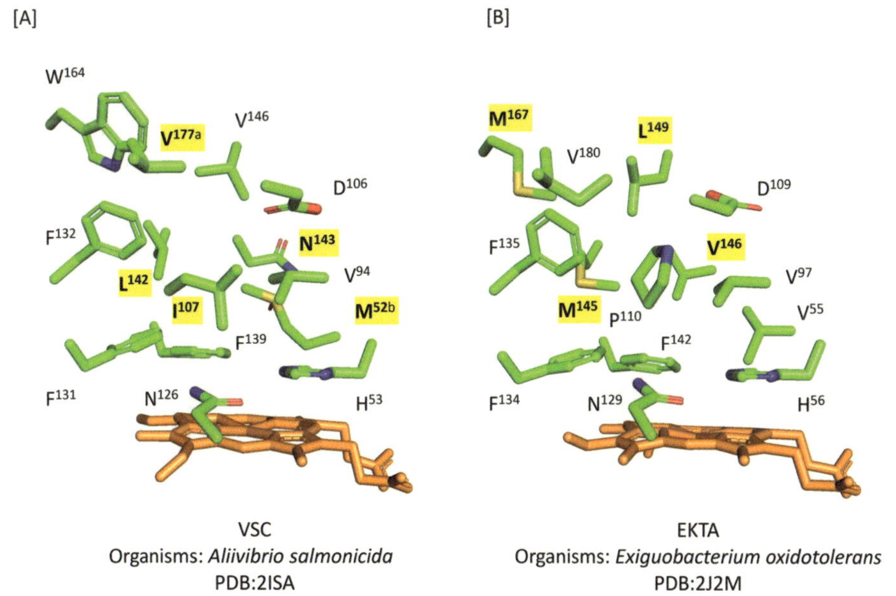

Figure 2.
Structural model of narrow main channels of catalases of VSC [A] and EKTA [B]. Each characteristic amino acid residues are indicated by yellow marker. Number for amino acid residues was accordance with ***Figure 1****. The amino acid residues of narrow main channels in VSC are the same as VKTA. [a]This amino acid residue is substituted to "T" in PKTA. [b]This amino acid residue is modified as S-dioxymethionine.*

variations in amino acid residues, except D^{109}, define the size of the bottleneck structure and the reaction rate with substrates larger than H_2O_2. Based on the alignment of multiple catalases including other catalases derived from other species belonging to the genus *Exiguobacterium*, there are several common amino acid residues between EKTA and *Exiguobacterium enclense* catalase (M^{145}, V^{146}, L^{149} and M^{167}). Owing to the lower volumes of these residues compared with the corresponding residues in other catalases, these residues are thought to be related to the genus-specific efficiency catalytic reactions in the presence of high concentrations of H_2O_2.

In contrast, M^{64}, I^{119}, L^{154}, N^{155} and T^{158} are specific amino acid residues in the narrow main channel of PKTA. These amino acid residues are corresponding to M^{60}, I^{115}, L^{150}, N^{151} and V^{154} in VKTA and catalases from *Proteus mirabilis*, *Aliivibrio salmonicida*, *Psychrobacter phenylpyruvicus* and *Psychrobacter cryohalolentis* catalases. Although the activities of the latter two catalases are not known, the other three catalases exhibit high catalytic efficiency for H_2O_2 [40]. Therefore, these residues are specific to the catalase of Proteobacteria and affect the efficiency of these catalases.

8. Relationship between catalase phylogeny and the main channel structure of catalases

The clade 1 catalase EKTA exhibits a higher ratio (b/a = 1.4) of the compound I formation rate using peracetic acid (a) to catalase activity using H_2O_2 (b) than the clade 3 catalase PKTA (b/a = 0.0056) [29]. Although the size of the bottleneck of PKTA is unknown, the difference in the catalytic characteristics can be attributed to the seize of the bottleneck, which this can be ascertained from the amino acid residues in the bottleneck. In addition to EKTA and PKTA, the b/a ratio was estimated using the clade I catalases, *Pseudomonas syringae* catalase (PSCF) and *Deinococcus radiodurans* catalase and the clade 3 catalases BLC and MLC. Differences in the b/a ratio are related to the intensity of the degree of the extended branch in the phylogenetic tree of catalase (**Table 1** and **Figure 3**). This indicates that catalases from H_2O_2-tolerant bacteria evolved in different directions depending on the bacterial taxonomic phylogenetic position. Thus, the phylogenetic position can be

	EKTA	PKTA	VKTA
Bottle neck structure			
BN2–BN4	L^{149}, **M167**, I^{180}	V^{158}, **W176**, T^{189}	V^{154}, **W172**, V^{185}
The size of BN2–BN4	164.6, **167.7**, 164.9	150.6, **231.7**, 120.0	150.6, **231.7**, 139.1
Enzymatic feature			
b/a ratio[a]	**1.4**	**0.0056**	ND
Kinetic parameters for H_2O_2			
V_{max} (/s)	1.5×10^{6} [b]	2.4×10^{5} [c]	8.0×10^{5} [b]
K_m (mM)	40[b]	75[c]	35[b]
k_{cat}/K_m (/M/s)	3.8×10^{7} [b]	3.2×10^{6} [c]	2.3×10^{7} [b]
Cellular features			
Percentage of catalase in cell extract	**6.5%**	**10%**	1.8%
Location of isolation	Upstream of the drain (**6–38 mM** H_2O_2)	Upstream of the drain (**6–38 mM** H_2O_2)	Downstream of the drain (1.5–6 mM H_2O_2)
Involved bacteria	Gram positive	Gram negative	Gram negative

DOI: http://dx.doi.org/10.5772/intechopen.95489

	EKTA	PKTA	VKTA
Phylogeny			
Clade	1	3	3
Extended of phylogenetic position	**Yes**	**Yes**	**Yes**
Purified catalase activity (U/mg)[c]			
Catalase activity of cell extract (U/mg)[d]	**28,000**	**20,000**	7,300

[a]*The ratio of compound I formation rate using peracetic acid (a) to catalase activity using H_2O_2 (b).*
[b]*Determined by spectrophotometry.*
[c]*Determined by oxygen electrode analysis.*
[d]*Standard reaction conditions of 30 mM H_2O_2 at pH 7.*

Table 1.
Summary of the characteristics of catalases from H_2O_2-tolerant bacteria.

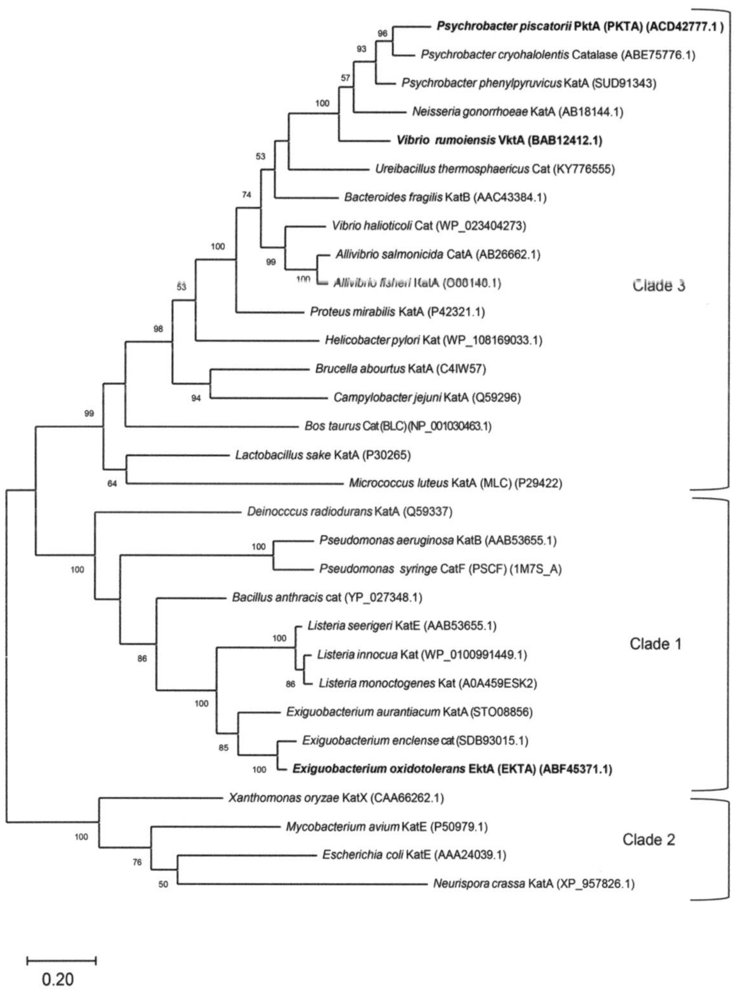

Figure 3.
Phylogenetic position of catalases clades 1–3. The phylogenetic tree was constructed using the Maximum Likelihood method and JTT matrix-based model [41]. Multiple alignments of the sequences were performed using the MUSCLE program [42]. The numbers in the branches indicate bootstrap percentages based on 500 replicates. Bar, 0.20 changes per amino acid position. Evolutionary analyses were conducted in MEGA X [13].

ascertained based on the amino acid sequences of catalase from *Exiguobacterium* spp. and *Psychrobacter* spp. However, it has been difficult to discriminate clade 1 and clade 3 catalase except phylogenetic position based on amino acid sequences. Indeed, these catalases can be discriminated based on differences in the catalytic efficiency for H_2O_2 according to the structure of the narrow main channel.

9. Environmental distribution and catalase function of H_2O_2-resistant bacteria

Results of a screening of bacterial strains adapted to high H_2O_2 environments (8°C, 6–38 mM H_2O_2), *E. oxidotolerans* T-2-2^T and *P. piscatorii* T-3^T and T-3-2 were isolated. Some microorganisms have been shown to thrive under extreme environments such as high and low temperatures and high and low pH. However, *Exiguobacterium* spp. and *Psychrobacter* spp. are known widely distributed in polar regions, permafrost, deep sea regions, temperate and tropical soils, and ordinary marine environments [43, 44]. Therefore, several strains belonging to the genera *Exiguobacterium* and *Psychrobacter* have been identified as psychrophilic or psychrotolerant bacteria. In addition to the cold-adapted variations of these genera, our studies revealed that there were variations in the H_2O_2 tolerance of these genera.

Although these genera exhibit common physiological characteristics and environmental distributions, phylogenetic positions are completely different from a taxonomical point of view [43]. Gram-positive *Exiguobacterium* belongs to the phylum Firmicutes, class Bacilli, and order Bacillales, whereas *Psychrobacter* belongs to the phylum Proteobacteria, class Gammaproteobacteria, order Pseudomonadales, family Moraxellaceae. Dias et al. analysed and compared four genomes of *Exiguobacterium* and *Psychrobacter* [44] and showed that *Psychrobacter* exhibited higher genomic plasticity, whereas *E. antarcticum* exhibited a large decrease in genomic content without changing its adaptability to cold environments. These results suggest that the H_2O_2 tolerance and molecular features of catalases and their productivities in H_2O_2-tolerant bacteria belonging to *Exiguobacterium* and *Psychrobacter* were related to the intrinsic genomic architectural dynamics of these taxa.

V. rumoiensis was isolated from an environment containing lower H_2O_2 concentration (1.5–6 mM) than the other two strains. The genus *Vibrio* and the closely related genus *Aliivibrio* are known for involving species of their pathogenicity and symbiosis with marine organisms. Thus, these organisms may have high capacity for adaptability to high H_2O_2 environment. Moreover, bacterial genome analysis of six bacterial species belonging to the rumoiensis clade revealed that there are ecogenomic signatures inferring the ongoing habit expansion in two strains (*V. rumoiensis* included) [45]. Thus, this microorganism may have adapted to environments containing high H_2O_2 by genomic altering specific characteristics.

10. Conclusion and future studies

It has been shown that completely different taxa of bacteria evolve catalases in different directions improving productivity of catalases in the same or similar environment (i.e., low temperature and high H_2O_2 concentration). Adaptations to environments with high concentration of H_2O_2 has been achieved by certain groups of bacteria, including psychrotolerant bacteria originating from marine environments, which are widely distributed and can survive under various environmental conditions (e.g., low temperature and high H_2O_2 concentration). This adaptability is observed in terms of enzymatic features, productivity and localisation of catalase.

Future studies are necessary to analyze the evolutionary process in more detail and determine the relationship of this evolutionary process with the functions of specific enzymes. Furthermore, detailed studies of the microbiota present in environments containing high H_2O_2 concentrations may provide insight into the mechanisms through which bacteria adapt to artificial extreme environments.

Acknowledgements

We greatly thank Professor Hidetoshi Matsuyama for his continues support in our study. We wish to thank Mr. Daisen Ichihashi, Mr. Hideaki Iwata, Mr. Fumihiko Takebe, and Mr. Hideyuki Kimoto for providing technical assistance.

Conflict of interest

The authors declare that the research was conducted in the absence of any commercial or financial relationships that could be construed as a potential conflict of interest.

Appendices and nomenclature

Website resources:
Catalase website (http://www.catalase.com/index.htm)
EMBEL-EBI Catalase
(http://pfam.xfam.org/family/PF00199#tabview=tab3)
Catalase (enzyme nomenclature designation [EC] 1.11.1.6)

Author details

Isao Yumoto[1,2]*, Yoshiko Hanaoka[1,2] and Isao Hara[1,3]

1 Bioproduction Research Institute, National Institute of Advanced Industrial Science and Technology (AIST), Sapporo, Japan

2 Graduate School of Agriculture, Hokkaido University, Japan

3 Simadzu Co. Ltd., Kyoto, Japan

*Address all correspondence to: i.yumoto@aist.go.jp

References

[1] Bolton JL, Trush MA, Penning TM, Dryhurt G, Monks TJ: Role of quinones in toxicology. Chem Res Toxicol. 2000;13:135-160. https://doi.org/10.1021/tx9902082

[2] Lin P-C, Türk K, Häse CC, Fritz G, Steuber J: Quinone reduction by the Na+–translocating NADH dehydrogenase promotes extracellular superoxide production in Vibrio cholerae. J Bacteriol. 2007; 189:3902-3908. doi: 10.1128/JB.01651-06

[3] Treberg JR, Quinlan CL, Brand MD: Evidence for two sites of superoxide production by mitochondrial NADH-ubiquinone oxidoreductase (Complex I). J Biol Chem. 2011;286:27103-27110. http://www.jbc.org/content/286/31/27103

[4] Yin Y, Yang S, Yu L, Yu CA: Reaction mechanism of superoxide generation during ubiquinol oxidation by the bc1 complex. J Biol Chem. 2011;285:17038-17045. http://www.jbc.org/content/285/22/17038

[5] Halliwell B, Gutteridge JMC Free Radical in Biology and Medicine, 3rd ed. Clarendon Press, 1999.

[6] Imlay JA, Linn S: DNA damage and oxygen radical toxicity. Science. 1988;240:1302-1309. https://science.sciencemag.org/content/240/4857/1302

[7] Rowe LA, Degtyareva N, Doetsch PW : DNA damage-induced reactive oxygen species (ROS) stress response in Saccharomyces cerevisiae. Free Radic Biol Med. 2008;45:1167-1177. https://www.sciencedirect.com/science/article/pii/S0891584908004267

[8] Katsuwon J, Anderson AJ: Characterization of catalase activities in root colonizing isolates of *Pseudomonas putida*. Can J Microbiol. 1992;38:1026-1032. https://www.nrcresearchpress.com/doi/abs/10.1139/m92-169#.Xf8kkkf7Rdg

[9] Rocha ER, Selby T, Coleman JP, Smith CJ: Oxidative stress response in an anaerobe, Bacteroides fragilis: A role for catalase in protection against hydrogen peroxide. J Bacteriol. 1996;178:6895-6903. https://jb.asm.org/content/178/23/6895

[10] Visick KL, Ruby EG: The periplasmic, group III catalase *Vibrio fischeri* is required for normal symbiotic competence and is induced both by oxidative stress and by approach to stationary phase. J Bacteriol. 1998;180:2087-2092. https://jb.asm.org/content/180/8/2087.short

[11] Zhou P, Li X, Huang I-H, Qi F: *Veillonella* catalase protects the growth of *Fusibacterium nucleatum* in microaerophilic and *Streptococcus gordonii*-resistant environments. Appl Environ Microbiol. 2017;83:e01079–e01017. https://pubmed.ncbi.nlm.nih.gov/28778894/

[12] Tanaka T, Kawasaki K, Daimon S, Kitagawa W, Yamamoto K, Tamaki H, Tanaka M, Nakatsu CH, Kamagata Y: A hidden pitfall in preparation of agar media undermines microorganism cultivability. Appl Environ Micobiol. 2014;80:7659-7666. https://aem.asm.org/content/80/24/7659.long

[13] Kumar S, Stecher G, Li M, Knyaz C, Tamura K; MEGA X: Molecular evolutionary genetics analysis across computing platforms. Mol Biol Evol. 2008; 35:1547-1549. https://academic.oup.com/mbe/article/35/6/1547/4990887

[14] Klotz MG, Klassen GR, Loewen PC: Phylogenetic relationships among prokaryotic and eukaryotic

catalases. Mol Biol Evol. 1997;14:951-958. https://academic.oup.com/mbe/article/14/9/951/1014674

[15] Zámocký M, Gasselhuber B, Furtmuller PG, Obinger C: Molecular evolution of hydrogen peroxide degrading enzymes. Arch Biochem Biophys. 2012;525:131-144. https://www.sciencedirect.com/science/article/pii/S0003986112000410

[16] Jones P, Middlemiss DN: Formation of compound I by the reaction of catalase with peroxoacetic acid. Biochem J. 1972;130:411-415. https://portlandpress.com/biochemj/article-abstract/130/2/411/6043/Formation-of-compound-I-by-the-reaction-of

[17] Deisseroth A and Dounce AL: Catalase: Physical and chemical properties, mechanism of catalysis, and physiological role. Physiol Rev.1970;50:319-375.

[18] Schonbaum GR, Chance B Catalase, in The enzymes (Boyer, P. D., Ed.) Academic Press; 1976. p 363-408.

[19] Yumoto I, Yamazaki K, Kawasaki K, Ichise N, Morita N, Hoshino T, Okuyama H: Isolation of *Vibrio* sp. S-1 exhibiting extraordinarily high catalase activity. J Ferment Bioeng. 1998;85:113-116. https://www.sciencedirect.com/science/article/abs/pii/S0922338X97803649

[20] Yumoto I, Iwata H, Sawabe T, Ueno K, Ichise N, Matsuyama H, Okuyama H, Kawasaki K: Characterization of a facultatively psychrophilic bacterium, *Vibrio rumoiensis* sp. nov., that exhibits high catalase activity. Appl Environ Microbiol. 1999;65:67-72. https://aem.asm.org/content/65/1/67

[21] Ichise N, Morita N, Hoshino T, Kawasaki K, Yumoto I, Okuyama H: A mechanism of resistance to hydrogen peroxide in *Vibrio rumoiensis* S-1. Appl. Environ. Microbiol. 1999;65:73-79. https://aem.asm.org/content/65/1/73

[22] Ichise N, Morita N, Kawasaki K, Yumoto I, Okuyama H; Gene cloning and expression of the catalase from the hydrogen peroxide-resistant bacterium *Vibrio rumoiensis* S-1 and its subcellular localization. J Biosci Bioeng. 2000;90:530-534. https://www.sciencedirect.com/science/article/pii/S1389172301800359

[23] Ichise N, Hirota K, Ichihashi D, Nodasaka Y, Morita N, Okuyama H, Yumoto I; H_2O_2 tolerance of *Vibrio rumoiensis* S-1^T is attributable to the cellular catalase activity. J Biosci Bioeng. 2008;106:39-45. https://www.sciencedirect.com/science/article/pii/S1389172308701397

[24] Yumoto I, Ichihashi D, Iwata H, Istokovics A, Ichise N, Matsuyama H, Okuyama H, Kawasaki K; Purification and characterization of a catalase from the facultative psychrophilic bacterium *Vibrio rumoiensis* S-1^T exhibiting high catalase activity. J Bacteriol. 2000;182:1903-1909. https://jb.asm.org/content/182/7/1903

[25] Yumoto I, Hishinuma-Narisawa M, Hirota K, Shingyo T, Takebe F, Nodasaka Y, Matsuyama H, Hara I; *Exiguobacterium oxidotolerans* sp. nov., a novel alkaliphile exhibiting high catalase activity. Int J Syst Evol Microbiol. 2004;54:2013-2017. https://www.microbiologyresearch.org/content/journal/ijsem/10.1099/ijs.0.63129-0

[26] Hara I, Ichise N, Kojima K, Kondo H, Ohgiya S, Matsuyama H, Yumoto I; Relationship between the size of the bottleneck 15 Å away from iron in the main channel and reactivity of catalase corresponding to the molecular size of substrates. Biochemistry. 2007;46:11-22. https://pubs.acs.org/doi/abs/10.1021/bi061519w

[27] Takebe F, Hara I, Matsuyama H, Yumoto I; Effect of H_2O_2 under low- and high-aeration-level conditions on growth and catalase activity in *Exiguobacterium oxidotolerans* T-2-2^T. J Biosci Bioeng. 2007;104:464-469. https://www.sciencedirect.com/science/article/pii/S1389172308700045

[28] Hanaoka Y, Takebe F, Nodasaka Y, Hara I, Matsuyama H, Yumoto I; Growth-dependent catalase localization in *Exiguobacterium oxidotolerans* T-2-2^T reflected by catalase activity of cells. PLoS ONE. 2013;8:e76862. https://journals.plos.org/plosone/article?id=10.1371/journal.pone.0076862

[29] Hanaoka Y, Yumoto I; Manipulation of culture conditions for extensive extracellular catalase production by *Exiguobacterium oxidotolerans* T-2-2^T Ann Microbiol. 2015;65:1183-1187. https://link.springer.com/article/10.1007/s13213-014-0943-7

[30] Dastager SG, Mawlankar R, Sonalkar VV, Thorat MN, Mual P, Verma A, Krishnamurthi S, Tang SK, Li WJ; Exiguobacterium enclense sp. nov., isolated from sediment. Int J Syst Evol Microbiol. 2015; 65:1611-1616. doi: 10.1099/ijs.0.000149.

[31] Lei F, Cui C, Zhao H, Tang X, Zhao M; Phylogenetic diversity and biotechnological potentials of marine bacteria from continental slope of eastern Arabian Sea. J Genet Eng Biotechnol. 2018; 16:253-258. doi: 10.1016/j.jgeb.2018.06.002.

[32] Yumoto I, Hara I Psychrotolerant bacteria and environmental H_2O_2-resistant adaptation of their catalases. In: Yumoto I (ed) Cold-adapted microorganisms. Caister Academic Press; 2013. p 137-158.

[33] Yumoto I, Hirota K, Kimoto H, Nodasaka Y, Matsuyama H, Yoshimune K; *Psychrobacter piscatorii* sp. nov., a psychrotolerant bacterium exhibiting high catalase activity isolated from an oxidative environment. Int J Syst Evol Microbiol. 2010;60:205-208. https://www.microbiologyresearch.org/content/journal/ijsem/10.1099/ijs.0.010959-0

[34] Kimoto H, Matsuyama H, Yumoto I, Yoshimune K; Heme content of recombinant catalase from *Psychrobacter* sp. T-3 altered by host *Escherichia coli* growth condition. Protein Express Purif. 2008;59: 357-359.

[35] Kimoto H, Yoshimune K, Matsuyama H, Yumoto I; Characterization of catalase from psychrotolerant *Psychrobacter piscatorii* T-3 exhibiting high catalase activity. Int J Mol Sci. 2012;13:1733-1746. https://www.mdpi.com/1422-0067/13/2/1733

[36] Romanenko LA, Schumann P, Rohde M, Lysenko AM, Mikhailov VV, Stackebrandt E; *Psychrobacter submarinus* sp. nov. and *Psychrobacter marincola* sp. nov., psychrophilic halophiles from marine environments. Int J Syst Evol Microbiol. 2002;52:1291-1297. doi: 10.1099/00207713-52-4-1291.

[37] Switala J, Loewen PC; Diversity of properties among catalases. Arch Biochem Biophys. 2002; 401:145-154. https://www.sciencedirect.com/science/article/abs/pii/S0003986102000498

[38] Harpaz Y, Gerstein M, Chothia C; Volume changes on protein folding. Structure. 1994;15:641-649. https://www.sciencedirect.com/science/article/abs/pii/S0969212600000654

[39] Hanaoka Y, Kimoto H, Yoshimune K, Hara I, Matsuyama H, Yumoto I; Relationship between main channel structure of catalases and the evolutional direction in cold adapted hydrogen peroxide-tolerant *Exiguobacterium* and *Psychrobacter*. Indian J Microbiol. 2020;60:353-362. https://link.springer.com/article/10.1007/s12088-020-00878-3

[40] Lorentzen MS, Moe E, Jouve HM, Willassen NP; Cold adapted feature of *Vibrio salmonicida* catalase: characterization and comparison to the mesophilic counterpart from *Proteus mirabilis*. Extremophiles. 2006;10:427-440. https://link.springer.com/article/10.1007/s00792-006-0518-z

[41] Jones D.T., Taylor W.R., and Thornton J.M.; The rapid generation of mutation data matrices from protein sequences. Comput Appl Biosci. 1992;8: 275-282.

[42] Edgar RC; A multiple sequence alignment method with reduced time and space complexity. BMC Bioinformatics. 2004;5:113. https://bmcbioinformatics.biomedcentral.com/articles/10.1186/1471-2105-5-113

[43] Rodrigues DF, da C Jesus E, Ayala-Del-Río HL, Pellizari VH, Gilichinsky D, Sepulveda-Torres L, Tiedje JM; Biogeography of two cold-adapted genera: *Psychrobacter* and *Exiguobacterium*. ISME J. 2009; 3:658-665. https://www.nature.com/articles/ismej200925

[44] Dias LM, Folador ARC, Oliveira AM, Ramos RTJ, Silva A, Baraúna RA; Genomic architecture of the two cold-adapted genera *Exguibacterium* and *Psychrobacter*: evidence of functional reduction in the *Exgiguobacterium antarcticum* B7 genome. Genome Biol Evol. 2018;10:731-741. https://academic.oup.com/gbe/article/10/3/731/4846359

[45] Tanaka M, Kumakura D, Mino S, Doi H, Ogura Y, Hayashi T, Yumoto I, Cai M, Zhou Y.-G, Gomez-Gil B, Araki T, Sawabe T; Genomic characterization of closely related species in the Rumoiensis clade infers ecogenomic signatures to non-marine environments. Environ Microbiol. 2020; 22: 3205-3217. https://sfamjournals.onlinelibrary.wiley.com/doi/abs/10.1111/1462-2920.15062

Chapter 25

Antioxidant Properties of Metabolites from New Extremophiles Microalgal Strain (Southern, Tunisia)

Sana Gammoudi, Ines Dahmen-Ben Moussa, Neila Annabi-Trabelsi, Habib Ayadi and Wassim Guermazi

Abstract

With the demand for bioproducts that can provide benefits for biotechnology sectors like pharmaceuticals, nutraceuticals, and cosmeceuticals, the exploration of microalgal products has turned toward extremophiles. This chapter is intended to provide an insight to most important molecules from halotolerant species, the cyanobacteria *Phormidium versicolor* NCC-466 and *Dunaliella* sp. CTM20028 isolated from Sfax Solar Saltern (Sfax) and Chott El Djerid (Tozeur), Tunisia. These microalgae have been cultured in standard medium with a salinity of 80 PSU. The *in vitro* antioxidant activities demonstrated that extremolyte from *Dunaliella* and *Phormidium* as, phycocaynin, lipids, and polyphenol compound presents an important antioxidant potential.

Keywords: microalgae, halophile, biomolecule, antioxidant properties

1. Introduction

The primary producers of oxygen in aquatic environments are algae, especially planktonic microalgae. They play an important role in carbon dioxide (CO_2) recycling through photosynthesis [1]. Microalgae have been divided into ten groups, which refer to the color of the cell including: Cyanobacteria, blue-green algae; Chlorophyta, green algae; Rhodophyta, red algae; Glaucophyta; Euglenophyta; Haptophyta; Cryptophyta; photosynthetic Stramenopiles; Dinophyta; and Chlorarachniophyta [2]. Cyanobacteria are much closer to bacteria in terms of structure and their cells lack both nucleus and chloroplasts. Cyanobacteria are also known as a source of pigments, chlorophyll (a), phycocyanin, phycoerythrin, xanthophyll, and ß-carotene. Microalgae are widely distributed in nature and adapted to different environments from fresh to hypersaline water ecosystems. Salt lakes in arid regions (sabkhas) and solar salterns are an examples of high salty environments inhabited by extremely halophilic microorganisms that include halophilic Archaea (halobacteria), halophilic cyanobacteria, and green algae [3–5]. These microorganisms must have specific adaptive strategies for surviving in high salinity conditions to prevent the loss of cellular water under high osmolarity in hypersaline conditions [6]. Halophiles generally develop two basic mechanisms: (i) halobacteria and microalgae accumulate KCl (potassium chloride) in their cells to maintain high intracellular salt concentrations, osmotically at least equivalent to the external concentrations (the "salt-in" strategy); (ii) other halophiles produce or accumulate low molecular weight compounds (osmolyte or compatible solute) that have osmotic potential.

Microalgae provide many biotechnology applications in various industrial sectors such as food, cosmetics, pharmaceuticals, energy and environmental industries. Hyperhalophilic microalgae and their bioproducts, has gained a great deal of attention in the last decade. They are well known for their production of high value products such as β-carotene, lipids, and omega 3 fatty acids.

There are high demands for novel lead molecules for new classes of pharmaceutical and research biochemicals, and in combination, these drivers have led to an increased interest in microalgae and cyanobacteria as sources of both bioactive natural products.

Cyanobacteria species contain potential products for medicinal [7] and energy applications [8]. Some of this group has secondary metabolites that can potentially be used as therapeutic agents, such as antivirals, immunomodulators, inhibitors, cytostastics and antioxidants [9]. Several natural compounds such as vitamin C, tocopherol, and numerous plant extracts have been commercialized as natural antioxidants to fight against oxidative stress associated with various chronic diseases including atherosclerosis, diabetes mellitus, neurodegenerative disorders, and certain types of cancer [10]. Antioxidants are a crucial defense against free radical-induced damage [11].

Microalgae are abundant in nature and can be used as a renewable source of natural antioxidants [12]. Free radicals including reactive oxygen species (ROS), such as superoxide (O2•−), hydroxyle (OH•) and Hydrogen Peroxide (H_2O_2), and reactive nitrogen species (RNS) are generated during normal cellular metabolism. These free radicals are highly reactive species and play a dual role in humans as both beneficial and toxic compounds depending on their concentration. At low or moderate concentration, these reactive species exert beneficial effects on cellular redox signaling and immune function. At high concentration, however, these radical species produce oxidative stress, a harmful process that can lead to cell death through oxidation of protein, lipid, and DNA [11, 13].

A number of microalgae have been used in the commercial production of pigments with antioxidant properties, for example: astaxanthin from *Haematococcus pluvialis*, ß carotene from *Dunaliella salina*, as well as phycobiliproteins from *Arthrosphira* and *Phorphyridium* [12]. The review here in is about antioxidant capacity of the majors compounds extracted from new strain of hyperhalophilic microalgae (*Dunaliella* sp.) from salt lake Chott El-Djerid and cyanobacteria (*Phormidium versicolor*) from Sfax Solar Saltern (Tunisia).

2. Methods of cultivation and antioxidant assays

2.1 Isolation and principal production of the culture of new highly halophilic microalgae strains

Although most species of green algae (Chlorophyceae) are moderately halophilic, a few of them, including *Dunaliella salina*, are extremely halophilic species [3]. They are responsible for most of the primary production in hypersaline environments [4]. *Dunaliella salina* is the most important species of the genus for beta-carotene production. Several investigations have demonstrated that *D. salina* produces more than 10% of the dry weight [14]. Lutein, chlorophyll, and other pigments and carotenoids are also produced by the genus of *Dunaliella*, under the same stressful environmental conditions [15]. Lipids for aquaculture, human nutrition, and biodiesel production have also been investigated in *Dunaliella* species [16].

Dunaliella sp. CTM 20028 have been isolated for the first time from Chott El-Djerid (Southern Tunisia) with a mean salinity of 142 PSU [17]. Chott El-Djerid (5. 000 km^2) consists of salty shallow pools and marshes, and it is covered by a large salt pan during the dry season (June to August). The water emerges into the Chott El-Djerid trough a thinclay aquiclude of Quaternary age [18]. This generally allows temporary flooding of the Chott during winter. The climate of the area is arid-saharian with a mean annual rainfall between 80 and 140 mm and mean temperature of 21 °C. The elevation of the Chott surface is controlled by the position of the water table and the associated capillary fringe [19].

After acclimatation and purification, *Dunaliella* sp. was cultured in optimized f/2 Provasoli medium. Culture was carried out in 200 ml flask at 31 °C, 21 rad/s agitation and 54 mmol photon/m^2/s continuous illumination intensity supplied by cool-white fluorescence tubes and in a saturated atmosphere to 0.1 v/v/m CO2.

Cyanobacteria *Phormidium versicolor* NCC466 have been isolated from hypersaline ponds (75 PSU) of Sfax Solar Saltern (Central Tunisia). The solar saltern studied is located in the central-eastern coast of Sfax (Tunisia, 34°39'N and 10°42′E), and consists of a series of shallow interconnected ponds (20–70 cm depth) extending over an area of 1.500 ha. The salinity of water ponds varied from 45 to 450 PSU. The morphometric characteristics of the Saltern were reported elsewhere [20]. This Saltern show high microalgae diversity, 13 diatoms, 26 Dinoflagellates, 5 cyanobacteria and 2 Chlorophyceae [5]. *Phormidium versicolor* was identified according to its internal transcribed spacer sequence based on the rDNA sequence (GenBank accession number NCC 466). It was grown in 250 mL Erlenmeyer flasks in batch containing 100 mL of a modified BG11 medium. The flasks were placed in homeothermic incubator at 25 °C under a light intensity of 100 μM photons m^{-2} s^{-1}, with a 14/10 h light/dark cycle for 11 days.

2.2 Extraction of metabolite and in vitro antioxidant evaluation

Total lipids were extracted at the end of the exponential phase of growth of *Dunaliella*'s cells according to the method of [21]. The phycocyanin pigment was isolated from *P. versicolor* using the method developed by [22]. However, the phenolic and total flavonoids content were determined in ethanolic extract according to [23, 24], respectively.

2.2.1 In vitro free radical scavenging and antioxidant assays

The antioxidant potential of the lipid extract (LE) of *Dunaliella* from Chott El-Djerid in batch culture was assessed on the basis of the 2,2-Diphenylpicrylhydrazyl (DPPH) and superoxide anion radical-scavenging activities. When DPPH radicals encounter a proton donating substrate, such as an antioxidant, the radicals would be scavenged and the absorbance would be reduced [25]. Antioxidant potential of C-PC was evaluated by Superoxide (O2•−) scavenging, Hydroxyl (OH•) and Nitric oxide (NO) scavenging capacity. Moreover, the ability of C-phycocyanin to inhibit the lipid peroxidation was assessed using the method described by [26].

The free radical scavenging capacity of phenolic and flavonoids compounds extracted from *P. versicolor* was assessed through DPPH, NO and 2,2-azino-bis-(3-ethylbenzothiazoline-6-sulfonic acid (ABTS) tests. The antioxidant activities of polyphenol were expressed as IC50, defined as the concentration of the these compounds required causing a 50% decrease in initial DPPH, NO and ABTS concentration.

3. Lipid antioxidant properties of *Dunaliella* sp. from Chott El-Djerid

Lipid compounds such as wax, fat, fat-soluble vitamins, oil, triacylglycerols, phospholipids, co-enzymes (ubiquinone), pigments (carotenoids), and more, could be found in plants or animals. Lipids are formed from long-chain hydrocarbons and sometimes contain other functional groups of oxygen, phosphorus, nitrogen, and sulfur. They are insoluble in water, but soluble in organic solvents such as chloroform, hexane, and ether. As invascular plants, microalgae produce both polar and neutral lipids. There is a wide range of bio-based lipid products that can be harvested from microalgal biomass. Microalgae lipids offer great potential in terms of biotechnology applications (e.g. food, food supplements, energy, cosmetics, and pharmaceuticals). In functional food, the use of microalgal lipids has already been established as an industry. The type and quality of the lipid products depend on microalgae species, culture conditions, and recovery methods.

The present study is the first comprehensive *in vitro* study revealing the protective effect of the lipidic extract (LE) of the *Dunaliella* sp. from Chott El-Djerid [17]. The in vitro antioxidant activity demonstrated that LE presents an important antioxidant potential. The DPPH radical-scavenging activity was investigated at different concentrations from 0.1 to 3 mg/mL of the LE. LE exhibited an interesting radical scavenging activity that was concentration dependent (**Figure 1A**). The IC50 value obtained was about 0.1 ± 0.02 mg/mL which, is only 1.4 times higher than those of control, ascorbic acid and BHT. The antioxidant effect of *Dunaliella* sp. lipid extract was assessed at aconcentration of 1, 2, and 3 mg/mL. The results show that the concentration of 2 and 3 mg/mL of *Dunaliella* sp. Lipid extract indicate a high radical scavenging ability compared with the ascorbic acid and BHT and that of 1 mg/mL of LE presents high activity compared with BHT as positive standard.

The low IC50 indicates the higher free radical-scavenging ability of *Dunaliella* sp.-LE, which contained a high amount of essential fatty acid [17]. In addition, these authors reported that *Dunaliella* sp.-LE exhibited a strong NBT (Nitroblue-terazolium) photoreduction inhibition. Omega-3 EFAs is well documented for the

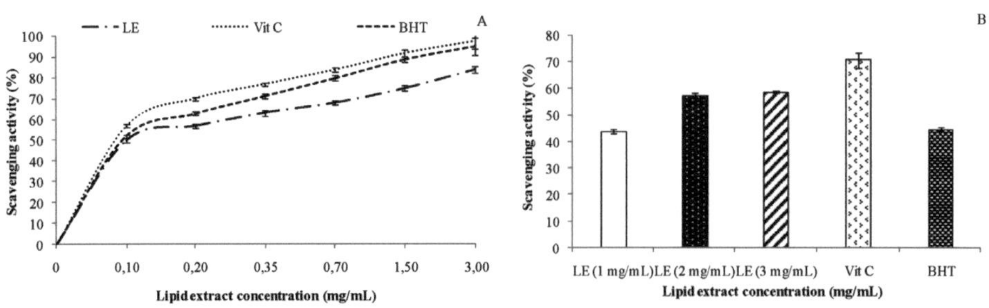

Figure 1.
Antioxidant activities of Dunaliella salina *lipid extract (LE) determined by two methods: DPPH-scavenging activity (A) and superoxide anion scavenging (B) and compared with synthetic antioxidants: Vitamin C (Vit C) and BHT. Data are presented as mean ± SD [17].*

attenuation of oxidant mediated organ damage induced by various xenobiotics and disease states [27]. Moreover [17], stated that LE of *D. salina* from Chott El-Djerid enhance the anticoxidant effect against Ni-induced toxicity by in vitro and in vivo test.

4. Phycocyanin pigments from *Phormidium versicolor* NCC466 from Sfax solar saltern

Phycocyanin (C-PC) isa hetero-oligomer consisting of a grouping of subunits that are organized into complexes called « phycobilisomes » [28]. C-PC possess a number of unique properties that make it useful colorant, including a higher molecular absorbance, fluorescence quantum yields, stable oligomers, and high photosatbility [29]. Phycocyanin has primarily been used as natural dye; however, it is increasingly being used as nutraceuticals or in ither biotechnological applications [29]. However, to the best of our knowledge, the antioxidant capacity of *P. versicolor* phycocyanin fraction (C-PC) has not been proved.

P. versicolor phycocyanin had a strong ability to scavenge free radicals (**Figure 2**). The ability of C-PC to scavenge the O2• – and OH• radicals were measured and compared with that of the positive control (ascorbic acid and BHT) (**Figure 2(a)** and **(b)**). C-PC presented the highest scavenging activity against O2• – and OH• radicals ((87.42 and 88.75% at 1 mg. mL^{-1}), respectively). Phycocyanin fractions isolated from cyanobacteria species were reported to be very efficient free radical

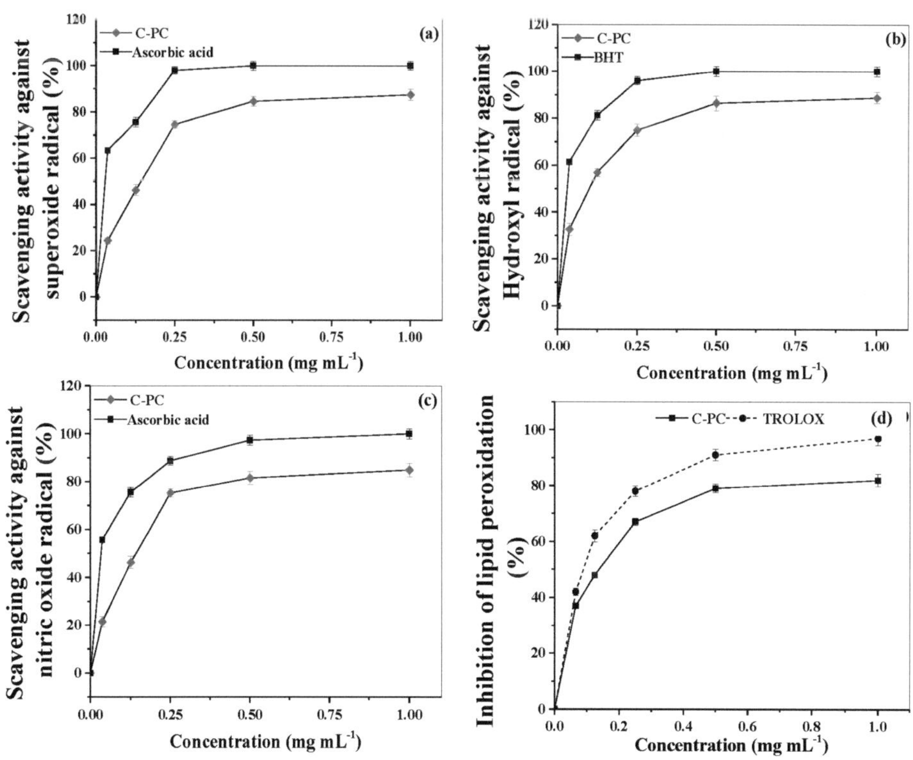

Figure 2.
Antioxidant activity of C-PC extract on (a) superoxide radical, (b) hydroxyl radical, (c) nitric oxide radical and (d) inhibition of lipid peroxidation. BHT, ascorbic acid, TROLOX were used as standard. Values are presented as mean ± SD (n = 3).

scavengers and exhibit the highest antioxidant activity [30]. All phycocyanin extracts showed fairly moderate to high scavenging capacity against free radicals. As for nitric oxide radical (NO•), the C-PC showed a strong NO• scavenging activity reaching up to 84.87% (**Figure 2c**).

Several studies showed that phycocyanin isolated from cyanobacteria species exhibited strong antioxidant properties and can be protected cells against oxidative stress [31, 32]. Moreover, in vitro studies suggest that phycocyanin of *Spirulina* enhance antioxidant enzyme activity and inhibit lipid peroxidation in cells. The effect of *P. versicolor* phycocyanin (C-PC) on ferrous sulfate induced lipid peroxidation *in vitro* was illustrated in **Figure 2d**. Indeed, the inhibition rats of lipid peroxidation of C-PC varied between 37.65 and 82.31%.

The results here in suggested that administration of C-PC in reaction mixture significantly inhibited lipid peroxidation. The present finding revealed that C-PC had a strong effect and had antagonized action against ferrous sulfate induced lipid peroxidation *in vitro*. In this regards, Thangam et al. [33] showed that phycocyanin isolated from *Oscillatoria tenuis* possesses excellent antioxidant activity against DPPH radical, OH• and nitric oxide. Similarly, Ou et al. [31] indicated that *Spirulina maxima* phycocyanin protects human hepatocyte cell line L02 against H_2O_2 induced lipid damage. C-PC from halophilic *P. versicolor* could be used to produce a natural antioxidant complement or added to healthy food products.

5. Antioxidant properties of polyphenolic compounds from *P. versicolor* NCC466

Polyphenols represent a group of chemical compounds emerging from a common intermediate, phenylalanine, or a close forerunner, shikimic acid [34]. Polyphenols are able to protect cells from oxidative stress by various mechanisms; they can chelate transition metal ions, can inhibit lipid peroxidation by trapping the lipid alkoxyl radical, or can directly scavenge molecular species of active oxygen [34]. Flavonoids are a class of phenolic metabolites that have strong chelating and antioxidant properties [34]. Their tendency to inhibit free radical-mediated events is controlled by their chemical structure. This structure–activity relationship has been well established *in vitro* as previously reported [35, 36]. *P. versicolor* exhibited a high amount of phenolics and flavonoids reaching 408 ± 18.8 mg GAE g^{-1} FW and 13,67 ± 0.788 mg QEq g^{-1} FW, respectively (**Table 1**). These amounts are signficantly higher than those recorded in *Dunaliella salina* from Sfax Solar Saltern [37]. These later recorded 0.086 ± 0.002 mg GAE g^{-1} FW and 0.006 ± 0.0001 mg QEq g^{-1} FW respectively for phenolics and flavonoids. Total antioxidant capacity (TAC) of phenolics and flavonoids extracted from *P. versicolor* are high about 0.94 ± 0.02 mg Eq g-1 FW. The IC50 concentrations DPPH, ABTS and NO scanvenging were low (0.007 to 0.031 mg. l^{-1}), suggested a high antioxidant activity of polyphenols and flavonoids extract from *P. versicolor* on the ROS (**Table 1**).

Antioxidant test	***Polyphenols and flavonoids extract***	***Standard***
DPPH (mg. l^{-1})	0.031 ± 0.08	0.077 ± 0.06 (BHT)
ABTS (mg. l^{-1})	0.015 ± 0.01	0.098 ± 0.02 (TROLOX)
NO (mg. l^{-1})	0.007 ± 0.03	0.094 ± 0.01 (Vit C)

Table 1.
Antioxydant capacity (IC50 concentrations) of phenolics and flavonoids metabolites extracted from P. versicolor *NCC466. BHT, Trolox and vitamin C represent the standard.*

6. Conclusion

News hyerhalophilic microlagae strains, *Dunaliella* sp. and *Phormidium versicolor* NCC466 are rich in lipid and phycocyanin even secondary metabolite such polyphenloic compounds. Scavenging activity tests indicated that these extremoplytes have an excellent capacity as natural antioxidant.

Acknowledgements

This study was supported by the Ministry of Higher Education and Scientific Research of Tunisia. We thank Dr. Mohammad Ali from Institute for Scientific Research (Kuwait) for correcting the English language.

Author details

Sana Gammoudi[1], Ines Dahmen-Ben Moussa[2], Neila Annabi-Trabelsi[1], Habib Ayadi[1] and Wassim Guermazi[1]*

1 Laboratory of Marine Biodiversity and Environment, Department of Life Sciences, Faculty of Sciences, University of Sfax Tunisia, CP, Tunisia

2 Laboratory of Environmental Bioprocesses, Centre of Biotechnology of Sfax, University of Sfax, Sfax, Tunisia

*Address all correspondence to: wassim016@yahoo.fr

References

[1] Chisti Y. Microalgae as sustainable cell factories. Environmental Engineering and Management Journal. 2006;5:261-274.

[2] Graham LE, Graham J, Wilcox LW. Algae. Wilbur B. editor. 2nd ed. San Francisco: Pearson Education; 2009. 100p.

[3] Grant WD, Gemmel RT, McGenity TJ. Halophiles. In: Horikoshi K, Grant, WD, editors. Extremophiles: Microbial Life in Extreme Environments. Wiley-Liss; 1998. p. 93-132.

[4] Oren A. A hundred years of *Dunaliella* research1905-2005. Aquatic Biosystems. 2005 ;1:1-14. DOI: 10.1186/1746-1448-1-2

[5] Ayadi H, Elloumi J, Guermazi W, Bouain A, hammami M, Giraudoux P, Aleya L. Fatty acids composition in relation to the microorganisms in the Sfax solar saltern, Tunisia. Acta protozoologica. 2008; 47:189-203

[6] Oren A. Bioenergetic aspect of halophilism. Microbiology and Molecular Biology Reviews. 1999;63:334-348.DOI: 10.1128/MMBR.63.2.334-348.1999.

[7] Rastogi RP, Sinha RP. Biotechnological and industrial significance of cyanobacterial secondary metabolites. Biotechnology Advances. 2009;27:521-539. DOI:10.1016/j.biotechadv.2009.04.009

[8] Angermayr SA, Hellingwerf KJ, Lindblad P, de Mattos MJT. Energy biotechnology with cyanobacteria. Current Opinion in Biotechnology. 2009;20:257-263. DOI:10.1016/j.copbio.2009.05.011

[9] Smith JL, Boyer GL, Zimba PV. A review of cyanobacterial odorous and bioactive metabolites: Impacts and management alternatives in aquaculture. Aquaculture. 2008;280:5-20. DOI:10.1016/j.aquaculture.2008.05.007.

[10] Vadlapudi V. Antioxidant activities of marine algae: a review. In: Cappasso A, editor. Medicinal plants as antioxidant agents: understanding their mechanism of action and therapeutic efficacy. Research Signpost: Kerala; 2012. p. 189-203.

[11] Sen S, Chakraborty R. The role of antioxidants in human health. In: Hepel M, Andreescu S, editors. Oxidative stress: diagnostics, prevention, and therapy. American Chemical Society: Washington, D.C; 2011.p 1-37.

[12] Spolaore P, Joannis-Cassan C, Duran E, Isambert A. Commercial applications of microalgae. Journal of Bioscience and Bioengineering. 2006;101:87-96. DOI:10.1263/jbb.101.87

[13] Pham-Huy LA, He H, Pham-Huy C. Free radicals, antioxidants in disease and health. International Journal of Biomedical Science. 2008;4:89-95.

[14] Olmos-Soto J, Paniagua-Michel J, Contreras R, Trujillo L. Molecular identification of β-carotene hyperproducing strain of *Dunaliella* from saline environment using species-specific oligonucleotides. Biotechnology Letters. 2002; 24:365-369.DOI: 10.1023/A:1014516920887

[15] Skjanes K, Rebours C, Lindblad P. Potencial for green microalgae to producer hydrogen, pharmaceuticals and other high value products in a combined process. Critical Reviews in Biotechnology. 2013;33:172-215. DOI: 10.3109/07388551.2012.681625

[16] Da Silva CM, Gomez ADA, Couri S. Morphological and chemical aspect of *Chlorella pyrenoidosa*, *Dunaliella*

tertiolecta, *Isochrysis galbana* and *Tetraselmis gracilis* microalgae. Natural Science. 2013;5:783-791.DOI: 10.4236/ns.2013.57094

[17] Dahmen-Ben Moussa I, Bellassoued K, Athmouni K, Naifar M, Chtourou H, Ayadi, H., Makni-Ayadi F, Sayadi S, El Feki A, Dhouib, A. Protective effect of *Dunaliella* sp., lipid extract rich in polyunsaturated fatty acids, on hepatic and renal toxicity induced by nickel in rats. Toxicology Mechanisms and Methods. 2016; 26(3):221-230. DOI:10.3109/15376516.2016.1158340

[18] Roberts CR, Mitchell CW. Spring mounds in southernTunisia. In: Frostick L, Reid, I editors. Desert Sediments: Ancient and Modern. Geol. Soc. London, Special Publications;1987. p. 321-334.

[19] Swezey CS. The role of climate in the creation and destruction of continental stratigraphic records: an example from the northern margin of the Sahara Desert. In: Climate Controls on Stratigraphy. SEPM Special Publication; 2003. p. 207-225.

[20] Elloumi J, Carrias JF, Ayadi H, Sime-Ngando T, Boukhris M, Bouain A. Composition and distribution of planktonic ciliates from ponds of different salinity in the solar saltwork of Sfax, Tunisia. Estuarine, Coastal and Shelf Science.2006;67:21-29.DOI: 10.1016/j.ecss.2005.10.011

[21] Bligh EG, Dyer WJ. A rapid method of total lipid extraction and purification. Canadian Journal of Biochemistry and Physiology. 1959;37:911-917.

[22] Silveira ST, Burkert JFdM, Costa JAV, Burkert CAV, Kalil SJ. Optimization of phycocyanin extraction from *Spirulina platensis* using factorial design. Bioresource Technology. 2007; 98 (8): 1629-1634. DOI: 10.1016/j.biortech.2006.05.050.

[23] Hajimahmoodi M, Faramarzi MA, Mohammadi N, Soltani N, Oveisi MR, Nafissi-Varcheh N. Evaluation of antioxidant properties and total phenolic contents of some strains of microalgae. Journal of Applied Phycology. 2010; 22:43-50. DOI: 10.1007/s10811-009-9424-y

[24] Kim Dk, Jeong SW, Lee CY. Antioxidant capacity of phenolic phytochemicals from various cultivars of plums. Food Chemistry. 2003;81:321-326. DOI: 10.1016/S0308-8146(02)00423-5

[25] Fakhfakh N, Ktari N, Haddar A, Hamza Mnif I., Dahmen I, Nasri M. Total solubilisation of the chicken feathers by fermentation with a keratinolytic bacterium, *Bacillus pumilus* A1, and the production of protein hydrolysate with high antioxidative activity. Process Biochemistry. 2011;46:1731-1737.DOI: 10.1016/j.procbio.2011.05.023.

[26] Halliwell B. Free radicals, reactive oxygen species and human disease: a critical evaluation with special reference to atherosclerosis. British Journal of Experimental Pathology. 1989; 70(6):737-757.

[27] Fayez AM, Awad AS, El-Naa MM, Kenawy SA, El-Sayed ME. Beneficial effects of thymoquinone and omega-3 on intestinal ischemia/reperfusion induced renal dysfunction in rats. Bulletin of Faculty of Pharmacy, Cairo University. 2014;52:171-177.

[28] Wiedenmann J. Marine proteins. In: Oceans and Human Health. Risks and Remedies from the Sea. Walsh PJ, Smith SL, Fleming LE, Solo-Gabriele HM, Gerwick WH, editors. Academic Press: St. Louis, MO; 2008. p. 469-495.

[29] Becker W. Microalgae in human and animal nutrition. In: Richmond A, editor. Handbook of Microalgal Culture: Biotechnology and Applied Phycology:

Blackwell Publishing Ltd, Oxford; 2004. p.312-351.

[30] Bermejo P, Piñero E, Villar ÁM. Iron-chelating ability and antioxidant properties of phycocyanin isolated from a protean extract of *Spirulina platensis*. Food Chemistry. 2008;110:436-445. DOI: 10.1016/j.foodchem.2008.02.021

[31] Ou Y, Zheng S, Lin L, Jiang Q, Yang X. Protective effect of C-phycocyanin against carbon tetrachloride-induced hepatocyte damage in vitro and in vivo. Chemico-Biological Interactions. 2010;185 (2):94-100. DOI: 10.1016/j.cbi.2010.03.013.

[32] Niu YJ, Zhou W, Guo J, Nie ZW, Shin KT, Kim NH, Lv WF, Cui XS. C-Phycocyanin protects against mitochondrial dysfunction and oxidative stress in parthenogenetic porcine embryos. Scientific Reports. 2017;7(1):16992. DOI: 10.1038/s41598-017-17287-0.

[33] Thangam R, Suresh V, Princy WA, Rajkumar M, SenthilKumar N, Gunasekaran P, Rengasamy R, Anbazhagan C, Kaveri K, Kannan S. C-Phycocyanin from *Oscillatoria tenuis* exhibited an antioxidant and in vitro antiproliferative activity through induction of apoptosis and G0/G1 cell cycle arrest. Food Chemistry. 2013;140(1-2):262-272.DOI: 10.1016/j.foodchem.2013.02.060

[34] Rodrigo R, Libuy M. Modulation of Plant Endogenous Antioxidant Systems by Polyphenols. In: Watson RR, editor. Polyphenols in Plants Isolation, Purification and Extract Preparation. ISBN: 978-0-12-397934-6

[35] Heim KE, Tagliaferro A, Bobiya D. Flavonoid antioxidants: chemistry, metabolism and structure–activity relationships. Journal of Nutritional Biochemistry. 2002;13:572-584. DOI: 10.1016/s0955-2863(02)00208-5

[36] Amić D, Davidović-Amić D, Beslo D, Rastija V, Lucić B, Trinajstic N. SAR and QSAR of the antioxidant activity of flavonoids. Curr Med Chem. 2007;14:827-845. DOI: 10.2174/092986707780090954.

[37] Belghith T, Athmouni K, Bellassoued K, El Feki A, Ayadi H. Physiological and biochemical response of *Dunaliella salina* to cadmium pollution. Journal of Applied Phycology. 2015;28(2):991-999. DOI: 10.1007/s10811-015-0630-5.

Chapter 26

Endogenous Enzymatic Antioxidant Defense and Pathologies

Atika Eddaikra and Naouel Eddaikra

Abstract

Oxidative stress is an important component of various diseases. It manifests as an imbalance caused by an excessive production of reactive oxygen species (ROS) which are associated with a deficit of antioxidant activity. This deficit can be the consequence of genetic factors, environmental ones, metabolic imbalance, toxicity or direct attacks by the accumulation of free radicals. These can induce metabolic dysfunction affecting biological macromolecules in their structures or activities. From a physiological perspective, the neutralization of free radicals is ensured by enzymatic, antioxidant and non-enzymatic defense systems. In the present chapter, we will focus on the endogenous enzymatic antioxidant defense system such as superoxide dismutase (SOD), catalase (CAT), glutathione peroxidase (GPxs), thio redoxin (Trx) and paraxonase which play an important role in homeostatic redox balance. Also, we will review this set of antioxidants enzymes within different pathological states such as diabetes, cancer, autoimmune diseases, cardiovascular, Alzheimer's, Parkinson's or parasitic diseases such as Leishmaniasis and Malaria.

Keywords: oxidative stress, antioxidant defense, ROS, enzymatic antioxidant, pathology

1. Introduction

Oxidative stress is defined as an imbalance between the production of reactive oxygen species (ROS) and cellular antioxidant capacities. ROS have long been considered toxic by-products of normal oxygen metabolisms and they are implicated in various pathologies. Yet, their controlled production is an essential mechanism of cell signaling that participates in the maintenance of cell homeostasis [1].

As a concept in redox biology and medicine, Oxidative stress was formulated in 1985 [2]. Currently, as of late 2020, approximately 14,216 publications are presented for the term oxidative stress and 3,775 are associated with the term antioxidant defense in PubMed. An important component of various diseases, oxidative stress can also be said to be the result of a biological inability to detoxify reactive intermediates [3]. A large number of methods, such as DNA oxidation, have been developed and used in almost all diseases to measure its extent and nature. Findings confirm the fact that the paradox of ROS, as these are both toxic products of metabolism, and molecules essential for cell signaling and regulation. A moderate and controlled production of ROS can lead to a reversible oxidation of the surrounding molecules.

IntechOpen

In such a case, ROS act as correct second messengers. Conversely, an overproduction of ROS or a deficit in defense mechanisms can lead to the appearance of stress which causes non-specific and irreversible oxidation of biological molecules, engendering dysfunction [1, 4]. The production of free radicals occurs continuously in cells as a result of common metabolic processes. However, at high concentrations, whether from endogenous pathological stimuli (hyper-LDLemia, hypertension, diabetes, etc.) or exogenous sources (environmental pollutants, smoking, etc.), they can lead to cell death and disease states via the deterioration of molecular and cellular constituents of the arterial wall [5]. Such a stress can be limited by antioxidant systems, followed by a rapid return to a physiological redox state. It can also be prolonged, resulting in the creation of a new redox balance of a higher and permanent oxidizing level, similar to the one that can be found in chronic pathologies [6].

It is well established that oxidative stress is the main pathophysiological component of many human or animal. It participates in pathogenesis as well as the inflammation with which it is often associated. In several serious diseases, especially those related to aging, oxidative stress is often the original triggering factor. This is the case for cancers, eye pathologies (cataracts and macular degeneration), neurodegenerative diseases (ataxias, lateral sclerosis, Alzheimer's disease). Familial amyotrophic lateral sclerosis is the most illustrative example, since it is caused by a defect in the antioxidant enzyme superoxide dismutase gene. In other diseases, oxidative stress plays only a secondary role in the onset of the pathology, but participates nonetheless in immune or vascular complications. This is the case for infectious diseases such as AIDS, septic shock, diabetes, Parkinson's disease or kidney failure [7]. This is also the case with parasitic diseases. Studies suggest the hypothesis that cellular environments, lifestyle, genetic factors (genetic polymorphism) and metabolic state such as hyperglycemia are stimulants that trigger stress. They have shown that when the antioxidant defense is diminished or absent, the biological environment can no longer counter or adapt to the new physiological situation, and a cascade of ROS production reaction is triggered inducing both immune and metabolic imbalance, as well as structural and functional altercations of proteins involved in antioxidant defense. In the present chapter, we are interested in elements of the endogenous enzymatic antioxidant defense system, such as superoxide dismutase (SOD), catalase (CAT), glutathione peroxidase (GPxs), thioredoxin (Trx) and paraxonase which play a role important in the homeostatic redox balance. We will discuss the association of endogenous enzymatic defense with certain pathologies such as neurodegenerative diseases, autoimmune diseases such as diabetes, cancer, cardiovascular diseases, parasitic diseases.

2. Antioxidant defense mecanisms

The production of free radicals in living systems is continuous [8]. Oxygen (or dioxygen, O_2) is an essential gas to life. It can become reactive, forming superoxide ($O_2^{\bullet -}$). It is likely to cause damaging effects in the human body via the formation of free radicals and reactive oxygen species (ROS) [9]. These are much more toxic than oxygen itself [10]. However, O_2 toxicity and "free radical theory" has already been proposed in the literature to explain the aging process [11].

Antioxidant enzymes play a key role in detoxifying free radicals and reducing oxidative stress. They are the basis of the scavenging of reactive oxygen species (ROS) [12].

Electrons released by the mitochondrial electron transport chain (Mito-ETC) and produced by NADPH oxidases (NOX) are the main source of endogenous

DOI: http://dx.doi.org/10.5772/intechopen.95504

reactive oxygen species. Coupled with molecular oxygen, they give rise to the primary free radical and the precursor of the remaining species - superoxide ($O_2^{\bullet-}$). When in reaction with a short-lived nitric oxide ($NO^{\bullet}$), the superoxide forms a highly reactive peroxynitrate ($ONOO^-$) capable of modifying the structure and function of proteins. Superoxide dismutase (SOD) converts superoxide to hydrogen peroxide (H_2O_2), which can be converted in several ways. In the presence of transition metal ions like Fe^{2+} (Fenton reaction) or in the context of a reaction with superoxide, H_2O_2 forms a highly reactive hydroxyl radical ($OH^{\bullet}$) which damages lipids, proteins. DNAHydrogen peroxide (H_2O_2) can also be implicated in the oxidation reaction of monomeric glutathione (GSH) to glutathione disulfide (GSSG), or that of reduced thioredoxin (Trx red) to oxidized thioredoxin (Trx ox) catalyzed by glutathione peroxidase (GPX) or peroxidases involved in the renewal of thioredoxin (Trx). The reduced glutathione pool is restored by glutathione reductase (GR) which reduces oxidized glutathione via the use of NADPH. Thanks to the thiol groups in the cysteine (Cys) residues, glutathione and thioredoxin participate in the reduction of oxidized proteins. Their synthesis and renewal take place under tight homeostatic control creating a system responsible for the reduction of proteins sensitive to oxidation–reduction in the event of oxidative stress (**Figure 1**). Permeable H_2O_2 is involved in the signaling process and is degraded by catalase, glutathione peroxidase and peroxiredoxin3. Efficient regulation of mitochondrial H_2O_2 via endogenous antioxidant pathways is therefore an essential mechanism for maintaining physiological redox signaling and homeostasis [13, 14].

The mitochondria is not only one of the main sources of intracellular ROS, it is above all the main target. ROS can have a direct effect on mitochondrial activity. An induced alteration of mtDNA can alter the functioning of the respiratory chain and

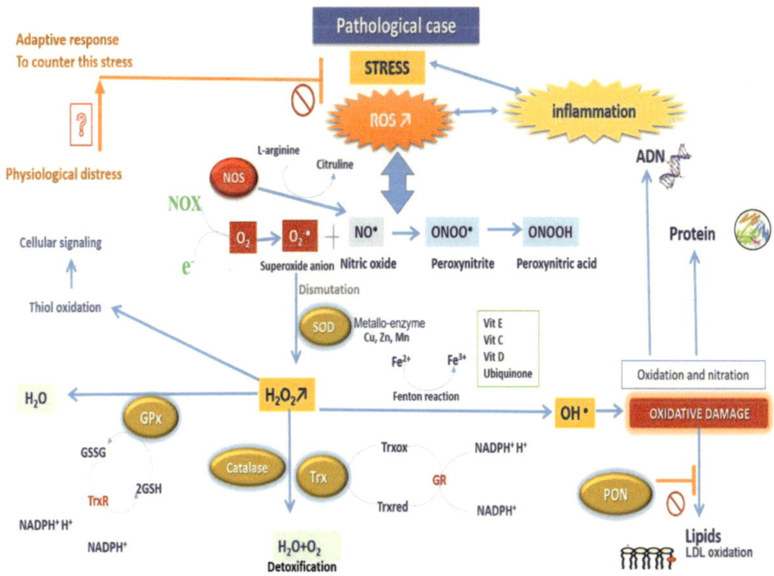

Figure 1.
Defense mechanisms of antioxidants. e-: electron; GPxs: glutathione peroxidase, GR: Glutathione reductase, GSH: Glutathione, GSSG: Glutathione disulfide ; H_2O_2 : Hydrogen peroxide, iNOS: nitric oxide synthase; LDL: low density lipoprotein; $NO^{\bullet}$: Nitric oxide ; NOS : nitricoxide synthase ; NOX: NADPH oxidases; NADP: Nicotinamide Adenine Dinucleotide Phosphate; O_2: Dioxygen; $O_2^{\bullet-}$: Superoxide anion; $OH^{\bullet}$: Hydroxyl radical; $ONOO^{\bullet}$: Peroxynitrite; ONOOH: Peroxynitrite acid; PON: Paraxonase; ROS: reactive oxygenated species; SOD: superoxide dismutase; Trx ox: oxidized thioredoxin ; Trx red: reduced Thioredoxin ; Trx: thioredoxin; Cu: copper Fe: iron; Zn: zinc; Mn: manganese;Vit: vitamin.

trigger a vicious cycle that increases ROS production and oxidative mitochondrial damage. Likewise, increased oxidation of mitochondrial membrane phospholipids could alter mitochondrial function [15].

3. Endogenous antioxidant enzymes

3.1 Superoxide dismutases

Superoxide dismutase (SOD) is a metalloprotein, representing one of the first lines of defense against the deleterious effects of free radicals. Thus, SODs are able to eliminate the superoxide anion $O_2^{\bullet -}$ by a disproportionation reaction, forming, with two superoxides, one molecule of oxygen and one molecule of hydrogen peroxide H_2O_2. In humans, 3 isoenzymes are described: cytosolic SOD1 (Cu/Zn-SOD), mitochondrial SOD2 (Mn-SOD) and extracellular SOD3 (Cu/Zn-SOD) [9, 16, 17]. These different forms of SOD elicit similar functions, but the characteristics of their quaternary protein structures, their chromosomal locations, their requirements for metal cofactors, their gene distributions and their cellular compartmentalisation are different from one another [18, 19].

SOD1, or CuZn-SOD (EC 1.15.1.1) was the first enzyme to be characterized. It consists of a copper and zinc-containing homodimer found almost exclusively in intracellular cytoplasmic spaces [20]. The SOD2, or Mn-SOD (EC 1.15.1.1), exists in the form of a tetramer containing manganese. It is a 222 amino acid protein with an N-terminal signal sequence of 24 amino acids. This enzyme is found exclusively in the mitochondrial matrix [21]. SOD3, or EC-SOD (EC 1.15.1.1), is a tetramer containing copper and zinc. It is found exclusively in the extracellular spaces. It is secreted by smooth muscle cells and constitutes the major antioxidant system of the arterial wall: its expression and secretion are increased by vasoactive factors (histamine, endothelin 1, angiotensin II) and decreased by homocysteine [9].

3.2 Catalase

Human catalase [CAT; EC 1.11.1.6] is an endogenous antioxidant enzyme of approximately 60 kDa. Its protein structure takes the form of a tetramer composed of a complex of 4 identical subunits, each containing 527 amino acid residues and a heme group with Fe_3^+ [22, 23]. Catalase has been mapped on chromosome 11p13. It converts the hydrogen peroxide "H_2O_2" of reactive oxygen species into water "H_2O" and oxygen "O_2" thus reducing the toxic effects of hydrogen peroxide [24].

3.3 Glutathion peroxydase

Glutathione peroxidases (GPx; EC 1.11.1.19) are a family of phylogenetically related oxidoreductases distributed in all living domains. GPx is a tetrameric selenoprotein, containing seleno-cysteine (Sec) in the active site [25]. It catalyzes the reduction of organic hydroperoxides (-ROOH) into alcohol and water groups using reduced glutathione (GSH) as a cosubstrate. It can also catalyze the reduction of hydrogen peroxide (H_2O_2) to H_2O and oxygen by oxidation of GSH reduced to its disulfide (GSSG). Oxidized glutathione (GSSG) can be reduced to GSH by the enzyme GSH reductase (GR), via the use of NADPH as a reducing substrate [26, 27]. Thus, GPxs protect against oxidative damage and are involved in the detoxification of hydrogen peroxide [28].

3.4 Paraxonase

The paraoxonase (PON) (EC:3.1.1.2) gene family includes three proteins, PON1, PON2 and PON3. PON1 and PON3 are both associated with high density lipoprotein (HDL) particles and exert anti-oxidant and anti-inflammatory properties [29]. The PON gene is located on the long arm of chromosome 7 in humans [30, 31]. PON proteins are all associated with high density lipoprotein (HDL) particles and exert anti-oxidant, anti-inflammatory and lipo-lactonase activities [29]. All PON proteins are involved in the pathogenesis of several inflammatory diseases including atherosclerosis, Alzheimer's disease, Parkinson's disease, diabetes and cancer. PON1 is found exclusively extracellular and associated only with high density lipoprotein (HDL) particles in the circulation, and partly confers the anti-oxidant and anti-inflammatory properties associated with HDL. Studies have shown that intracellular PON proteins; PON2 and PON3 are associated with mitochondria and membranes associated with mitochondria, modulate mitochondria-dependent superoxide production and prevent apoptosis. In addition, it has been shown that the overexpression of the PON2 and PON3 genes protects the mitochondria from mitochondrial dysfunction [31].

3.5 Thioredoxine

The thioredoxin (Trx) system is one of the central antioxidant systems in mammalian cells, maintaining a reducing environment by catalyzing the flow of electrons from nicotinamide adenine dinucleotide phosphate to Trx reductase in Trx, which reduces its target proteins using highly conserved thiol groups. Thioredoxin (Trx) is a 12 kD oxidoreductase enzyme containing a dithiol-disulfide active site. It is ubiquitous and found in many organisms, from plants and bacteria to mammals. It is located on chromosome 9 in the cytogenic position 9q31.3 [32]. The redox cascade of the Trx system is initiated by $NADPH^{+}$. H^{+} is generated by the pentose phosphate pathway. $NADPH^{+}H^{+}$ reduces oxidized Trx reductase (TrxR), which regenerates the pool of reduced Trx. Reduced Trx helps maintain a reducing environment for a number of different proteins [33]. In mammalian cells, there are two isoforms of Trx, a cytosolic Trx1 isoform which under certain circumstances can be transferred into the nucleus and secreted out of the cell, and the mitochondrial isoform Trx2. Unless explicitly stated otherwise. There is also a truncated form of Trx (Trx80) which has no redox properties and is not reduced by Trx reductase [33]. Trx, as an antioxidant, maintains the balance of redox status bound to thiol and also plays a central role in the regulation of redox signaling. Trx detects and responds to environmental oxidative stress1. The ROS generated by cellular respiration, metabolism and immune response, then modulates the redox status, function and activity of its target signaling proteins. Deregulation of such a Trx system affects various cellular functions and outcomes such as cell survival and death, leading to human diseases including cancer and inflammation [34]. Thioredoxin reductase (rxRs) are oxidoreductases necessary for the reduction of the active disulfide site in Trx and responsible for maintaining the pool of reduced and active Trx. Additionally, TrxR is a selenoprotein, and selenium is required for its expression and activity [33].

4. Pathologies

4.1 Neurodegenerative diseases

Aging is a major risk factor for several common neurodegenerative diseases, including Parkinson's disease (PD), amyotrophic lateral sclerosis (ALS),

Alzheimer's disease (AD) and Huntington's disease (HD). Recent studies have implicated mitochondrial dysfunction and oxidative stress in the aging process and also in the pathogenesis of neurodegenerative diseases. In the brain and other tissues, aging is associated with progressive impairment of mitochondrial function and increased oxidative damage. Three phenomena leading to oxidative stress in the brain, and implicated in neurodegenerative diseases, include inhibition of mitochondrial metabolism, neuronal excitotoxicity, and neuroinflammation [35].

4.1.1 Parkinson disease

Oxidative stress is an important factor in the Parkinson's disease (PD) pathogenesis. The main source of oxidative stress in the genesis of PD is the activation of glial cells and dopaminergic neuronal death of the substantia nigra [36, 37]. The oxidative imbalance involved in the neurodegenerative processes of PD appears to be a multifactorial phenomenon triggered by factors such as aging of the brain, genetic predisposition, mitochondrial dysfunction, free radical production and environmental toxins [37, 38]. Some studies suggest that although the accumulation of ROS plays a key role in the initiation and acceleration of cell death in PD, it is not the only cause of cell death in this disorder [39].

The activities of SOD, CAT, glutathione peroxidase (GSH-Px) and glucose-6-phosphate dehydrogenase (G6PD) have been reported to be significantly lower in patients with PD [36, 37]. The production of superoxide has also been found to increase considerably when the flow of electrons is inhibited at the level of the mitochondrial complex I or III complex [35, 40, 41].

4.1.2 Alzheimer's disease

Oxidative stress plays a role in Alzheimer's disease (AD), an age-related multifactorial disease leading to loss of cognitive functions [42]. It is characterized by a loss of synapses, an increase in the number of senile plaques (SP) and extracellular amyloid rich in beta-peptide (Aβ). Metal ions can bind to beta amyloid peptide (Aβ) to produce ROS. Thus, the damaged Aβ during the production of ROS, causes cellular toxicity and oxidation of neuronal membrane biomolecules and leads to disruption of membrane integrity [43]. It has been reported that oxidative stress may play a role in the pathogenesis of dementia AD and cerebral ischemia that causes vascular dementia (DV) [43]. The presence of early oxidative damage in mild cognitive impairment in amnesia (aMCI) has been shown to exist before clinical dementia in AD develops [44].

It has been reported that the neurodegenerative process of this disease is linked to a cyclical process between impaired energy metabolism, associated with lactate production and oxidative stress. Indeed, a decrease in complex IV activity and mitochondrial DNA mutations has been identified in patients with AD [40]. In addition, oxidative stress may be an early event in AD etiology, since markers of oxidation appear in mild cognitive impaired regions of the brain [42]. A strong association between low serum CAT, SOD, GPx and PON1 activity and the risk of AD has been reported.

4.2 Cardiovascular diseases

Cardiovascular disease is a group of disorders affecting heart and blood vessels. In a physiological state, ROS are modulators of signal transduction pathways and gene expression involved in vascular homeostasis. The cells of the vascular wall exhibit a physiological redox state that can be disrupted under many pathophysiological circumstances, causing oxidative stress that is deleterious to the cells concerned and their vascular functions. The causes of this imbalance are multiple, and overlap at least partially the classic cardiovascular risk factors: arterial hypertension, hypercholesterolemia, diabetes, etc. These risk factors are at the origin of stimuli responsible for an abnormal production of ROS, in particular by activation of NADPH oxidases and of the mitochondrial respiratory chain, a decrease in the bioavailability of NO to vasodilator effects. The pro-oxidant imbalance leads to the formation of oxidized LDL and multiple cell dysfunctions: release of pro-inflammatory factors and factors promoting cell proliferation, process of apoptosis and/or necrosis [6].

Several causes can produce an oxidative alteration which ultimately affects gene expression. Extracellular signals (cytokines emitted during inflammation, for example) are transmitted at the membrane level by receptors. These activate oxidases, thus generating H_2O_2, which acts as a second messenger. Likewise, an influx of xenobiotics can activate oxidative metabolism and lead to an overproduction of H_2O_2. The resulting modification of the "intracellular redox potential" will modulate the activity of certain transcription factors, and lead to a modification of gene expression [45] which as a result is partly responsible for the lowering of the defense of antioxidant enzymes.

4.3 Auto-immune diseases

Autoimmune disease is a pathological condition characterized by the breakdown of the self-tolerance of the immune system in the body in which genetic and environmental factors are involved. Immunological processes against tissues and organs lead to increased oxidative stress, and in turn, an imbalance of oxidative stress worsens the pathobiology of the disease. This is for example the case in type1 diabetes, multiple sclerosis or rheumatoid arthritis, systemic lupus erythematosus (SLE) and Sjögren syndrome (SS) [46]. Here, we will look at the oxidative stress and antioxidant defense relationship in type 1 diabetes (T1D).

T1D is a multifactorial disease and results from the destruction of insulin-secreting beta cells induced by an autoimmune process [47] with a strong inflammatory component [48]. Usually T1D is triggered by individuals with a specific genetic predisposition [49]. It is now clear that environmental factors play an important role in the development of this disease [50]. T1D involves the generation of pro-inflammatory cytokines and reactive oxygen species (ROS) [1]. The generation of free radicals potentiates the pathogenesis by promoting the destruction of cellular components, tissue damage and inflammation [51].

There is an inherent association with stress and the synthesis of reactive oxygen species (ROS) by immune cells to directly induce the destruction of B cells in the pancreas. However, recent evidence has shown that ROS can not only function as effector molecules involved in the pathogenesis of pancreatic β cells, but can also promote activation of innate and adaptive immune pathways in T1D [52]. Several previous studies have shown that hyperglycemia is associated with a decrease in oxidative defense. This confirms the hypothesis that hyperglycemia is at the origin of the production of reactive species and the decline in antioxidant defense [53, 54]. On the other hand, another study, carried out on endothelial cells of human origin, shows that high concentrations of glucose increase the activities of anti-oxidant enzymes (SOD, catalase, glutathione-peroxidase) as well as their cellular overexpression. This is evidence of an oxidative stress response resulting from high glucose levels [55]. It has been reported in poorly balanced diabetic patients that erythrocyte SOD is often reduced when the glycation level is high. This results in a reduction of enzyme's activity. Experimental evidence has shown that exposure to high concentrations of hydrogen peroxide can damage beta cells in the pancreas [56].

4.4 Cancer

It is becoming increasingly evident that ROS play an important role in the biology of tumorigenesis. Cancer cells increase ROS production to activate localized pro-tumorigenic signaling, and balance the increase in ROS with high antioxidant activity to maintain redox balance. Nevertheless, mutations associated with different types of cancer are often cited as the cause in the increased production of ROS. Hypoxia, activation of oncogenes, mutations in mitochondrial DNA, and loss of tumor suppressors have all been shown to lead to increased mitochondrial ROS-dependent tumorigenesis. Several tumor suppressors such as the "guardian of the genome" P53 have been shown to have ROS inhibitory functions. In about 50% of cancers, the tumor suppressor p53 is lost or mutated [57].

Several studies have shown that there is a strong relationship between inflammation, oxidative stress and cancer. The evolution of tumor metastases depends on an oxidative environment and inflammation, thus contributing to long-term cell damage and promoting carcinogenesis. Alterations in PON status encompassing genotype, activity and/or expression have been demonstrated in cancer patients, as well as in various cancer cells in vitro [58]. In recent years, overexpression of PON2 and PON3 has been observed in cancer cells and it has been proposed that both enzymes may be involved in tumor survival and resistance to stress. In addition, a lower activity of serum PON1 has been reported in cancer patients [58, 59]. Huang et al. found that PON3 is involved in multi-drug resistance in esophageal cancer (CE). Drug resistance prevents effective treatment of cancers [60]. As a result, blocking the antioxidant defense in tumors decreases their ability to balance oxidative stress and results in cell death [61]. Indeed, several clinical studies on several types of cancer have reported low levels of activity of antioxidant enzymes such as SOD, GSH and CAT in groups of patients with prostate cancer [62], breast cancer [63] et malignant lymphoma in children [64]. Also, another study showed that MCF-7 breast cancer cells chronically exposed to ascorbate/menadione become resistant (Resox cells) by primarily increasing catalase activity. These data suggest that chromatin remodeling is a major regulatory process controlling the expression of catalase in breast cancer cells when developing resistance to oxidative stress [65].

4.5 Parasitic diseases

Infectious diseases are often associated with oxidative stress and an inflammatory response. Infection and inflammation trigger a cascade of reactions in the host, known as the acute-phase response. Neglected diseases due to the parasitic protozoa *Leishmania*, *Trypanosoma* and *Plasmodium* affect millions of people worldwide, and the lack of suitable treatments has promoted an ongoing drug discovery effort to identify novel nontoxic and cost-effective chemotherapies. Leishmaniasis and Malaria are the most important neglected tropical diseases, with a disease burden of 0.2 to 0.4 million cases with a mortality rate of 20,000 to 40,000 reported per year for visceral leishmaniasis [66] and 214 million cases for malaria in 2015 and mortality of 1 to 2 million every year [67].

DOI: http://dx.doi.org/10.5772/intechopen.95504

4.5.1 Oxidative stress and malaria

In response to infection caused by *Plasmodium* parasites, the natural host defense mechanism is activated with involvement of phagocytes (macrophages and neutrophils). These, in turn, generate large amounts of ROS and RNS, causing an imbalance between the formation of oxidizing species and the activity of antioxidants. This imbalance is what triggers oxidative stress, which is an important mechanism of human hosts in response to infections and, in the case of Malaria, can lead to the death of the parasites [68]. *Plasmodium* spp. are global pathogens with a complex life cycle alternating between female Anopheles mosquitoes and vertebrate hosts that require the formation of unique zoite forms to invade different cell types at specific stages. Once sporozoites enter the host, they infect hepatocytes, and this is followed by the asexual cycle in the blood. Sexual forms that develop during the blood stage are ingested by a feeding mosquito, completing the cycle [69].

Plasmodium digests hemoglobin within its acidic food vacuole and releases toxic ferriprotoporphyrin IX (FP) and ROS [70]. Normally FP polymerizes to hemozoin but can also react with O_2 to form ROS, superoxide radical ($O_2^{\bullet-}$) that can be reduced to H_2O_2 by SOD. H_2O_2 can further be reduced to H_2O by either thioredoxin-dependent peroxidase (TPx) or GST in the parasite or by GST, TPx, GPx, and CAT in the host cell. ROS can react with lipids and proteins forming oxidized lipids or proteins. During the redox reactions, GSH and TrxSH become oxidized to GSSG and thioredoxin disulfide (TrxS2). Both GSSG and TrxS2 are reduced back by GR and TrxR, respectively. GSH is also synthesized in a pathway involving c-glutamyl-cysteinyl ligase (cGCL) and glutathione synthetase (GSH synt). NADPH is recycled by the pentose phosphate pathway under enzymes glucose-6-phosphate dehydrogenase (G6PD) and 6-phosphogluconate dehydrogenase (6PGD) [71].

4.5.2 Leishmania implementation and oxidative stress

Leishmaniosis are group of parasitic of neglected tropical diseases endemic in 98 countries. *Leishmania* spp. are intracellular parasitic protozoa with a complex digenetic life cycle requiring a susceptible vertebrate host and a permissive *phlebotomus* insect vector, which allow their transmission. The disease manifestations are from self-healing cutaneous lesion to visceral pathology depending on complex interactions between the parasite and the host immune system. The parasite *Leishmania* use Trojan horse strategy when it is transmitted into the circulation system of the mammals after the vector sandfly blood meal. The promastigote motile form is phagocytized by macrophages and subsequently transform into the nonmotile amastigote form. The obligatory intracellular amastigotes reside within phagolysosomal vacuoles and adopt sophisticated mechanisms that enable them to avoid the hostile defense system of their host organism. The interplay between the parasite and its host is a complex process, in which the paramount interest of the parasite is to restrict the immune and microbicidal activities of the macrophage, while keeping it alive as a nutritional Source [72].

Phagocytosis of microbes leads to a burst of $O_2^{\bullet-}$ production through activation of NADPH oxidase [73, 74]. Once inside the host cell, ROS and RNS are the cellular major arms against *Leishmania*. NO is synthesized by nitricoxide synthase (NOS) during the conversion of l-arginine to l-citrulline, while $O_2^{\bullet-}$ and other ROS are generated by the membrane-bound NADPH-dependent oxidases (NOX) [75].

To deal with this avalanche of oxidative stress molecules and host immune response, *Leishmania* has developed several immune evasion strategies to avoid a certain death by oxidative stress. NO production by nitric oxide synthase iNOS is disturbed by highlighting the efficiency of this effect or mechanism. *Leishmania* parasites are particularly efficient at disrupting signals that lead to the activation and differentiation of CD4+ Th1cells, such as IL-12 and CD40 signaling [76, 77]. *Leishmania* does not express GSH/GR, but its redox metabolism relies on the glutathione conjugate N1,N8-bis(L-γ-glutamyl-L-hemicystinylglycyl) spermidine, also known as trypanothione (T(SH)2). Trypanothione disulfide (TS2) is generated when T(SH)2 reduces ROS [78]. Trypanothione reductase (TRs) have structural analogies with GRs and are also members of the NADPH-dependent flavoprotein oxidoreductase family. TR uses NADPH as an electron donor for the reduction of $T(S)_2$ [77, 79].

Leishmania does not express catalase and classical selenium-containing glutathione peroxidases, two major hydroperoxide-eliminating enzymes generally present in eukaryotes (Krauth-Siegel & comini, 2008). Instead, these organisms' hydroperoxide metabolism was found to depend on tryparedoxin (TXN) and peroxiredoxin (PRX) belonging to the peroxiredoxin family of enzymes and are pivotal for $T(SH)_2$ to reduce H_2O_2 [80, 81]. Overexpression of peroxidases in *Leishmania* demonstrated its protective action against oxidative stress, ROS-induced programmed cell death, and protein damage [82, 83]. The combined hydroperoxide and ONOO- metabolizing activities of 2-Cys peroxiredoxins are also likely to account for the increased infectivity of Leishmania mutants overexpressing a cytosolic peroxiredoxin, in an ex vivo model of infection [84].

5. Conclusion

The moderate and controlled production of ROS can lead to a reversible oxidation of the surrounding molecules: the ROS then act as true second messengers. Conversely, an overproduction of ROS or a deficit in defense systems leads to the appearance of stress which causes a non-specific and irreversible oxidation of biological molecules, leading to a loss of function [4]. In addition, it is obvious to emphasize that individuals do not have the same antioxidant potential depending on their eating habits, their lifestyle, their genetic characteristics or the environment in which they live. As a result, the antioxidant defense may be different from one individual to another. In order to counter the ROS attack and adjust the redox balance, a repair process is set up for each pathological situation. As a result, endogenous defense induces several signaling mechanisms to adapt to the new physiological situation.

Conflict of interest

The authors declare no conflict of interest.

Abbreviations

6PGD	6-phosphogluconate dehydrogenase
AD	Alzheimer's disease
ALS	Amyotrophic Lateral Sclerosis
aMCI	cognitive impairment in amnesia
Aβ	beta-peptide
CAT	catalase
cGCL	c-glutamyl-cysteinyl ligase

DOI: http://dx.doi.org/10.5772/intechopen.95504

FP	ferriprotoporphyrin IX
G6PD	glucose-6-phosphate dehydrogenase
GPxs	glutathione peroxidase
GR	Glutathione reductase
GSH synt	glutathione synthetase
GSH	Glutathione
GSSG	Glutathione disulfide
H_2O_2	Hydrogen peroxide
HD	Huntington's disease
HDL	High Density Lipoprotein
iNOS	nitric oxide synthase
LDL	low density lipoprotein
Mito-ETC	Mitochondrial- Electron Transport Chain
mtDNA	mitochondrial DNA
$NO^{\bullet}$	Nitric oxide
NOS	nitricoxide synthase
NOX	NADPH oxidases
$O_2{}^{\bullet -}$	Superoxide
O_2	Dioxygen
$OH^{\bullet}$	Hydroxyl radical
$ONOO^{\bullet}$	Peroxynitrate
PD	Parkinson's disease
PON	paraxonase
$ROOH^{-}$	Hydroperoxides
ROS	reactive oxygenated species
SLE	Systemic lupus erythematosus
SOD	superoxide dismutase
SS	Sjögren syndrome
T(SH)2	trypanothione
$T(SH)_2$	trypanothione.
T1D	Type 1 diabetes
TP53	tumor protein 53
TRs	trypanothione reductase
TRs	trypanothione reductase
Trx ox	oxidized thioredoxin
Trx red	reduced Thioredoxin
Trx	thioredoxin
TrxR	Trx Reductase
TS2	Trypanothione disulfide
TS_2	Trypanothione disulfide
β cells	beta cells

Author details

Atika Eddaikra[1,2*] and Naouel Eddaikra[3]

1 Department of Cellular Biology and Physiology, Faculty of Nature and Life, Saad Dahlab University, Blida, Algeria

2 Structural Bioinformatics, Molecular Modeling and Drug Design, Bioinformatics Laboratory, Applied Microbiology and Biomolecules, M'Hamed Bougara University, Boumerdes, Algeria

3 Department of Parasitology, Laboratory of Parasitic Eco-epidemiology and Population Genetics, Institute Pasteur of Algeria, Route du petit Staoueli, Algiers, Algeria

*Address all correspondence to: aeddaikra@yahoo.fr

References

[1] Migdal C, Serres M. Espèces réactives de l'oxygène et stress oxydant. Medecine/Sciences 2011;27:405-412.

[2] Sies H. Hydrogen peroxide as a central redox signaling molecule in physiological oxidative stress: Oxidative eustress. Redox Biol 2017;11:613-619.

[3] Kim TH, Hong JM, Oh B, et al. Genetic association study of polymorphisms in the catalase gene with the risk of osteonecrosis of the femoral head in the Korean population. Osteoarthr Cartil 2008;16:1060-1066.

[4] Carrière A, Galinier A, Fernandez Y, et al. Les espèces actives de l'oxygène: Le yin et le yang de la mitochondrie. Medecine/Sciences 2006;22:47-53.

[5] Amir Aslani B, Ghobadi S. Studies on oxidants and antioxidants with a brief glance at their relevance to the immune system. Life Sci 2016;146:163-173.

[6] Beaudeux J-L, Peynet J, Bonnefont-Rousselot D, et al. Cellular sources of reactive oxygen and nitrogen species. Roles in signal transcription pathways. Ann Pharm Fr 2006;64:373-381.

[7] Favier A. Stress oxydant Stress oxydant et pathologies humaines. Ann Pharm Fr 2006;64:390-396.

[8] Goudable J, Favier A. Radicaux libres oxygénés et antioxydants. Nutr Clin Métabolisme 1997;11:115-120.

[9] Haleng et al. Le stress oxydant. no date;

[10] Gardès-Albert M, Bonnefont-Rousselot D, Abedinzadeh Z, et al. Espèces réactives de l'oxygène. Comment l'oxygène peut-il devenir toxique? Actual Chim 2003;269:91-96.

[11] Alfonso-Prieto M, Biarnés X, Vidossich P, et al. The Molecular Mechanism of the Catalase Reaction. J Am Chem Soc 2009;131:11751-11761.

[12] Leverve X. Stress oxydant et antioxydants? Cah Nutr Diet 2009;44:219-224.

[13] Forman HJ, Maiorino M, Ursini F. Signaling functions of reactive oxygen species. Biochemistry 2010;49:835-842.

[14] Angelova PR, Abramov AY. Role of mitochondrial ROS in the brain: from physiology to neurodegeneration. FEBS Lett 2018;592:692-702.

[15] Echtay KS, Esteves TC, Pakay JL, et al. A signalling role for 4-hydroxy-2-nonenal in regulation of mitochondrial uncoupling. EMBO J 2003;22:4103-10.

[16] Candas D, Li JJ. MnSOD in oxidative stress response-potential regulation via mitochondrial protein influx. Antioxid Redox Signal 2014;20:1599-617.

[17] Chistiakov AD, Savost'anov K V., Turakulov RI, et al. A new type 1 diabetes susceptibility locus containing the catalase gene (chromosome 11p13) in a Russian population. Diabetes Metab Res Rev 2004;20:219-224.

[18] Miao L, St Clair DK. Regulation of superoxide dismutase genes: implications in disease. Free Radic Biol Med 2009;47:344-56.

[19] Bresciani G, Cruz IBM, De Paz JA, et al. The MnSOD Ala16Val SNP: Relevance to human diseases and interaction with environmental factors. Free Radic Res 2013;47:781-792.

[20] Banks CJ, Andersen JL. Mechanisms of SOD1 regulation by post-translational modifications. Redox Biol 2019;26:101270.

[21] Zelko IN, Mariani TJ, Folz RJ. Superoxide dismutase multigene family: A comparison of the CuZn-SOD (SOD1), Mn-SOD (SOD2), and EC-SOD (SOD3) gene structures, evolution, and expression. Free Radic Biol Med 2002;33:337-349.

[22] Ogata M, Mizugaki J. Properties of Residual Catalase in the Erythroeytes of Japanese-Type Acatalasemia. 1979;338:329-338.

[23] Kodydková J, Vávrová L, Kocík M, et al. Human catalase, its polymorphisms, regulation and changes of Its activity in different diseases. Folia Biol (Czech Republic) 2014;60:153-167.

[24] Ahn J, Nowell S, McCann SE, et al. Associations between catalase phenotype and genotype: Modification by epidemiologic factors. Cancer Epidemiol Biomarkers Prev 2006;15:1217-1222.

[25] Kang DH, Kang SW. Targeting cellular antioxidant enzymes for treating atherosclerotic vascular disease. Biomol Ther 2013;21:89-96.

[26] Toppo S, Flohé L, Ursini F, et al. Catalytic mechanisms and specificities of glutathione peroxidases: Variations of a basic scheme. Biochim Biophys Acta - Gen Subj 2009;1790:1486-1500.

[27] Ursini F, Maiorino M, Forman HJ. Redox homeostasis: The Golden Mean of healthy living. Redox Biol 2016;8:205-215.

[28] Lubos E, Kelly NJ, Oldebeken SR, et al. Glutathione peroxidase-1 deficiency augments proinflammatory cytokine-induced redox signaling and human endothelial cell activation. J Biol Chem 2011;286:35407-35417.

[29] Bacchetti T, Ferretti G, Sahebkar A. The role of paraoxonase in cancer. Semin Cancer Biol 2019;56:72-86.

[30] Primo-Parmo SL, Sorenson RC, Teiber J, et al. The human serum paraoxonase/arylesterase gene (PON1) is one member of a multigene family. Genomics 1996;33:498-507.

[31] Devarajan A, Shih D, Reddy ST. Inflammation, infection, cancer and all that...the role of paraoxonases. Adv Exp Med Biol 2014;824:33-41.

[32] Heppell-Parton A, Cahn A, Bench A, et al. Thioredoxin, a mediator of growth inhibition, maps to 9q31. Genomics 1995;26:379-381.

[33] Lee S, Kim SM, Lee RT. Thioredoxin and thioredoxin target proteins: From molecular mechanisms to functional significance. Antioxidants Redox Signal 2013;18:1165-1207.

[34] Matsuzawa A. Thioredoxin and redox signaling: Roles of the thioredoxin system in control of cell fate. Arch Biochem Biophys 2017;617:101-105.

[35] Golden TR, Patel M. Catalytic Antioxidants and Neurodegeneration. 2009;11:.

[36] Dias V, Junn E, Mouradian MM. The role of oxidative stress in parkinson's disease. J Parkinsons Dis 2013;3:461-491.

[37] Percário S, Da Silva Barbosa A, Varela ELP, et al. Oxidative Stress in Parkinson's Disease: Potential Benefits of Antioxidant Supplementation. Oxid Med Cell Longev 2020;2020:.

[38] Zhou C, Huang Y, Przedborski S. Oxidative stress in Parkinson's disease: A mechanism of pathogenic and therapeutic significance. Ann N Y Acad Sci 2008;1147:93-104.

[39] Trist BG, Hare DJ, Double KL. Oxidative stress in the aging substantia nigra and the etiology of Parkinson's disease. Aging Cell 2019;18:.

[40] Bowling AC, Beal MF. Bioenergetic and oxidative stress in neurodegenerative diseases. Life Sci 1995;56:1151-1171.

[41] Schapira AHV, Cooper JM, Dexter D, et al. Mitochondrial Complex I Deficiency in Parkinson's Disease. J Neurochem 1990;54:823-827.

[42] Cheignon C, Tomas M, Bonnefont-Rousselot D, et al. Oxidative stress and the amyloid beta peptide in Alzheimer's disease. Redox Biol 2018;14:450-464.

[43] Casado Á, Encarnación López-Fernández M, Concepción Casado M, et al. Lipid peroxidation and antioxidant enzyme activities in vascular and alzheimer dementias. Neurochem Res 2008;33:450-458.

[44] Di Domenico F, Pupo G, Giraldo E, et al. Oxidative signature of cerebrospinal fluid from mild cognitive impairment and Alzheimer disease patients. Free Radic Biol Med 2016;91:1-9.

[45] Morel Y, Barouki R. Influence du stress oxydant sur la régulation des gènes. Médecine/Sciences 1998;14:713.

[46] Ramani S, Pathak A, Dalal V, et al. Oxidative Stress in Autoimmune Diseases: An Under Dealt Malice. Curr Protein Pept Sci 2020;21:611-621.

[47] Barcala Tabarrozzi AE, Castro CN, Dewey RA, et al. Cell-based interventions to halt autoimmunity in type 1 diabetes mellitus. Clin Exp Immunol 2013;171:135-146.

[48] Cabrera SM, Chen Y-G, Hagopian WA, et al. Blood-based signatures in type 1 diabetes. Diabetologia 2016;59:414-25.

[49] Bluestone JA, Herold K, Eisenbarth G. Genetics, pathogenesis and clinical interventions in type 1 diabetes. Nature 2010;464:1293-300.

[50] Castro-Correia C, Maia ML, Norberto S, et al. Can Antioxidative Status Be Involved in Type 1 Diabetes? J Clin Med Res 2017;9:998-1001.

[51] Pradeep DCD, Vegi K, Kutty AVM. Protein carbonyl content as a stable Oxidative stress marker in Type II Diabetes . Int J Biol Med Res 2012;3:2362-2365.

[52] Padgett LE, Broniowska KA, Hansen PA, et al. The role of reactive oxygen species and proinflammatory cytokines in type 1 diabetes pathogenesis. Ann N Y Acad Sci 2013;1281:16-35.

[53] Eddaikra A, Amroun H, Raache R, et al. Clinical variables and ethnicity may influenced by polymorphism of CAT −262C/T and MnSOD 47C/T antioxidant enzymes in Algerian type1 diabetes without complications. Gene 2018;670:182-192.

[54] Eddaikra A, Touil Boukoffa C. Polymorphism of MnSOD 47C/T antioxidant enzymes and type 1 diabetes. In: Diabetes. Elsevier; 2020. p. 107-115.

[55] Bonnefont-Rousselot D, Peynet J, Beaudeux JL, et al. Stress oxydant, fonctions vasculaires et athérosclérose. Nutr Clin Metab 2002;16:260-267.

[56] Góth L, Nagy T. Inherited catalase deficiency: Is it benign or a factor in various age related disorders? Mutat Res - Rev Mutat Res 2013;753:147-154.

[57] Sullivan LB, Chandel NS. Mitochondrial reactive oxygen species and cancer. Cancer Metab 2014;2:.

[58] Bacchetti T, Sartini D, Pozzi V, et al. Exploring the role of Paraoxonase-2 in

bladder cancer: Analyses performed on tissue samples, urines and cell cultures. Oncotarget 2017;8:28785-28795.

[59] Utangaç MM, Yeni E, Savaş M, et al. Mesane kanserinde paraoksanaz ve arilesteraz aktivitesi. Turk Urol Derg 2017;43:147-151.

[60] Huang D, Wang Y, He Y, et al. Paraoxonase 3 is involved in the multi-drug resistance of esophageal cancer 11 Medical and Health Sciences 1112 Oncology and Carcinogenesis. Cancer Cell Int 2018;18:1-11.

[61] Sznarkowska A, Kostecka A, Meller K, et al. Inhibition of cancer antioxidant defense by natural compounds. Oncotarget 2017;8:15996-16016.

[62] Ahmed Amar SA, Eryilmaz R, Demir H, et al. Determination of oxidative stress levels and some antioxidant enzyme activities in prostate cancer. Aging Male 2019;22:198-206.

[63] Kangari P, Farahany TZ, Golchin A, et al. Enzymatic antioxidant and lipid peroxidation evaluation in the newly diagnosed breast cancer patients in Iran. Asian Pacific J Cancer Prev 2018;19:3511-3515.

[64] Galleze A, Kocyigit A, Cherif N, et al. Assessment of oxidative/anti-oxidative markers and DNA damage profile induced by chemotherapy in algerian children with lymphoma. Drug Chem Toxicol 2020;43:169-173.

[65] Glorieux C, Calderon PB. Catalase, a remarkable enzyme: Targeting the oldest antioxidant enzyme to find a new cancer treatment approach. Biol Chem 2017;398:1095-1108.

[66] Alvar J, Vélez ID, Bern C, et al. Leishmaniasis worldwide and global estimates of its incidence. PLoS One 2012;7:.

[67] Geneva: World Health Organization. World malaria report 2019. 2019.

[68] Percário S, Moreira DR, Gomes BAQ, et al. Oxidative stress in Malaria. Int J Mol Sci 2012;13:16346-16372.

[69] Cowman AF, Healer J, Marapana D, et al. Malaria: Biology and Disease. Cell 2016;167:610-624.

[70] Postma NS, Mommers EC, Eling WMC, et al. Oxidative stress in malaria; implications for prevention and therapy. Pharm World Sci 1996;18:121-129.

[71] Kavishe RA, Koenderink JB, Alifrangis M. Oxidative stress in malaria and artemisinin combination therapy: Pros and Cons. FEBS J 2017;284:2579-2591.

[72] Shapira M, Zinoviev A. Leishmania parasites act as a Trojan horse that paralyzes the translation system of host macrophages. Cell Host Microbe 2011;9:257-259.

[73] Babior BM. Phagocytes and oxidative stress. Am J Med 2000;109:33-44.

[74] Minakami R, Sumimoto H. Phagocytosis-coupled activation of the superoxide-producing phagocyte oxidase, a member of the NADPH oxidase (Nox) family. Int J Hematol 2006;84:193-198.

[75] Cecílio P, Pérez-Cabezas B, Santarém N, et al. Deception and manipulation: The arms of Leishmania, a successful parasite. Front Immunol 2014;5:1-16.

[76] Mougneau E, Bihl F, Glaichenhaus N. Cell biology and immunology of Leishmania. Immunol Rev 2011;240:286-296.

[77] Olekhnovitch R, Bousso P. Induction, Propagation, and Activity of Host Nitric Oxide: Lessons from Leishmania Infection. Trends Parasitol 2015;31:653-664.

[78] Van Assche T, Deschacht M, Da Luz RAI, et al. Leishmania-macrophage interactions: Insights into the redox biology. Free Radic Biol Med 2011;51:337-351.

[79] Krauth-siegel RL, Enders B, Henderson GB, et al. Trypanothione reductase from. 1987;128:123-128.

[80] Castro H, Tomás AM. Peroxidases of trypanosomatids. Antioxidants Redox Signal 2008;10:1593-1606.

[81] Romao S, Castro H, Sousa C, et al. The cytosolic tryparedoxin of Leishmania infantum is essential for parasite survival. Int J Parasitol 2009;39:703-711.

[82] Dolai S, Yadav RK, Pal S, et al. Leishmania major ascorbate peroxidase overexpression protects cells against reactive oxygen species-mediated cardiolipin oxidation. Free Radic Biol Med 2008;45:1520-1529.

[83] Dolai S, Yadav RK, Pal S, et al. Overexpression of mitochondrial Leishmania major ascorbate peroxidase enhances tolerance to oxidative stress-induced programmed cell death and protein damage. Eukaryot Cell 2009;8:1721-1731.

[84] Barr SD, Gedamu L. Role of peroxidoxins in Leishmania chagasi survival. Evidence of an enzymatic defense against nitrosative stress. J Biol Chem 2003;278:10816-10823.

Chapter 27

Role of Secondary Metabolites to Attenuate Stress Damages in Plants

Masuma Zahan Akhi, Md. Manjurul Haque and Md. Sanaullah Biswas

Abstract

Plants are constantly facing various threats posed by the biotic and abiotic stressors. To survive in these challenged environment, plants evolve a variety of defense mechanism. Among the various phytochemicals, secondary metabolites (SMs) accumulate higher amount under stressful conditions and initiate signaling functions to up-regulation of defense responsive genes. SMs ensures the survival, persistence and competitiveness of the plant against the threat generated under stressful conditions. Therefore, the signaling functions of SMs to protect the plant from biotic and abiotic stressors are getting importance in the recent times. In this chapter the contribution of SMs to protect the plant from specific environmental stresses has been discussed.

Keywords: reactive oxygen species, environmental stress, biotic and abiotic stress, plant tolerance and adaptation, programmed cell death

1. Introduction

A hundred years ago it is reported that primary metabolites (carbohydrates, proteins, amino acids, vitamins, acetone, ethanol, etc.), are involved in various life functions in plants such as cell division, growth and development, photosynthesis, respiration, and reproduction [1]. However, Kossel was the first to define the secondary metabolites (SMs) as opposed to the primary ones and then concept of SMs has been introduced in plant biology [2]. The term metabolite is usually confined to tiny molecules and products of metabolism. Plants produce unlimited and manifold assortment of organic compounds, the great majority of which do not take part in growth and development immediately. These substances commonly referred to as SMs, often are differentially distributed among limited taxonomic groups within the plant kingdom [3]. In the last decade SMs, low molecular compounds occurring in all living organisms while mostly distributed in plants, became a subject of dramatically increasing interest relevant to their outstanding practical implication for medicinal, nutritive and cosmetic purposes, as well as to their undebatable importance in plant stress physiology [4].

Recent advances of SMs research on plant stress physiology suggesting its involvement to the mitigating detrimental effects of various stressors [5, 6]. In addition to the protective functions of SMs, they also act as defending molecules of primary metabolites such as proteins and nucleic acids from stress-induced damages [7, 8]. Therefore, physiological modifications such as secondary metabolism adjustment, ion and water balance, minimization of oxidative damage etc. occurred in plant body which can provide the phenotypic response of stress tolerance directly or indirectly. The stress response could also be a growth inhibition or cell death [9–11], which will depend upon how many and which kind of genes are up- or down-regulated [12]. However, most of the cases secondary metabolism adjustment play an important role in defense mechanism either increasing or decreasing their production in plant body. In this chapter the role and involvement of SMs in regulation of various biotic and abiotic stresses in plants has been discussed.

2. Plant responses to stress factors

Plants throughout their life cycle are subjected to various forms of biotic and abiotic stresses, as a sessile organism plants lack the ability to escape from that danger areas. Plants express responses to stress conditions in three ways. Some plants avoid the stress altogether (e.g. ephemeral, short-lived, desert plants), some show susceptibility to stress which may ultimately lead to plant death and some show resistant capacity [13]. To defend themselves against diverse stresses, plants have evolved complicated and highly regulated systems. To cope with these challenging environment plants evolve some efficient mechanism such as adjustment in photosynthetic rates, stomatal conductance, transpiration, cell wall architecture, remodeling of membrane structure, alterations in cell cycle and division rates with overall effect on general growth to fine-tune physiology and metabolism of bioactive compounds [14]. Initiation of stress and defense responses are mediated by signaling processes and pathways which trigger the primary metabolism that provides biosynthetic intermediates for secondary metabolism in plant body. These include the stress responsive system and the inducible defense system which depends on inducible activation of massive defense-related genes, suit of molecular and cellular process as well as inducible production of diverse defense-related SMs [15]. Plant accumulate a large number of SMs from primary metabolites in cells, and the production of that metabolites are regarded as an adaptive capacity in coping with stressful constraints during challenging environment [16–18].

3. Mechanism of stress adaptation in plant

Generally, a stress signal transduction pathway comprises the following key steps: (i) signal perception; (ii) signal transduction; and (iii) stress response. The first step in the activation of signaling cascade for any given stress is the recognition of stress signals via receptors located on the membrane of plant cell. Recently a few research works indicated that various plasma membrane proteins like COLD1 (Chilling Tolerance Divergence-1) [19], CNGCs (cyclic nucleotide nucleotide-gated channel), GLR (glutamate-receptor like) channel, histidine kinases, calcium channel are the main sensors for stress signaling. After recognition, the receptors transmit the signal into downstream through phytohormones and second messengers such as Ca^{2+} and ROS [20]. The second messengers, like ROS, trigger the activation of another set of ROS-modulated protein kinases (PKs) and protein phosphatases (PPs), including MAPK (mitogen-activated protein kinase) cascades, CDPKs (calcium-dependent protein kinases), CBLs (calcineurin-B-like proteins), CIPK (CBL-interacting protein kinase), and many other PKs as well as PPs such as some PP2Cs (protein phosphatase 2Cs). Subsequently, these PKs and PPs deliver the information downstream and trigger a series of phosphorylation or dephosphorylation of transcription factors (TFs), that finally culminates either directly in the expression of functional genes involved in cellular protection, or indirectly in the expression of regulatory genes participating in signaling cascades and transcriptional regulation of gene expression.

In addition of the enzymatic (such as superoxide dismutase, catalase, ascorbate peroxidase) and non-enzymatic antioxidants (such as ascorbic acid, reduced glutathione, α-tocopherol, carotenoids, flavonoids), primary metabolites including sugars, amino acids contribute to cellular homeostasis to adapt under stressful conditions [21]. Recently, the research advances supporting that products of secondary metabolism are important to alleviate toxic effects of stresses [5] through expression of stress responsive genes. Therefore, in presence of stress signals accumulated various species of SMs are critically important for adaptation and tolerance to the altering environment.

4. Generation and diversity of secondary metabolites in plants

Plant SMs are classified into four major categories. These four categories include (i) terpenes (such as carotenoids, sterols, cardiac glycosides and plant volatiles), (ii) phenolics (such as lignans, phenolic acid, tannins, coumarins, lignins, stilbenes and flavonoids), (iii) nitrogen containing compounds (such as cyanogenic glycosides, alkaloids, and glucosinolates) and (iv) sulfur containing compounds (such as glutathione, phytoalexins, thionins, defensins and lectins) [22, 23]. But on the basis of biosynthesis pathways plant SMs are usually classified into three chemically distinct groups [24]. The diverse chemical structures of the SMs determine their functions to the medicine and stress adaptation. Three major categories are (i) terpenes derived from mevalonic acid pathway [25] and methyl erythritol phosphate pathway [26], (ii) phenolics derived from malonic acid pathway or a few case shikimic acid pathway [27], (iii) N (Nitrogen) and S (Sulfur) containing compounds via tricarboxylic acid cycle or sometimes via shikimic acid pathway. Among the pathways of SMs accumulation, shikimic acid, mevalonic acid, phenylpropanoic acid and methyl erythritol phosphate pathways are highly regulated under stress stimuli.

5. Terpenes for stress responses in plant

Plants produce various types of SMs, many of which have been subsequently exploited by humans for their beneficial roles in a diverse array of biological functions [28]. Terpenes are one of the diverse species of SMs contribute to the various biological process in plants. Terpenoids are terpenes with an oxygen moiety and additional structural rearrangements. Therefore, these two terms of terpenes and terpenoids are used interchangeably. Terpenoids have their roles in plant defense against biotic and abiotic stresses or they are treated as signal molecules to attract the insects for pollination. The first step of terpenoid biosynthesis is generation of C5 unit like as isopentenyl diphosphate (IPP) or dimethylallyl diphosphate (DMAPP). On the basis of C5 units, we can classify the terpenoids as C5 (hemiterpenes), C10 (monoterpenes), C15 (sesquiterpenes), C20 (diterpenes), C25 (sesterpenes), C30 (triterpenes), C40 (tetraterpenes), C40 (polyterpenes) [29–31].

5.1 Terpenes for biotic stress responses

The rate of terpene emission in *Pinus sylvestris subsp. nevadensis* is increased due to attack of the caterpillar of Pine Processionary Moth (PPM). PPM is the main defoliator of pine tree in the mediterranean region. The emission rates of terpenes are higher in attacked branches of trees than non-attacked trees. That indicates, terpenes are toxic volatile compounds accumulate in plant to provide sufficient defense mechanism [32]. Terpenoids can serve as repellents and reduce larval feeding and oviposition by herbivores [33, 34]. Isoprene is volatile organic compound and belongs to the terpenoids group. *Manduca sexta* caterpillars were released to the transgenic tobacco plants containing isoprene synthase gene and the wild type of which does not emit isoprene. This study showed that isoprene-emitting transgenic tobacco plants deters *Manduca sexta* from feeding [35].

In attack of root feeding herbivore, plant produce various types of metabolites such as sesquiterpene lactone taraxinic acid β-D glucopyranosyl ester (TA-G) [36]. The main function of these compounds is to protect the plant against below ground herbivore attack. Dandelion (*Taraxacum officinale*) is known to release secondary metabolite-rich latex from wounded roots which help to protect this plant from its native root feeding enemy, larvae of the common cockchafer beetle (*Melolontha melolontha*). A study showed that TA-G-deficient lines lost more main and side root mass than control lines after 10 d of feeding by *M. melolontha* relative to undamaged control plants [37].

5.2 Terpenes for abiotic stress responses

Under abiotic stress conditions volatile terpenes alleviate the effects of oxidative stress either through direct reactions with oxidant intercellularly, and alteration of ROS signaling. The amphipathic nature of isoprene enhances hydrophobic interactions between membrane proteins and lipids [38] which prevents membrane disintegration and protein disintegration. In response to oxidative stimuli, membrane bound SMs such as such as tocopherol and carotenoids (zeaxanthin, neoxanthin, and lutein) acts as antioxidants and may directly scavenge ROS in response to photoinhibition [39–43]. Singlet oxygen generated under oxidative stress considered is one of the strong oxidants also removed by the isoprenoids [44]. Oleuropein, a member of terpene family SMs, found higher amount of accumulation in leaves and roots of olive tree in response to salinity stress. The increase accumulation of oleuropein under salinity stress protect the olive tree from the oxidative stress [45]. The reason behind this relationship is that oleuropein acts as a glucose-reservoir for osmoregulation or high energy-consuming processes required for plant adaptation to salinity. Furthermore, oleuropein may act as an additional constituent of the antioxidant defense system of olive trees. Although most studies showed plant tolerant mechanism largely depends on the functions of non-volatiles antioxidant compounds. However, various volatiles organic compounds of the terpenes family have been connected in the protection to abiotic stresses, in particular photooxidative stress, heat stress and ozone stress. In response to ozone and heat stress, plant emitting isoprene alleviate ROS accumulation and protected plant from oxidative damages. Grapevines are not isoprene emitting plants but other volatiles isoprenoids such as monoterpenes emitter grapevine clone showed tolerance to heat stress [46].

Among the terpenes, isoprene (C5) and monoterpene hydrocarbons ameliorate abiotic stress in a number of plant species via membrane stabilization and direct antioxidant effects. Besides antioxidants properties of isoprene and monoterpene hydrocarbons they also rapid react with ozone to reduce its toxicity. A transgenic tobacco (*Nicotiana attenuata*) overexpressing a maize terpene synthase gene (ZmTPS10) might protected plants from intermitted heat stress by the accumulation of sesquiterpene hydrocarbons (C15) (E)-ß-farnesene and (E)-α-bergamotene [47–49]. Rice seedlings exposed to UV-B radiation and hydrogen peroxide accumulated higher amount of dozens of monoterpenes such as limonene, sabinene and myrcene to adapt in the altering environment [50].

Zealexins and kauralexins are two acidic terpenoid phytoalexins mediate biotic damages caused by insect and pathogen in aboveground part of maize plants. Recently it is showed that terpenoid phytoalexins also protect root damages under abiotic stress factors such as drought and salinity stress. Wild type maize plant accumulated terpenoid phytoalexins are positively correlated with the biomass accumulation of the plants. On the other side, mutant maize deficient with kauralexin synthesis are sensitive to water deficit condition [51]. Carnosic acid (CA), a diterpene protect Labiatae species from water stress-induced oxidative damages in combination with that of other low-molecular weight antioxidants (α-tocopherol and ascorbate) in chloroplasts [52]. These findings suggest that terpenes protect plants from biotic and abiotic stress damages due to their antioxidant properties or direct quenching of oxidants.

6. Phenolics for stress responses in plant

Phenolics are one of the most ubiquitous groups of SMs which are synthesize in plants and possess biological properties like antifeedant [53], antioxidant, anti-apoptosis, anti-aging, anticarcinogenic, anti-inflammation, and cell proliferation activity. Phenolics consist of an aromatic ring with one or more hydroxyl groups. Coumarin, furano-coumarins, lignin, flavonoids, isoflavonoids and tanins are the available forms of phenolics. Phenolics are often produced and accumulated in the sub-epidermal layers of plant tissues exposed to stress and pathogen attack [54]. The concentration of a particular phenolic compound within a plant tissue is dependent on season and may also vary at different stages of growth and development [55]. Several internal and external factors, including trauma, wounding, drought and pathogen attack, affect the synthesis and accumulation of phenolics [56, 57].

6.1 Phenolics for biotic stress responses

Phenolics are ubiquitous SMs in plants serves as a protective agent, inhibitors, natural animal toxicants and pesticides against invading herbivores, nematodes, phytophagous insects, and fungal and bacterial pathogens [58, 59]. Among the phenolic compounds coumarins are simple phenolic widespread in vascular plants and appear to function in different capacities in various plant defense mechanisms against insect herbivores and fungi. Several studies in many different plant species have shown that coumarins can accumulate in response to infection by a diversity of pathogens, including viruses, bacteria, fungi and oomycetes. The extent and timing of coumarin accumulation in plant parts have been associated with the level of disease resistance [60, 61]. The phenolic compounds ferulic acid and protocatecuic acid are accumulated increasingly in rice by the fungal attack to reduce mycotoxin. The accumulation of these two phenolics are positively correlated with *p*-coumaric acid and 4-hydroxybenzoic acid to protect plant from mycotoxin [62].

6.2 Phenolics for abiotic stress responses

The accumulation of phenolics in plant tissues is considered as an adaptive response of plants to adverse environmental conditions. In response to various external stimuli plant cell increases accumulation of phenolic substances. Therefore, the degree of interactions between plants and their changing environments has been a major driving force behind the emergence of specific natural products. For example, cold stress increases phenolic production into the cell wall in winter rye (*Secale cereale*) either as suberin or lignin. Lignification and suberin deposition increase resistance to cold stress. These cell wall thickenings protect the plant from freezing stress. An increase in cell wall thickening could reduce cell collapse during freezing-induced dehydration and mechanical stress, thus providing freezing resistance to the plant [63]. Inhibition of root growth was recorded due to the accumulation of soluble phenolics and higher lignification in cucumber. Soluble phenolic compounds increased with time at chilling temperature but after rewarming these were decreased slightly. The decreased level in both organs (hypocotyl and root) after rewarming may suggest their important role in protection of both soybean organs against chilling injury. These compounds may participate in auxin metabolism, change membrane permeability, influence respiration and oxidative phosphorylation or protein synthesis [64].

Metabolic name of phenol	Nature of response	Abiotic stress	Plant species	Reference
Coniferyl alcohol, ferulic acid and p-coumaric	Increase accumulation and tolerance level	Nutrient deficiency	Reviewed in various plant species	Ahagnar et al. [72]
Chlorogenic acid, apigenin and luteolin	Increase accumulation and tolerance level	Drought stress	*Capsicum annuum L.*	Rodríguez-Calzada et al. [73]
Chlorogenic acid, rutin, hyperoside, isoquercetine, quercitrine and quercetine	Increased accumulation and tolerance level	Salinity	*Hypericum pruinatum*	Caliskan et al. [74]
Protocatecuic acid	Increased tolerance level	Salinity *S. macrosiphon*	Valifard et al. [67]	
Flavonols and hydroxycinnamic acids	Increase accumulation and tolerance level	Heat stress, salinity stress	*Solanum lycopersicon cv. Boludo*	Martinez et al. [75]
Chlorogenic acid	Increased accumulation	Full sunlight	*V. myrtillus*	Alqahtani et al. [68]
Caffeic acid, p-coumaric acid and ferulic acid	Decreased accumulation and tolerance level	Drought	*Vitis vinifera* L.	Kro'l et al. [76]
Flavonoids, isoflavonoids	Increased accumulation, become drought resistant	Drought *Arabidopsis thaliana*	Nakabayashi et al. [66]	
Quercetin	Increased level of deposition provide protection from damaging light	UV	*F. esculentum*	Regvar *et al.* [65]
Catechin and quercetin	Increased accumulation and become resistant against heavy metal	Heavy metal	*Zea mays L*	Michalak [69]
Lignin or suberin	Increased deposition and become freezing resistant	Cold stress/free zing	*Secale cereal*	Griffith and Yaish [63]

Table 1.
Nature of responses of phenolic compounds to abiotic stress in some plant species.

Exposure of ambient solar UV-B radiation to plants in open fields adversely affects macromolecules through the generation of ROS. At the same time, plants synthesize phenolic compounds, which act as a screen inside the epidermal cell layer to defend themselves from this damaging radiation and by adjusting the antioxidant systems at both the cell and whole organism level. A comparative accumulation of phenolics were measured after UV irradiation in buckwheat genotypes (*Fagopyrum esculentum and F. tataricum*) and found a specific increase of quercetin concentration in *F. esculentum* [65]. Drought is the major abiotic stress that affects plant growth and development and causes losses in agricultural production. As has been reported by several studies, phenolics content increased in plants under water scarcity to improve drought tolerance in *Arabidopsis thaliana* [66]. Tolerant and sensitive rice cultivars to salinity showed variable amount of phenolic compounds. A large increase of total phenolics and the content of protocatechuic acid was found in tolerant varieties, whereas in contrast, a markedly reduce was found in the susceptible cultivar [67]. In addition, the content of flavonoids and chlorogenic acid are positively correlated to the growth-lighting condition in Australian *Centella asiatica* (L.) *Urb* [68].

Certain flavonoids exhibit the ability to provide heavy metal stress protection by transition metals chelation (e.g., Fe, Cu, Ni, Zn), which generates hydroxyl radical via Fenton's reaction revealed that the chelation of these metals in the soil may be an effective form of defense against the effects of high metals concentration toxicity. The biosynthesis of phenolic compounds that are precursors of lignin intensifies under stress conditions [69]. Research on corn plants (*Zea mays* L.) confirmed this phenomenon when grown on soil contaminated with aluminum ions and root exudates were found with high levels of catechin and quercetin. Phenolic compounds also contribute to reduce heavy metal toxicity in plants. Cadmium metal-stressed *Brassica juncea* plants accumulated higher amount of rutin polyphenol than untreated plants to prevent oxidative damages [70]. Phenolic compounds were related to the antioxidant activity, and they play a major role in stabilizing lipid peroxidation. Actually during stress condition plants become potentially active and by releasing phenolic substance, modulating the activities of antioxidants, enzyme activities, and radicals scavenging activities demonstrated their active participation in oxidative stress management [71]. Some other evidences of nature of responses of phenolic compounds to abiotic stress in some plant species are summarized in **Table 1**.

7. N and S containing SMs for stress responses in plant

A large family of N and S containing SMs found in approximately 20% of the species of vascular plants, most frequently in the herbaceous dicot and relatively a few in monocots and gymnosperms. They include alkaloids, cyanogenic glucosides, non-protein amino acids phytoalexins, thionine, defensins and allinin. Most of them are biosynthesized from common amino acids.

7.1 N and S containing SMs for biotic stress responses

Alkaloids are nitrogenous organic SMs that have been shown to have antimicrobial activity (such as quinolones, metronidazole, or others) through inhibiting enzyme activity or other mechanisms. Squalamine, a polyamine alkaloid, acts through a detergent-like mechanism of action against gram-negative bacteria, leading to the disruption of their outer membranes, and it depolarizes gram-positive bacterial membranes [77].

Phytoalexins are S containing SMs, in response to fungal and bacterial pathogen, other forms of stress such as mechanical damages accumulate in the infection sites. The accumulation of phytoalexins limit the spreading of pathogen by inducing cell death known as hypersensitive response (HR) in a diverse group of plants. Defensins, thionins and lectins S-rich SMs accumulate in pathogen attack and external injury. These compounds also showed broad range of inhibition of microbial pathogen such as fungi and bacteria [78]. Glucosinolates are sulfur-rich SMs, widely synthesized in all vegetable and oilseed species of the order Brassicales (*Brassica oleracea*). The enzyme myrosinase (thioglucosidase) are stored in special myrosinase cells. When the tissue damage is commenced due to insect feeding, this enzyme comes into contact with glucosinolates and hydrolyses indole glucosinolates to produce nitriles and unstable isothiocyanates and aliphatic glucosinolates to produce volatile and pungent isothiocyanates. These products have toxic properties that inhibits growth (antibiosis) and act as feeding deterrents (antixenosis) against a range of insects; from leaf chewing lepidopteran larvae to phloem-feeding aphids [79]. Glucosinolate accumulation by the attack of diamondback moth insect on cabbage protect the plant by creating toxicity [80].

7.2 N and S containing SMs for abiotic stress responses

Alkaloids are N containing SMs also trigger adaption mechanism of plants. The concentration of four kind of alkaloids such as vindoline, catharanthine, vinblastine and vincristine significantly increased with the increasing saline concentration but the total dry weight to some extent were decreased. The reduction in plant growth may be an adaptive response to salt stress which allows the conservation of energy, thereby launching the appropriate defense response and also reducing the risk of heritable damage [81]. To adapt in the water scarcity stress *Senecio jacobaea*, *Senecio aquaticus*, and their hybrids increased the accumulation of pyrrolizidine alkaloids (PAs) [82]. The influence of drought stress changes the contents of alkaloids such as narkotine, morphine, codeine in *Papaver somniferum*. The comparison to the control group demonstrated that alkaloids narkotine and morphine trigger tolerance mechanism of plants [83]. The contents of alkaloids such as vindoline, catharanthine and vinblastine were significantly increased in the seedling leaves of *Catharanthus roseus* under short exposure of heat stress. Therefore, accumulation of alkaloids species under stressful conditions are critically important to adapt in the altering environments.

8. Conclusion

Plant tolerance to stresses is jointly controlled by the plants' anatomy, physiology, biochemistry, genetics, development and evolution. In addition to the primary metabolites, in response to various stresses either biotic and abiotic plants start to synthesize SMs in their cell. As a result, some physiological modification such as metabolic adjustment, ion and water balance, regulation of stomatal conductance, activation of different types of antioxidant and enzyme occurs which help the plant to increase tolerance level. Plant tolerance and adaptation mechanism to stressful conditions are mainly adjusted by the modifying primary metabolism pathway. According to the aforementioned data, SMs functions on stress adaptation are established in the recent year. Therefore, manipulating the generation and action of SMs and the activity of genes responsible for the accumulation of SMs are critically important to enhance the tolerance level and adaptability of plants under stressful conditions.

Author details

Masuma Zahan Akhi[1], Md. Manjurul Haque[2] and Md. Sanaullah Biswas[1*]

1 Department of Horticulture, Bangabandhu Sheikh Mujibur Rahman Agricultural University, Gazipur, Bangladesh

2 Department of Environmental Science, Bangabandhu Sheikh Mujibur Rahman Agricultural University, Gazipur, Bangladesh

*Address all correspondence to: sanaullah@bsmrau.edu.bd

References

[1] Bourgaud F, Gravot A, Milesi S, Gontier E. Production of plant secondary metabolites: A historical perspective. Plant Science. 2001;161:839-851. DOI: 10.1016/S0168-9452(01)00490-3

[2] Kossel A, Ueber Schleim und schleimbildende Stoffe1. DMW-Deutsche Medizinische Wochenschrift. 1891;17:1297-1299

[3] Jain C, Khatana S, Vijayvergia R. Bioactivity of secondary metabolites of various plants: a review. International Journal of Pharmaceutical Science and Research. 2019;10:494-504. DOI: 10.13040/IJPSR.0975-8232.10.494-04

[4] Edreva A, Velikova V, Tsonev T, Dagnon S, Gürel A, Aktaş L, Gesheva E. Stress-protective role of secondary metabolites: diversity of functions and mechanisms. General and Applied Plant Physiology. 2008;34:67-78

[5] Chrysargyris A, Papakyriakou E, Petropoulos SA, Tzortzakis N. The combined and single effect of salinity and copper stress on growth and quality of *Mentha spicata* plants. Journal of Hazardous Materials. 2019;368:584-593. DOI: 10.1016/j.jhazmat.2019.01.058

[6] Austen N, Lake JA, Phoenix G, Cameron DD. The regulation of plant secondary metabolism in response to abiotic stress: interactions between heat shock and elevated CO2. Frontiers in Plant Science. 2019;10:1463. DOI: 10.3389/fpls.2019.01463

[7] Ahmad S, Nadeem S, Muhammad N. Boundary layer flow over a curved surface imbedded in porous medium. Communications in Theoretical Physics. 2019;71:344. DOI: 10.1088/0253-6102/71/3/344

[8] Piasecka A, Jedrzejczak-Rey N, Bednarek P. Secondary metabolites in plant innate immunity: conserved function of divergent chemicals. New Phytologist. 2015;206:948-964. DOI: 10.1111/nph.13325

[9] Mano J, Biswas MS, Sugimoto K. Reactive carbonyl species: a missing link in ROS signaling. Plants. 2019; 8:391. DOI: 10.3390/plants8100391

[10] Biswas MS, Mano J. Lipid peroxide-derived short-chain carbonyls mediate hydrogen peroxide-induced and salt-induced programmed cell death in plants. Plant Physiology. 2015;168: 885-898. DOI: 10.1104/pp.115.256834

[11] Biswas MS, Mano, J. Reactive carbonyl species activate caspase-3-like protease to initiate programmed cell death in plants. Plant and Cell Physiology. 2016;57:1432-1442. DOI: 10.1093/pcp/pcw053

[12] Kurutas EB, Ozturk P. The evaluation of local oxidative/nitrosative stress in patients with pityriasis versicolor: a preliminary study. Mycoses. 2016;59:720-725. DOI: 10.1111/myc.12522

[13] Shimizu-Sato S, Tanaka M, Mori H. Auxin–cytokinin interactions in the control of shoot branching. Plant Molecular Biology. 2009;69:429. DOI: 10.1007/s11103-008-9416-3

[14] Atkinson NJ, Urwin PE. The interaction of plant biotic and abiotic stresses: from genes to the field. Journal of Experimental Botany. 2012;63:3523-3543. DOI: 10.1093/jxb/ers100

[15] Jones JD, Dangl JL. The plant immune system. Nature. 2006;444: 323-329. DOI:10.1038/nature0528

[16] Akula R, Ravishankar GA. Influence of abiotic stress signals on secondary metabolites in plants. Plant Signaling

and Behavior. 2011;6:1720-1731. DOI: 10.4161/psb.6.11.17613

[17] Narayani M, Srivastava S. Elicitation: a stimulation of stress in in vitro plant cell/tissue cultures for enhancement of secondary metabolite production. Phytochemistry Reviews. 2017;16:1227-1252. DOI: 10.1007/s11101-017-9534-0

[18] Caretto S, Linsalata V, Colella G, Mita G, Lattanzio V. Carbon fluxes between primary metabolism and phenolic pathway in plant tissues under stress. International Journal of Molecular Sciences. 2015;16:26378-26394. DOI: 10.3390/ijms161125967

[19] Ma Y, Dai X, Xu Y, Luo W, Zheng X, Zeng D, Pan Y, Lin X, Liu H, Zhang D, Xiao J. COLD1 confers chilling tolerance in Rice. Cell. 2015;160:1209-1221. DOI: 10.1016/j.cell.2015.01.046.

[20] Mahajan S, Pandey GK, Tuteja N. Calcium-and salt-stress signaling in plants: shedding light on SOS pathway. Archives of Biochemistry and Biophysics. 2008;471:146-158. DOI: 10.1016/j.abb.2008.01.010

[21] Ahanger MA, Bhat JA, Siddiqui MH, Rinklebe J, Ahmad P. Integration of silicon and secondary metabolites in plants: a significant association in stress tolerance. Journal of Experimental Botany. 2020;71:6758-6774. DOI: 10.1093/jxb/eraa291

[22] Ashraf MA, Iqbal M, Rasheed R, Hussain I, Riaz M, Arif MS. Environmental stress and secondary metabolites in plants: an overview. In Plant metabolites and regulation under environmental stress. Academic Press. 2018;153-167. DOI: 10.1016/B978-0-12-812689-9.00008-X

[23] Mazid M, Khan TA, Mohammad F. Role of secondary metabolites in defense mechanisms of plants. Biology and Medicine. 2011;3:232-249

[24] Harborne JB. Classes and functions of secondary products from plants. Chemicals from Plants. 1999;26:1-25. DOI:10.1142/9789812817273_0001

[25] Kumar SR, Shilpashree HB, Nagegowda DA. Terpene moiety enhancement by overexpression of geranyl (geranyl) diphosphate synthase and geraniol synthase elevates monomeric and dimeric monoterpene indole alkaloids in transgenic Catharanthus roseus. Frontiers in Plant Science. 2018;9:942. DOI: 10.3389/fpls.2018.00942

[26] González-Cabanelas D, Hammerbacher A, Raguschke B, Gershenzon J, Wright LP. Quantifying the metabolites of the methylerythritol 4-phosphate (MEP) pathway in plants and bacteria by liquid chromatography–triple quadrupole mass spectrometry. Methods in Enzymology. Academic Press. 2016;576:225-249. DOI: 10.1016/bs.mie.2016.02.025

[27] Santos-Sánchez NF, Salas-Coronado R, Hernández-Carlos B, Villanueva-Cañongo C. Shikimic acid pathway in biosynthesis of phenolic compounds. Plant Physiological Aspects of Phenolic Compounds. Intech Open. 2019; DOI: 10.5772/intechopen.83815

[28] Balandrin MF, Klocke JA, Wurtele ES, Bollinger WH. Natural plant chemicals: sources of industrial and medicinal materials. Science. 1985;228:1154-1160. DOI: 10.1126/science.3890182

[29] Boncan DA, Tsang SS, Li C, Lee IH, Lam HM, Chan TF, Hui JH. Terpenes and Terpenoids in Plants: Interactions with Environment and Insects. International Journal of Molecular Sciences. 2020;21:7382. DOI: 10.3390/ijms21197382

[30] Ashour M, Wink M, Gershenzon J. Biochemistry of terpenoids: monoterpenes, sesquiterpenes and

diterpenes. Annual Plant Reviews Online. 2018;15:258-303. DOI: 10.1002/9781119312994.apr0427

[31] Martin JJ, Pitera DJ, Withers ST, Newmann JD, Keasling JD. Engineering a mevalonate pathway in *Escherichia coli* for production of terpenoids. Nature Biotechnology. 2003;21:796-802. DOI: 10.1038/nbt833

[32] Castells AA. The role of terpenes in the defensive responses of conifers against herbivores and pathogens. Universitat Autònoma de Barcelona; 2015.

[33] Unsicker SB, Kunert G, Gershenzon J. Protective perfumes: the role of vegetative volatiles in plant defense against herbivores. Current Opinion in Plant Biology. 2009;12:479-485. DOI: 10.1016/j.pbi.2009.04.001

[34] Maffei ME. Sites of synthesis, biochemistry and functional role of plant volatiles. South African Journal of Botany. 2010;76:612-631. DOI: 10.1016/j.sajb.2010.03.003

[35] Laothawornkitkul J, Paul ND, Vickers CE, Possell M, Taylor JE, Mullineaux PM, Hewitt CN. Isoprene emissions influence herbivore feeding decisions. Plant, Cell & Environment. 2008;31:1410-1415. DOI: 10.1111/j.1365-3040.2008.01849.x

[36] Huber M, Triebwasser-Freese D, Reichelt M, Heiling S, Paetz C, Chandran JN, Bartram S, Schneider B, Gershenzon J, Erb M. Identification, quantification, spatiotemporal distribution and genetic variation of major latex secondary metabolites in the common dandelion (*Taraxacum officinale* agg.). Phytochemistry. 2015;115:89-98. DOI: 10.1016/j.phytochem.2015.01.003

[37] Huber M, Epping J, Schulze Gronover C, Fricke J, Aziz Z, Brillatz T, Swyers M, Köllner TG, Vogel H, Hammerbacher A, Triebwasser-Freese D. A latex metabolite benefits plant fitness under root herbivore attack. PLOS Biology. 2016;14:1002332. DOI: 10.1371/journal.pbio.1002332

[38] Sharkey TD, Yeh S. Isoprene emission from plants. Annual Review of Plant Biology. 2001;52:407-436. DOI: 10.1146/annurev.arplant.52.1.407

[39] Goh CH, Ko SM, Koh S, Kim YJ, Bae HJ. Photosynthesis and environments: photoinhibition and repair mechanisms in plants. Journal of Plant Biology. 2012;55:93-101. DOI: 10.1007/s12374-011-9195-2

[40] Havaux M, Eymery F, Porfirova S, Rey P, Dörmann P. Vitamin E protects against photoinhibition and photooxidative stress in Arabidopsis thaliana. The Plant Cell. 2005;17:3451-3469. DOI: 10.1105/tpc.105.037036

[41] Havaux M, Niyogi KK. The violaxanthin cycle protects plants from photooxidative damage by more than one mechanism. Proceedings of the National Academy of Sciences. 1999;96:8762-8767. DOI: 10.1073/pnas.96.15.8762

[42] Dall'Osto L, Fiore A, Cazzaniga S, Giuliano G, Bassi R. Different roles of α-and β-branch xanthophylls in photosystem assembly and photoprotection. Journal of Biological Chemistry. 2007;282:35056-35068. DOI: 10.1074/jbc.M704729200

[43] Peng L, Ma J, Chi W, Guo J, Zhu S, Lu Q, Lu C, Zhang L. LOW PSII ACCUMULATION1 is involved in efficient assembly of photosystem II in Arabidopsis thaliana. The Plant Cell. 2006;18:955-969. DOI: 10.1105/tpc.105.037689

[44] Velikova V, Edreva A, Loreto F. Endogenous isoprene protects Phragmites australis leaves against singlet oxygen. Physiologia

Plantarum. 2004;122:219-225. DOI: 10.1111/j.0031-9317.2004.00392.x

[45] Petridis A, Therios I, Samouris G, Tananaki C. Salinity-induced changes in phenolic compounds in leaves and roots of four olive cultivars (*Olea europaea* L.) and their relationship to antioxidant activity. Environmental and Experimental Botany. 2012;79:37-43. DOI: 10.1016/j.envexpbot.2012.01.007

[46] Bertamini M, Grando MS, Zocca P, Pedrotti M, Lorenzi S, Cappellin L. Linking monoterpenes and abiotic stress resistance in grapevines. BIO Web of Conferences. 2019;13:01003. DOI: 10.1051/bioconf/20191301003

[47] Palmer-Young EC, Veit D, Gershenzon J, Schuman MC. The Sesquiterpenes (E)-ß-Farnesene and (E)-α-Bergamotene quench ozone but fail to protect the wild tobacco Nicotiana attenuata from ozone, UVB, and Drought Stresses. PLOS One. 2015;10:0127296. DOI: 10.1371/journal.pone.0127296

[48] Loreto F, Mannozzi M, Maris C, Nascetti P, Ferranti F, Pasqualini S. Ozone quenching properties of isoprene and its antioxidant role in leaves. Plant Physiology. 2001;126:993-1000. DOI: 10.1104/pp.126.3.993

[49] Shu Y, Atkinson R. Rate constants for the gas-phase reactions of O3 with a series of terpenes and OH radical formation from the O3 reactions with sesquiterpenes at 296±2 K. International Journal of Chemical Kinetics. 1994;26:1193-1205. DOI: 10.1002/kin.550261207

[50] Lee GW, Lee S, Chung MS, Jeong YS, Chung BY. Rice terpene synthase 20 (OsTPS20) plays an important role in producing terpene volatiles in response to abiotic stresses. Protoplasma. 2015;252:997-1007. DOI: 10.1007/s00709-014-0735-8

[51] Vaughan MM, Christensen S, Schmelz EA, Huffaker A, Mcauslane HJ, Alborn HT, Romero M, Allen LH, Teal PE. Accumulation of terpenoid phytoalexins in maize roots is associated with drought tolerance. Plant, Cell & Environment. 2015;38:2195-2207. DOI: 10.1111/pce.12482

[52] Munné-Bosch S, Alegre L. Drought-induced changes in the redox state of α-tocopherol, ascorbate, and the diterpene carnosic acid in chloroplasts of Labiatae species differing in carnosic acid contents. Plant Physiology. 2003;131:1816-1825. DOI: 10.1104/pp.102.019265

[53] Dar AS, Rather BA, Wani AR, Ganie MA. Resistance against Insect pests by plant phenolics and their derivative compounds. Chemical Science Review and Letters. 2017;6:1073-1081

[54] Clé C, Hill LM, Niggeweg R, Martin CR, Guisez Y, Prinsen E, Jansen MA. Modulation of chlorogenic acid biosynthesis in Solanum lycopersicum; consequences for phenolic accumulation and UV-tolerance. Phytochemistry. 2008;69:2149-2156. DOI: 10.1016/j.phytochem.2008.04.024

[55] Dar SA. Screening of brinjal genotypes/verities against brinjal shoot and fruit borer. [thesis] Division of Entomology. SKUAST-K, Srinager, Kashmir; 2012

[56] Naikoo MI, Dar MI, Raghib F, Jaleel H, Ahmad B, Raina A, Khan FA, Naushin F. Role and regulation of plants phenolics in abiotic stress tolerance: an overview. In Plant signaling molecules. 2019;157-168. Woodhead Publishing. DOI: 10.1016/B978-0-12-816451-8.00009-5

[57] Kefeli VI, Kalevitch MV, Borsari B. Phenolic cycle in plants

and environment. Journal of Cell and Molecular Biology. 2003;2:13-18

[58] Isah T. Stress and defense responses in plant secondary metabolites production. Biological Research. 2019; 52: 39. DOI: 10.1186/s40659-019-0246-3

[59] Thakur AV, Ambwani S, Ambwani TK, Ahmad AH, Rawat DS. Evaluation of phytochemicals in the leaf extract of Clitoria ternatea Willd. through GC-MS analysis. Tropical Plant Research. 2018;5:200-206. DOI: 10.22271/tpr.2018.v5.i2.025

[60] Stringlis IA, De Jonge R, Pieterse CM. The age of coumarins in plant–microbe interactions. Plant and Cell Physiology. 2019;60:1405-14019. DOI: 10.1093/pcp/pcz076

[61] Tortosa M, Cartea ME, Rodríguez VM, Velasco P. Unraveling the metabolic response of Brassica oleracea exposed to Xanthomonas campestris pv. campestris. Journal of the Science of Food and Agriculture. 2018;98:3675-3683. DOI: 10.1002/jsfa.8876

[62] Giorni P, Rastelli S, Fregonara S, Bertuzzi T. Monitoring Phenolic Compounds in Rice during the Growing Season in Relation to Fungal and Mycotoxin Contamination. Toxins. 2020;12:341. DOI: 10.3390/toxins12050341

[63] Griffith M, Yaish MW. Antifreeze proteins in overwintering plants: a tale of two activities. Trends in Plant Science. 2004;9:399-405. DOI: 10.1016/j.tplants.2004.06.007

[64] Posmyk MM, Bailly C, Szafrańska K, Janas KM, Corbineau F. Antioxidant enzymes and isoflavonoids in chilled soybean (*Glycine max* (L.) Merr.) seedlings. Journal of Plant Physiology. 2005;162:403-412. DOI: 10.1016/j.jplph.2004.08.004

[65] Regvar M, Bukovnik U, Likar M, Kreft I. UV-B radiation affects flavonoids and fungal colonisation in *Fagopyrum esculentum* and *F. tataricum*. Open Life Sciences. 2012;7:275-283. DOI: 10.2478/s11535-012-0017-4

[66] Nakabayashi R, Yonekura-Sakakibara K, Urano K, Suzuki M, Yamada Y, Nishizawa T, Matsuda F, Kojima M, Sakakibara H, Shinozaki K, Michael AJ. Enhancement of oxidative and drought tolerance in Arabidopsis by overaccumulation of antioxidant flavonoids. The Plant Journal. 2014;77:367-379. DOI: 10.1111/tpj.12388

[67] Valifard M, Mohsenzadeh S, Kholdebarin B. Salinity effects on phenolic content and antioxidant activity of Salvia macrosiphon. Iranian Journal of Science and Technology. Transactions A: Science. 2017;41:295-300. DOI: 10.1007/s40995-016-0022-y

[68] Alqahtani A, Tongkao-on W, Li KM, Razmovski-Naumovski V, Chan K, Li GQ. Seasonal variation of triterpenes and phenolic compounds in Australian *Centella asiatica* (L.) Urb. Phytochemical Analysis. 2015;26:436-443. DOI: 10.1002/pca.2578

[69] Michalak A. Phenolic compounds and their antioxidant activity in plants growing under heavy metal stress. Polish Journal of Environmental Studies. 2006;15: 523-530.

[70] Kapoor D. Antioxidative defense responses and activation of phenolic compounds in *Brassica juncea* plants exposed to cadmium stress. International Journal of Green Pharmacy. 2016;10:228-234. DOI: 10.22377/IJGP.V10I04.760

[71] Gill SS, Tuteja N. Reactive oxygen species and antioxidant machinery in abiotic stress tolerance in crop plants. Plant Physiology and Biochemistry. 2010;48: 909-930. DOI: 10.1016/j.plaphy.2010.08.016

[72] Ahanger MA, Bhat JA, Siddiqui MH, Rinklebe J, Ahmad P. Integration of

silicon and secondary metabolites in plants: a significant association in stress tolerance. Journal of Experimental Botany. 2020;71:6758-6774. DOI: 10.1093/jxb/eraa291

[73] Rodríguez-Calzada T, Qian M, Strid Å, Neugart S, Schreiner M, Torres-Pacheco I, Guevara-González RG. Effect of UV-B radiation on morphology, phenolic compound production, gene expression, and subsequent drought stress responses in chili pepper (*Capsicum annuum* L.). Plant Physiology and Biochemistry. 2019;134:94-102. DOI: 10.1016/j.plaphy.2018.06.025

[74] Caliskan O, Radusiene J, Temizel KE, Staunis Z, Cirak C, Kurt D, Odabas MS. The effects of salt and drought stress on phenolic accumulation in greenhouse-grown *Hypericum pruinatum*. Italian Journal of Agronomy. 2017;12. DOI: 10.4081/ija.2017.918.

[75] Martınez V, Mestre TC, Rubio F, Girones-Vilaplana A, Moreno DA, Mittler R, Rivero RM. Accumulation of Flavonols over Hydroxycinnamic acids favors oxidative damage protection under abiotic stress. Frontiers in Plant Science. 2016;7:838. DOI: 10.3389/fpls.2016.00838

[76] Król A, Amarowicz R, Weidner S. Changes in the composition of phenolic compounds and antioxidant properties of grapevine roots and leaves (*Vitis vinifera* L.) under continuous of long-term drought stress. Acta Physiologia Plantarum. 2014;36:1491-1499. DOI: 10.1007/s11738-014-1526-8.

[77] Alhanout K, Malesinki S, Vidal N, Peyrot V, Rolain JM, Brunel JM. New insights into the antibacterial mechanism of action of squalamine. Journal of Antimicrobial Chemotherapy. 2010;65:1688-1693. DOI: 10.1093/jac/dkq213

[78] Pagare S, Bhatia M, Tripathi N, Pagare S, Bansal YK. Secondary metabolites of plants and their role: Overview. Current Trends in Biotechnology and Pharmacy. 2015;9:293-304.

[79] Santolamazza-Carbone S, Sotelo T, Velasco P, Cartea ME. Antibiotic properties of the glucosinolates of Brassica oleracea var. acephala similarly affect generalist and specialist larvae of two lepidopteran pests. Journal of Pest Science. 2016;89:195-206. DOI: 10.1007/s10340-015-0658-y

[80] Robin AH, Hossain MR, Park JI, Kim HR, Nou IS. Glucosinolate profiles in cabbage genotypes influence the preferential feeding of diamondback moth (*Plutella xylostella*). Frontiers in Plant Science. 2017;8:1244. DOI: 10.3389/fpls.2017.01244

[81] Jing-Yan WA, Zhao-Pu LI. Alkaloid accumulation in Catharanthus roseus increases with addition of seawater salts to the nutrient solution. Pedosphere. 2010;20:718-724. DOI: 10.1016/S1002-0160(10)60062-8

[82] Kirk H, Vrieling K, Van Der Meijden E, Klinkhamer PG. Species by environment interactions affect pyrrolizidine alkaloid expression in Senecio jacobaea, Senecio aquaticus, and their hybrids. Journal of Chemical Ecology. 2010;36:378-387. DOI: 10.1007/s10886-010-9772-8

[83] Yang L, Wen KS, Ruan X, Zhao YX, Wei F, Wang Q. Response of plant secondary metabolites to environmental factors. Molecules. 2018;23:762. DOI: 10.3390/molecules23040762

Chapter 28

Valorization of Natural Antioxidants for Nutritional and Health Applications

Pedro Ferreira-Santos, Zlatina Genisheva, Claudia Botelho, Cristina Rocha and José António Teixeira

Abstract

The significant increase in the world population age, 47 years in 1950 to 73 years in 2020, resulted in an increase in aging related diseases as well as in degenerative diseases. In consequence, researchers have been focusing in the development of new therapies, with a particular emphasis on the use of compounds with antioxidant properties, namely phytochemicals, such as polyphenols and carotenoids. Several *in vitro* and *in vivo* studies have demonstrated the phytochemicals antioxidant capacity. Their use is broad, as they can be part of food supplements, medicine and cosmetics. The health benefit of antioxidant phytochemicals is an indisputable question. Phytochemical properties are highly influenced by the natural matrix as well as by extraction process, which have a key role. There are several extraction methods that can be applied depending on the chemical properties of the bioactive compounds. There is a wide range of solvents with different polarities, which allows a selective extraction of the desired target family of compounds. Greener technologies have the advantage to reduce extraction time and solvent quantity in comparison to the most traditional methods. This chapter will focus on the different green extraction strategies related to the recovery of antioxidant bioactive compounds from natural sources, their nutritional and health potential.

Keywords: bioactive compounds, antioxidants, green technologies, oxidative stress, health benefits

1. Introduction

Nowadays, the awareness for the need to have a healthier lifestyle results in a higher consumption of natural organic food products and nutritionally rich antioxidants rather than synthetic and processed foods. In the past decade, an increased interest in the exploitation of natural ingredients to be used in the food and food products was observed. Researchers from all over the world are focusing on alternative sources of healthy nutrients promoting a safer and convenient diet. There is not clear evidence that synthetic antioxidants have toxic effects, although, consumer's interest is moving towards the natural products. Moreover, synthetic antioxidants and preservatives in food may lead to lipid peroxidation and deterioration of food flavor and quality [1]. Therefore, organic and sustainable processes, the identification of new phytochemicals with attractive biological activities, such as antioxidant, anticancer, antimicrobial, among others, are a hot topic among food researchers as well as for food industry aiming to develop new functional and therapeutic products.

Natural antioxidants are mainly derived from food, plants and other living organisms, such as fruits, vegetables, flowers, cereals, mushrooms, macro and micro-algae, spices and traditional medicinal herbs [2]. It is known that exogenous antioxidants have a strong potential to inhibit oxidative stress, preventing the lipid peroxidation process, and restore the cellular homeostasis [3]. Indeed, most of the antioxidant products shown to act as potential therapeutic agents. The consumption of antioxidants is highly important not only in prevention but also as an adjunct in the treatment of various human pathologies associated with oxidative stress, such as diabetes, aging, neurological, cardiovascular, and cancer [4]. In this sense, beneficial health effects of antioxidants are directly linked to regular daily intake and bioavailability.

The issues created by the increase of the human population, together with a reduction in renewable resources, is reflected in the increase of the global demand for reuse of industrial biowastes, as well as increasing the use of underexploited resources. The growing demand for new or alternative bioactive molecules obtained by green and sustainable processes, and decreasing the quantity of biowastes are premises for the development of conscious approaches for the valorization of phytochemicals from natural sources [5, 6]. Additionally, the development and optimization of efficient and intensified process for the recovery and isolation of high value phytochemicals are important.

The current chapter is focused on appreciation of different green extraction strategies related to the recovery of high value bioactive compounds from natural sources, their potential antioxidant activity, and possible nutritional and health applications.

2. Green approach in the extraction of antioxidant compounds

The recovery of antioxidant biomolecules or extracts is an important step to enable the reuse of natural resources for subsequent application in pharmaceutical, cosmetic products, food enrichment and preservatives, supplements and nutraceuticals.

Usually, bioactive phytochemicals are obtained using solid–liquid extraction, the unit operation, and depends on several factors, including the applied extraction technique, the parameters associated with the technique (such as temperature, time, pH and the extraction solvent), and the raw materials composition [7]. Extraction process is composed by 4 essential steps: (1) raw material pre-treatment (drying, grinding, *etc.*) to increase surface contact area and solvent penetration; (2) extraction with appropriated solvent; (3) post-treatment of the obtained liquid extract (filtration, concentration, purification, *etc.*); (4) solvent removal and its reuse [8].

The extraction process, when it is not optimized, is often time and energy consuming, induces the use of huge amount of water or petroleum-based solvents (harmful for environment and consumers) and generates large quantity of waste [9]. Moreover, the resulting extract may not be safe for the consumers, as it may contain residual solvents, contaminants from raw material, or denatured compounds due to extreme extraction conditions [5]. In this sense, the extraction processes intensification/optimization is necessary. The goal of an intensified process is to obtain greater extraction efficiency, high-quality and safe extracts while reducing extraction time, energy consumption, number of unit operations, amount

Extraction technology	Concept	Advantages	Disadvantages	References
Microwave assisted extraction (MAE)	Microwaves are electromagnetic fields in the range of 300 MHz to 300 GHz. The solvent penetrates into the solid matrix by diffusion leading to cell disruption and releasing the compounds of interest from a matrix to a solvent.	Lower time of extraction; low solvent volume; effective, uniform and selective heating.	High extraction pressure might modify the chemical structures of the compounds; low penetration of radiation in bulk products; equipment more expensive.	[5, 19]
Ultrasound assisted extraction (UAE)	Ultrasound is a sound wave of 20 kHz to 100 MHz. This process produces a phenomenon called cavitation, which means that the production, growth, and collapse of the bubbles to form pores that facilitate the cell wall disruption and increased the release of intracellular compounds into the extraction medium.	Fast; low solvent usage; lower extraction temperatures; preserving heat-sensitive compounds; eco-friendly and cheap process.	Energy intensive; dificult to scale up.	[20, 21]
Pressurized liquid extraction (PLE)	This technology is based on the use of liquid solvents at temperature and pressure values above the atmospheric boiling point and below the critical point values, decreasing the viscosity of the solvent, promoting accelerated dissolution kinetics, and increasing the solutes' solubility. The process disrupts the matrix, which increases the mass transfer of the analyte from the solvent sample	Rapid extraction; reduced organic solvent consumption.	Requires sophisticated instrumentation; possible degradation of thermolabile compounds.	[22, 23]
Supercritical fluid extraction (SFE)	Supercritical extraction is characterized by changes in temperature and pressure which transform the gas in supercritical fluid.	Fast; selective extraction; no residual solvents.	High cost; energy intensive; low polarity; type of co-solvent affects the efficiency of the extraction of antioxidant compounds.	[23, 24]
High hydrostatic pressure (HHP)	This technology applys very high pressures (100–1000 MPa) at 0 °C to less than 100 °C for a short period of time. Improves mass transfer rates and increases the secondary metabolite diffusion according to phase transitions.	Time efficient, requires less solvent, convenient, eco-friendly, safe and energy efficient; does not generate waste; pure and microbiologically safe products; absence of heating, avoiding compound denaturation and ensuring the extraction of thermo-sensitive components.	Variable efficiency; high processing costs.	[25–28]

Extraction technology	Concept	Advantages	Disadvantages	References
Enzyme assisted extraction (EAE)	The matrix and enzyme solution are loaded into an extraction vessel and placed in a thermostated water bath at the certain temperature and time.	Moderate extraction conditions; eco-friendly; selectivity due to the specificity of enzymes.	Expensive cost of enzymes; activity of enzymes varying with the environmental factors; filtration and cleanup step required; time consuming.	[3, 7, 23]
Pulsed electric field (PEF)	The material is placed between two electrodes. The pulse amplitude varies from 100–300 V/cm to 20–80 kV/cm. The treatment is conducted at room temperature or slightly higher. The principle of PEF extraction is to induce the electroporation of the cell membrane, thereby increasing the extraction yield.	Improves extraction and diffusion; cell permeability; minimize loss of heat sensitive molecules; selectivity of extracted compounds.	High control of parameters associated with the process (energy input, strength, pulses, temperature, and raw material properties, *e.g.* conductivity).	[5, 9, 29, 30]
High voltage electrical discharges (HVED)	It is an effective method to damage the cell structure and the extraction of valuable cellular compounds. The first step is the formation and propagation of a coil of a needle electrode and the formation of gaseous cavities. The second stage occurs when the streamer reaches the electrode plate (phase decomposition).	Efficiency of cell destruction; low solvent consumption; low operating temperature and temperature rise.	Free radicals production, which can react with antioxidant compounds, thus decreasing their bioactivy; lower selectivy; scale-up difficulties.	[19, 22, 31]
Ohmic heating (OH)	Non-pulsed electrotechnology centered on the conversion of electric energy into thermal energy based in the Joule effect (heat is generated inside a conductive matrix). The voltage applied in the OH process normally varies between 400 and 4000 V (electric field from 0.001 to 1 kV/cm).	Fast and homogeneous heating; reduction of energy consumption and times; low water and organic solvents use; low waste generation; selectivity of extracted compounds; improves extraction and diffusion by cell permeability.	High control of parameters associated with the process (similar to PEF and HVED).	[9, 32, 33]

Table 1.
Geen technologies for the extraction of antioxidant compounds from natural sources.

of water and organic solvents in the process, environmental impact, economic costs and quantity of waste generated [8].

In the last decades, the growing interest in the global ecological footprint reduction, bioeconomy control and consumer safety, has propel the implementation of innovative and clean alternatives in the food, chemical, cosmetic and pharmaceutical industries, following the principles of green chemistry and green engineering [10, 11].

Among the various extraction factors, solvents play an important role in extraction efficiency. The reduction of hazardous solvents is also considered one of the priorities of international policies [12]. A suitable solvent is able to obtain safe and high-quality ingredients and to preserve the biological effects of the extracted compounds. Furthermore, it should be recyclable and reusable, preventing negative environmental effects.

Numerous solvents have been used for the extraction of antioxidants from foods, marine sources, medicinal plants and agroindustrial wastes [6]. The selection of solvents must be based on the chemical nature and polarity of the compounds to be extracted, since solvents with different polarities are necessary for the isolation of compounds with different chemical structure [5]. For example, most of the phenolics, flavanoids and anthocyanins are hydrosoluble antioxidants. The polar and medium polar solvents, such as water, ethanol, methanol, propanol, acetone and their aqueous mixtures, are widely used for their extraction [13–15]. Carotenoids are lipid-soluble antioxidants, and common organic solvents, such as the mixtures of hexane with acetone, ethanol, methanol, or mixtures of ethyl acetate with acetone, ethanol, methanol, have been used for extraction [16–18].

A number of new alternatives to conventional techniques (Soxhlet, heat reflux, infusion, distillation, *etc.*), have been proposed to extract target antioxidant compounds from various natural matrices. **Table 1** presents a summary of the concept, the many benefits of some innovative extraction technologies as well as challenges associated with its use in the recovery of antioxidant molecules.

In the following sections some examples of natural matrices used as sources of antioxidant compounds using clean and innovative processes will be reported.

3. Natural sources of antioxidants

Fruits and vegetables are highly recommended dietary contents, widely known for their health-promoting effects and nutritious values. They got an essential place as conventional foods in the history because of their high amount of minerals, specifically electrolytes; vitamins, mainly vitamins C and E. Several studies are also demonstrating their high phytochemical contents eith antioxidant properties. Antioxidants obtained from plants, vegetables and fruits are mostly of terpenes, polyphenols, phytosterols, peptides, vitamins and minerals (**Figure 1**) [34, 35]. Antioxidant minerals, such as iron, zinc, selenium, copper, and manganese, act as cofactor of many antioxidant enzymes, absence of which may certainly disturb the activity of their enzymatic scavenging activity [2].

It has been argued that agri-food residues generated by the use of plants and their derivatives might have a negative impact on the environment when they are discarded. In developed countries, 42% of food waste is produced by households, while 39% losses occur in the food manufacturing industry, 14% in food service sector and remaining 5% in retail and distribution [36]. Waste from parts of plants such as peel, leaves, stem, seed, and roots generated from agriculture, to industrial manufacturing and processing [2]. They constitute a low-cost source of antioxidant molecules, which exhibit other biological activities, like antidiabetic, anti-obesity, antihypertensive, anticancer, and antimicrobial [13, 37, 38].

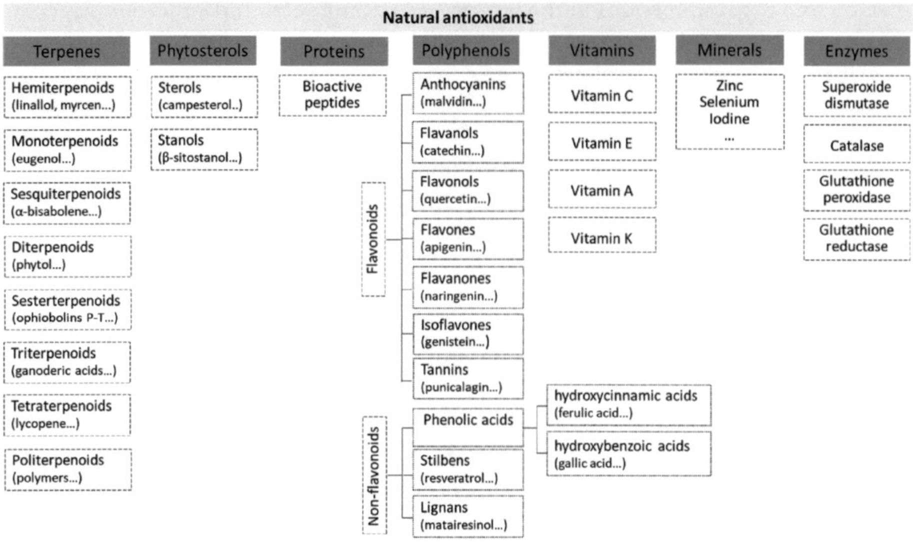

Figure 1.
Classification of natural antioxidants.

Marine biodiversity is another underexploited source of natural products. Marine resources are gaining the attention of industries such as foods, pharmaceuticals, nutraceuticals, and cosmetics because they have several interesting antioxidant molecules and other attractive biotechnological compounds (*e.g.* polysaccharides, pigments, proteins, *etc.*), making these resources a profound and renewable source to investigate novel molecules. Currently, more than 30000 structurally diverse secondary metabolites have been isolated from marine sources [39].

Algae are considered the richest source of active compounds with antioxidant activity (and other biological activities). They can be used as nutraceuticals, food additives and cosmetics. Algae are composed by a complex group of photosynthetic organisms with simple reproductive organs, which can be multicellular, known as macroalgae or seaweeds, and unicellular named as microalgae [40]. Algae produce various secondary metabolites with many antioxidant activities such as pigments (phycobiliproteins, chlorophylls and carotenoids), polyphenols (bromophenols, flavonoids, phlorotannins and phenolic acids), vitamins (β-carotene and other carotenoids), a complex of B vitamins (B1, B2, B3, B5, B6, B7 and B12), vitamin C (ascorbic acid), vitamin D and vitamin E (α-tocopherol) [40, 41]. Sulfated polysaccharides are nonanimal compounds reported to have antioxidant activities, which can be obtained from marine algae and other marine organisms from the phaeophyta group [42]. These compounds may be used as hydrocolloids and as nutraceuticals in the food industry.

Iodine (an important mineral from seaweeds), is a key element for hormones related with the thyroid, helping in the metabolism regulation [43].

Marine sponges (family Aplysinellidae) are recognized as producers of bromotyrosine derivatives, displaying a myriad of biological and pharmacological potentialities [39]. Many biological compounds previously isolated from some other marine organisms such as fish, crustaceans, and their by-products present bioactive potential.

For the past few decades, researchers and industry have been focusing their work on the use of by-products or biowastes to obtain products with high added value, using innovative and environmentally friendly processes. These products can be used as (bio)functional additives, or as a therapeutic alternative in the prevention or treatment of cardiometabolic, cancer and neurodegenerative diseases [40, 42, 44, 45].

Sources	Compounds	Technologies (Solvents)	Bioactivities	References
Plants and by-products				
Passion fruit peel	Carotenoids Pectin	MAE,UAE (water, Olive oil sun flower oil)	Antioxidant Antimicrobial Anticancer	[46, 47]
Vine pruning	Polyphenols	OH, MAE, (water, ethanol)	Antioxidant Anticancer	[48, 49]
Grape skins	Anthocyanins Polyphenols	OH, MAE, UAE, EAE, PLE (water, eutectic solvents)	Antioxidant	[50–55]
Colored potato	Anthocyanins	OH (water)	Antioxidant Antimicrobial Anticancer Neuroprotective	[15]
Pine bark	Polyphenols	OH, MAE, UAE, SFE (CO_2, water, ethanol)	Antioxidant Anticancer Antimicrobial Antihyperglycemic	[13, 56–58]
Pine nuts	Polyphenols	PLE, UAE, MAE (water)	Antioxidant	[59]
Soy beans	Proteins Isoflavones	EAE, UAE, PLE (eutectic solvents, ionic liquid, water, methanol)	Antioxidant Cardioprotective Anticancer	[60–63]
Mentha	Polyphenols Essential oil	UAE, SFE, MAE, OH (water, ethanol, methanol)	Antioxidant	[64–66]
Tomato by products	Polyphenols Pectin Fatty acids Carotenoids	MAE, HHP, UAE, PEF, SFE, EAE (hexane, methanol, acetone, ethyl lactate)	Antioxidant Cardioprotective Antihypertensive Antidiabetic Anticancer	[67–71]
Apple peels	Pectin Polyphenols	UAE, SFE (water)	Antioxidant	[72, 73]
Apple seeds	Essential oils polyphenols	PFE, UAE, SFE (CO_2, water)	Antioxidant	[74–76]
Brewer's spent grains	Polyphenols, proteins	PEF, UAE, SFE (water, ethanol)	Antioxidant	[77–79]
Orange peel	Pectin Polyphenols	PEF, MAE (citric acid)	Antioxidant	[37, 80]
Moringa leaves	Polyphenols Vitamin C	PLE (water)	Antioxidant	[81]
Rapeseed oil Guava oil,	Phytosterols, Polyphenols Tocopherols	SFE (CO_2, Euctetic solvents)	Anticholesterolemic Antioxidant	[82, 83]
Roselle seeds Black sesame seeds	Phytosterols	SFE (CO_2, ethanol)	Anticholesterolemic Antioxidant	[84, 85]
Microalgae				
Spirulina platensis	Polyphenols Carotenoids Phycobiliproteins	OH; MAE; PEF; UAS; EAE (water, ethanol)	Antioxidant Antimicrobial Anticancer Anti-inflammatory	[86–95]
Heterochlorella luteoviridis	Carotenoids Lipids	OH; UAE (ethanol)	Antioxidant Anti-inflammatory	[96, 97]

Sources	Compounds	Technologies (Solvents)	Bioactivities	References
Chorella vulgaris	Carotenoids Polyphenols	PEF; SFE (CO_2, Water, water: ethanol)	Antioxidant Antimicrobial Anticancer Anti-inflammatory	[98–101]
Nannochloropsis spp	Carotenoids Chlorophylls Polyphenols Proteins Lipids	UAE; PEF; PLE (water, ethanol, dimethyl sulfoxide)	Antioxidant UV-protective Anti-inflammatory Anticancer	[102–104]
Phaeodactylum tricornutum	Proteins Pigments Lipids Carotenoids Chlorophylls Polyphenols	HVED; HHP; PLE, MAE (water, ethanol, chloroform: methanol)	Antioxidant	[17, 105]
Neochloris oleoabundans	Carotenoids	PLE (ethanol)	Antioxidant	[106]
Macroalgae				
Gracilaria	Sulfated polysaccharides	Maceration by liquid nitrogen (sodium acetate buffer)	Antioxidant	[42]
Laminaria ochroleuca	Fatty acids Polyphenols	PLE (hexane, ethyl acetate, ethanol and ethanol:water)	Antioxidant Anti-atherogenic	[107]
Ascophyllum nodosum *Laminaria japonica* *Lessonia trabeculate* *Lessonia nigrecens*	Polyphenols	MAE (70% methanol)	Antioxidant Anti-hyperglycemic	[108]
Fucus serratus *Laminaria digitata* *Gracilaria gracilis* *Codium fragile*	Polyphenols	PLE (water, ethanol/water, and methanol/water)	Antioxidant Antiproliferative	[40, 109]
Palmaria palmata	Proteins Peptides	EAE (water)	Antioxidant Cardioprotective Anti-inflammatory Anti-diabetic	[110, 111]
Gelidium pusillum	Phycobiliproteins	UAE (phosphate buffer)	Antioxidant Anticancer Anti-inflammatory	[112, 113]

MAE, Microwave assisted extraction; UAE, Ultrasound assisted extraction; PLE, Pressurized liquid extraction; SFE, Supercritical fluid extraction; HHP, High hydrostatic pressure; EAE, Enzyme assisted extraction; PEF, Pulsed electric field; HVED, High voltage electrical discharges; OH, Ohmic heating.

Table 2.
Green processes for antioxidants recovery from some plants, algae and by-products.

Table 2 shows some examples of bioactive molecules from natural sources (plants and their by-products and algae), as well as the type of technologies and solvents used in the extraction process.

Currently, phytochemicals are being used in several commercial applications, like nutraceuticals, food supplements, cosmetic products, food coloring agents, among others. As an example *Moringa Olifeira* extract is widely used in cosmetics or bath cosmetics [114]. Pycnogenol® is trade mark for the French pine bark extract, which is used as a food supplement with antioxidant properties [115]. Curcumin (Biocurcumax ®, BCM-95® CURCUGREEN®) is used as coloring agent for food and cosmetics, as well as a nutraceutical [116].

Multiple cosmetics companies use algae extracts and compounds in their formulations, as an active agent, or a moisturizer, excipient, gelling, thickening, dyes, pigments, preservatives, additives, aroma or fragrance agents. For example, *Gracilaria* species extracts are integrated into various commercial cosmetics, such as hydrogel soap from Sealaria® (Kfar Hess, Israel), facial mask by Balinique® (Miami, FL, USA), and hydrating cream by Thalasso® (Rosa Graf, Stamford, CT, USA). The *Chondrus crispus* extract enriched in sulphated polysaccharides, Gelcarin® (Dupont Nutrition and Biosciences, Wilmington, DEL, USA), to be used in various cosmetic products as gelling, thickener and stabilizer agent [43].

β-Carotene was the first high-value product commercially produced from a microalga *Dunaliella salina* with production starting in the 1980s by four producers—Koor Foods (Nature Beta Technology) in Israel, Western Biotechnology Ltd. and Betatene Ltd. in Australia, and Nutralite in the USA [117].

3.1 Enzymes

Antioxidant enzymes, such as superoxide dismutase (SOD), catalase (CAT), and glutathione peroxidase (GPx), are considered to be, the first line defense in the cells against reactive species like superoxide radical ($^{\cdot}O_2$). SOD, CAT and GPx are indispensable in the antioxidant defense of the body [118]. SOD is an endogenous enzyme and the most powerful antioxidant in the cell. As a metalloenzyme SOD requires a metal cofactor for its activity (iron,zinc or copper). It catalyzes the conversion of two molecules of $^{\cdot}O_2$ to hydrogen peroxide (H_2O_2). The level of superoxide dismutase decrease with the age. Moreover, the SOD deficiency was connected to a number of pathologies in both animals and humans. The daily intake of SOD supplement protect the immune system and slow down aging process. CAT is highly efficient antioxidant enzyme, located primarily in the peroxisomes but absent in mitochondria of mammalian cells. It catalyzes the reduction of H_2O_2 to water and molecular oxygen, completing the process initiated by SOD. In the mammalian mitochondria cells, where the catalase is absent, the breakdown of the hydrogen peroxide to water and oxygen is carried out by another enzyme the GPx. GPx is an intracellular enzyme, and its activity depends on the micronutrient cofactor selenium [118]. Cabbage, brussels sprouts, and broccoli are natural sources of these enzymes [118].

3.2 Proteins and peptides

The protein role in the antioxidant defense system is a result of their direct action as precursors of intracellular formation of glutathione [119]. The antioxidant potential of fruit and vegetable juices and grain products is comparable to the antioxidant potential of milk [119]. Plant proteins are considered the new source of antioxidant peptides [120]. Soy milk is soybean-derived product rich in bioactive peptides and isoflavones. It is one of the most popular milk-substitutes for individuals with lactose-intolerance [121]. Other known plant protein drinks substitutes of caw milk are rice milk and almond milk.

Bioactive peptides are present in many fermented and functional foods. The bioactive peptides usually have between 2 and 20 amino acids residues and exercise their activities only after being released from the main protein. Bioactive peptides can display different activities, e.g. antihypertensive, antioxidant, immunomodulatory, anti-inflammatory or antimicrobial, depending on the sequence and amino acid composition [122]. Agroindustrial by-products and wastes are being used as a source of bioactive peptides. Tomato seeds, containing 28% of protein, were subjected to fermentation to obtain different size of peptides [122]. Many times in fruit processing the main generated waste is the fruit stone. The alternatives for reutilization of these type of waste are few (as fertilizers or fuels). The cherry fruit stone contain high values of protein (up to 39%), and is considered a cheap source for production of bioactive peptides [123]. The obtained peptide fractions had high antioxidant or antihypertensive activities [123]. Phycobiliproteins are water soluble protein found in Rhodophyta (red algae), Cyanobacteria (*Spirulina*), and Cryptophyta (**Table 2**). These proteins are well known for their strong antioxidant and free-radical scavenging activities [124]. Phycobiliproteins are divided in three classes phycoerythrin, phycocyanin and allophycocyanin. These proteins constitute up to 60% of the total soluble cellular protein in microalgae [125]. Phycobiliproteins have high commercial value as natural colorants in the nutraceutical, cosmetic, and pharmaceutical industries [124].

Other wastes like, peel, leaves, stem, seeds and roots are generated during harvesting, post-harvesting or processing of plants. These wastes are low-cost source of antioxidant molecules like terpenes, polyphenols, phytosterols and peptides that can exhibit different biological activities including antidiabetic, anti-obesity, antihypertensive, anticancer, antiviral and antibacterial [126].

3.3 Terpenes

Terpenes also known as terpenoids or isoprenoids are antioxidant molecules formed by the condensation of two subunits of isoprene (C_5H_8). Moreover, the terpenes are classified on the basis of the number of isoprene units (**Figure 1**). Terpenes are the main constituents of essential oils (up to 90%) and are very diverse in structure and compounds. Carotenoids are a class of natural lipid-soluble pigments that are responsible for the red, yellow, and orange colors found in various plants and microorganisms. Carotenoids are tetraterpenes (C-40) classified in two groups xanthophylls (lutein, zeaxanthin, and β-cryptoxanthin) and carotenes (α-carotene, β-carotene, and lycopene). Carotenoids are beneficial for humans and animals demonstrating antioxidant, antidibetic, antihypertensive, anti-inflammatory and anticancer activities [33, 127–129].

3.4 Polyphenols

Polyphenol compounds are secondary metabolites produced in plants as a response to different stress conditions. Nowadays more than 8,000 polyphenols are known and more than a half correspond to the group of flavonoids. The main structure of the phenols is the benzene ring with different OH radicals. According to their chemical structure phenolic compounds can be divided in two major groups flavonoid and non-flavonoid. The non-flavonoid group includes the phenolic acids (hydroxybenzoic acids and hydroxycinnamic acids), stilbenes and lignans. The anthocyanins, flavanols, flavonols, flavones, flavanones, isoflavones and tannins are flavonoids [5].

Flavonoid consumption is associated with a reduced risk of coronary heart disease, stroke and cancer. Rich sources of polyphenol compounds in nature are fruits and vegetables, cereals, chocolate, olive oils and beverages such as tea and wine (**Table 2**). Polyphenols are known for their strong antioxidant properties [5].

The strength of their antioxidant activity depends on their interaction with other molecules. For example the absorption of polyphenols in human body is enchased when there is no sugar molecules attached with them. This means that tea polyphenol have higher absorption than fruit polyphenols because of the high sugar content. Normally from the total consumed amount of polyphenol only 15% -20% are absorbed in the human blood [2]. Moreover, studies demonstrated that the addition of milk to tea, a habit common in the United Kingdom, reduces the absorption of flavonols and diminish their antioxidant effect [130].

3.5 Vitamins

Vitamins obtained from fruit and vegetables also act as antioxidants. Examples are vitamin C and vitamin E. Vitamin C, that is ascorbic acid is powerful antioxidant found in citrus fruits and vegetables such as oranges, lemons, as well as tomatoes. Vitamin E is a fat-soluble vitamin found naturally in lipid-rich fruits and vegetables, such as olives, sun flower, and nuts [2].

3.6 Phytosterols

Phytosterols are natural bioactive compounds belonging to the group of triterpens. Humans must obtain phytosterols from plant-derived foods, such as nuts, seeds, cereals and legumes, vegetable oils, soybean oil, and sunflower oil (examples in **Table 2**) [126]. The most important and abundant phytosterols are β-sitosterol (carbon structure C-29), campesterol (C-28), and stigmasterol (C-29) [126, 131]. Phytosterols have chemical structures and functions similar to cholesterol, but differ from it by an extra methyl or ethyl group at C-24 or a double bond at the C-22 position [132]. Because of the similarity in the structure, phytosterols can reduce cholesterol absorption in the small intestine and thus decreasing blood cholesterol levels. Additional known bioactivities of the phytosterols are anticholesterolemic, antidiabetic, hepatoprotective, anticancer, antioxidant, antimicrobial and anti-inflammatory [131, 133].

4. Antioxidant actions of phytochemicals

4.1 *In vitro* evidence

Oxidation is a natural phenomenon of human cells. Several important biological processes need reactive oxygen species (ROS) like superoxide radicals, hydrogen peroxide, hydroxyl radicals and singlet oxygen [134, 135]. Without them, protein phosphorylation, activation of transcriptional factors, apoptosis or cell differentiation would not occur. The problem lays on the formation/degradation imbalance of ROS and/or reactive nitrogen species (RNS) [134, 135]. The cell has intrinsic mechanisms to protect itself from excess of ROS/RNS, but only to an extent. If the threshold levels are overcome, cellular structures can be damaged like protein [134–136], lipids [134, 135, 137], polysaccharides [134, 135, 138] and nucleic acids [134, 135, 139]. Several cell mechanisms of defense against oxidative stress have been described in the literature [140, 141]. These mechanisms can be divided into enzymatic and non-enzymatic. SOD, CAT, GPx, Thioredoxin (TRX), Peroxiredoxin (PRX), Glutathione transferase (GST) are endogenous enzymatic mechanisms, while All trans retinol 2 (Vitamin A), Ascorbic acid (Vitamin C) and α-Tocopherol (Vitamin E) are non-enzymatic endogenous antioxidant mechanism [141]. SOD catalyzes de dismutation of the superoxide anion free radical into molecular oxygen and hydrogen peroxide [141, 142] (Eqs. (1) and (2)). As described by Younus [142] this reaction is accompanied by an alternate oxidation–reduction of the metal ions present in the active site of SOD.

$$M^{(n+1)} - SOD + O_2^- \rightarrow M^{n+} - SOD + O_2 \quad (1)$$

$$M^{(n+)} - SOD + O_2^- + 2H^+ \rightarrow M^{(n+1)} - SOD + H_2O_2 \quad (2)$$

CAT can use iron or even manganese as a cofactor for its enzymatic reactions that will lead to the degradation or reduction of hydrogen peroxide to water molecules and oxygen. This enzyme competes the detoxification process that SOD initiated (Eqs. (3)-(5))[118, 143, 144].

$$2H_2O_2 \rightarrow O_2 + H_2O \quad (3)$$

$$H_2O_2 + Fe(III) - E \rightarrow H_2O + O = Fe(IV) - E(.+) \quad (4)$$

$$H_2O_2 + O = Fe(IV) - E(.+) \rightarrow H_2O + Fe(III) - E + O_2 \quad (5)$$

GTPx encompasses two independent reactions, the first one is the reduction of the enzyme by a hydroperoxide (Eq. (6)) followed by the oxidation to GSH [145].

$$2GSH + ROOH \rightarrow GSSG + 2ROH + H_2O \quad (6)$$

$$2GSH + H_2O_2 \rightarrow GSSG + 2H_2O \quad (7)$$

Trx system is composed by Trx and thioredoxin reductase and NADPH. It is described that Trx uses cysteines at position 32 and 35 for the enzymatic reaction. In the first reaction (Adenosine monophosphate + sulfite + thioredoxin disulphide = 5′-adenylyl+thioredoxin) [141, 146] the N-terminal cysteine of Trx acts on the disulphide bond of the substrate protein, leading to the formation a mixed disulphide bond between Trx and the substrate protein. Following the reaction to the C-terminal cysteine of Trx on the intermediate intermolecular disulphide bond, which will form in a disulphide bond in the oxidized Trx and the breakdown of the disulphide bond in the reduce substrate (Adenosine 3′,5′-bisphosphate + sulfite + thioredoxin disulphide = 3′-phosphoadenylyl sulphate+thioredoxin) [141, 146]. PRX are antioxidant enzyme with the ability to reduce hydroperoxides, organic hydroperoxides and peroxynitrite using Trx as electrons donor (Eq. 8) [141, 147].

$$2R`-SH + ROOH = R`-S-S-R` + H_2O + ROH \quad (8)$$

The presence of ROS initiates an autocatalytic chain lipid peroxidation of polyunsaturated acids, which leads to the formation of toxic electrophilic species and free radicals. This reaction may lead to the increase of 4-Hydroxynonenal (4HNE).

GST catalyze conjugation of lipid aldehydes like 4HNE, with GSH are the major defense against oxidative stress-induced cytotoxicity (Eq. (9)) [141, 148].

$$RX + GSH = HX + R - S - GSH \tag{9}$$

It is not clear if oxidative stress is the onset of degenerative diseases [149], but it is well known that it plays a significant role in their progression, like in the case of Alzheimer's disease or vascular dementia [150]. Oxidative stress is also involved in other diseases like cancer [151, 152], cardiovascular diseases [153], metabolic disorders [154], and even on aging [149, 155]. Therefore, it is necessary to lower the ROS/RNS concentration inside the cell to minimize the effect. Antioxidants can act by different chemical mechanism: hydrogen atom transfer (HAT), single electron transfer (SET) and the ability to chelate transition metals.

Most of the commercially available anti-inflammatory and antioxidant medication present side effects [156], therefore the interest in natural antioxidants has grown considerably for the past years, being the phytochemicals a group of interest.

The characterization of molecules with antioxidant potential is complex, due to the inherent complexity of the oxidative reactions that occurs in cells [156]. There are several methods to determine the antioxidant potential of a particular substrate. **Table 3** describes some of the chemical *in vitro* methods.

The chemical characterization of phytochemicals in terms of their antioxidant capacity is only the first step. It is necessary to perform a second screening using *ex vivo* models, like LDL-cholesterol assay [165, 166], supercoiled plasmid pBR322 DNA Model [166], Haemololysis inhibiton assay [167], 2′,7′-dichlorofluorescin diacetate (DCFH-DA) [168]

Several studies have been made regarding the antioxidative properties of phytochemicals, as an example Ferreira-Santos *et al.* [13] demonstrated that the presence of phytochemicals in *Pinus* bark has antioxidant properties. It has been shown that extracts of *Moringa oleifera* leaves significantly reduced the ROS production inducing by H_2O_2 in HEK-293 cells [169]. Dilworth *et al*. presented similar results, it was demonstrated that the presence of *Moring oleifera* extract results in a significant decrease of the ROS in HL60 cells after an oxidative insult [170]. Soybean peptide also demonstrated similar results, where HepG2 cells in the presence of this compound resulted in a significant decrease on ROS [171]. These are a few of the several studies that demonstrate the high potential of phytochemicals.

The third step is to evaluate these molecules *in vivo*. Pre-clinical tests using animal models and human clinical studies are required.

4.2 *In vivo* evidence

In the literature there are extensive studies regarding phytochemicals impact human health, particularly on the prevention of cardiovascular, metabolic, neurodegenerative and cancer diseases.

4.2.1 Cardiovascular and metabolic diseases

Cardiovascular diseases are associated with a multiple risk factors like hypercholesterolemia, hypertension, smoking, diabetes, poor diet, stress and physical inactivity. Usually, vegetables like spinach, citrus fruits, soybean oil, sprouts, peppers, cereals, spices, whole grain, honey, walnuts and black tea can significantly increase the hepatic antioxidant enzymes reduces the risk of cardiovascular diseases. Some

Method	Description	Determination	References
2,2-diphenyl-1-picrylhydrazyl (DPPH)	DPPH is a stable free radical that in contact with a substrate that can donate a hydrogen bond forms a non-radical molecule Diphenylpicrylhhydrazine. Scavenging activity mechanism.	Colorimetric	[1]
2,2`-azino-bis(3-ethylbenzothiazoline-6-sulphonic acid (ABTS)	In the presence of antioxidant $ABTS^{\cdot+}$ is reduce to ABTS resulting in a decrease in color. Scavenging activity mechanism.	Colorimetric	[157, 158]
$O_2^{\cdot-}$ scavenging activity	This assay is optimized for enzymatic antioxidants and relies on the competition kinetics of $O_2^{\cdot-}$ reduction of cytochrome C (probe) and $O_2^{\cdot-}$ scavenger (sample). Not suitable for non-enzymatic antioxidants. Scavenging activity mechanism.	Fluorescence	[1]
H_2O_2 scavenging activity	A common assay that claims to measure H_2O_2 scavenging capacity of dietary antioxidants uses horseradish peroxidase to oxidize scopoletin to a nonfluorescent product. In the presence of antioxidants the oxidation is inhibited. Scavenging activity mechanism.	Fluorescence	[1]
Ferric ion reducing antioxidant power (FRAP)	It is based on the ability of antioxidants to reduce ferric iron. The molecule 2,3,5-triphenyl-1,3,4-triaza-2-azoniacyclopenta-1,4-diene chloride (TPTZ) is reduce to the ferrous form at a low pH. This reduction will result in a color change. Reducing power mechanism.	Colorimetric	[158, 159]
Cupric ion reducing antioxidant capacity (CUPRAC)	bis(neocuproine)copper(II) chloride (Cu(II)-Nc) chromogenic oxidizing agent can react with a polyphenol. The reactive Ar-OH from the polyphenol are oxidized to quinones and Cu (II)-Nc reduced to a highly colored Cu (I)-Nc chelate.	Colorimetric	[158, 160]
Oxygen radical absorbance capacity (ORAC)	Assay is based on the oxidation of a fluorescent probe by peroxyl radicals by way of a hydrogen atom transfer (HAT) process. Peroxyl radicals are produced by a free radical initiator, which quenches the fluorescent probe over time. Antioxidants present in the assay work to block the peroxyl radical oxidation of the fluorescent probe until the antioxidant activity in the sample is depleted. The remaining peroxyl radicals destroy the fluorescence of the fluorescent probe.	Fluorescence	[161, 162]

Method	Description	Determination	References
Total radical-trapping antioxidant potential (TRAP)	It is based on the measurement of the fluorescence decay of R-phytocoerythrin during an oxidation reaction. Antioxidant activity mechanism.	Chemiluminescence quenching	[163, 164]
Thiobarbituric reactive substances (TBARS)	Lipid peroxidation inhibition.	Colorimetric Fluorescence	[1]

Table 3.
In vitro *assays to evaluate natural substrates antioxidant potential.*

specific fruits, vegetables or legumes can prevent cardiovascular disease induced by oxidative stress, due to presence of unique dietary antioxidant components [34].

Already in 1999, a study comprising approximately 100 000 patients in the US evaluated over a period of 7 years the outcome of flavonoid intake. The results demonstrated that flavonoid consumption was associated with lower risk of death with cardiovascular disease [172]. Patel *et al.* described that cohort studies clearly indicate that the consuption of plant-based foods decrease the prevalence of cardiovascular diseases [173]. Zhang *et al.* examinated the relation between soy food intake and the incidence of coronary heart disease in a cohort study of 75 000 and concluded that there is a clear evidence of soy food intake and reduce risk of coronary heart disease [174].

Hypertension is characterized by high blood pressure leading to cardiac and vascular problems. A study performed in hypertensive rats demonstrated that the intake of *Moringa oleifera* seed powder did not reduce blood pressure, but decreased nocturnal heart rate and improved cardiac diastolic function [175]. Another study, lycopene diet ameliorates metabolic syndrome, lowering blood pressure, maintains normal blood glucose and prevents insulin resistance, ameliorates hypertension, vascular function and improves oxidative stress [33].

Diabetes mellitus, a chronic metabolic disease, characterized by elevated levels of blood glucose and insufficiency in production and action of insulin is the seventh leading cause of death worldwide. Phytochemicals with antioxidant activity like cinnamic acids, coumarins, diterpenes, flavonoids, lignans, prophenylphenols, monoterpenes, tannins, triterpenes, *etc.* also proved beneficial to protect diabetes or protect diabetic complications [176].

4.2.2 Cancer

Similarly to cardiovascular diseases, the number of reports regarding the benefices of phytochemicals and cancer prevention and treatment are immense. Briefly, it has been reported that curcumin, a polyphenol compound that has anticancer properties, acting on cell cycle regulation, apoptosis, oncogene expression and metastasis [177]. The intake of green tea seem to help in the treatment of patients with low grade B-cell tumors [178, 179]. Another phytochemical that demonstrated positive results is *Panax ginseng (*responsible chemical groups, steroid glycosides and triterpene saponins*)*. Clinical trials demonstrated that *P. ginseng* decreases cancer incidence and inflammation, particularly that ginseng tea decreases the risk of pharynx, larynx, esophagus cancer among others [180]. Some of the reported flavonoids (*e.g.,* catechin, apigenin, kaempferol, quercetin, *etc*) are able to influence the deregulated processes during cancer development. Thus, flavonoids have beneficial effects on health and have the potential for the development of possible chemoprotective therapeutic agents for the treatment of cancer. Some dietary flavonoids have antitumor activity during *in vivo* studies and also repress angiogenesis. *In vitro* studies conclude the potential of flavonoid-induced modulation of kinases with apoptosis, vascularization, cell differentiation, cell proliferation, *etc* [181]. For example, flavonoids have shown a potential effect in breast cancer as potent inhibitors of aromatase, *i.e.,* cytochrome P450 enzyme complex. Quercetin has shown decreased cell proliferation in prostate cancer and cell apoptosis by downregulation of heat-shock protein 90 (HSP90) [182].

4.2.3 Neurodegenerative diseases

Neurodegenerative diseases are highly debilitating diseases associated to oxidative stress and inflammatory processes. Several studies have been performed to validate the benefices of phytochemicals on the several neurodegenerative diseases, like Alzheimer's, Parkinson's and multiple sclerosis. Flavonoids have a specific role in central nervous system maintaining homeostasis by effecting as antianxiety, anticonvulsant, by modulating neuronal oxidative metabolism, and neurotransmitters [183]. Epigallocatechin-3-galate, a polyphenol present in the tea leaves seems to delay neurons degeneration [184]. A commercial drug which has in its composition Epigallocatechin-3-galate demonstrated to reduce amyloid plaques on an Alzheimer disease model [185, 186]. Another study demonstrated that epigallocatechin-3-galate and tea prevented the loss of cells in substantia nigra in a Parkinson Disease model [187]. In a neuronal cell culture model SH-SY5Y cells, the presence of epigallocatechin-3-galate has a protective effect [187].

In vitro studies for Parkinson's, quercetin markedly reduced the apoptosis of pheochromocytoma (PC-12) cells and hippocampal neurons. It showed increased cell viability and inhibited ROS and MDA production in H2O2-induced toxicity in PC-12 cells [183].

Once again curcumin demonstrates to have a positive effect in Alzheimer's disease, as it can bind to amyloid plaques by inhibiting NF-κβ [188]. A different study demonstrated that ethanolic turmeric extract (*Curcuma longa* L.) prevented oxidative stress by decreasing the plasma and brain MDA levels and increasing the SOD, CAT, and GPx enzyme activities as well as GSH levels in the brain, showing neuroprotective effects [189].

Yang *et al.* [190] reported the neuroprotective effects of *Ginkgo biloba* extract (rich in flavonol glycosides and terpene trilactones) by preventive action on neuronal cell death and enhancement of the function of brain capillary endothelial monolayers.

As an example of a carotenoid action, astaxanthin has potent antioxidant, anti-inflammatory and neuroprotective properties. Wu and coworkers [191] suggested that astaxanthin could alleviate brain aging, which may be due to attenuating oxidative stress, ameliorating hippocampus damage and increasing brain derived neurotrophic factor levels, preventing age-related neurodegenerative diseases.

5. Conclusions and future perspectives

The use of green methodologies and extraction process optimization to obtain highly value molecules with antioxidant properties, like terpenes, polyphenolic, phytosterols, and bioactive peptides, has increased for the past years. The reduction of the environmental footprint and the ability to obtain safe products with high industrial interest is fundamental for the future.

Upon extraction and purification of the added value compounds it is possible to determine their antioxidant potential by several chemical and biological processes.

Plants, algae and by-products or waste products of the food industry are an invaluable source of active molecules with antioxidant properties. It is of upmost interest the discovery/development of new therapeutical molecules for the application in several diseases. Computer-aided drug screening techniques, animal models and clinical trials should be taken into account to further develop this field of research.

There are several natural bioactive compounds already used for the treatment of different diseases (in combination with the conventional drugs), demonstrating good results.

Overall, natural antioxidant obtained from plants and marine resources have high nutritional potential and reveal a fundamental role in promoting human health, as an alternative to synthetic products.

Acknowledgements

This chapter was funded by the Portuguese Foundation for Science and Technology (FCT) under the scope of the strategic funding of UIDB/04469/2020 unit and BioTecNorte operation (NORTE-01-0145-FEDER-000004) funded by the European Regional Development Fund under the scope of Norte2020 - Programa Operacional Regional do Norte. The chapter was also supported by the European Union's Horizon 2020 research and innovation programme under the Marie Skłodowska-Curie grant (MSCA-RISE; FODIAC; 778388). Pedro Santos is supported by a doctoral advanced training fellowship (call NORTE-69-2015-2015), funded under the scope of Norte2020 (NORTE-08-5369-FSE-000036).

Conflict of interest

The authors declare no conflict of interest.

Author details

Pedro Ferreira-Santos*, Zlatina Genisheva, Claudia Botelho, Cristina Rocha and José António Teixeira
CEB - Centre of Biological Engineering, University of Minho, Braga, Portugal

*Address all correspondence to: pedrosantos@ceb.uminho.pt

References

[1] Carocho M, Ferreira ICFR. A review on antioxidants, prooxidants and related controversy: Natural and synthetic compounds, screening and analysis methodologies and future perspectives. Food Chem Toxicol. 2013;51:15-25. Available from: http://dx.doi.org/10.1016/j.fct.2012.09.021

[2] Anwar H, Hussain G, Mustafa I. Antioxidants from Natural Sources. In: Shalaby E, Azzam G, editors. Antioxidants in Foods and Its Applications. London: InTechOpen; 2018. Available from: http://dx.doi.org/10.5772/intechopen.75961

[3] Xu DP, Li Y, Meng X, Zhou T, Zhou Y, Zheng J, et al. Natural antioxidants in foods and medicinal plants: Extraction, assessment and resources. Int J Mol Sci. 2017 Jan 5;18(1):96. Available from: http://dx.doi.org/10.3390/ijms18010096

[4] Zhang YJ, Gan RY, Li S, Zhou Y, Li AN, Xu DP, et al. Antioxidant phytochemicals for the prevention and treatment of chronic diseases. Molecules. 2015. 20(12): 21138-21156. Available from: http://dx.doi.org/10.3390/molecules201219753

[5] Ferreira-Santos P, Zanuso E, Genisheva Z, Rocha CMR, Teixeira JA. Green and Sustainable Valorization of Bioactive Phenolic Compounds from Pinus By-Products. Molecules. 2020;25(12):2931. Available from: https://doi.org/10.3390/molecules25122931

[6] Torres-Valenzuela LS, Ballesteros-Gómez A, Rubio S. Green Solvents for the Extraction of High Added-Value Compounds from Agri-food Waste. Food Eng Rev. 2019;12:83-100. Available from: https://doi.org/10.1007/s12393-019-09206-y

[7] Wen L, Zhang Z, Sun D-W, Sivagnanam SP, Tiwari BK. Combination of emerging technologies for the extraction of bioactive compounds. Crit Rev Food Sci Nutr. 2020 Jun 16;60(11):1826-1841. Available from: https://doi.org/10.1080/10408398.2019.1602823

[8] Chemat F, Abert-Vian M, Fabiano-Tixier AS, Strube J, Uhlenbrock L, Gunjevic V, et al. Green extraction of natural products. Origins, current status, and future challenges. TrAC Trends Anal Chem. 2019;118:248-263. Available from: https://doi.org/10.1016/j.trac.2019.05.037

[9] Rocha CMR, Genisheva Z, Ferreira-Santos P, Rodrigues R, Vicente AA, Teixeira JA, et al. Electric field-based technologies for valorization of bioresources. Bioresour Technol. 2018 Apr 1;254:325-339. Available from: https://doi.org/10.1016/j.biortech.2018.01.068

[10] Chemat F, Rombaut N, Meullemiestre A, Turk M, Périno S, Fabiano-Tixier A-S, et al. Review of Green Food Processing techniques. Preservation, transformation, and extraction. Innov Food Sci Emerg Technol. 2017;41:357-377. Available from: https://doi.org/10.1016/j.ifset.2017.04.016

[11] Soquetta MB, Terra L de M, Bastos CP. Green technologies for the extraction of bioactive compounds in fruits and vegetables. CYTA - J Food. 2018;16(1):400-12. Available from: https://doi.org/10.1080/19476337.2017.1411978

[12] Cvjetko Bubalo M, Vidović S, Radojčić Redovniković I, Jokić S. New perspective in extraction of plant biologically active compounds by green solvents. Food Bioprod Process. 2018 May 1;109:52-73. Available from: https://doi.org/10.1016/j.fbp.2018.03.001

[13] Ferreira-Santos P, Genisheva Z, Botelho C, Santos J, Ramos C, Teixeira JA, et al. Unravelling the Biological Potential of *Pinus pinaster* Bark Extracts. Antioxidants. 2020 Apr 20;9(4):334. Available from: https://doi.org/10.3390/antiox9040334

[14] Barba FJ, Grimi N, Vorobiev E. Evaluating the potential of cell disruption technologies for green selective extraction of antioxidant compounds from Stevia rebaudiana Bertoni leaves. J Food Eng. 2015;149:222-228. Available from: https://doi.org/10.1016/j.jfoodeng.2014.10.028

[15] Pereira RN, Rodrigues RM, Genisheva Z, Oliveira H, de Freitas V, Teixeira JA, et al. Effects of ohmic heating on extraction of food-grade phytochemicals from colored potato. LWT - Food Sci Technol. 2016;74:493-503. Available from: https://doi.org/10.1016/j.lwt.2016.07.074

[16] Andreou V, Dimopoulos G, Dermesonlouoglou E, Taoukis P. Application of pulsed electric fields to improve product yield and waste valorization in industrial tomato processing. J Food Eng. 2020 Apr 1;270:109778. Available from: https://doi.org/10.1016/j.jfoodeng.2019.109778

[17] Zhang R, Lebovka N, Marchal L, Vorobiev E, Grimi N. Multistage aqueous and non-aqueous extraction of bio-molecules from microalga Phaeodactylum tricornutum. Innov Food Sci Emerg Technol. 2020 Jun;62:102367. Available from: https://doi.org/10.1016/j.ifset.2020.102367

[18] Goula AM, Ververi M, Adamopoulou A, Kaderides K. Green ultrasound-assisted extraction of carotenoids from pomegranate wastes using vegetable oils. Ultrason Sonochem. 2017;34:821-830. Available from: http://dx.doi.org/10.1016/j.ultsonch.2016.07.022

[19] Carbonell-Capella JM, Šic Žlabur J, Rimac Brnčić S, Barba FJ, Grimi N, Koubaa M, et al. Electrotechnologies, microwaves, and ultrasounds combined with binary mixtures of ethanol and water to extract steviol glycosides and antioxidant compounds from *Stevia rebaudiana* leaves. J Food Process Preserv. 2017 Oct 1;41(5):e13179. Available from: http://doi.wiley.com/10.1111/jfpp.13179

[20] Okolie CL, Akanbi TO, Mason B, Udenigwe CC, Aryee ANA. Influence of conventional and recent extraction technologies on physicochemical properties of bioactive macromolecules from natural sources: A review. Food Res Int. 2019;116:827-839. Available from: https://doi.org/10.1016/j.foodres.2018.09.018

[21] Vinatoru M, Mason TJ, Calinescu I. Ultrasonically assisted extraction (UAE) and microwave assisted extraction (MAE) of functional compounds from plant materials. TrAC Trends Anal Chem. 2017;97:159-178. Available from: https://doi.org/10.1016/j.trac.2017.09.002

[22] Barba FJ, Zhu Z, Koubaa M, Sant'Ana AS, Orlien V. Green alternative methods for the extraction of antioxidant bioactive compounds from winery wastes and by-products: A review. Trends Food Sci Technol. 2016;49:96-109. Available from: http://dx.doi.org/10.1016/j.tifs.2016.01.006

[23] Bonifácio-Lopes T, Teixeira JA, Pintado M. Current extraction techniques towards bioactive compounds from brewer's spent grain–A review. Crit Rev Food Sci Nutr. 2020;60(16):2730-2741. Available from: https://pubmed.ncbi.nlm.nih.gov/31433199/

[24] Wrona O, Rafińska K, Mozenski C, Byszewski B. Supercritical fluid extraction of bioactive compounds from plant materials. J AOAC Int.

2017;100(6):1624-1635. Available from: http://dx.doi.org/10.5740/jaoacint.17-0232

[25] Andrés V, Mateo-Vivaracho L, Guillamón E, Villanueva MJ, Tenorio MD. High hydrostatic pressure treatment and storage of soy-smoothies: Colour, bioactive compounds and antioxidant capacity. LWT. 2016;69:123-130. Available from: https://doi.org/10.1016/j.lwt.2016.01.033

[26] Moreira SA, Silva S, Costa EM, Saraiva JA, Pintado M. Effect of high hydrostatic pressure extraction on biological activities of stinging nettle extracts. Food Funct. 2020;11(1):921-31. Available from: https://doi.org/10.1039/C9FO02442E

[27] Scepankova H, Martins M, Estevinho L, Delgadillo I, Saraiva JA. Enhancement of Bioactivity of Natural Extracts by Non-Thermal High Hydrostatic Pressure Extraction. 2018;73:253-67. Available from: https://doi.org/10.1007/s11130-018-0687-9

[28] Khan SA, Aslam R, Makroo HA. High pressure extraction and its application in the extraction of bio-active compounds: A review. J Food Process Eng. 2019;42(1):e12896. Available from: http://doi.wiley.com/10.1111/jfpe.12896

[29] Azmi AA bin, Sankaran R, Show PL, Ling TC, Tao Y, Munawaroh HSH, et al. Current application of electrical pre-treatment for enhanced microalgal biomolecules extraction. Vol. 302, Bioresource Technology. Elsevier Ltd; 2020. p. 122874.

[30] Puértolas E, Barba FJ. Electrotechnologies applied to valorization of by-products from food industry: Main findings, energy and economic cost of their industrialization. Food Bioprod Process. 2016;100:172-184. Available from: https://doi.org/10.1016/j.fbp.2016.06.020

[31] Li Z, Fan Y, Xi J. Recent advances in high voltage electric discharge extraction of bioactive ingredients from plant materials. Food Chem. 2019;277:246-260. Available from: https://doi.org/10.1016/j.foodchem.2018.10.119

[32] Sastry S. Ohmic heating and moderate electric field processing. Food Sci Technol Int. 2008;14(5):419-422. Available from: https://doi.org/10.1177/1082013208098813

[33] Ferreira-Santos P, Aparicio R, Carrón R, Montero MJ, Sevilla MÁ. Lycopene-supplemented diet ameliorates metabolic syndrome induced by fructose in rats. J Funct Foods. 2020;73:104098. Available from: https://doi.org/10.1016/j.jff.2020.104098

[34] Septembre-Malaterre A, Remize F, Poucheret P. Fruits and vegetables, as a source of nutritional compounds and phytochemicals: Changes in bioactive compounds during lactic fermentation. Food Res Int. 2018;104:86-99. Available from: https://doi.org/10.1016/j.foodres.2017.09.031

[35] Fidelis M, De Moura C, Kabbas T, Pap N, Mattila P, Mäkinen S, et al. Fruit seeds as sources of bioactive compounds: Sustainable production of high value-added ingredients from by-products within circular economy. Molecules. 2019;24(21):1-67. Available from: https://doi.org/10.3390/molecules24213854

[36] Mirabella N, Castellani V, Sala S. Current options for the valorization of food manufacturing waste: A review. J Clean Prod. 2014;65:28-41. Available from: https://doi.org/10.1016/j.jclepro.2013.10.051

[37] Luengo E, Álvarez I, Raso J. Improving the pressing extraction of polyphenols of orange peel by pulsed electric fields. Innov Food Sci Emerg Technol. 2013;17:79-84. Available

from: https://doi.org/10.1016/j.ifset.2012.10.005

[38] Fierascu RC, Fierascu I, Avramescu SM, Sieniawska E. Recovery of Natural Antioxidants from Agro-Industrial Side Streams through Advanced Extraction Techniques. Molecules. 2019;24(23). Available from: https://doi.org/10.3390/molecules24234212

[39] El-Demerdash A, Atanasov AG, Horbanczuk OK, Tammam MA, Abdel-Mogib M, Hooper JNA, et al. Chemical diversity and biological activities of marine sponges of the genus Suberea: A systematic review. Mar Drugs. 2019;17(2):115. Available from: https://doi.org/10.3390/md17020115

[40] Jimenez-Lopez C, Pereira AG, Lourenço-Lopes C, Garcia-Oliveira P, Cassani L, Fraga-Corral M, et al. Main bioactive phenolic compounds in marine algae and their mechanisms of action supporting potential health benefits. Food Chem. 2021;341:128262. Available from: https://doi.org/10.1016/j.foodchem.2020.128262

[41] Geada P, Rodrigues R, Loureiro L, Pereira R, Fernandes B, Teixeira JA, et al. Electrotechnologies applied to microalgal biotechnology – Applications, techniques and future trends. Renew Sustain Energy Rev. 2018;94:656-668. Available from: https://doi.org/10.1016/j.rser.2018.06.059

[42] Alencar POC, Lima GC, Barros FCN, Costa LEC, Ribeiro CVPE, Sousa WM, et al. A novel antioxidant sulfated polysaccharide from the algae Gracilaria caudata: In vitro and in vivo activities. Food Hydrocoll. 2019;90:28-34. Available from: https://doi.org/10.1016/j.foodhyd.2018.12.007

[43] Morais T, Cotas J, Pacheco D, Pereira L. Seaweeds Compounds: An Ecosustainable Source of Cosmetic Ingredients? Cosmet. 2021 Jan 15;8(1):8. Available from: https://doi.org/10.3390/cosmetics8010008

[44] Nagar S, Sharma N, Kumar S. C-Phycocyanin Extraction and Purification from Spirulina Platensis. 2018;8(2):60-3. Available from: https://doi.org/10.1007/s40502-014-0094-7

[45] Gontijo DC, Gontijo PC, Brandão GC, Diaz MAN, de Oliveira AB, Fietto LG, et al. Antioxidant study indicative of antibacterial and antimutagenic activities of an ellagitannin-rich aqueous extract from the leaves of Miconia latecrenata. J Ethnopharmacol. 2019;236:114-123. Available from: https://doi.org/10.1016/j.jep.2019.03.007

[46] Chutia H, Mahanta CL. Green ultrasound and microwave extraction of carotenoids from passion fruit peel using vegetable oils as a solvent: Optimization, comparison, kinetics, and thermodynamic studies. Innov Food Sci Emerg Technol. 2020;102547 (In Press). Available from: https://doi.org/10.1016/j.ifset.2020.102547

[47] Thu Dao TA, Webb HK, Malherbe F. Optimization of pectin extraction from fruit peels by response surface method: Conventional versus microwave-assisted heating. Food Hydrocoll. 2021;113:106475. Available from: https://doi.org/10.1016/j.foodhyd.2020.106475

[48] Jesus MS, Ballesteros LF, Pereira RN, Genisheva Z, Carvalho AC, Pereira-Wilson C, et al. Ohmic heating polyphenolic extracts from vine pruning residue with enhanced biological activity. Food Chem. 2020;316:126298. Available from: https://doi.org/10.1016/j.foodchem.2020.126298

[49] Jesus MS, Genisheva Z, Romaní A, Pereira RN, Teixeira JA, Domingues L. Bioactive compounds recovery optimization from vine pruning residues using conventional

heating and microwave-assisted extraction methods. Ind Crops Prod. 2019;132:99-110. Available from: https://doi.org/10.1016/j.indcrop.2019.01.070

[50] Pereira RN, Coelho MI, Genisheva Z, Fernandes JM, Vicente AA, Pintado ME, et al. Using Ohmic Heating effect on grape skins as a pretreatment for anthocyanins extraction. Food Bioprod Process. 2020;124. Available from: https://doi.org/10.1016/j.fbp.2020.09.009

[51] Kwiatkowski M, Kravchuk O, Skouroumounis GK, Taylor DK. Microwave-assisted and conventional phenolic and colour extraction from grape skins of commercial white and red cultivars at veraison and harvest. J Clean Prod. 2020;275:122671. Available from: https://doi.org/10.1016/j.jclepro.2020.122671

[52] Natolino A, Da Porto C. Kinetic models for conventional and ultrasound assistant extraction of polyphenols from defatted fresh and distilled grape marc and its main components skins and seeds. Chem Eng Res Des. 2020;156:1-12. Available from: https://doi.org/10.1016/j.cherd.2020.01.009

[53] Cvjetko Bubalo M, Ćurko N, Tomašević M, Kovačević Ganić K, Radojcic Redovnikovic I. Green extraction of grape skin phenolics by using deep eutectic solvents. Food Chem. 2016;200:159-166. Available from: https://doi.org/10.1016/j.foodchem.2016.01.040

[54] Fernández K, Vega M, Aspé E. An enzymatic extraction of proanthocyanidins from País grape seeds and skins. Food Chem. 2015;168: 7-13. Available from: https://doi.org/10.1016/j.foodchem.2014.07.021

[55] Stavikova L, Polovka M, Hohnová B, Karásek P, Roth M. Antioxidant activity of grape skin aqueous extracts from pressurized hot water extraction combined with electron paramagnetic resonance spectroscopy. Talanta. 2011;85(4):2233-2240. Available from: https://doi.org/10.1016/j.talanta.2011.07.079

[56] Ferreira-Santos P, Genisheva Z, Pereira RN, Teixeira JA, Rocha CMR. Moderate Electric Fields as a Potential Tool for Sustainable Recovery of Phenolic Compounds from Pinus pinaster Bark. ACS Sustain Chem Eng. 2019;7(9):8816-8826. Available from: https://doi.org/10.1021/acssuschemeng.9b00780

[57] Mellouk H, Meullemiestre A, Maache-Rezzoug Z, Bejjani B, Dani A, Rezzoug SA. Valorization of industrial wastes from French maritime pine bark by solvent free microwave extraction of volatiles. J Clean Prod. 2016;112:4398-4405. Available from: https://doi.org/10.1016/j.jclepro.2015.06.129

[58] Seabra IJ, Dias AMA, Braga MEM, de Sousa HC. High pressure solvent extraction of maritime pine bark: Study of fractionation, solvent flow rate and solvent composition. J Supercrit Fluids. 2012;62:135-148. Available from: https://doi.org/10.1016/j.supflu.2011.10.016

[59] Liazid A, Schwarz M, Varela RM, Palma M, Guillén DA, Brigui J, et al. Evaluation of various extraction techniques for obtaining bioactive extracts from pine seeds. Food Bioprod Process. 2010;88(2-3):247-252. Available from: https://doi.org/10.1016/j.fbp.2009.11.004

[60] Perović MN, Knežević Jugović ZD, Antov MG. Improved recovery of protein from soy grit by enzyme-assisted alkaline extraction. J Food Eng. 2020;276:109894. Available from: https://doi.org/10.1016/j.jfoodeng.2019.109894

[61] Bajkacz S, Adamek J. Evaluation of new natural deep eutectic solvents for

the extraction of isoflavones from soy products. Talanta. 2017;168:329-335. Available from: https://doi.org/10.1016/j.talanta.2017.02.065

[62] Magiera S, Sobik A. Ionic liquid-based ultrasound-assisted extraction coupled with liquid chromatography to determine isoflavones in soy foods. J Food Compos Anal. 2017;57:94-101. Available from: https://doi.org/10.1016/j.jfca.2016.12.016

[63] Lu W, Chen XW, Wang JM, Yang XQ, Qi JR. Enzyme-assisted subcritical water extraction and characterization of soy protein from heat-denatured meal. J Food Eng. 2016;169:250-258. Available from: https://doi.org/10.1016/j.jfoodeng.2015.09.006

[64] Patonay K, Szalontai H, Csugány J, Szabó-Hudák O, Kónya EP, Németh ÉZ. Comparison of extraction methods for the assessment of total polyphenol content and in vitro antioxidant capacity of horsemint (Mentha longifolia (L.) L.). J Appl Res Med Aromat Plants. 2019;15:100220. Available from: https://doi.org/10.1016/j.jarmap.2019.100220

[65] Shahsavarpour M, Lashkarbolooki M, Eftekhari MJ, Esmaeilzadeh F. Extraction of essential oils from Mentha spicata L. (Labiatae) via optimized supercritical carbon dioxide process. J Supercrit Fluids. 2017;130:253-260. Available from: https://doi.org/10.1016/j.supflu.2017.02.004

[66] Gavahian M, Farahnaky A, Farhoosh R, Javidnia K, Shahidi F. Extraction of essential oils from Mentha piperita using advanced techniques: Microwave versus ohmic assisted hydrodistillation. Food Bioprod Process. 2015;94:50-58. Available from: https://doi.org/10.1016/j.supflu.2017.02.004

[67] Baltacıoğlu H, Baltacıoğlu C, Okur I, Tanrıvermiş A, Yalıç M. Optimization of microwave-assisted extraction of phenolic compounds from tomato: Characterization by FTIR and HPLC and comparison with conventional solvent extraction. Vib Spectrosc. 2021;113. Available from: https://doi.org/10.1016/j.vibspec.2020.103204

[68] Ninčević Grassino A, Ostojić J, Miletić V, Djaković S, Bosiljkov T, Zorić Z, et al. Application of high hydrostatic pressure and ultrasound-assisted extractions as a novel approach for pectin and polyphenols recovery from tomato peel waste. Innov Food Sci Emerg Technol. 2020;64. Available from: https://doi.org/10.1016/j.ifset.2020.102424

[69] Pataro G, Carullo D, Falcone M, Ferrari G. Recovery of lycopene from industrially derived tomato processing by-products by pulsed electric fields-assisted extraction. Innov Food Sci Emerg Technol. 2020;63:102369. Available from: https://doi.org/10.1016/j.ifset.2020.102369

[70] Squillace P, Adani F, Scaglia B. Supercritical CO2 extraction of tomato pomace: Evaluation of the solubility of lycopene in tomato oil as limiting factor of the process performance. Food Chem. 2020;315:126224. Available from: https://doi.org/10.1016/j.foodchem.2020.126224

[71] Catalkaya G, Kahveci D. Optimization of enzyme assisted extraction of lycopene from industrial tomato waste. Sep Purif Technol. 2019;219:55-63. Available from: https://doi.org/10.1016/j.seppur.2019.03.006

[72] Shivamathi CS, Moorthy IG, Kumar RV, Soosai MR, Maran JP, Kumar RS, et al. Optimization of ultrasound assisted extraction of pectin from custard apple peel: Potential and new source. Carbohydr Polym. 2019;225:115240. Available from: https://doi.org/10.1016/j.carbpol.2019.115240

[73] Massias A, Boisard S, Baccaunaud M, Leal Calderon F, Subra-Paternault P. Recovery of phenolics from apple peels using CO2 + ethanol extraction: Kinetics and antioxidant activity of extracts. J Supercrit Fluids. 2015;98:172-182. Available from: https://doi.org/10.1016/j.supflu.2014.12.007

[74] Wang L, Boussetta N, Lebovka N, Vorobiev E. Cell disintegration of apple peels induced by pulsed electric field and efficiency of bio-compound extraction. Food Bioprod Process. 2020;122:13-21. Available from: https://doi.org/10.1016/j.fbp.2020.03.004

[75] Panadare DC, Gondaliya A, Rathod VK. Comparative study of ultrasonic pretreatment and ultrasound assisted three phase partitioning for extraction of custard apple seed oil. Ultrason Sonochem. 2020;61:104821. Available from: https://doi.org/10.1016/j.ultsonch.2019.104821

[76] Montañés F, Catchpole OJ, Tallon S, Mitchell KA, Scott D, Webby RF. Extraction of apple seed oil by supercritical carbon dioxide at pressures up to 1300 bar. J Supercrit Fluids. 2018;141:128-136. Available from: https://doi.org/10.1016/j.supflu.2018.02.002

[77] Li W, Yang H, Coldea TE, Zhao H. Modification of structural and functional characteristics of brewer's spent grain protein by ultrasound assisted extraction. Lwt. 2020;110582. (In Press) Available from: https://doi.org/10.1016/j.lwt.2020.110582

[78] Martín-García B, Tylewicz U, Verardo V, Pasini F, Gómez-Caravaca AM, Caboni MF, et al. Pulsed electric field (PEF) as pre-treatment to improve the phenolic compounds recovery from brewers' spent grains. Innov Food Sci Emerg Technol. 2020;64:102402. Available from: https://doi.org/10.1016/j.ifset.2020.102402

[79] Spinelli S, Conte A, Lecce L, Padalino L, Del Nobile MA. Supercritical carbon dioxide extraction of brewer's spent grain. J Supercrit Fluids. 2016;107:69-74. Available from: https://doi.org/10.1016/j.supflu.2015.08.017

[80] Hosseini SS, Khodaiyan F, Yarmand MS. Optimization of microwave assisted extraction of pectin from sour orange peel and its physicochemical properties. Carbohydr Polym. 2016;140:59-65. Available from: https://doi.org/10.1016/j.carbpol.2015.12.051

[81] Nuapia Y, Cukrowska E, Tutu H, Chimuka L. Statistical comparison of two modeling methods on pressurized hot water extraction of vitamin C and phenolic compounds from Moringa oleifera leaves. South African J Bot. 2020;129:9-16. Available from: https://doi.org/10.1016/j.sajb.2018.09.001

[82] Narváez-Cuenca CE, Inampues-Charfuelan ML, Hurtado-Benavides AM, Parada-Alfonso F, Vincken JP. The phenolic compounds, tocopherols, and phytosterols in the edible oil of guava (Psidium guava) seeds obtained by supercritical CO2 extraction. J Food Compos Anal. 2020;89:103467. Available from: https://doi.org/10.1016/j.jfca.2020.103467

[83] Jafarian Asl P, Niazmand R, Jahani M. Theoretical and experimental assessment of supercritical CO2 in the extraction of phytosterols from rapeseed oil deodorizer distillates. J Food Eng. 2020;269:109748. Available from: https://doi.org/10.1016/j.jfoodeng.2019.109748

[84] Nyam KL, Tan CP, Lai OM, Long K, Che Man YB. Optimization of supercritical fluid extraction of phytosterol from roselle seeds with a central composite design model. Food Bioprod Process. 2010;88(2-3):239-246.

Available from: https://doi.org/10.1016/j.fbp.2009.11.002

[85] Botelho JRS, Medeiros NG, Rodrigues AMC, Araújo ME, Machado NT, Guimarães Santos A, et al. Black sesame (Sesamum indicum L.) seeds extracts by CO2 supercritical fluid extraction: Isotherms of global yield, kinetics data, total fatty acids, phytosterols and neuroprotective effects. J Supercrit Fluids. 2014;93:49-55. Available from: https://doi.org/10.1016/j.supflu.2014.02.008

[86] Izadi M, Fazilati M. Extraction and purification of phycocyanin from spirulina platensis and evaluating its antioxidant and anti-inflammatory activity. Asian J Green Chem. 2018;2(4):364-379. Available from: https://doi.org/10.22034/AJGC.2018.63597

[87] İlter I, Akyıl S, Demirel Z, Koç M, Conk-Dalay M, Kaymak-Ertekin F. Optimization of phycocyanin extraction from Spirulina platensis using different techniques. J Food Compos Anal. 2018;70:78-88. Available from: https://doi.org/10.1016/j.jfca.2018.04.007

[88] Martínez JM, Luengo E, Saldaña G, Álvarez I, Raso J. C-phycocyanin extraction assisted by pulsed electric field from Artrosphira platensis. Food Res Int. 2017;99:1042-1047. Available from: https://doi.org/10.1016/j.foodres.2016.09.029

[89] Jaeschke DP, Mercali GD, Marczak LDF, Müller G, Frey W, Gusbeth C. Extraction of valuable compounds from Arthrospira platensis using pulsed electric field treatment. Bioresour Technol. 2019;283:207-212. Available from: https://doi.org/10.1016/j.biortech.2019.03.035

[90] Ferreira-Santos P, Nunes R, De Biasio F, Spigno G, Gorgoglione D, Teixeira JA, et al. Influence of thermal and electrical effects of ohmic heating on C-phycocyanin properties and biocompounds recovery from Spirulina Platensis. LWT. 2020;109491. Available from: https://doi.org/10.1016/j.lwt.2020.109491

[91] Pagels F, Guedes AC, Amaro HM, Kijjoa A, Vasconcelos V. Phycobiliproteins from cyanobacteria: Chemistry and biotechnological applications. Biotechnol Adv. 2019;37(3):422-443. Available from: https://doi.org/10.1016/j.biotechadv.2019.02.010

[92] Goiris K, Muylaert K, Fraeye I, Foubert I, De Brabanter J, De Cooman L. Antioxidant potential of microalgae in relation to their phenolic and carotenoid content. J Appl Phycol. 2012;24(6):1477-1486. Available from: https://doi.org/10.1007/s10811-012-9804-6

[93] Czerwonka A, Kaławaj K, Sławińska-Brych A, Lemieszek MK, Bartnik M, Wojtanowski KK, et al. Anticancer effect of the water extract of a commercial Spirulina (Arthrospira platensis) product on the human lung cancer A549 cell line. Biomed Pharmacother. 2018;106:292-302. Available from: https://doi.org/10.1016/j.biopha.2018.06.116

[94] Alshuniaber MA, Krishnamoorthy R, AlQhtani WH. Antimicrobial activity of polyphenolic compounds from Spirulina against food-borne bacterial pathogens. Saudi J Biol Sci. 2021 Jan 1;28(1):459-64. Available from: https://doi.org/10.1016/j.sjbs.2020.10.029

[95] Chittapun S, Jonjaroen V, Khumrangsee K, Charoenrat T. C-phycocyanin extraction from two freshwater cyanobacteria by freeze thaw and pulsed electric field techniques to improve extraction efficiency and purity. Algal Res. 2020;46:101789. Available from: https://doi.org/10.1016/j.algal.2020.101789

[96] Jaeschke DP, Menegol T, Rech R, Mercali GD, Marczak LDF. Carotenoid and lipid extraction from Heterochlorella luteoviridis using moderate electric field and ethanol. Process Biochem. 2016;51(10):1636-1643. Available from: https://doi.org/10.1016/j.procbio.2016.07.016

[97] Jaeschke DP, Rech R, Marczak LDF, Mercali GD. Ultrasound as an alternative technology to extract carotenoids and lipids from Heterochlorella luteoviridis. Bioresour Technol. 2017 Jan 1;224:753-757. Available from: https://doi.org/10.1016/j.biortech.2016.11.107

[98] 't Lam GP, Postma PR, Fernandes DA, Timmermans RAH, Vermuë MH, Barbosa MJ, et al. Pulsed Electric Field for protein release of the microalgae *Chlorella vulgaris* and Neochloris oleoabundans. Algal Res. 2017;24:181-7. Available from: https://doi.org/10.1016/j.algal.2017.03.024

[99] Postma PR, Pataro G, Capitoli M, Barbosa MJ, Wijffels RH, Eppink MHM, et al. Selective extraction of intracellular components from the microalga Chlorella vulgaris by combined pulsed electric field-temperature treatment. Bioresour Technol. 2016;203:80-88. Available from: https://doi.org/10.1016/j.biortech.2015.12.012

[100] Cho H-S, Oh Y-K, Park S-C, Lee J-W, Park J-Y. Effects of enzymatic hydrolysis on lipid extraction from Chlorella vulgaris. Renew Energy [Internet]. 2013 Jun;54:156-160. Available from: http://dx.doi.org/10.1016/j.renene.2012.08.031

[101] Wang HM, Pan JL, Chen CY, Chiu CC, Yang MH, Chang HW, et al. Identification of anti-lung cancer extract from Chlorella vulgaris C-C by antioxidant property using supercritical carbon dioxide extraction. Process Biochem. 2010;45(12):1865-1872. Available from: https://doi.org/10.1016/j.procbio.2010.05.023

[102] Parniakov O, Apicella E, Koubaa M, Barba FJ, Grimi N, Lebovka N, et al. Ultrasound-assisted green solvent extraction of high-added value compounds from microalgae Nannochloropsis spp. Bioresour Technol. 2015;198:262-267. Available from: http://dx.doi.org/10.1016/j.biortech.2015.09.020

[103] Parniakov O, Barba FJ, Grimi N, Marchal L, Jubeau S, Lebovka N, et al. Pulsed electric field assisted extraction of nutritionally valuable compounds from microalgae Nannochloropsis spp. using the binary mixture of organic solvents and water. Innov Food Sci Emerg Technol. 2015;27:79-85. Available from: https://doi.org/10.1016/j.ifset.2014.11.002

[104] Gallego R, Bueno M, Chourio AM, Ibáñez E, Saldaña MDA, Herrero M. Use of high and ultra-high pressure based-processes for the effective recovery of bioactive compounds from Nannochloropsis oceanica microalgae. J Supercrit Fluids. 2021;167:105039. Available from: https://doi.org/10.1016/j.supflu.2020.105039

[105] Gilbert-López B, Barranco A, Herrero M, Cifuentes A, Ibáñez E. Development of new green processes for the recovery of bioactives from Phaeodactylum tricornutum. Food Res Int. 2017;99:1056-1065. Available from: https://doi.org/10.1016/j.foodres.2016.04.022

[106] Castro-Puyana M, Herrero M, Urreta I, Mendiola JA, Cifuentes A, Ibáñez E, et al. Optimization of clean extraction methods to isolate carotenoids from the microalga Neochloris oleoabundans and subsequent chemical characterization using liquid chromatography tandem mass spectrometry. Anal Bioanal Chem. 2013;405(13):4607-4616. Available

from: https://doi.org/10.1007/s00216-012-6687-y

[107] Otero P, López-Martínez MI, García-Risco MR. Application of pressurized liquid extraction (PLE) to obtain bioactive fatty acids and phenols from Laminaria ochroleuca collected in Galicia (NW Spain). J Pharm Biomed Anal. 2019;164:86-92. Available from: https://doi.org/10.1016/j.jpba.2018.09.057

[108] Yuan Y, Zhang J, Fan J, Clark J, Shen P, Li Y, et al. Microwave assisted extraction of phenolic compounds from four economic brown macroalgae species and evaluation of their antioxidant activities and inhibitory effects on α-amylase, α-glucosidase, pancreatic lipase and tyrosinase. Food Res Int. 2018;113:288-297. Available from: https://doi.org/10.1016/j.foodres.2018.07.021

[109] Heffernan N, Smyth TJ, FitzGerald RJ, Soler-Vila A, Brunton N. Antioxidant activity and phenolic content of pressurised liquid and solid-liquid extracts from four Irish origin macroalgae. Int J Food Sci Technol. 2014;49(7):1765-1772. Available from: http://doi.wiley.com/10.1111/ijfs.12512

[110] Mæhre HK, Jensen IJ, Eilertsen KE. Enzymatic pre-treatment increases the protein bioaccessibility and extractability in dulse (palmaria palmata). Mar Drugs. 2016;14(11):196. Available from: https://doi.org/10.3390/md14110196

[111] Pimentel FB, Alves RC, Harnedy PA, FitzGerald RJ, Oliveira MBPP. Macroalgal-derived protein hydrolysates and bioactive peptides: Enzymatic release and potential health enhancing properties. Trends Food Sci Technol. 2019;93:106-124. Available from: https://doi.org/10.1016/j.tifs.2019.09.006

[112] Mittal R, Tavanandi HA, Mantri VA, Raghavarao KSMS. Ultrasound assisted methods for enhanced extraction of phycobiliproteins from marine macro-algae, Gelidium pusillum (Rhodophyta). Ultrason Sonochem. 2017;38:92-103. Available from: https://doi.org/10.1016/j.ultsonch.2017.02.030

[113] Kissoudi M, Sarakatsianos I, Samanidou V. Isolation and purification of food-grade C-phycocyanin from Arthrospira platensis and its determination in confectionery by HPLC with diode array detection. J Sep Sci. 2018;41(4):975-981. Available from: https://doi.org/10.1002/jssc.201701151

[114] Nizioł-ŁUkaszewska Z, Furman-Toczek D, Bujak T, Wasilewski T, Hordyjewicz-Baran Z. Moringa oleifera L. Extracts as Bioactive Ingredients That Increase Safety of Body Wash Cosmetics. Dermatol Res Pract. 2020;2020. Available from: https://doi.org/10.1155/2020/8197902

[115] Schoonees A, Visser J, Musekiwa A, Volmink J. Pycnogenol ® for the treatment of chronic disorders. In: Cochrane Database of Systematic Reviews. John Wiley & Sons, Ltd; 2012;2:CD008294. Available from: https://doi.org/10.1002/14651858.CD008294.pub3

[116] Kunnumakkara AB, Bordoloi D, Padmavathi G, Monisha J, Roy NK, Prasad S, et al. Curcumin, the golden nutraceutical: multitargeting for multiple chronic diseases. British Journal of Pharmacology. 2017;174(11):1325-48. Available from: https://doi.org/10.1111/bph.13621

[117] Borowitzka MA. High-value products from microalgae-their development and commercialisation. J Appl Phycol. 2013;25(3):743-756. Available from: https://doi.org/10.1007/s10811-013-9983-9

[118] Ighodaro OM, Akinloye OA. First line defence antioxidants-superoxide dismutase (SOD), catalase (CAT)

and glutathione peroxidase (GPX): Their fundamental role in the entire antioxidant defence grid. Alexandria J Med. 2018;54(4):287-293. Available from: https://doi.org/10.1016/j.ajme.2017.09.001

[119] Caroprese M, Ciliberti MG, Albenzio M, Marino R, Santillo A, Sevi A. Role of antioxidant molecules in milk of sheep. Small Rumin Res. 2019;180:79-85. Available from: https://doi.org/10.1016/j.smallrumres.2019.07.011

[120] Wen C, Zhang J, Zhang H, Duan Y, Ma H. Plant protein-derived antioxidant peptides: Isolation, identification, mechanism of action and application in food systems: A review. Trends Food Sci Technol. 2020;105:308-322. Available from: https://doi.org/10.1016/j.tifs.2020.09.019

[121] Eslami O, Shidfar F. Soy milk: A functional beverage with hypocholesterolemic effects? A systematic review of randomized controlled trials. Complement Ther Med. 2019;42:82-88. Available from: https://doi.org/10.1016/j.ctim.2018.11.001

[122] Moayedi A, Mora L, Aristoy MC, Safari M, Hashemi M, Toldrá F. Peptidomic analysis of antioxidant and ACE-inhibitory peptides obtained from tomato waste proteins fermented using Bacillus subtilis. Food Chem. 2018;250:180-187. Available from: https://doi.org/10.1016/j.foodchem.2018.01.033

[123] García MC, Endermann J, González-García E, Marina ML. HPLC-Q-TOF-MS Identification of Antioxidant and Antihypertensive Peptides Recovered from Cherry (Prunus cerasus L.) Subproducts. J Agric Food Chem. 2015;63(5):1514-1520. Available from: https://doi.org/10.1021/jf505037p

[124] Pereira T, Barroso S, Mendes S, Amaral RA, Dias JR, Baptista T, et al. Optimization of phycobiliprotein pigments extraction from red algae Gracilaria gracilis for substitution of synthetic food colorants. Food Chem. 2020;321:126688. Available from: https://doi.org/10.1016/j.foodchem.2020.126688

[125] Sonani RR, Singh NK, Kumar J, Thakar D, Madamwar D. Concurrent purification and antioxidant activity of phycobiliproteins from Lyngbya sp. A09DM: An antioxidant and anti-aging potential of phycoerythrin in Caenorhabditis elegans. Process Biochem. 2014;49(10):1757-1766. Available from: https://doi.org/10.1016/j.procbio.2014.06.022

[126] Lizárraga-Velázquez C, Leyva-López N, Hernández C, Gutiérrez-Grijalva EP, Salazar-Leyva J, Osuna-Ruíz I, et al. Antioxidant Molecules from Plant Waste: Extraction Techniques and Biological Properties. Processes. 2020;8:1-44. Available from: https://doi.org/10.3390/pr8121566

[127] Park WS, Kim HJ, Li M, Lim DH, Kim J, Kwak SS, et al. Two classes of pigments, carotenoids and c-phycocyanin, in spirulina powder and their antioxidant activities. Molecules. 2018;23(8):1-11. Available from: https://doi.org/ 10.3390/molecules23082065

[128] Toh DWK, Sutanto CN, Loh WW, Lee WY, Yao Y, Ong CN, et al. Skin carotenoids status as a potential surrogate marker for cardiovascular disease risk determination in middle-aged and older adults. Nutr Metab Cardiovasc Dis. 2020;(In Press). Available from: https://doi.org/10.1016/j.numecd.2020.10.016

[129] Mohamadnia S, Tavakoli O, Faramarzi MA. Enhancing production of fucoxanthin by the optimization of culture media of the microalga Tisochrysis lutea. Aquaculture. 2021;533:736074. Available from: https://doi.org/10.1016/j.aquaculture.2020.736074

[130] Cloetens L, Panee J, Åkesson B. The antioxidant capacity of milk - The application of different methods in vitro and in vivo. Cell Mol Biol. 2013;59(1):43-57. Available from: https://pubmed.ncbi.nlm.nih.gov/24200020/

[131] Miras-Moreno B, Sabater-Jara AB, Pedreno MA, Almagro L. Bioactivity of Phytosterols and Their Production in Plant in Vitro Cultures. J Agric Food Chem. 2016;64(38):7049-7058. Available from: https://doi.org/10.1021/acs.jafc.6b02345

[132] Kritchevsky D, Chen SC. Phytosterols—health benefits and potential concerns: a review. Nutrition Research. 2005;25(5):413-428. Available from: https://doi.org/10.1016/j.nutres.2005.02.003

[133] Ferreira-Santos P, Carrón R, Recio I, Sevilla MÁ, Montero MJ. Effects of milk casein hydrolyzate supplemented with phytosterols on hypertension and lipid profile in hypercholesterolemic hypertensive rats. J Funct Foods. 2017;28:168-176. Available from: https://doi.org/10.1016/j.jff.2016.11.020

[134] Pizzino G, Irrera N, Cucinotta M, Pallio G, Mannino F, Arcoraci V, et al. Oxidative Stress: Harms and Benefits for Human Health. Oxid Med Cell Longev. 2017;2017. Available from: https://doi.org/10.1155/2017/8416763

[135] Turrens JF. Mitochondrial formation of reactive oxygen species. Journal of Physiology. 2003;552(2):335-344. Available from: https://doi.org/10.1113/jphysiol.2003.049478

[136] Stadtman ER, Levine RL. Protein oxidation. In: Annals of the New York Academy of Sciences. New York Academy of Sciences; 2000. p. 191-208.

[137] Rubbo H, Parthasarathy S, Barnes S, Kirk M, Kalyanaraman B, Freeman BA. Nitric oxide inhibition of lipoxygenase-dependent liposome and low-density lipoprotein oxidation: Termination of radical chain propagation reactions and formation of nitrogen-containing oxidized lipid derivatives. Arch Biochem Biophys. 1995;324(1):15-25. Available from: https://doi.org/10.1006/abbi.1995.9935

[138] Kaur H, Halliwell B. Evidence for nitric oxide-mediated oxidative damage in chronic inflammation Nitrotyrosine in serum and synovial fluid from rheumatoid patients. FEBS Lett. 1994;350(1):9-12. Available from: https://doi.org/10.1016/0014-5793(94)00722-5

[139] Ledoux SP, Driggers WJ, Hollensworth BS, Wilson GL. Repair of alkylation and oxidative damage in mitochondrial DNA. Mutat Res - DNA Repair. 1999;434(3):149-159. Available from: https://doi.org/10.1016/s0921-8777(99)00026-9

[140] Surai PF, Kochish II, Fisinin VI, Kidd MT. Antioxidant defence systems and oxidative stress in poultry biology: An update. Antioxidants. 2019; 8(7):235. Available from: https://doi.org/10.3390/antiox8070235

[141] Birben E, Sahiner UM, Sackesen C, Erzurum S, Kalayci O. Oxidative stress and antioxidant defense. World Allergy Organ J. 2012;5(1):9-19. Available from: https://doi.org/10.1097/WOX.0b013e3182439613

[142] Younus H. Therapeutic potentials of superoxide dismutase. Int J Health Sci (Qassim). 2018;12(3):88-93. Available from: https://www.ncbi.nlm.nih.gov/pmc/articles/PMC5969776/

[143] Marklund SL. Extracellular superoxide dismutase and other superoxide dismutase isoenzymes in tissues from nine mammalian species. Biochem J. 1984;222(3):649-55.

Available from: https://doi.org/10.1042/bj2220649

[144] Chelikani P, Fita I, Loewen PC. Diversity of structures and properties among catalases. Cell Mol Life Sci. 2004;61(2):192-208. Available from: https://doi.org/ 10.1007/s00018-003-3206-5

[145] Dworzański J, Strycharz-Dudziak M, Kliszczewska E, Kiełczykowska M, Dworzańska A, Drop B, et al. Glutathione peroxidase (GPx) and superoxide dismutase (SOD) activity in patients with diabetes mellitus type 2 infected with Epstein-Barr virus. PLoS One. 2020;15(3):e0230374. Available from: https://doi.org/10.1371/journal.pone.0230374

[146] Lee S, Kim SM, Lee RT. Thioredoxin and thioredoxin target proteins: From molecular mechanisms to functional significance. Antioxid Redox Signal. 2013;18(10):1165-1207. Available from: https://doi.org/10.1089/ars.2011.4322

[147] Trivedi A, Singh N, Bhat SA, Gupta P, Kumar A. Redox Biology of Tuberculosis Pathogenesis. Adv Microb Physiol. 2012;60:263-324. Available from: https://doi.org/10.1016/B978-0-12-398264-3.00004-8

[148] Singhal SS, Singh SP, Singhal P, Horne D, Singhal J, Awasthi S. Antioxidant role of glutathione S-transferases: 4-Hydroxynonenal, a key molecule in stress-mediated signaling. Toxicol Appl Pharmacol. 2015;289(3):361-370. Available from: https://doi.org/10.1016/j.taap.2015.10.006

[149] Liguori I, Russo G, Curcio F, Bulli G, Aran L, Della-Morte D, et al. Oxidative stress, aging, and diseases. Clin Interv Aging. 2018;13:757-772. Available from: https://doi.org/10.2147/CIA.S158513

[150] Luca M, Luca A, Calandra C. The Role of Oxidative Damage in the Pathogenesis and Progression of Alzheimer's Disease and Vascular Dementia. V Oxid Med Cell Longev. 2015; 2015: 504678. Available from: https://doi.org/10.1155/2015/504678

[151] Hayes JD, Dinkova-Kostova AT, Tew KD. Oxidative Stress in Cancer. Cancer Cell. 2020;38(2):167-197. Available from: https://doi.org/10.1016/j.ccell.2020.06.001

[152] Reuter S, Gupta SC, Chaturvedi MM, Aggarwal BB. Oxidative stress, inflammation, and cancer: How are they linked? Free Radic Biol Med. 2010; 49(11):1603-1616. Available from: https://doi.org/10.1016/j.freeradbiomed.2010.09.006

[153] Pignatelli P, Menichelli D, Pastori D, Violi F. Oxidative stress and cardiovascular disease: New insights. Kardiol Pol. 2018;76(4):713-722. Available from: https://doi.org/10.5603/KP.a2018.0071

[154] Sharifi-Rad M, Anil Kumar N V., Zucca P, Varoni EM, Dini L, Panzarini E, et al. Lifestyle, Oxidative Stress, and Antioxidants: Back and Forth in the Pathophysiology of Chronic Diseases. Front Physiol. 2020;11:694. Available from: https://doi.org/10.3389/fphys.2020.00694

[155] Finkel T, Holbrook NJ. Oxidants, oxidative stress and the biology of ageing. Nature. 2000;408(6809):239-247. Available from: https://doi.org/10.1038/35041687

[156] Chakrabarti S, Jahandideh F, Wu J. Food-derived bioactive peptides on inflammation and oxidative stress. Biomed Res Int. 2014;2014:608979. Available from: https://doi.org/10.1155/2014/608979

[157] Seeram NP, Henning SM, Niu Y, Lee R, Scheuller HS, Heber D. Catechin

and caffeine content of green tea dietary supplements and correlation with antioxidant capacity. J Agric Food Chem. 2006;54(5):1599-1603. Available from: https://doi.org/10.1021/jf052857r

[158] Alam MN, Bristi NJ, Rafiquzzaman M. Review on in vivo and in vitro methods evaluation of antioxidant activity. Saudi Pharm J. 2013;21(2):143-52. Available from: https://doi.org/10.1016/j.jsps.2012.05.002

[159] Benzie IFF, Strain JJ. Ferric reducing/antioxidant power assay: Direct measure of total antioxidant activity of biological fluids and modified version for simultaneous measurement of total antioxidant power and ascorbic acid concentration. Methods Enzymol. 1999;299:15-27. Available from: https://doi.org/10.1016/s0076-6879(99)99005-5

[160] Apak R, Güçlü K, Özyürek M, Çelik SE. Mechanism of antioxidant capacity assays and the CUPRAC (cupric ion reducing antioxidant capacity) assay. Microchim Acta.2008;160:413-419. Available from: https://doi.org/10.1007/s00604-007-0777-0

[161] Prior RL. Oxygen radical absorbance capacity (ORAC): New horizons in relating dietary antioxidants/bioactives and health benefits. J Funct Foods. 2015;18:797-810. Available from: http://dx.doi.org/10.1016/j.jff.2014.12.018

[162] Huang D, Ou B, Hampsch-Woodill M, Flanagan JA, Prior RL. High-throughput assay of oxygen radical absorbance capacity (ORAC) using a multichannel liquid handling system coupled with a microplate fluorescence reader in 96-well format. J Agric Food Chem. 2002;50(16):4437-4444. Available from: https://doi.org/10.1021/jf0201529

[163] Moharram H, Youssef M. Methods for Determining the Antioxidant Activity: A Review. Alexandria J Food Sci Technol. 2014;11(1):31-42.

[164] Číž M, Čížová H, Denev P, Kratchanova M, Slavov A, Lojek A. Different methods for control and comparison of the antioxidant properties of vegetables. Food Control. 2010;21(4):518-523. Available from: https://doi.org/10.1016/j.foodcont.2009.07.017

[165] Shahidi F, Zhong Y. Measurement of antioxidant activity. J Funct Foods. 2015;18:757-781. Available from: http://dx.doi.org/10.1016/j.jff.2015.01.047

[166] Chandrasekara A, Shahidi F. Bioactivities and antiradical properties of millet grains and hulls. J Agric Food Chem. 2011;59(17):9563-9571. Available from: http://doi.org/10.1021/jf201849d

[167] Gião MS, Leitão I, Pereira A, Borges AB, Guedes CJ, Fernandes JC, et al. Plant aqueous extracts: Antioxidant capacity via haemolysis and bacteriophage P22 protection. Food Control. 2010;21(5):633-638. Available from: https://doi.org/10.1016/j.foodcont.2009.08.014

[168] Wolfe KL, Rui HL. Cellular antioxidant activity (CAA) assay for assessing antioxidants, foods, and dietary supplements. J Agric Food Chem. 2007;55(22):8896-8907. Available from: https://doi.org/10.1021/jf0715166

[169] Vongsak B, Mangmool S, Gritsanapan W. Antioxidant Activity and Induction of mRNA Expressions of Antioxidant Enzymes in HEK-293 Cells of Moringa oleifera Leaf Extract. Planta Med. 2015;81(12-13):1084-1089. Available from: https://doi.org/10.1055/s-0035-1546168

[170] Dilworth LL, Stennett D, Omoruyi FO. Effects of Moringa oleifera Leaf Extract on Human Promyelocytic Leukemia Cells Subjected to Oxidative Stress. J Med Food. 2020;23(7):728-734.

Available from: https://doi.org/ 10.1089/jmf.2019.0192

[171] Yi G, Din JU, Zhao F, Liu X. Effect of soybean peptides against hydrogen peroxide induced oxidative stress in HepG2 cells: Via Nrf2 signaling. Food Funct. 2020;11(3):2725-37. Available from: https://doi.org/10.1039/C9FO01466G

[172] McCullough ML, Peterson JJ, Patel R, Jacques PF, Shah R, Dwyer JT. Flavonoid intake and cardiovascular disease mortality in a prospective cohort of US adults. Am J Clin Nutr. 2012 Feb;95(2):454-464. Available from: https://doi.org/10.3945/ajcn.111.016634

[173] Patel H, Chandra S, Alexander S, Soble J, Williams KA. Plant-Based Nutrition: An Essential Component of Cardiovascular Disease Prevention and Management. Curr Cardiol Rep. 2017;19(10):104. Available from: https://doi.org/10.1007/s11886-017-0909-z

[174] Zhang X, Shu XO, Gao YT, Yang G, Li Q, Li H, et al. Soy food consumption is associated with lower risk of coronary heart disease in Chinese women. J Nutr. 2003;133(9):2874-2878. Available from: https://doi.org/10.1093/jn/133.9.2874

[175] Randriamboavonjy JI, Loirand G, Vaillant N, Lauzier B, Derbré S, Michalet S, et al. Cardiac protective effects of moringa oleifera seeds in spontaneous hypertensive rats. Am J Hypertens. 2016;29(7):873-881. Available from: https://doi.org/10.1093/ajh/hpw001

[176] Bacanli M, Dilsiz SA, Başaran N, Başaran AA. Effects of phytochemicals against diabetes. In: Advances in Food and Nutrition Research. Academic Press Inc. 2019.89:209-38. Available from: https://doi.org/10.1016/bs.afnr.2019.02.006

[177] Wilken R, Veena MS, Wang MB, Srivatsan ES. Curcumin: A review of anti-cancer properties and therapeutic activity in head and neck squamous cell carcinoma. Mol Cancer. 2011;10:12. Available from: https://doi.org/10.1186/1476-4598-10-12

[178] Shanafelt TD, Lee YK, Call TG, Nowakowski GS, Dingli D, Zent CS, et al. Clinical effects of oral green tea extracts in four patients with low grade B-cell malignancies. Leuk Res. 2006;30(6):707-712. Available from: https://doi.org/10.1016/j.leukres.2005.10.020

[179] Hosseini A, Ghorbani A. Cancer therapy with phytochemicals: evidence from clinical studies. Avicenna J phytomedicine. 2015;5(2):84-97. Available from: https://pubmed.ncbi.nlm.nih.gov/25949949/

[180] Yun T-K, Choi S-Y, Yun HY. Epidemiological Study on Cancer Prevention by Ginseng: Are All Kinds of Cancers Preventable by Ginseng? J Korean Med Sci. 2001;19-27. Available from: https://doi.org/10.3346/jkms.2001.16.S.S19

[181] Patil VM, Masand N. Anticancer Potential of Flavonoids: Chemistry, Biological Activities, and Future Perspectives. In: Studies in Natural Products Chemistry. Elsevier. 2018;59:401-30. Available from: https://doi.org/10.1016/B978-0-444-64179-3.00012-8

[182] Aalinkeel R, Bindukumar B, Reynolds JL, Sykes DE, Mahajan SD, Chadha KC, et al. The dietary bioflavonoid, quercetin, selectively induces apoptosis of prostate cancer cells by down-regulating the expression of heat shock protein 90. Prostate. 2008;68(16):1773-89. Available from: http://doi.wiley.com/10.1002/pros.20845

[183] Kavitha R V., Kumar JR, Egbuna C, Ifemeje JC. Phytochemicals as therapeutic interventions in neurodegenerative diseases. In:

Phytochemicals as Lead Compounds for New Drug Discovery. Elsevier. 2019;161-178. Available from: https://doi.org/10.1016/B978-0-12-817890-4.00010-X

[184] Velmurugan BK, Rathinasamy B, Lohanathan BP, Thiyagarajan V, Weng CF. Neuroprotective role of phytochemicals. Molecules. 2018;23(10):2485. Available from: https://doi.org/10.3390/molecules23102485

[185] Walker JM, Klakotskaia D, Ajit D, Weisman GA, Wood WG, Sun GY, et al. Beneficial effects of dietary EGCG and voluntary exercise on behavior in an Alzheimer's disease mouse model. J Alzheimer's Dis. 2015;44(2):561-572. Available from: https://doi.org/10.3233/JAD-140981

[186] Wobst HJ, Sharma A, Diamond MI, Wanker EE, Bieschke J. The green tea polyphenol (−)-epigallocatechin gallate prevents the aggregation of tau protein into toxic oligomers at substoichiometric ratios. FEBS Lett. 2015;589(1):77-83. Available from: https://doi.org/10.1016/j.febslet.2014.11.026

[187] Koh SH, Kim SH, Kwon H, Park Y, Kim KS, Song CW, et al. Epigallocatechin gallate protects nerve growth factor differentiated PC12 cells from oxidative-radical-stress-induced apoptosis through its effect on phosphoinositide 3-kinase/Akt and glycogen synthase kinase-3. Mol Brain Res. 2003;118(1-2):72-81. Available from: https://doi.org/10.1016/j.molbrainres.2003.07.003

[188] Zhang C, Browne A, Child D, Tanzi RE. Curcumin decreases amyloid-β peptide levels by attenuating the maturation of amyloid-β precursor protein. J Biol Chem. 2010;285(37):28472-28480. Available from: https://doi.org/10.1074/jbc.M110.133520

[189] Yuliani S, Mustofa, Partadiredja G. The neuroprotective effects of an ethanolic turmeric (*Curcuma longa* L.) extract against trimethyltin-induced oxidative stress in rats. Nutr Neurosci. 2019;22(11):797-804. Available from: https://doi.org/10.1080/1028415X.2018.1447267

[190] Yang X, Zheng T, Hong H, Cai N, Zhou X, Sun C, et al. Neuroprotective effects of Ginkgo biloba extract and Ginkgolide B against oxygen–glucose deprivation/reoxygenation and glucose injury in a new in vitro multicellular network model. Front Med. 2018;12(3):307-318. Available from: https://doi.org/10.1007/s11684-017-0547-2

[191] Wu W, Wang X, Xiang Q, Meng X, Peng Y, Du N, et al. Astaxanthin alleviates brain aging in rats by attenuating oxidative stress and increasing BDNF levels. Food Funct. 2014;5(1):158-66. Available from: https://doi.org/ 10.1039/c3fo60400d

Chapter 29

Recent Advances in Antioxidant Capacity Assays

Andrei Florin Danet

Abstract

This work presents a survey of the important antioxidant capacity/activity assays applied for a diversity of samples including plant extracts, foods, biological material, etc. The published materials are critically discussed, emphasizing the recent findings in the field. New and emergent antioxidant capacity assays, such as nanoparticles-based assay, are also presented. The discussion includes chemical-based methods as well as biochemical and cellular assays. Chemical methods detailed are radical/ROS-based scavenging assays (the trolox equivalent antioxidant capacity (TEAC/ABTS), 2,2-diphenyl-1-picrylhydrazyl (DPPH), oxygen radical absorbance capacity (ORAC) assays, chemiluminescence methods, total radical-trapping antioxidant parameter (TRAP), total oxy radical scavenging capacity (TOSC), and β-carotene bleaching assays), non-radical redox potential-based assays (ferric reducing antioxidant power (FRAP), cupric reducing antioxidant capacity (CUPRAC), nanoparticle-based methods and electrochemical methods), metal chelation capacity and total phenolic content tests. The biochemical-based assays and *in vivo* assays discussed include the oxidation of low density lipoprotein (LDL), the thiobarbituric acid reactive substances (TBARS) and the cellular antioxidant activity (CAA) assays. While a direct link between the antioxidant capacity and health benefits is still a matter of debate, the antioxidant testing methodologies presented in this chapter remain valuable for the high efficiency and cost-effective evaluation of antioxidants, from compound discovery to quality control.

Keywords: antioxidant, total antioxidant capacity, reactive species, phenolic compounds, antioxidant assay, phytochemicals, food analytical method

1. Introduction

Antioxidants are classified in two categories: (1) primary or chain-breaking antioxidants, especially acting by scavenging reactive oxygen species/reactive nitrogen species (ROS/RNS) and (2) secondary or preventive antioxidants, that suppress the oxidation promoters such as metal ions, singlet oxygen, pro-oxidative enzymes and other antioxidants, commonly operating by transition metal ion chelation [1]. An antioxidant may operate directly or indirectly: directly by scavenging ROS/RNS species or by inhibiting their generation, indirectly, e.g., by up-regulating endogenous antioxidant defenses [2, 3]. Antioxidants can be also classified as enzymatic and non-enzymatic antioxidants. In the present review we shall discuss only the non-enzymatic antioxidants. The efficacy of an antioxidant depends on its antioxidant activity and/or its antioxidant capacity.

IntechOpen

It should be stated from the very beginning that antioxidant activity and antioxidant capacity are two different terms. The antioxidant activity is linked to rate constant of an antioxidant against a specified free radical, whereas the antioxidant capacity represents the number of moles of a specified free radical, scavenged by an individual antioxidant present in the analyzed mixture [4]. Antioxidant activity is related especially to the reaction kinetics, whereas antioxidant capacity is related to the thermodinamics of the process regarding the oxidative conversion of an antioxidant and is connected with equilibrium constant of the process [5].

The antioxidant assays can target a specific compound (e.g., ascorbic acid, vitamin E, uric acid, etc.) or the total antioxidant capacity (TAC) given by the combined antioxidant capacities of all substances in a sample.

Antioxidant assays include direct and indirect methods. Direct assays are competitive, in which the produced reactive species simultaneously attack a „probe" and the antioxidant. Indirect assays are non-competitive, the redox reactions being simulated using an artificial probe, whose structural changes are measured by different techniques (spectroscopy, electrochemistry, or other methods).

The most common assays for TAC comprise: (i) the measurement of oxygen radical antioxidant capacity (ORAC) using different fluorescent probes [6], (ii) the Trolox equivalent antioxidant capacity based on 2,2′-azino-bis(3-ethylbenzothiazoline-6-sulphonic acid) (ABTS) (TEAC/ABTS) [7], (iii) the 2,2-diphenyl-1-picrylhydrazyl (DPPH) assay [8], (iv) the ferric reducing antioxidant power (FRAP) test [9], (v) the cupric reducing antioxidant capacity (CUPRAC) assay [10] and (vi) Folin–Ciocalteu's phenol reagent reducing capacity (for the content of total phenolics) [11, 12].

Extensive reviews regarding the methods for assaying antioxidant capacity/activity could be found in literature [1, 5, 6, 13–19] and a book has also been published recently [20] with a focus on the measurement of antioxidant activity and capacity. Several papers have discussed the advantages and disadvantages of different antioxidant assays, with a focus on method selection for specific requirements [14–16, 21, 22].

There are numerous research articles in literature pertaining to the evaluation of antioxidant methodology. However very few discuss the mechanistic steps involved in the respective reactions [23, 24]. In depth evaluation of ORAC, ABTS and DPPH methods were comprehensively presented [25]. Some important antioxidant assays in terms of mechanisms and kinetics of the involved reactions were evaluated [6, 14], while the mechanisms, advantages and disadvantages of different antioxidant assays were also described in [18, 26, 27].

A review of the main methods for monitoring the antioxidant capacity/activity of lipid-containing samples was presented in [28]. In addition, the determination of the antioxidant capacity of lipids via the flow injection analysis (FIA) coupled with chemiluminescence detection was specifically discussed in [29].

The role of antioxidants from a pharmaceutical perspective is presented in [30] and a review of the methodologies for the determination of biological antioxidant capacity *in vitro* is presented in [31].

Compiled information about antioxidants in terms of the chemistry, legislation and their application in foods as preservatives can be found in [32]. The extrapolation of laboratory data relative to the antioxidants' function and their implications on food production and human health, etc. is critically discussed in [33].

Some recent reviews [13, 34, 35] commented on the advance, applications, advantages and disadvantages of total antioxidant capacity assays. The contentions and limitations of some largely used antioxidant assays, hints for suitable assay selection, emerging techniques in antioxidant testing and future perspectives are provided in [5].

An interesting discussion is presented in [36] about the development of several TAC databases of foods, the development of methods for evaluating TAC in the diet, the application of TAC databases in epidemiological studies, the application of TAC methods to biological fluids and the correlation between consumption of antioxidant rich-foods and the plasma TAC. The advantages and disadvantages of different TAC assays were also summarized.

Unfortunately many studies on TAC have reported disparate results regarding antioxidant capacity measured on the same material in different laboratories even by using the same analytical method, or in a particular laboratory by using different methods. Such discrepancies could be explained by the fact that the employed methods evaluate different things under various conditions, e.g., some measurements are done in homogenous solutions, other in suspensions, some methods evaluate hydrogen atom transfer capacity, other evaluate electron transfer capacity, etc.

Consequently, developing standardized antioxidant capacity methods might reduce the results spreading. A basic rationale to develop standardized antioxidant capacity methods for food, being provided in [37], which considered three candidates assays for standardization, i.e., ORAC, TEAC/ABTS and Folin Ciocalteu method.

Radicals are usually quenched by two mechanisms [6, 25], i.e., by transferring either an electron (ET) or a hydrogen atom (HAT) to transform the radical to a more stable species, albeit sometimes the mentioned mechanisms may not be well distinguished [37]. Consequently antioxidant capacity measurements may be in large, categorized as electron transfer (ET)- and hydrogen atom transfer, (HAT)-based assays.

In **ET–electron transfer assays,** one or more electrons are transferred to reduce the compounds of interest according to the following reaction schemes:

$$ROO^{\bullet} + AH / ArOH \rightarrow ROO^{-} + AH^{\bullet+} / ArOH^{\bullet+} + H_2O \rightarrow A^{\bullet} / ArO^{\bullet} + H_3O^{+} \quad (1)$$

$$ROO^{-} + H_3O^{+} \rightarrow ROOH + H_2O \quad (2)$$

$$M(III) + AH / ArOH \rightarrow AH^{\bullet+} / ArOH^{\bullet+} + M(II) \quad (3)$$

HAT–hydrogen atom transfer assays involve the transfer of a H atom to the target radical and eventual secondary quenching by radical recombination, as follows:

$$ROO^{\bullet} + AH / ArOH \rightarrow ROOH + A^{\bullet} / ArO^{\bullet} \quad (4)$$

$$ROO^{\bullet} + A^{\bullet} \rightarrow ROOA \quad (5)$$

where AH = any antioxidant with donatable H, ArOH = phenol or polyphenol, M = redox-active metal.

As can be seen from the chemical reactions written above, regardless of the mechanism involved (ET or HAT), antioxidants scavenge ROS/RNS generating the same end products indifferent to mechanism involved, albeit kinetics and influence of system parameters, particularly solvent and pH, and potential for side reactions vary [37]. Moreover, HAT and proton coupled ET reactions may occur concurrently and the main mechanism in a particular system is determined by antioxidant properties and structure, partition coefficient, solvent, etc. [37].

The ET-based methods evaluate an antioxidant's reducing capacity (also of the probe for monitoring the reaction). Mainly HAT-based methods measure competitive reaction kinetics, and the determination is effected taking into account the kinetic curves. HAT-based assays mostly involve a synthetic free radical source, an oxidizable probe, and an oxidant. An elaborate description of antioxidant mechanisms is well presented in several review papers [6, 13–16, 38].

Antioxidant capacity is expressed as equivalents of a reference antioxidant such as trolox, gallic acid, etc., or antioxidant inhibition against oxidation of the probe (generated by ROS). Oxidation of the probe is determined by different detection techniques, such as: spectrophotometric, fluorimetric, chemiluminescent, EPR, amperometric methods, cyclic voltammetry, etc.

A classification of the methods for the assessment of antioxidant capacity/activity discussed in this work is presented in **Table 1**.

Classifications		**Assays**	**References**
Chemical based assays			
Radical/ROS-based scavenging assays	HAT/ET assays (Mixed mode)	TEAC/ABTS assay	[1, 15, 18, 24, 34]
		DPPH assay	[1, 15, 34]
	HAT assay	ORAC assay	[1, 15, 25, 37]
		Chemiluminescence methods	[29, 37, 39, 40]
		TRAP assay	[13, 15, 41]
		TOSC assay	[15, 42]
		β-Carotene bleaching assay	[15, 34, 43]
Non-radical redox potential-based assays	ET assay	FRAP assay	[13, 15, 20, 34]
		CUPRAC assay	[21, 35, 44]
		Nanoparticles based assays	[15, 45–47]
		• colorimetric detection, AuNPs- and AgNPs-based assays	[15, 45–47]
		• electrochemical detection, AuNPs-based assays	[15, 45–47]
		• magnetic NPs-based assays	[48]
		Electrochemical methods	[49–51]
		• cyclic voltammetry (CV) based assays	[52, 53]
		• diferential pulse voltammetry (DPV) based assays	[54]
		• Square wave voltammetry (SWV) based assays	[55]
		• Amperometry, biamperometry-based assays	[56–58]
		Metal chelation capacity	[13, 59]
		Total phenolic content (TPC)	[60, 61]
Biochemical based assays and *in vivo* assays		Oxidation of low density lipoproteins (LDL) assay	[18, 62]
		The thiobarbituric acid reactive substances (TBARS) assay	[18, 63, 64]
		Cellular antioxidant activity assay	[18, 65, 66]

Table 1.
Classifications of antioxidant capacity/activity assays.

2. Chemical based assays

2.1 Radical/ROS scavenging assays

2.1.1 Scavenging ability toward stable free radicals ABTS•+ and DPPH•

2,2′-azino-bis(3-ethylbenzothiazole-6-sulphonate) radical cation, ABTS•+ and 2,2-diphenyl-1-picrylhydrazyl, DPPH• are colored and stable free radicals that have been largely used to measure antioxidant capacity. DPPH• is commercially available, but ABTS•+ must be produced from the oxidation of ABTS with chemical reagents such as $K_2S_2O_8$, MnO_2, etc. ABTS•+ is soluble in aqueous and in alcoholic media (λ_{max} 734 nm), while DPPH• is soluble in different organic solvents (λ_{max} 517 nm, in ethanol). The chemical structures of ABTS•+ and DPPH• are presented in **Figure 1**.

The trolox equivalent antioxidant capacity (TEAC/ABTS) assay based on the use of ABTS•+ radical cation and DPPH• radical-based (DPPH) assay are among the most used antioxidant capacity assays.

In TEAC/ABTS assays, the antioxidant capacity is evaluated as the capability of analyzed sample to diminish the color intensity after reacting with the ABTS•+ radical. This assay can be employed for lipophilic as well as hydrophilic compounds. The assay is technically simple, being widely applied for screening and habitual determinations. Most often, ABTS•+ is produced by oxidation of ABTS with $K_2S_2O_8$. The reaction of antioxidants with ABTS•+ is quite fast. Generally, the measurements are done after a fixed period of time. The TEAC/ABTS assays were recently investigated with regards to their basic chemistry, reaction stoichiometry and the reaction pathways behind the ABTS/potassium persulfate decolorization assay [24].

A recent review [67] of TEAC/ABTS assays gives a comprehensive insight into this approach for evaluating the antioxidant capacity, including different methods of ABTS•+ generation, experimental design, and quantification strategies, as well as TEAC value data collection obtained using a diversity of samples. Other recent reviews regarding both ABTS/TEAC and DPPH assays can be found in [1, 5, 18, 34].

A comprehensive critical evaluation of the TEAC/ABTS, DPPH, and oxygen radical absorbance capacity (ORAC) assays, presented in [25] discusses the different methods, the intrinsic mechanisms of reactions, the advantages and disadvantages, the limitations and recommendations for applications of the methods.

The TEAC method has several advantages:

- It allows the assessment of a plethora of synthetic as well as natural antioxidants (phenols, peptides, thiols, indols, flavonoids, aminoacids, carotenoids, tocopherols, vitamin C, etc.).

- It can be applied over a large pH range.

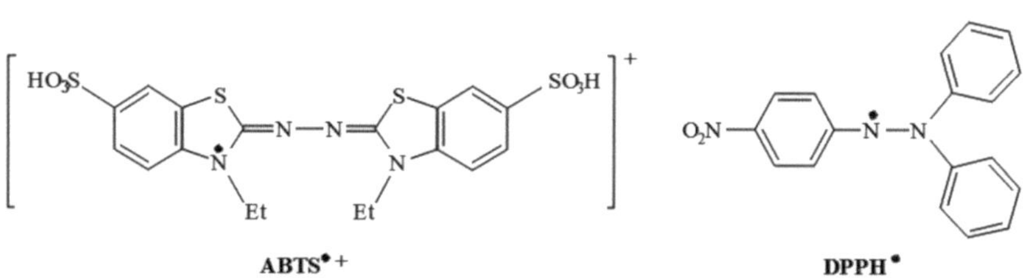

Figure 1.
Chemical structures of 2,2′-azino-bis(3-ethylbenzothiazole-6-sulphonate) radical cation, ABTS•+ and 2,2-diphenyl-1-picrylhydrazyl, DPPH• radical.

- The solubility of $ABTS^{\bullet+}$ in buffered and organic media enables measurement of both hydrophilic and lipophilic antioxidant activities.

- ABTS is affordable and easy to use.

Disadvantages of TEAC include:

- For some antioxidants different TEAC values may be obtained, depending on the way in which $ABTS^{\bullet+}$ is generated and on the measurement time interval selected.

- $ABTS^{\bullet+}$ (the same is applicable for $DPPH^{\bullet}$) is a metastable radical that does not exist in nature, being a "non-physiological" radical.

- The results of the assays depend on the reaction time. Some antioxidants react very fast and completely while other react slowly or combine a mix of fast and slow reactions [68].

- In the TEAC the molecular size and steric hindrance is an important characteristic. The accessibility of polyphenolics with bulky substituents to the radical cation ABTS is sterically restricted.

The DPPH assay is low-cost and simple and consequently has been largely used in laboratory settings for many applications. The assay is based on measuring the decrease of the absorbance of $DPPH^{\bullet}$ radical (at a wavelength of 517 nm) as a result of its reaction with antioxidants from the sample. This method was criticized for lacking standardization in different stages of the analytical process [37].

The criticism regarding DPPH assay is expressed even harder in [25]:"The DPPH reaction has been used as if it is a simplistic chemical "black box" – reagents are mixed and a number is generated, and the chemistry occurring between is ignored." In fact, antioxidant reactions with DPPH reagent are actually complex and reaction curves show multiple reactivity patterns [69]. DPPH reactions are very sensitive to the reaction medium, such as: water and solvent, pH, light exposure, dissolved oxygen, pH, etc. [69, 70].

The disadvantages of DPPH assay consist of the following:

- The evaluation of antioxidant capacity by the change in $DPPH^{\bullet}$ absorbance has to be carefully evaluated since the absorbance of $DPPH^{\bullet}$ after reaction with an analyzed sample may be diminished by some other factors (pH, O_2, light, type of solvent, etc.).

- Fixed-time assays may undervalue the radical scavenging capacities of slow-reacting antioxidants.

- Since the ionization of phenols – and consequently the reaction rates – are highly influenced by solvent composition and pH, the DPPH assay is not adequate to ranking antioxidant compounds and natural extracts.

In essence, the significant shortcomings of both TEAC/ABTS and DPPH assays are related to the intricacy of the mechanisms of reaction with antioxidants, the big influence of the experimental conditions on the obtained results, and the important difference between $DPPH^{\bullet}$ and $ABTS^{\bullet+}$ chemical structures and those of free radicals existing in biological systems.

2.1.2 Oxygen radical absorbance capacity (ORAC) assay

The ORAC method determines the radical chain breaking capacity of antioxidants by measuring the blocking-up of peroxyl radical generated oxidation. The peroxyl radical reacts with a probe (usually fluorescent) to form a non-fluorescent product, and the process can be monitored with a good sensitivity by fluorescence. Antioxidant capacity is determined by measuring rate and amount of product generated over time. Competition between reaction of probe and antioxidants with the $ROO^{\bullet}$ radical (or other ROS/RNS) constitute the premise of the assay.

Peroxyl radicals ($ROO^{\bullet}$) are the main free radicals that act in lipid oxidation in biological environment under physiological circumstances and in foods. For this reason, ORAC assay could be considered to have a biological concern as a reference for antioxidant efficacy. Commonly, 2,2′-azo bis(2-methylpropionamidine) hydrochloride (AAPH) is employed as $ROO^{\bullet}$ source that generates peroxyl radical at a known rate at incubation in aqueous media. The reactions involved in ORAC assay are as follows:

$$\mathrm{AAPH} + \mathrm{O_2} \rightarrow 2\mathrm{ROO}^{\bullet} + \mathrm{N_2} \tag{6}$$

$$\mathrm{ROO}^{\bullet} + \mathrm{Probe}_{\mathrm{fluorescent}} \rightarrow \mathrm{ROOH} + \mathrm{Oxidised\ Probe}_{\mathrm{non-fluorescent}} \tag{7}$$

$$\mathrm{ROO}^{\bullet} + \mathrm{AH} \rightarrow \mathrm{ROOH} + \mathrm{A}^{\bullet} \tag{8}$$

$$\mathrm{ROO}^{\bullet} + \mathrm{A}^{\bullet} \rightarrow \mathrm{ROOA} \tag{9}$$

The antioxidant capacity is measured by a diminished rate and through the quantity of product generated over time. A set of fluorescence decay curves can be obtained with or without antioxidants. The difference in the area under the curves (AUC) between the curves recorded in the presence and in the absence of the oxidant is considered to be a marker of the peroxyl radical scavenging capacity. Usually trolox (a standard antioxidant) is employed as reference and the obtained ORAC

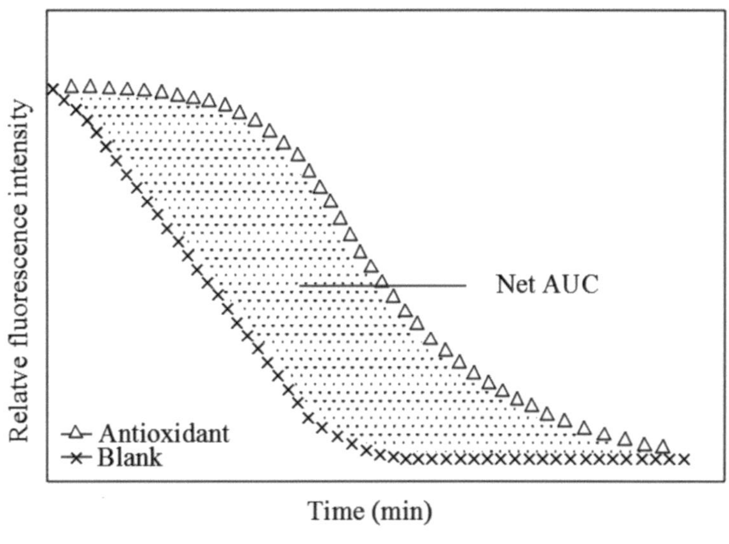

Figure 2.
ORAC antioxidant capacity of a sample expressed as the net AUC.

values are provided as trolox equivalents of the tested antioxidants. Data are shown as micromoles of trolox equivalents (TE) per liter or per gram of sample (µmol of TE/L or µmol of TE/g). The ORAC antioxidant capacity of a sample shown as the net area under the curve (AUC) is presented in **Figure 2**.

ORAC assay is a HAT-based method because it measures the capacity of hydrogen atom donating ability of antioxidants. β-phycoerythrin (β-PE), a protein obtained from *Porphyridium cruentum*, was employed as the fluorescent probe in the first studies. However, the use of β-PE in antioxidant assays has several shortcomings and can cause false ORAC values. The currently preferred fluorescent probes are fluorescein and dichlorofluorescein diacetate [37], as they are more stable and less reactive. Nevertheless, fluorescein may undergo undesired fluorescence quenching and side reactions [71] and other fluorescent probes have been suggested in consequence.

In order to measure both hydrophilic as well as lipophilic antioxidants the initial ORAC assay was modified using a solution of 50% acetone/50% water (v/v) and 7% randomly methylated β-cyclodextrin as a solubility enhancer of the antioxidants [72, 73].

The ORAC method has the utility to be a simple and standardized assay, however, secondary reactions can occur, affecting the reported results. For example, it was reported that antioxidant-metal reactions could result in a smaller concentration of antioxidants and hence to a depreciation of the ORAC value [74].

The ORAC method can be readily automated and it is perhaps the most largely recognized of all the antioxidant methods.

2.1.3 Chemiluminescence methods

The fundamental chemistry of chemiluminescence measurements of antioxidants is based on the reaction of ROS/RNS species with special reagents to generate species in an excited state that light up (chemiluminescence). The chemical compounds that react with the initiating reactive species diminish the light generation. Hence, generally, chemiluminescence measurements for antioxidant capacity assay are based on competitive reactions. By changing the oxidant initiator (e.g., $O_2^{\bullet}$, $HO^{\bullet}$, $ROO^{\bullet}$, $ONOO^-$, HOCl, $^1O_2$, etc.) it is possible to measure the capacity of quenching of different ROS/RNS by an antioxidant [37]. Chemiluminescence is a highly sensitive analytical method. The detection limit is very low, below that of most chemical methods. The mainly used chemiluminescence reagents are luminol [37, 75–79], lucigenin [39], pholasin (a bioluminescent protein) [80] and peroxyoxalate [81]. Luminol is the main commonly employed aqueous chemiluminescent reagent. Luminol reacts with an oxidizing agent, hydrogen peroxide (in presence of a catalyst) to yield 3-aminophthalate in an excited electronic state, which emits light. Antioxidants can quench the produced ROS (by hydrogen peroxide) and diminish hydrogen peroxide-induced chemiluminescence.

Chemiluminescence method has been automated in flow-based assays, e.g., flow injection analysis (FIA) [29, 76, 79, 82], sequential injection analysis (SIA) [83, 84], multi-syringe FIA (MS-FIA) and multi commutation.

A review on antioxidant assays with chemiluminescence detection is presented in [40] and other more general reviews of antioxidant assays including methods with chemiluminescence detection are presented in [1, 16, 17].

The methods for the determination of lipid hydroperoxides and of the antioxidant capacity of lipids by using flow injection analysis with chemiluminescence reagents are reviewed in [29].

The TAC of some *Rosmarinus officinalis* L. (rosemary) extracts was measured by an in batch analytical method based on Co(II)-ethylendiaminetetraacetic acid

(EDTA)-induced luminol-hydrogen peroxide chemiluminescence (luminol/Co(II) EDTA/H_2O_2) [75]. The method allows for TAC determination in the range 10^{-5}–2.5 10^{-3} moles L^{-1} of gallic acid equivalent. The same in batch method was applied for the TAC determination of fruit juices and noncarbonated soft drinks [77] and fruit seeds extracts [85].

The luminol/Co(II)EDTA/H_2O_2 system with chemiluminescence detection was used also in a flow injection analysis (FIA) method for the total antioxidant capacity determination of wines [79] and culinary and medicinal plants extracts [76].

Amperometric TAC measurements of several plant extracts using an electrochemical gold nanozyme-sensor based on the enzyme-like catalytic activity of gold nanoparticles [58] were associated with those obtained from a chemiluminescence method reported in [75]. A good correlation has been found between the two methods (Pearson's correlation coefficient of 0.958).

A new microfluidic chemiluminescence method for fast determination of the TAC of apple and pomegranate juices and honey samples was reported in [86]. The method is based on the $NaHCO_3$-H_2O_2-Co^{2+} chemiluminescence reaction.

A chemiluminescence-sensing platform for the determination of natural antioxidants and imaging of their tissue distribution is reported in [87]. The chemiluminescence radiation is emitted upon the redox reaction of antioxidants (e.g., L-ascorbic acid) with quinones (e.g., menadione), in the presence of luminol.

Different chemiluminescent system that allow the evaluation of both hydrophilic and lipophilic antioxidants by using the same method were reported. Thus, lucigenin–hydrogen peroxide chemiluminescence in 2-propanol has been proposed to measure the activity of both hydrophilic and lipophilic antioxidants [88].

A peroxyoxalate–hydrogen peroxide–imidazol–fluorophore system was applied in the evaluation of antioxidants in olive oils and honey samples. The system relies on a furan dicarboxylate derivative as fluorophore [81].

2.1.4 Other radical/ROS scavenging assays

Total radical trapping antioxidant parameter (TRAP) assay. This method generally measures the antioxidant's capability to interfere with the reaction between $ROO^\bullet$ (usually generated from AAPH) and a probe. It is relatively complex and laborious to perform [39 [37]. An early review of TRAP assay is presented in [89].

A TRAP assay for measuring total plasma antioxidant capacity used R-phycoerythrin (red protein pigments from the cells of red algae) as a fluorescent probe and AAPH, as $ROO^\bullet$ radical generator [41]. Fluorescence quenching was measured in absence and in presence of the analyzed antioxidant samples. The quantification of antioxidants is based on the duration of the lag phase.

Initiators for $ROO^\bullet$ radicals have been produced selectively by azides, enzymes (e.g., horseradish peroxidase) [90], or H_2O_2-hemin [91], etc. Some of the probes used in TRAP assays include fluorescein, dichlorofluorescein diacetate [92], R-phycoerythrin [93] and luminol [90].

It was reported that an important limitation of the TRAP assay is the use of the lag phase for determination of antioxidant capacity because not all antioxidants have a clear lag phase [94].

Total oxy radical scavenging capacity (TOSC) assay. The assay is based on the determination of antioxidants particularly toward three strong oxidants ($^\bullet OH$, $ROO^\bullet$, and $ONOO^-$) [15, 42]. In TOSC assay the oxidation of α-keto-γ-methiolbutyric acid (KMBA) to ethylene by ROS and ethylene formation was determined by head space gas chromatography relative to a reference reaction. The antioxidants compete with KMBA for ROS and the formation of ethylene is inhibited.

The most important drawback of this assay is the long reaction time (hundreds of minutes) and the necessity of several chromatographic analyses for each experiment [21].

β-Carotene bleaching assay. This assay employs an aqueous emulsion of linoleic acid and β-carotene, which is discolored under the influence of the radicals generated through the spontaneous oxidation of the fatty acid, owing to exposure to dissolved O_2, promoted by thermal induction. The measurements are done typically at 50 °C. Quantification is based on varying the rate at which β-carotene absorbance decays (at a wavelength of about 470–490 nm) in the presence of increasing concentrations of the antioxidant or prooxidant under evaluation. The decolorization is due to the breaking of π-conjugation by the addition reaction of radicals into a C=C bond of β-carotene [34]. The antioxidant capacity/activity is calculated in terms of % inhibition with regard to the reference.

An investigation of the experimental conditions that influence β-carotene bleaching assay is presented in [43] and in [95]. The β-carotene bleaching assay can screen both lipophilic and hydrophilic samples. It is sensitive to temperature, oxygen, pH and solvent effects and is time-consuming (an assay last hundreds of minutes).

2.2 Non-radical redox potential-based assays

2.2.1 Ferric reducing antioxidant power (FRAP) and cupric reducing antioxidant capacity (CUPRAC) assays

Ferric reducing antioxidant power (FRAP) and cupric reducing antioxidant capacity (CUPRAC) assays were reviewed in several recent papers [13, 14, 20, 21, 34, 35].

FRAP assay is based on antioxidants to reduce the ferric 2,4,6-tripyridyl-s-triazine complex $[Fe^{3+}-(TPTZ)_2]^{3+}$ to the blue colored ferrous complex, $[Fe^{2+}-(TPTZ)_2]^{2+}$ in acidic medium (pH 3.6). Measuring the increase in absorption at 593 nm monitors this reduction. The antioxidant capacity is expressed as μM Fe^{2+} equivalents or as a standard antioxidant equivalents. The FRAP assay is conducted at acidic pH 3.6 in order to prevent iron precipitation.

The reaction detects compounds with redox potentials lower than 0.7 V so FRAP is an adequate screen for the capacity to maintain redox status in cells or tissues. FRAP cannot measure compounds that act by radical quenching (H transfer), specifically bio-thiols (such as glutathione) and proteins [96]. For this reason the method is rather inadequate to measure the antioxidant capacity of intracellular fluids and human plasma/serum [97, 98].

Because the redox potential of $[Fe^{3+}-(TPTZ)_2]^{3+}$ is similar to $ABTS^{\bullet+}$ potential (0.68 V), similar compounds react in both the FRAP and TEAC assays. The FRAP mechanism is totally electron transfer and not mixed ET and HAT, and so in association with other antioxidant methods can be very useful in differentiating preponderant mechanisms with different antioxidants [37].

FRAP really determine only the reducing capacity based upon the ferric ion, which is not relevant to antioxidant capacity physiologically and mechanistically. However, in contrast to other assays of TAC, the FRAP method is simple, fast, inexpensive and robust and does not necessitate special equipment.

Cupric reducing antioxidant capacity (CUPRAC) assay. The method measures the reducing power of antioxidants to convert cupric (Cu^{2+}) to cuprous (Cu^{+}) ion. The copper reducing ability is measured by complexation of Cu^{+} with bathocuproine (2,9-dimethyl-4,7-diphenyl-1,10-phenanthroline) or neocuproine (2,9-dimethyl-1,10-phenanthroline) the corresponding complexes having absorption maximum at 490 nm and 450 nm, respectively [99]. **Figure 3** presents the cupric reducing antioxidant capacity (CUPRAC) reaction mechanism.

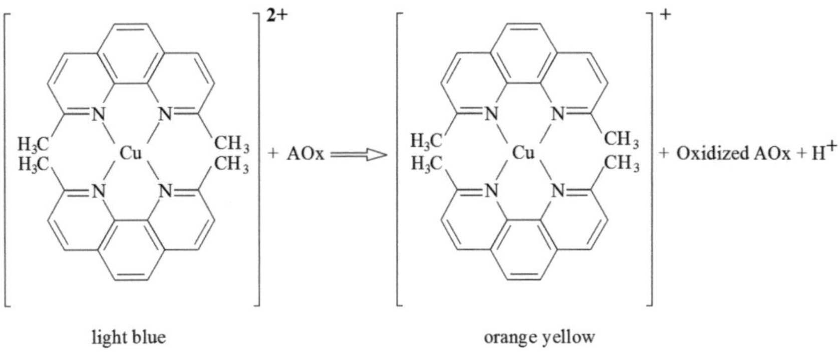

Figure 3.
Cupric reducing antioxidant capacity (CUPRAC) reaction mechanism.

FRAP and CUPRAC have comparable values with TEAC values (with some exceptions) since similar redox potential probes are employed in the assay. The original CUPRAC assay has been modified in order to allow analysis of different samples, e.g., acetone/water medium containing methyl-β-cyclodextrin has been employed for simultaneous assay of hydrophilic and lipophilic antioxidants [100].

In another modified CUPRAC assay, an optical sensor containing immobilized CUPRAC reagent Cu^{2+}–neocuproine complex onto a perfluorosulfonate cation-exchange polymer (Nafion) membrane matrix was developed. The measurements of absorbance were done at 450 nm [101].

CUPRAC assay is more selective due to its lower redox potential than that of redox couples like Ce^{4+}/Ce^{3+} and Fe^{3+}/Fe^{2+} [102]. The CUPRAC assay have been discussed in a comprehensive review in [44].

2.2.2 Nanoparticles based assays

For the determination of antioxidants, nanoparticles (NPs) can be employed as electrochemical or colorimetric probes, components in chemical and biological detection systems, and for radical generation. Several reviews regarding TAC determination by using NPs can be found in literature [18, 45–47, 103].

Chemical reduction-based nanotechnological assays of colorimetric TAC measurements make use of the generation or growth of noble metal nanoparticles (AuNPs, AgNPs, etc.) upon reaction of Au^{3+} or Ag^{+} salts with antioxidant. The strong visible light absorption at a specific wavelength results from the surface plasmon resonance absorption of metal nanoparticles.

In a pioneering work, reported in [104] the antioxidant capacity of several phenolic acids was determined from the formation and growth of gold nanoparticles (AuNPs). The same experimental approach was employed in [105] to evaluate the antioxidant capacity of chrysanthemum extracts and tea beverages.

A comparison of a AgNPs-based method for TAC assays in different rapeseed varieties with those of several spectrophotometric methods (total phenolic with Folin–Ciocalteu reagent, FRAP and DPPH assays) was performed in [106]. A significant correlation (r: 0.59–0.91) was found between the spectrophotometric methods and the nanoparticle-based assay.

Another interesting alternative, an optoelectonic tongue based on an array of gold and silver nano-particles for analysis of a diversity of natural, synthetic and biological antioxidants is described in [107].

A portable nanoparticle based-assay for rapid and sensitive measurement of food antioxidants was proposed in [108] based on the use of immobilized ceria (cerium oxide) nanoparticles. Due to the reversible oxidation state of cerium Ce^{3+}/Ce^{4+} on the NPs surface, nanoceria is capable of changing redox states and surface properties after interaction with antioxidants.

Furthermore, a novel chemical sensing array, based on metal oxide nanoparticles (i. e., cerium oxide, titanyl oxalate, TiO_2, Fe_2O_3, ZrO_2, ZnO and SiO_2) immobilized onto cellulose, was described as a portable and cheap paper-based colorimetric assay for polyphenol detection and field evaluation of antioxidant containing samples [109].

Last but not least, a novel method was proposed in [110] for evaluating the composition of mixtures of natural polyphenolic compounds by using an array of nano-oxides sensors and by chemometric analysis of the experimental data.

Some spectrometric and electrochemical nanomaterial-based assays for antioxidant assessment are presented in **Table 2**.

The nanoparticle-based assays to evaluate antioxidant capacity of natural products embody a novel and promising domain melding nanoscience with food and health research [18, 47].

	Antioxidant	Nano-material	Detection principle	Real samples	Reference
Spectro-metric	Total polyphenols in fat-rich samples	AuNPs	Detection of polyphenols in organic medium without extraction, by AuNPs formation at 540 nm	Chocolate, olive oil	[111]
	Polyphenols in food	AuNPs	Detection of polyphenol-mediated AuNPs formation from extracts via LSPR* by UV- visible spectroscopy at 540 nm	Tea, apple, pear, wine, honey	[112]
	Polyphenols	AuNPs	Au reduction, mild conditions, LSPR* detection	Fruit extracts	[113]
	Polyphenols	AgNPs	AgNPs seed-growth, LSPR* detection	Fruit juices, olive oils	[114]
	Polyphenols	AgNPs	AgNPs seed-growth, LSPR* detection	Ginger	[115]
	Total catechins evaluation	RhNPs	RhNPs LSPR* shifting	Teas	[116]
	Polyphenols	CdTe QDs**	CdTe QDs** fluorescence quenching inhibition	Teas	[117]
	Polyphenols	Graphene QDs	Graphene QDs fluorescence quenching	Olive oil extracts	[118]
	Phenolic acids	AuNPs on paper	Reduction of gold ions to AuNPs on paper sensors and measurement of the resultant color intensity	Tea, red wine	[119]

	Antioxidant	Nano-material	Detection principle	Real samples	Reference
	Flavonoids	Fluorescent gold nanocluster	Fluorescence quenching of gold nanoclusters imbedded into the cavity of bovine serum albumin tertiary structure	Serum, plasma, pharmaceutical analysis	[120]
Electro-chemical	*tert*-butylhydroquinone (TBHQ) and butylated hydroxyanisole (BHA)	Nano-carbon black	Measurements in the presence of the cationic surfactant CPB*** by square wave voltammetry using a carbon black paste electrode	Food samples and biodiesel	[121]
	Gallic acid	$NiAl_2O_4$ glassy carbon nano-composite	Cyclic voltammetry and amperometry with a $NiAl_2O_4$ glassy carbon working electrode	Food samples	[122]
	Flavonoids (myricetin and rutin)	Single-walled carbon nanohorns	Based on host–guest supramolecular recognition concept	Human serum	[123]
	Antioxidant capacity	Multi-walled carbon nanotubes	Chronocoulometry at glassy carbon electrode modified with multi-walled carbon nanotubes	Red/white wine	[124]
	Antiioxidant capacity (o-diphenols)	Cerium (IV)oxide NPs	Polyphenols oxidation at quinones, quinones reduction at screen printed carbon electrode-CeO_2(IV) NPs	Red/white wine	[125]

*Laser surface plasmon resonance.
**Quantum dots.
***Cetylpyridinium bromide.

Table 2.
Spectrometric and electrochemical nanomaterial-based assays for antioxidant assessment.

2.2.3 Electrochemical methods

Electrochemical techniques emerged as an alternative strategy for a quick, precise, and cost-effective determination of the TAC of different samples, e.g., foods and beverages, plant extracts, etc. They circumvent some of the drawbacks of spectrophotometric methods such as long analyses and sample preparation time, the use of expensive reagent and undefined reaction time. These methods also enable the quantification of the antioxidant compounds, with very good sensitivity [126, 127] and sometimes, they permit determinations in the presence of compounds that interfere in other methods, such as the case of ascorbic acid in juice [128].

Electrochemical methods for antioxidant capacity/activity evaluation have been reviewed in [129] and more recently in [14, 49–51, 130]. The most commonly used electrochemical techniques for antioxidant assays in different samples are cyclic voltammetry, differential pulse voltammetry, square wave voltammetry and amperometry.

Cyclic voltammetry (CV) [131]. The half-wave potential ($E_{1/2}$) of the registered cyclic voltammogram indicates a specific constituent in the analyzed sample (its ability to donate electrons) whereas the maximum current intensity indicates the concentration of a constituent. Antioxidants with similar structures have similar electron donating abilities and therefore similar half-wave potentials in cyclic voltammetry. Thus, when present in mixtures, they contribute globally to the observed features of the sample cyclic voltammogram.

Cyclic voltammetry has been widely used for evaluating the TAC of low-molecular weight antioxidants present in biological fluids, animal plasma, plants and fruits [52].

In [53] the results obtained for the TAC determination of 10 different fruit tea infusions using spectrophotometric methods (TEAC/ABTS, FRAP, DPPH and Folin–Ciocalteu's reagent total phenolic content) and by applying the CV method were reported comparatively.

In addition, CV has been used to measure the antioxidant capacity of a diversity of samples such as different winemaking by-products (pomace, skins, seeds, and stems) [132], propolis [133], edible oils [134] and berry fruits [135], among others.

Differential pulse voltammetry (DPV) has been applied for TAC assay of white and red wines [54] by using gallic acid as reference. The elaborated method is based on gallic acid electro-oxidation at carbon nanotubes-modified carbon paste electrode, at 350 mV (vs. Ag/AgCl) in 0.1 M phosphate buffer solution (pH = 2.50). The method enabled a reliable evaluation of the TAC for red and white wine samples, when glucose and ascorbic acid do not interfere.

Square wave voltammetry (SWV) has been used to analyze catechins in green and black teas [55] obtaining a detection limit of 40 nM for epigallocatechin gallate in green teas.

A databank of the content of antioxidants in food products was created based on amperometric measurements [56]. The antioxidants were quantified in 1140 food products, beverages, etc.

Amperometric, CV and DPV measurements using an electrochemical gold nanozyme-sensor [58] (based on the enzyme-like catalytic activity of gold nanoparticles), were used to evaluate the TAC of several plant extracts. The results of the amperometric measurements were compared to those from a chemiluminescence method for TAC assays [75] and a good correlation was found.

Biamperometric determinations are based on the reaction of the analyte with a redox pair such as I_2/I^-, Fe^{3+}/Fe^{2+}, $DPPH^•/DPPH$, $[Fe(CN)_6]^{3-}/[Fe(CN)_6]^{4-}$. $DPPH^•/DPPH$ biamperometry was used in the analysis of fruit juices for the determination of their TAC, using two identical Pt electrodes [57] and for tea, wine and coffee using glassy carbon electrodes [136].

Analytical characteristics of some electrochemical methods applied for the determination of antioxidants or total antioxidant capacity are presented in **Table 3**.

Electrochemical measurements of antioxidant capacity are redox-based methods with many advantages over conventional chemical assays since they are rapid and simple and do not require special chemical reagents or complicated sample preparation. Thus, they allow analysis of colored samples that do not permit direct evaluation by spectrophotometric techniques (e.g., wine and fruit juice) [150]. Electrochemical techniques allow also a large number of experimental parameters to be easily controlled and to register important information from a sample (e.g., the half-wave potential, the voltammetric charge, peak current intensity, etc.) that helps characterize different compounds from a sample [53]. These methods can be used to evaluate samples of whatever lipophilicity or hydrophilicity [151].

DOI: http://dx.doi.org/10.5772/intechopen.96654

Electrochemical method	Electrode	Antioxidants	LOD/Linear range	Real samples	References
Cyclic voltammetry	Iridium-containing carbon (Ir-C)	Caffeic acid	0.0–25.0 mg L^{-1}	Wine	[137]
	Graphite Carbon microspheres Carbon nanotubes	Vanillic acid	2.85 μM 3.82 μM 4.13 μM/ 10–400 μM	Artificial wine solutions	[138]
	Glassy carbon	Curcumin	4.1×10^{-6} M	Spices	[139]
	Carbon ink chemically modified electrode containing $[Cu(neocuproine)_2]\ (NO_3)_2$	Trolox Gallic acid Ascorbic acid	2.51×10^{-5} M - -	Teas	[140]
	Glassy carbon electrode	TAC*	2–80 μmol L^{-1} trolox	Berry fruits	[135]
	Glassy carbon disc electrod	(+)-catechin as standard	0.0078 to 1 mM	Food grade oenological tannins	[141]
Differential pulse voltammetry	Carbon paste platinum	Ascorbic acid	0.02 mM/0.07–20 mM; 0.087 mM/ 0.31–20 mM	Fruit juices and wines	[142]
	Carbon nanotubes modified carbon paste	TAC* (vs gallic acid)	3.0×10^{-7} M/ 5.0×10^{-7}- 5.0×10^{-5} M	Red and white wines	[54]
	Dropping mercury	Gallic acid	0.3 μM/ 1.0–50 μM	Fruit juices	[143]
	Glassy carbon electrode surface activated by *in situ* chemical oxidation	Tertiary butyl hydroquinone	67 nM/ 1.0 μM – 1.1 mM	Jatropha biodiesel	[144]
Square wave voltammetry	4-[(4-decyloxyphenyl)- ethynyl]-1- methylpyridinium iodide modified glassy carbon	Total phenolic compounds (vs caffeic acid)	9.0×10^{-7} mol L^{-1}/ 9.9×10^{-7}- 3.8×10^{-5} mol L^{-1}	Total polyphenol content of Yerba mate extracts	[145]

Electrochemical method	Electrode	Antioxidants	LOD/Linear range	Real samples	References
	Screen printed electrode modified with CeNPs. (CeNPs/C/SPE)	Gallic acid Caffeic acid Quercetin *t*-resveratrol	7.0 μM 10.0 μM 9.0 μM 8.0 μM	White/red wines	[146]
Amperometry	Biosensor based on peroxidase-modified carbon paste	*t*-resveratrol Caffeic acid	0.023 mg L^{-1}/ 0.05–52 mg L^{-1} 0.020 mg L^{-1}/ 0.06–69 mg L^{-1}	Wine	[147]
Amperometry (flow injection)	Carbon nanotube modified-glassy carbon electrode	Gallic acid Catechin Quercetin Caffeic acid Trolox TAC* (vs trolox)	0.04 μM 0.02 μM 0.03 μM 0.08 μM 0.04 μM	Thai vegetables/herbs	[148]
Amperometry (flow injection)	Glassy carbon/carbon nanotubes/polyethyleneimine electrode	Caffeic acid, gallic acid Ferulic acid *p*-coumaric acid	< 0.1 μM/ 10^{-7}–10^{-4} M	Wines	[149]

Total antioxidant capacity.

Table 3.
Analytical characteristics of some electrochemical methods applied for the determination of antioxidants or total antioxidant capacity.

A disadvantage of the electrochemical methods of antioxidant capacity determination in complex media is the difficulty to analyze the macromolecules with antioxidant proprieties.

2.3 Metal chelating assay

Metal chelation capacity is evaluated by measuring the chelating effect of antioxidants for metal ions. Fe^{2+} ions are known to enhance lipid peroxidation trough Fenton reaction and also by decomposing lipid hydroperoxides into peroxyl and alkoxy radicals, which are more reactive. By Fenton reaction (written below), the ferrous ions produce $^{\bullet}OH$ radicals, which are highly reactive, and contribute appreciably to oxidative stress. The resulting hydroxy radicals cause damage to proteins, carbohydrates, cellular lipids and nucleic acids leading to cellular damage.

$$Fe^{2+} + H_2O_2 \rightarrow Fe^{3+} + OH^- + {}^{\bullet}OH \quad (10)$$

Numerous metal ions such as Cu^+, Ti^{3+}, Cr^{2+}, and Co^{2+} and their complexes in their lower oxidation states react with H_2O_2 in a similar manner as Fe^{2+}, and the mixtures of these metal ions with H_2O_2 were named "Fenton-like" reagents [96].

Metal chelation capability could be used as an indicator of antioxidant capacity. Chelating agents stabilizing the oxidized form of the metal ions are effective as secondary antioxidants.

Commonly, metal chelation capacity is evaluated by determining the chelating effect of antioxidants for ferrous ion [59]. The evaluation of the metal-chelating activity of an antioxidant is based on the absorbance measurement of Fe^{2+}-ferrozine complex in presence and in absence of the analyzed sample. The decrease in absorbance of the solution after the introduction of test sample is related to the metal chelation capacity of the sample. The measurements are performed spectrophotometrically at 562 nm [13]. Ethylenediaminetetraacetic acid (EDTA) is generally used as a standard metal chelator. Metal chelation capability of different samples is expressed as EDTA equivalents.

In [38] the results obtained at the determination of metal chelation capacity for a number of antioxidants and extracts are presented. A study regarding the standardization of the experimental protocols to evaluate the capability to chelate Fe^{2+} (employing ferrozine as chromogenic reagent) and Cu^{2+} (employing pyrocatechol violet as the chromogen agent) is presented in [152]. This study used 96-well microplates and analyzed Brazilian coffees (n = 20).

2.4 Total phenolic content (TPC)

Total phenolic content (TPC) or Folin–Ciocalteu reducing (FCR) assay is an important parameter of total antioxidant capacity (TAC) and largely employed for evaluation of a diversity of samples. The TPC assay has been used for a long period as a measure of total phenolic content in natural products [37]. In this method, TPC values are evaluated as equivalents of gallic acid or another phenolic compound, e.g., caffeic acid, catechin, ferrulic acid, etc.

The Folin Ciocalteu reagent contains phosphomolybdic/phosphotungstic acid complexes, with added lithium sulfate and bromine, in strong basic medium (5–10% aqueous Na_2CO_3, pH 10–12) to generate the phenolate anion [153]. The TPC method is based on the measurement of the blue-colored chromophore (λ_{max} = 620–765 nm) generated as a result of reduction of Folin Ciocalteu reagent with phenols from the sample [154]. The reduction site is considered the molybdenum centre in the complex (Mo^{6+} ion is reduced to Mo^{5+} by phenols).

TPC assay is operationally simple, reproducible and convenient for evaluation of total phenolic for a variety of samples because the reagent is commercially available.

However many non-phenolic compounds e.g., ascorbic acid, aromatic amines, sulfur dioxide, some metal ions (Cu^+ and Fe^{2+}), etc. can interfere by reducing Folin Ciocalteu reagent. Several methodologies have been studied to increase the selectivity of the TPC method for total phenolic determinations in plant extracts [60].

A critical review of the methods for the assays of TPC in food matrices is presented in [61]. The review focuses on the most used methods to measure by UV-Vis spectrometry the TPC, *o*-diphenols, flavonoids, flavonols, anthocyanins, and tannins. Examples of application of TPC assay for winemaking byproducts (seeds, skins, stems, and pomace) and in Venezuelean propolis are given in [155, 156], respectively.

The TPC assay is still widely employed. However solid phase extraction (SPE) was considered as clean-up step in only a few cases. When SPE was employed, the SPE-FCR assay presented excellent reproducibility [157].

TPC assays are low-cost, simple, do not require expensive equipment and they are used largely to evaluate a big diversity of samples.

3. Biochemical-based assays and *in vivo* assays

3.1 Oxidation of low density lipoprotein (LDL) assay

A review of this assay alongside other assays measuring lipid oxidation can be found in [62]. The oxidation of LDL generated by ROS/RNS was studied long ago. ROS play an very important role in the initiation, propagation and termination reactions of the LDL lipid peroxidation. The lipid peroxidation processes could be followed by different methods, e.g., UV spectrophotometry and/or chemiluminiscence techniques. As an initiator of LDL oxidation is commonly employed cupric sulfate. By using a spectrophotometric methods the formation of diene conjugates at 234 nm is measured. By using a chemiluminescence methods the emitted radiation is measured as a result of the formation of oxidative products. By mixing a cupric sulfate solution with LDL sample, the kinetic profiles correspond to the occurrence of a lag phase owing to the existence of endogenous antioxidants such as coenzyme Q and vitamin E in the LDL particle. Following the lag time, the peroxidation of lipids is measured as an growth of the analytical signal (absorbance or chemiluminescence intensity) that finally, after minutes or hours, hit a plateau. By adding an antioxidant to the reaction mixture the lag time is enhanced. The antioxidant capacity is evaluated by measuring of the lag time. The most important advantage of this method is the employment of a biological significant target.

3.2 The thiobarbituric acid reactive substances (TBARS) assay

Two review dedicated exclusively to TBARS assays are presented in [63, 64]. Important aspects of the TBARS assay such as state-of-the-art of the method, determination in physiological systems, assays in food systems and the employment of TBARS in antioxidant evaluation studies are presented in [63].

The thiobarbituric reactive substances (TBARS) assay is frequently used to evaluate lipid peroxidation. The method is based on the reaction of malondialdehyde (MDA) generated as an advanced product of unsaturated lipid degradation under the influence of ROS/RNS, with thiobarbituric acid (TBA) under acidic conditions and at high temperature (100 °C) [158]. It is obtained a characteristic colored product [MDA-$(TBA)_2$] which is measured spectrophotometrically at

532 nm. MDA is a marker of oxidative stress. It is formed from polyunsaturated fatty acids (PUFA) with at least three double bonds in their molecule. This method is not a selective assay for lipid peroxidation products because TBA reacts with a diversity of aldehydes, not only those generated in the lipid peroxidation process [14]. The lack of specificity of the method is emphasized by the designation: thiobarbituric acid reactive substances (TBARS). MDA formation is the most largely employed method for lipid peroxidation evaluation. The method was significantly enhanced by coupling with HPLC. Several food components such as sugar degradation products, proteins and Maillard browning products affect the measurements. The thiobarbituric acid reactive substances (TBARS) method is widely employed to evaluate antioxidant activity and lipid oxidation in a diversity of samples.

3.3 Cellular antioxidant activity (CAA) assay

Cellular-based antioxidant activity assays (CAA) are performed within the cell medium and are presumed to be biologically more appropriate than the respective chemical assays owing to their better representation of the physico-chemical characteristics of the medium [159]. At the cellular level the antioxidant outcome is not confined only to reactive species scavenging, but imply also gene expression, modulation of redox cell signaling and upregulation of detoxifying or antioxidant enzymes. Moreover, in order to assay antioxidant capacity/activity it is very important to take into consideration some features regarding the bioavailability of an antioxidant such as the uptake, the partitioning in membranes and the metabolism. CAA assay is very useful for the evaluation of a new antioxidant because the change of the redox state at the cellular level (caused by the antioxidant) is strongly influenced by the different cell components.

The principle of CAA is presented in **Figure 4**. The cell-permeable non-polar 2′,7′-dichlorofluorescin diacetate (DCFH-DA) is used as a fluorescence probe. Within the cells this molecule is deacetylated by cellular esterases generating a polar molecule, 2′,7′-dichlorofluorescin (DCFH) which is captured in the cells. Afterwards, peroxyl radicals produced inside the cells from 2, 2′-azo bis(2-amidinopropane) dihydrochloride (AAPH) which cross easily the cellular membrane oxidize DCFH to form dichlorofluorescein (DCF) which is fluorescent. The fluorescence intensity generated within the cells is related with the extent of oxidation. The molecules with antioxidant properties scavenge peroxyl radicals and will decrease the generation of fluorescence. Consequently, the antioxidant activity of a sample can be evaluated by assessing the decrease in the cellular fluorescence.

Several reviews were published regarding this topic [18, 65, 66]. Based on the CAA concept introduced in [160], CAA was used to determine the antioxidant capacity of dietary supplements, foods and phytochemicals in cell cultures [159]. In this study, human hepatocarcinoma HepG2 cells were loaded with the redox sensor DCFH which is oxidized to fluorescent DCF by the $ROO^{\bullet}$ resulted from the thermal decomposition of AAPH. Antioxidants diminish the fluorescent radiation emitted by DCF. CAA is expressed as μmoles of quercetin equivalents per 100 μmol of tested pure compound or per 100 g product (vegetables, fruits, etc.). Several cell sorts have been employed for the CAA assay beyond HepG2, e.g., Caco-2 matured differentiated intestinal cells [161], human gastric adenocarcinoma cell line AGS [162], etc.

Cellular oxidative stress can also be elicited by exposing cell cultures to H_2O_2 (in the mM range) and then measuring fluorimetrically the oxidation of the probe (DCFH) [163].

Saccharomyces cerevisiae cells were employed in a CAA assay to measure antioxidant capacity of different types of products in living systems [164]. Pretreatment of

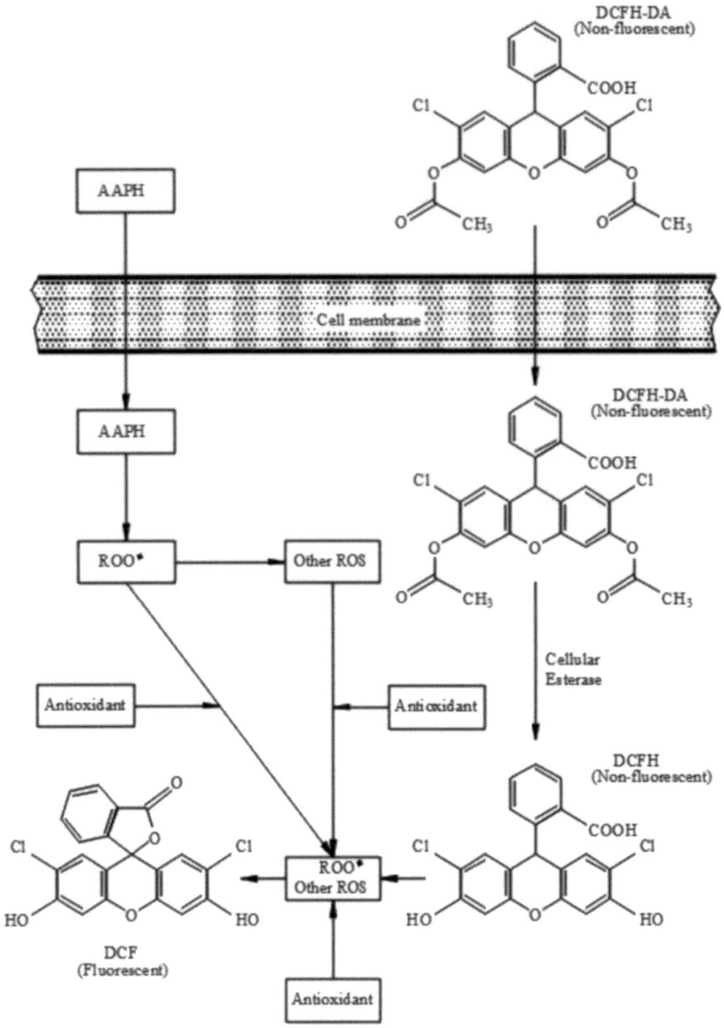

Figure 4.
Schematic presentation of cellular antioxidant activity assay. DCFH-DA, _ dichlorofluorescin diacetate; DCFH, 2′,7′-dichlorofluorescin; DCF, dichlorofluorescein; AAPH, 2, 2′-azo bis(2-amidinopropane) dihydrochloride.

the cells with different flavonoids [164] or mixtures of polyphenols [165] partially diminished the damage generated by H_2O_2.

S. cerevisiae as a model organism system for the antioxidant activity assessment of dietary natural products is reviewed in [65].

An investigation of antioxidant activities of 44 types of dark teas using the DPPH, ABTS, FRAP assays, and CAA assay (by using HepG2 cells) is reported in [166]. Correlation analysis indicated that there was a significant positive correlation between the levels of epigallocatechin gallate and the antioxidant activities evaluated using the ABTS and FRAP assays.

The CAA assay is an adequate and very good technique to measure the performance of antioxidants against oxidative stress. In this manner it is evaluated the capacity of a compound or a mixture of compounds to exercise an antioxidant response at the cellular level and to reduce intracellular oxidative stress, not just its capability as a reducing agent or its ROS/RNS scavenging ability. The CAA methodology is closer to a biological approach, and an antioxidant is regarded as a compound useful to modulate the redox state of the cell.

It is indicated to evaluate the antioxidant capacity of a sample by employing several chemical methods and CAA assays. The antioxidant capacities evaluated by CAA assays are not related well with their chemical values because the two types of methods are affected by very distinct factors.

4. Conclusions

Many studies were published concerning the antioxidant capacity of different products. However, with all these research efforts, a direct link between a food TAC value and health benefits was not found [12].

Taking into account the vast material published in the literature the following conclusion regarding the antioxidat assays can be drawn [14, 15]:

- The expression "total antioxidant capacity" (TAC) correspond to the cooperant effect of antioxidants existing in a sample (cumulative and maybe synergistic/antagonistic). It is a more adequate term to express the total antioxidant capability of a sample than the summation of individual antioxidant constituents.

- It is a stringent need to standardize the TAC assays and to formulate the results of measurements as equivalents of a standard material so that to enable relevant comparison between different methods and different samples [18].

- Most methods developed for TAC evaluation are not based on well detailed investigations of the chemical system involved in measurements (antioxidants interactions, pH, effect of solvents, kinetics, etc.) [16, 19].

- Many in vitro antioxidant methods are accomplished at pH values far from physiological pH and cannot have much sense for in *vivo* determinations of antioxidant effect.

- It is very useful to add a cellular-based assay to assess the analyzed sample capability to generate a cellular antioxidant response, in addition to its ability as a good scavenger of ROS/RNS [18].

- Potential mutual action of antioxidants (i.e., synergistic or antagonistic effects) or prooxidant actions of antioxidants (e.g., under the influence of the composition of the medium) should be taken into account [16, 167].

- For testing natural compounds it is necessary to employ several *in vitro* chemical-based assay that measures various facets of the reactivity of the antioxidants toward ROS/RNS [18]. Including a CAA assay is highly recommended [20].

Taking into account our evaluation regarding the state-of-the-art in the field of antioxidant capacity/activity assays we consider that the assessment regarding this subject expressed in [25] is correct, namely:" Twenty five years of antioxidant screening have NOT resolved issues of assay chemistry, standardization, and reporting; provided significant insight into chemical mechanisms and factors controlling antioxidant action; clearly connected *in vitro* assay chemistry to *in vivo* actions; established rate constants for reaction of antioxidants with radicals that are relevant in foods and biological tissues;...".

The *in vitro* antioxidant assays and the determination of total phenolic content employing colorimetric methods are not only used for the evaluation of potential beneficial effects of different products. There are also used for the quality control of natural products and foods [166, 168] where the antioxidant capacity of commercial samples, evaluated by *in vitro* assays, can be collated against reference materials. Hence, trends can be very valuable for comparing samples from the same materials. In food technology, *in vitro* antioxidant methods and TPC assay may be useful to assess, e.g., the antioxidant actions of herbal extracts on lipid-rich foods, the effects of processing steps on the stability of phenolic compounds from herbal extracts [168] employed to counteract lipid oxidation, or to obtain more antioxidant compounds from raw materials. In the area of active packaging, radical scavenging assays can contribute to assessing efficiency of antioxidant packaging formulations [169]. The *in vitro* methodologies for antioxidant and TPC assays are applied in routine quality control programs by food companies in many countries [170, 171]. The methodologies for antioxidant and TPC assays can be considered valuable high-throughput, low cost tools used to evaluate and find antioxidant sources and for quality control of foods and natural products.

Acknowledgements

This work was supported by a grant of the Romanian Ministry of Education and Research, CCCDI - UEFISCDI, project number PN-III-P2-2.1-PED-2019-3945, contract 362 PED, within PNCDI III.

Author details

Andrei Florin Danet
Faculty of Chemistry, University of Bucharest, Bucharest, Romania

*Address all correspondence to: andrei.danet@g.unibuc.ro

References

[1] Shahidi F, Zhong Y. Measurement of antioxidant activity. Journal of Functional Foods. 2015;18:757-781. DOI: 10.1016/j.jff.2015.01.047

[2] Halliwell B. Antioxidant characterization - methodology and mechanism. Biochemical Pharmacology. 1995;49(10):1341-1348. DOI: 10.1016/0006-2952(95)00088-h

[3] Halliwell B, Murcia MA, Chirico S, Aruoma OI. Free-radicals and antioxidants in food and in vivo -what they do and how they work Critical Reviews in Food Science and Nutrition. 1995;35(1-2):7-20. DOI: 10.1080/10408399509527682

[4] Amarowicz R, Pegg RB, Rahimi-Moghaddam P, Barl B, Weil JA. Free-radical scavenging capacity and antioxidant activity of selected plant species from the Canadian prairies. Food Chemistry. 2004;84(4):551-562. DOI: 10.1016/s0308-8146(03)00278-4

[5] Apak R. Current Issues in Antioxidant Measurement. Journal of Agricultural and Food Chemistry. 2019;67(33):9187-9202. DOI: 10.1021/acs.jafc.9b03657

[6] Huang DJ, Ou BX, Prior RL. The chemistry behind antioxidant capacity assays. Journal of Agricultural and Food Chemistry. 2005;53(6):1841-1856. DOI: 10.1021/jf030723c

[7] Re R, Pellegrini N, Proteggente A, Pannala A, Yang M, Rice-Evans C. Antioxidant activity applying an improved ABTS radical cation decolorization assay. Free Radical Biology and Medicine. 1999;26(9-10):1231-1237. DOI: 10.1016/s0891-5849(98)00315-3

[8] Brand-Williams W, Cuvelier ME, Berset C. Use of free-radical method to evaluate antioxidant activity Food Science and Technology-Lebensmittel-Wissenschaft & Technologie. 1995;28(1):25-30. DOI:

[9] Benzie IFF, Strain JJ. The ferric reducing ability of plasma (FRAP) as a measure of "antioxidant power": The FRAP assay. Analytical Biochemistry. 1996;239(1):70-76. DOI: 10.1006/abio.1996.0292

[10] Apak R, Guclu K, Ozyurek M, Celik SE. Mechanism of antioxidant capacity assays and the CUPRAC (cupric ion reducing antioxidant capacity) assay. Microchimica Acta. 2008;160(4):413-419. DOI: 10.1007/s00604-007-0777-0

[11] Berker KI, Olgun FAO, Ozyurt D, Demirata B, Apak R. Modified Folin-Ciocalteu Antioxidant Capacity Assay for Measuring Lipophilic Antioxidants. Journal of Agricultural and Food Chemistry. 2013;61(20):4783-4791. DOI: 10.1021/jf400249k

[12] Pellegrini N, Vitaglione P, Granato D, Fogliano V. Twenty-five years of total antioxidant capacity measurement of foods and biological fluids: merits and limitations. Journal of the Science of Food and Agriculture. 2020;100(14):5064-5078. DOI: 10.1002/jsfa.9550

[13] Gulcin I. Antioxidants and antioxidant methods: an updated overview. Archives of Toxicology. 2020;94(3):651-715. DOI: 10.1007/s00204-020-02689-3

[14] Apak R, Ozyurek M, Guclu K, Capanoglu E. Antioxidant Activity/Capacity Measurement. 1. Classification, Physicochemical Principles, Mechanisms, and Electron Transfer (ET)-Based Assays. Journal of Agricultural and Food Chemistry. 2016;64(5):997-1027. DOI: 10.1021/acs.jafc.5b04739

[15] Apak R, Ozyurek M, Guclu K, Capanoglu E. Antioxidant Activity/Capacity Measurement. 2. Hydrogen Atom Transfer (HAT)-Based, Mixed-Mode (Electron Transfer (ET)/HAT), and Lipid Peroxidation Assays. Journal of Agricultural and Food Chemistry. 2016;64(5):1028-1045. DOI: 10.1021/acs.jafc.5b04743

[16] Apak R, Ozyurek M, Guclu K, Capanoglu E. Antioxidant Activity/Capacity Measurement. 3. Reactive Oxygen and Nitrogen Species (ROS/RNS) Scavenging Assays, Oxidative Stress Biomarkers, and Chromatographic/Chemometric Assays. Journal of Agricultural and Food Chemistry. 2016;64(5):1046-1070. DOI: 10.1021/acs.jafc.5b04744

[17] Bunaciu AA, Danet AF, Fleschin S, Aboul-Enein HY. Recent Applications for in Vitro Antioxidant Activity Assay. Critical Reviews in Analytical Chemistry. 2016;46(5):389-399. DOI: 10.1080/10408347.2015.1101369

[18] Lopez-Alarcon C, Denicola A. Evaluating the antioxidant capacity of natural products: A review on chemical and cellular-based assays. Analytica Chimica Acta. 2013;763:1-10. DOI: 10.1016/j.aca.2012.11.051

[19] Niki E. Assessment of Antioxidant Capacity in vitro and in vivo. Free Radical Biology and Medicine. 2010;49(4):503-515. DOI: 10.1016/j.freeradbiomed.2010.04.016

[20] Apak R, Capanoglu E, Shahidi F, editors. Measurement of Antioxidant Activity & Capacity: Recent Trends and Applications. 1st ed. Chichester: Wiley; 2018. DOI: 10.1002/9781119135388

[21] Amorati R, Valgimigli L. Advantages and limitations of common testing methods for antioxidants. Free Radical Research. 2015;49(5):633-649. DOI: 10.3109/10715762.2014.996146

[22] Amorati R, Valgimigli L. Methods To Measure the Antioxidant Activity of Phytochemicals and Plant Extracts. Journal of Agricultural and Food Chemistry. 2018;66(13):3324-3329. DOI: 10.1021/acs.jafc.8b01079

[23] Shivakumar A, Kumar MSY. Critical Review on the Analytical Mechanistic Steps in the Evaluation of Antioxidant Activity. Critical Reviews in Analytical Chemistry. 2018;48(3):214-236. DOI: 10.1080/10408347.2017.1400423

[24] Ilyasov IR, Beloborodov VL, Selivanova IA, Terekhov RP. ABTS/PP Decolorization Assay of Antioxidant Capacity Reaction Pathways. International Journal of Molecular Sciences. 2020;21(3):article number 1131. DOI: 10.3390/ijms21031131

[25] Schaich KM, Tian X, Xie J. Hurdles and pitfalls in measuring antioxidant efficacy: A critical evaluation of ABTS, DPPH, and ORAC assays. Journal of Functional Foods. 2015;14:111-125. DOI: 10.1016/j.jff.2015.01.043

[26] Karadag A, Ozcelik B, Saner S. Review of Methods to Determine Antioxidant Capacities. Food Analytical Methods. 2009;2(1):41-60. DOI: 10.1007/s12161-008-9067-7

[27] Moon JK, Shibamoto T. Antioxidant Assays for Plant and Food Components. Journal of Agricultural and Food Chemistry. 2009;57(5):1655-1666. DOI: 10.1021/jf803537k

[28] Antolovich M, Prenzler PD, Patsalides E, McDonald S, Robards K. Methods for testing antioxidant activity. Analyst. 2002;127:183-198. DOI: 10.1039/b009171p

[29] Danet AF, Badea-Doni M. Determination of Lipid Oxidation by Chemiluminescence Reagents. In: RuizCapillas C, Nollet LML, editors. Flow Injection Analysis of Food Additives. Boca Raton: CRC Press; 2016. p. 623-638. DOI: 10.1201/b19644

[30] Ratnam DV, Ankola DD, Bhardwaj V, Sahana DK, Kumar MNVR. Role of antioxidants in prophylaxis and therapy: A pharmaceutical perspective. Journal of Controlled Release. 2006;113(3):189-207. DOI: 10.1016/j.jconrel.2006.04.015

[31] MacDonald-Wicks LK, Wood LG, Garg ML. Methodology for the determination of biological antioxidant capacity in vitro: a review. Journal of the Science of Food and Agriculture. 2006;86(13):2046-2056. DOI: 10.1002/jsfa.2603

[32] Carocho M, Morales P, Ferreira ICFR. Antioxidants: Reviewing the chemistry, food applications, legislation and role as preservatives. Trends in Food Science & Technology. 2018;71:107-120. DOI: 10.1016/j.tifs.2017.11.008

[33] Munialo CD, Naumovski N, Sergi D, Stewart D, Mellor DD. Critical evaluation of the extrapolation of data relative to antioxidant function from the laboratory and their implications on food production and human health: a review. International Journal of Food Science and Technology. 2019;54(5):1448-1459. DOI: 10.1111/ijfs.14135

[34] Sadeer NB, Montesano D, Albrizio S, Zengin G, Mahomoodally MF. The Versatility of Antioxidant Assays in Food Science and Safety-Chemistry, Applications, Strengths, and Limitations. Antioxidants. 2020;9(8):article number 709. DOI: 10.3390/antiox9080709

[35] Ivanova A, Gerasimova E, Gazizullina E. Study of Antioxidant Properties of Agents from the Perspective of Their Action Mechanisms. Molecules. 2020;25(18):article number 4251. DOI: 10.3390/molecules25184251

[36] Pellegrini N, Del Rio D, Colombi B, Bianchi M, Brighenti F. Application of the 2,2 '-azinobis(3-ethylbenzothiazoline-6-sulfonic acid) radical cation assay to a flow injection system for the evaluation of antioxidant activity of some pure compounds and beverages. Journal of Agricultural and Food Chemistry. 2003;51(1):260-264. DOI: 10.1021/jf020657z

[37] Prior RL, Wu XL, Schaich K. Standardized methods for the determination of antioxidant capacity and phenolics in foods and dietary supplements. Journal of Agricultural and Food Chemistry. 2005;53(10):4290-4302. DOI: 10.1021/jf0502698

[38] Shahidi F, Zhong Y. Lipid oxidation and improving the oxidative stability. Chemical Society Reviews. 2010;39(11):4067-4079. DOI: 10.1039/b922183m

[39] Christodouleas D, Papadopoulos K, Calokerinos AC. Determination of Total Antioxidant Activity of Edible Oils as well as Their Aqueous and Organic Extracts by Chemiluminescence. Food Analytical Methods. 2011;4(4):475-484. DOI: 10.1007/s12161-010-9189-6

[40] Hirayama O, Takagi M, Hukumoto K, Katoh S. Evaluation of antioxidant activity by chemiluminescence. Analytical Biochemistry. 1997;247(2):237-241. DOI: 10.1006/abio.1997.2053

[41] Ghiselli A, Serafini M, Maiani G, Azzini E, Ferroluzzi A. A FLUORESCENCE-BASED METHOD FOR MEASURING TOTAL PLASMA ANTIOXIDANT CAPABILITY. Free Radical Biology and Medicine. 1995;18(1):29-36. DOI: 10.1016/0891-5849(94)00102-p

[42] Senthilmohan ST, Davis BM, Wilson PF, McEwan MJ. Improved peroxyl radical scavenging TOSC assay to quantify antioxidant capacity using SIFT-MS. Redox Report.

2009;14(5):197-204. DOI: 10.1179/135100009x12525712409571

[43] Prieto MA, Rodriguez-Amado I, Vazquez JA, Murado MA. beta-Carotene Assay Revisited. Application To Characterize and Quantify Antioxidant and Prooxidant Activities in a Microplate. Journal of Agricultural and Food Chemistry. 2012;60(36):8983-8993. DOI: 10.1021/jf302218g

[44] Ozyurek M, Guclu K, Tutem E, Baskan KS, Ercag E, Celik SE, et al. A comprehensive review of CUPRAC methodology. Analytical Methods. 2011;3(11):2439-2453. DOI: 10.1039/c1ay05320e

[45] Alarcon-Angeles G, Alvarez-Romero GA, Merkoci A. Emerging Nanomaterials for Analytical Detection. Biosensors for Sustainable Food - New Opportunities and Technical Challenges, Comprehensive Analytical Chemistry. 74. Amsterdam: Elsevier; 2016. p. 195-246. DOI:10.1016/bs.coac.2016.03.022

[46] Della Pelle F, Compagnone D. Nanomaterial-Based Sensing and Biosensing of Phenolic Compounds and Related Antioxidant Capacity in Food. Sensors. 2018;18(2):article number 462. DOI: 10.3390/s18020462

[47] Vasilescu A, Sharpe E, Andreescu S. Nanoparticle-Based Technologies for the Detection of Food Antioxidants. Current Analytical Chemistry. 2012;8(4):495-505. DOI: 10.2174/157341112803216780

[48] Yu ZY, Li HJ, Lu JH, Zhang XM, Liu NK, Zhang X. Hydrothermal synthesis of Fe2O3/graphene nanocomposite for selective determination of ascorbic acid in the presence of uric acid. Electrochimica Acta. 2015;158:264-270. DOI: 10.1016/j.electacta.2015.01.131

[49] Sochor J, Dobes J, Krystofova O, Ruttkay-Nedecky B, Babula P, Pohanka M, et al. Electrochemistry as a Tool for Studying Antioxidant Properties. International Journal of Electrochemical Science. 2013;8(6):8464-8489. DOI:

[50] Pisoschi AM, Cimpeanu C, Predoi G. Electrochemical Methods for Total Antioxidant Capacity and its Main Contributors Determination: A review. Open Chemistry. 2015;13(1):824-856. DOI: 10.1515/chem-2015-0099

[51] Hoyos-Arbelaez J, Vazquez M, Contreras-Calderon J. Electrochemical methods as a tool for determining the antioxidant capacity of food and beverages: A review. Food Chemistry. 2017;221:1371-1381. DOI: 10.1016/j.foodchem.2016.11.017

[52] Chevion S, Roberts MA, Chevion M. The use of cyclic voltammetry for the evaluation of antioxidant capacity. Free Radical Biology and Medicine. 2000;28(6):860-870. DOI: 10.1016/s0891-5849(00)00178-7

[53] Piljac-Zegarac J, Valek L, Stipcevic T, Martinez S. Electrochemical determination of antioxidant capacity of fruit tea infusions. Food Chemistry. 2010;121(3):820-825. DOI: 10.1016/j.foodchem.2009.12.090

[54] Souza LP, Calegari F, Zarbin AJG, Marcolino-Junior LH, Bergamini MF. Voltammetric Determination of the Antioxidant Capacity in Wine Samples Using a Carbon Nanotube Modified Electrode. Journal of Agricultural and Food Chemistry. 2011;59(14):7620-7625. DOI: 10.1021/jf2005589

[55] Novak I, Seruga M, Komorsky-Lovric S. Characterisation of catechins in green and black teas using square-wave voltammetry and RP-HPLC-ECD. Food Chemistry. 2010;122(4):1283-1289. DOI: 10.1016/j.foodchem.2010.03.084

[56] Yashin YI, Nemzer BV, Ryzhnev VY, Yashin AY, Chernousova NI, Fedina PA.

Creation of a Databank for Content of Antioxidants in Food Products by an Amperometric Method. Molecules. 2010;15(10):7450-7466. DOI: 10.3390/molecules15107450

[57] Pisoschi A, Cheregi M, Danet A. Total Antioxidant Capacity of Some Commercial Fruit Juices: Electrochemical and Spectrophotometrical Approaches. Molecules. 2009;14(1):480-493. DOI: 10.3390/molecules14010480

[58] David M, Serban A, Radulescu C, Danet AF, Florescu M. Bioelectrochemical evaluation of plant extracts and gold nanozyme-based sensors for total antioxidant capacity determination. Bioelectrochemistry. 2019;129:124-134. DOI: 10.1016/j.bioelechem.2019.05.011

[59] Gulcin I, Sat IG, Beydemir S, Kufrevioglu OI. Evaluation of the in vitro antioxidant properties of broccoli extracts (Brassica oleracea L.). Italian Journal of Food Science. 2004;16(1):17-30. DOI:

[60] Carlos Sanchez-Rangel J, Benavides J, Basilio Heredia J, Cisneros-Zevallos L, Jacobo-Velazquez DA. The Folin-Ciocalteu assay revisited: improvement of its specificity for total phenolic content determination. Analytical Methods. 2013;5(21):5990-5999. DOI: 10.1039/c3ay41125g

[61] Granato D, Santos JS, Maciel LG, Nunes DS. Chemical perspective and criticism on selected analytical methods used to estimate the total content of phenolic compounds in food matrices. Trac-Trends in Analytical Chemistry. 2016;80:266-279. DOI: 10.1016/j.trac.2016.03.010

[62] Barriuso B, Astiasaran I, Ansorena D. A review of analytical methods measuring lipid oxidation status in foods: a challenging task. European Food Research and Technology. 2013;236(1):1-15. DOI: 10.1007/s00217-012-1866-9

[63] Ghani MA, Barril C, Bedgood DR, Jr., Prenzler PD. Measurement of antioxidant activity with the thiobarbituric acid reactive substances assay. Food Chemistry. 2017;230:195-207. DOI: 10.1016/j.foodchem.2017.02.127

[64] Guillen-Sans R, Guzman-Chozas M. The thiobarbituric acid (TBA) reaction in foods: A review. Critical Reviews in Food Science and Nutrition. 1998;38(4):315-330. DOI: 10.1080/10408699891274228

[65] Meng D, Zhang P, Li S, Ho C-T, Zhao H. Antioxidant activity evaluation of dietary phytochemicals using Saccharomyces cerevisiae as a model. Journal of Functional Foods. 2017;38:36-44. DOI: 10.1016/j.jff.2017.08.041

[66] Yang C, Shahidi F, Tsao R. Biomarkers of oxidative stress and cellular-based assays of indirect antioxidant measurement. In: Apak R, Capanoglu E, Shahidi F, editors. Measurement of Antioxidant Activity & Capacity: Recent Trends and Applications. Chichester: Wiley; 2018. p. 165-186. DOI:10.1002/9781119135388.ch9

[67] Cano A, Arnao MB. ABTS/TEAC (2,2'-azino-bis(3-ethylbenzothiazoline-6-sulfonic acid)/Trolox (R)-Equivalent Antioxidant Capacity) radical scavenging mixed-mode assay. In: Apak R, Capanoglu E, Shahidi F, editors. Measurement of Antioxidant Activity & Capacity: Recent Trends and Applications. Chichester: Wiley; 2018. p. 117-139. DOI:10.1002/9781119135388.ch7

[68] Zheng L, Zhao MM, Xiao CQ, Zhao QZ, Su GW. Practical problems when using ABTS assay to assess the radical-scavenging activity of

peptides: Importance of controlling reaction pH and time. Food Chemistry. 2016;192:288-294. DOI: 10.1016/j.foodchem.2015.07.015

[69] Xie J, Schaich KM. Re-evaluation of the 2,2-Diphenyl-1-picrylhydrazyl Free Radical (DPPH) Assay for Antioxidant Activity. Journal of Agricultural and Food Chemistry. 2014;62(19):4251-4260. DOI: 10.1021/jf500180u

[70] Ozcelik B, Lee JH, Min DB. Effects of light, oxygen, and pH on the absorbance of 2,2-diphenyl-1-picrylhydrazyl. Journal of Food Science. 2003;68(2):487-490. DOI: 10.1111/j.1365-2621.2003.tb05699.x

[71] Apak R, Gorinstein S, Bohm V, Schaich KM, Ozyurek M, Guclu K. Methods of measurement and evaluation of natural antioxidant capacity/activity (IUPAC Technical Report). Pure and Applied Chemistry. 2013;85(5):957-998. DOI: 10.1351/pac-rep-12-07-15

[72] Huang DJ, Ou BX, Hampsch-Woodill M, Flanagan JA, Deemer EK. Development and validation of oxygen radical absorbance capacity assay for lipophilic antioxidants using randomly methylated beta-cyclodextrin as the solubility enhancer. Journal of Agricultural and Food Chemistry. 2002;50(7):1815-1821. DOI: 10.1021/jf0113732

[73] Wu XL, Gu LW, Holden J, Haytowitz DB, Gebhardt SE, Beecher G, et al. Development of a database for total antioxidant capacity in foods: a preliminary study. Journal of Food Composition and Analysis. 2004;17(3-4):407-422. DOI: 10.1016/j.jfca.2004.03.001

[74] Nkhili E, Brat P. Reexamination of the ORAC assay: effect of metal ions. Analytical and Bioanalytical Chemistry. 2011;400(5):1451-1458. DOI: 10.1007/s00216-011-4884-8

[75] Popa C, Farcasanu I, Jipa S, Zaharescu T, Danet A. Chemiluminescence Determination of the Total Antioxidant Capacity of Rosemary Extract. Revista De Chimie. 2012;63(7):715-719. DOI:

[76] Popa C-V, Lungu L, Savoiu M, Bradu C, Dinoiu V, Danet AF. Total antioxidant activity and phenols and flavonoids content of several plant extracts. International Journal of Food Properties. 2012;15(3):691-701. DOI: 10.1080/10942912.2010.498545

[77] Popa CV, Danet AF, Jipa S, Zaharescu T. Determination of Total Antioxidant Capacity of Some Fruit Juices and Noncarbonated Soft Drinks by a FIA-CL Method. Revista De Chimie. 2012;63(10):978-983. DOI:

[78] Lungu L, Popa C, Savoiu M, Danet A, Dinoiu V. Antioxidant Activity of Brassica Oleracea L., Allium Cepa L. and Beta Vulgaris L. Extracts. Revista De Chimie. 2010;61(10):911-914. DOI:

[79] Popa C, Danet A, Jipa S, Zaharescu T. Determination of Total Antioxidant Activity of Wines Using a Flow Injection Method with Chemiluminescence Detection. Revista De Chimie. 2010;61(1):11-16. DOI:

[80] Weingerl V, Strlic M, Kocar D. Evaluation of chemiluminometric method for determination of polyphenols in wine Analytical Letters. 2011;44(7):1310-1322. DOI: 10.1080/00032719.2010.512674

[81] Zargoosh K, Ghayeb Y, Aeineh N, Qandalee M. Evaluation of Antioxidant Capacity of Hydrophilic and Hydrophobic Antioxidants Using Peroxyoxalate Chemiluminescence Reaction of the Novel Furandicarboxylate Derivative. Food Analytical Methods. 2014;7(2):283-290. DOI: 10.1007/s12161-013-9625-5

[82] Giokas DL, Vlessidis AG, Evmiridis NP. On-line selective

detection of antioxidants free-radical scavenging activity based on Co(II)/EDTA-induced luminol chemiluminescence by flow injection analysis. Analytica Chimica Acta. 2007;589(1):59-65. DOI: 10.1016/j.aca.2007.02.041

[83] Fassoula E, Economou A, Calokerinos A. Development and validation of a sequential-injection method with chemiluminescence detection for the high throughput assay of the total antioxidant capacity of wines. Talanta. 2011;85(3):1412-1418. DOI: 10.1016/j.talanta.2011.06.037

[84] Chladkova G, Kunovska K, Chocholous P, Polasek M, Sklenarova H. Automatic screening of antioxidants based on the evaluation of kinetics of suppression of chemiluminescence in a luminol-hydrogen peroxide system using a sequential injection analysis setup with a flow-batch detection cell. Analytical Methods. 2019;11(19):2531-2536. DOI: 10.1039/c9ay00160c

[85] Popa C-V, Cristea N-I, Farcasanu I-C, Danet AF. Total Antioxidant Capacity of Some Fruit Seeds Extracts. Revista De Chimie. 2013;64(12):1377-1380.

[86] Iranifam M, Al Lawati HAJ. Monitoring the antioxidant capacity in honey and fruit juices using a microfluidic device with a NaHCO3-H2O2-Co2+ chemiluminescence reaction. Food Chemistry. 2019;297:article number 124930. DOI: 10.1016/j.foodchem.2019.05.204

[87] Kishikawa N, El-Maghrabey M, Nagamune Y, Nagai K, Ohyama K, Kuroda N. A Smart Advanced Chemiluminescence-Sensing Platform for Determination and Imaging of the Tissue Distribution of Natural Antioxidants. Analytical Chemistry. 2020;92(10):6984-6992. DOI: 10.1021/acs.analchem.0c00044

[88] Christodouleas D, Fotakis C, Papadopoulos K, Yannakopoulou E, Calokerinos AC. Development and validation of a chemiluminogenic method for the evaluation of antioxidant activity of hydrophilic and hydrophobic antioxidants. Analytica Chimica Acta. 2009;652(1-2):295-302. DOI: 10.1016/j.aca.2009.08.012

[89] Ghiselli A, Serafini M, Natella F, Scaccini C. Total antioxidant capacity as a tool to assess redox status: Critical view and experimental data. Free Radical Biology and Medicine. 2000;29(11):1106-1114. DOI: 10.1016/s0891-5849(00)00394-4

[90] Whitehead TP, Thorpe GHG, Maxwell SRJ. Enhanced chemiluminescence assay for antioxidant capacity in biological-fluids Analytica Chimica Acta. 1992;266(2):265-277. DOI: 10.1016/0003-2670(92)85052-8

[91] Bastos E, Romoff P, Eckert C, Baader W. Evaluation of antiradical capacity by H2O2-hemin-induced luminol chemiluminescence. Journal of Agricultural and Food Chemistry. 2003;51(25):7481-7488. DOI: 10.1021/jf0345189

[92] Valkonen M, Kuusi T. Spectrophotometric assay for total peroxyl radical-trapping antioxidant potential in human serum. J Lipid Res. 1997;38(4):823-833. DOI:

[93] Delange RJ, Glazer AN. Phycoerythrin fluorescence-based assay for peroxy-radicals - a screen for biologically relevant protective agents. Analytical Biochemistry. 1989;177(2):300-306. DOI: 10.1016/0003-2697(89)90056-0

[94] Somogyi A, Rosta K, Pusztai P, Tulassay Z, Nagy G. Antioxidant measurements. Physiological Measurement. 2007;28(4):R41-R55. DOI: 10.1088/0967-3334/28/4/r01

[95] Lage MAP, Garcia MAM, Alvarez JAV, Anders Y, Curran TP. A new microplate procedure for simultaneous assessment of lipophilic and hydrophilic antioxidants and pro-oxidants, using crocin and beta-carotene bleaching methods in a single combined assay: Tea extracts as a case study. Food Research International. 2013;53(2):836-846. DOI: 10.1016/j.foodres.2012.11.026

[96] Ou BX, Huang DJ, Hampsch-Woodill M, Flanagan JA, Deemer EK. Analysis of antioxidant activities of common vegetables employing oxygen radical absorbance capacity (ORAC) and ferric reducing antioxidant power (FRAP) assays: A comparative study. Journal of Agricultural and Food Chemistry. 2002;50(11):3122-3128. DOI: 10.1021/jf0116606

[97] Cekic SD, Kara N, Tutem E, Baskan KS, Apak R. Protein-incorporated serum total antioxidant capacity measurement by a modified CUPRAC (cupric reducing antioxidant capacity) method Analytical Letters. 2012;45(7):754-763. DOI: 10.1080/00032719.2011.653901

[98] Bean H, Radu F, De E, Schuler C, Leggett RE, Levin RM. Comparative evaluation of antioxidant reactivity within obstructed and control rabbit urinary bladder tissue using FRAP and CUPRAC assays. Molecular and Cellular Biochemistry. 2009;323(1-2):139-142. DOI: 10.1007/s11010-008-9972-5

[99] Apak R, Guclu K, Ozyurek M, Karademir SE. Novel total antioxidant capacity index for dietary polyphenols and vitamins C and E, using their cupric ion reducing capability in the presence of neocuproine: CUPRAC method. Journal of Agricultural and Food Chemistry. 2004;52(26):7970-7981. DOI: 10.1021/jf048741x

[100] Ozyurek M, Bektasoglu B, Guclu K, Gungor N, Apak R. Simultaneous total antioxidant capacity assay of lipophilic and hydrophilic antioxidants in the same acetone-water solution containing 2% methyl-beta-cyclodextrin using the cupric reducing antioxidant capacity (CUPRAC) method. Analytica Chimica Acta. 2008;630(1):28-39. DOI: 10.1016/j.aca.2008.09.057

[101] Bener M, Ozyurek M, Guclu K, Apak R. Development of a Low-Cost Optical Sensor for Cupric Reducing Antioxidant Capacity Measurement of Food Extracts. Analytical Chemistry. 2010;82(10):4252-4258. DOI: 10.1021/ac100646k

[102] Apak R, Guclu K, Demirata B, Ozyurek M, Celik SE, Bektasoglu B, et al. Comparative evaluation of various total antioxidant capacity assays applied to phenolic compounds with the CUPRAC assay. Molecules. 2007;12(7):1496-1547. DOI: 10.3390/12071496

[103] Vilela D, Cristina Gonzalez M, Escarpa A. Nanoparticles as analytical tools for in-vitro antioxidant-capacity assessment and beyond. Trac-Trends in Analytical Chemistry. 2015;64:1-16. DOI: 10.1016/j.trac.2014.07.017

[104] Scampicchio M, Wang J, Blasco AJ, Arribas AS, Mannino S, Escarpa A. Nanoparticle-based assays of antioxidant activity. Analytical Chemistry. 2006;78(6):2060-2063. DOI: 10.1021/ac052007a

[105] Liu Q, Liu H, Yuan Z, Wei D, Ye Y. Evaluation of antioxidant activity of chrysanthemum extracts and tea beverages by gold nanoparticles-based assay. Colloids and Surfaces B-Biointerfaces. 2012;92:348-352. DOI: 10.1016/j.colsurfb.2011.12.007

[106] Szydlowska-Czerniak A, Tulodziecka A. Comparison of a silver nanoparticle-based method and the modified spectrophotometric methods for assessing antioxidant capacity of rapeseed varieties. Food Chemistry.

2013;141(3):1865-1871. DOI: 10.1016/j.foodchem.2013.04.111

[107] Bordbar MM, Hemmateenejad B, Tashkhourian J, Nami-Ana SF. An optoelectronic tongue based on anarray of gold and silver nanoparticles for analysis of natural, synthetic and biological antioxidants. Microchimica Acta. 2018;185(10):article number 493. DOI: 10.1007/s00604-018-3021-1

[108] Sharpe E, Frasco T, Andreescu D, Andreescu S. Portable ceria nanoparticle-based assay for rapid detection of food antioxidants (NanoCerac). Analyst. 2013;138(1):249-262. DOI: 10.1039/c2an36205h

[109] Sharpe E, Bradley R, Frasco T, Jayathilaka D, Marsh A, Andreescu S. Metal oxide based multisensor array and portable database for field analysis of antioxidants. Sensors and Actuators B-Chemical. 2014;193:552-562. DOI: 10.1016/j.snb.2013.11.088

[110] Popa CV, Vasilescu A, Litescu SC, Albu C, Danet AF. Metal Nano-Oxide based Colorimetric Sensor Array for the Determination of Plant Polyphenols with Antioxidant Properties. Analytical Letters. 2020;53(4):627-645. DOI: 10.1080/00032719.2019.1662430

[111] Della Pelle F, Cristina Gonzalez M, Sergi M, Del Carlo M, Compagnone D, Escarpa A. Gold Nanoparticles-based Extraction-Free Colorimetric Assay in Organic Media: An Optical Index for Determination of Total Polyphenols in Fat-Rich Samples. Analytical Chemistry. 2015;87(13):6905-6911. DOI: 10.1021/acs.analchem.5b01489

[112] Vilela D, Cristina Gonzalez M, Escarpa A. Gold-nanosphere formation using food sample endogenous polyphenols for in-vitro assessment of antioxidant capacity. Analytical and Bioanalytical Chemistry. 2012;404(2):341-349. DOI: 10.1007/s00216-012-6084-6

[113] Vilela D, Castaneda R, Cristina Gonzalez M, Mendoza S, Escarpa A. Fast and reliable determination of antioxidant capacity based on the formation of gold nanoparticles. Microchimica Acta. 2015;182(1-2):105-111. DOI: 10.1007/s00604-014-1306-6

[114] Ozyurek M, Gungor N, Baki S, Guclu K, Apak R. Development of a Silver Nanoparticle-Based Method for the Antioxidant Capacity Measurement of Polyphenols. Analytical Chemistry. 2012;84(18):8052-8059. DOI: 10.1021/ac301925b

[115] Teerasong S, Jinnarak A, Chaneam S, Wilairat P, Nacapricha D. Poly(vinyl alcohol) capped silver nanoparticles for antioxidant assay based on seed-mediated nanoparticle growth. Talanta. 2017;170:193-198. DOI: 10.1016/j.talanta.2017.04.009

[116] Gatselou V, Christodouleas DC, Kouloumpis A, Gournis D, Giokas DL. Determination of phenolic compounds using spectral and color transitions of rhodium nanoparticles. Analytica Chimica Acta. 2016;932:80-87. DOI: 10.1016/j.aca.2016.05.029

[117] Hemmateenejad B, Shamsipur M, Khosousi T, Shanehsaz M, Firuzi O. Antioxidant activity assay based on the inhibition of oxidation and photobleaching of L-cysteine-capped CdTe quantum dots. Analyst. 2012;137(17):4029-4036. DOI: 10.1039/c2an35588d

[118] Benitez-Martinez S, Valcarcel M. Graphene quantum dots as sensor for phenols in olive oil. Sensors and Actuators B-Chemical. 2014;197:350-357. DOI: 10.1016/j.snb.2014.03.008

[119] Choleva TG, Kappi FA, Giokas DL, Vlessidis AG. Paper-based assay of antioxidant activity using analyte-mediated on-paper nucleation of gold nanoparticles as colorimetric probes.

Analytica Chimica Acta. 2015;860:61-69. DOI: 10.1016/j.aca.2014.12.025

[120] Peng J, Su Y, Huang F-Q, Zuo Q, Yang L, Li J, et al. A simple and rapid fluorescent approach for flavonoids sensor based on gold nanoclusters. Journal of Colloid and Interface Science. 2019;539:175-183. DOI: 10.1016/j.jcis.2018.12.042

[121] Angelis PN, Mendonca JdC, da Rocha LR, Capelari TB, Prete MC, Segatelli MG, et al. Feasibility of a Nano-Carbon Black Paste Electrode for Simultaneous Voltammetric Determination of Antioxidants in Food Samples and Biodiesel in the Presence of Surfactant. Electroanalysis. 2020;32(6):1198-1207. DOI: 10.1002/elan.201900479

[122] Sivakumar M, Pandi K, Chen S-M, Yadav S, Chen T-W, Veeramani V. Highly Sensitive Detection of Gallic Acid in Food Samples by Using Robust NiAl2O4 Nanocomposite Materials. Journal of the Electrochemical Society. 2019;166(2):B29-B34. DOI: 10.1149/2.0121902jes

[123] Ran X, Yang L, Zhang J, Deng G, Li Y, Xie X, et al. Highly sensitive electrochemical sensor based on beta-cyclodextrine-gold@3, 4, 9, 10-perylene tetracarboxylic acid functionalized single-walled carbon nanohorns for simultaneous determination of myricetin and rutin. Analytica Chimica Acta. 2015;892:85-94. DOI: 10.1016/j.aca.2015.08.046

[124] Ziyatdinova G, Kozlova E, Budnikov H. Chronocoulometry of wine on multi-walled carbon nanotube modified electrode: Antioxidant capacity assay. Food Chemistry. 2016;196:405-410. DOI: 10.1016/j.foodchem.2015.09.075

[125] Andrei V, Sharpe E, Vasilescu A, Andreescu S. A single use electrochemical sensor based on biomimetic nanoceria for the detection of wine antioxidants. Talanta. 2016;156:112-118. DOI: 10.1016/j.talanta.2016.04.067

[126] Ceballos C, Fernandez H. Synthetic antioxidants in edible oils by square-wave voltammetry on ultramicroelectrodes. Journal of the American Oil Chemists Society. 2000;77(7):731-735. DOI: 10.1007/s11746-000-0118-1

[127] Medeiros RA, Rocha-Filho RC, Fatibello-Filho O. Simultaneous voltammetric determination of phenolic antioxidants in food using a boron-doped diamond electrode. Food Chemistry. 2010;123(3):886-891. DOI: 10.1016/j.foodchem.2010.05.010

[128] Sousa WR, da Rocha C, Cardoso CL, Silva DHS, Zanoni MVB. Determination of the relative contribution of phenolic antioxidants in orange juice by voltammetric methods. Journal of Food Composition and Analysis. 2004;17(5):619-633. DOI: 10.1016/j.jfca.2003.09.013

[129] Blasco AJ, Crevillen AG, Gonzalez MC, Escarpa A. Direct electrochemical sensing and detection of natural antioxidants and antioxidant capacity in vitro systems. Electroanalysis. 2007;19(22):2275-2286. DOI: 10.1002/elan.200704004

[130] Ivanova AV, Gerasimova EL, Brainina KZ. Potentiometric Study of Antioxidant Activity: Development and Prospects. Critical Reviews in Analytical Chemistry. 2015;45(4):311-322. DOI: 10.1080/10408347.2014.910443

[131] Wang J. Analytical electrochemistry. 2nd ed. Chichester: Wiley-WCH; 2001. 203 p. DOI: 10.1021/ed078p457.2

[132] Jara-PalaciosMJ,Escudero-GileteML, Hernandez-Hierro JM, Heredia FJ, Hernanz D. Cyclic voltammetry to evaluate the antioxidant potential in winemaking by-products. Talanta. 2017;165:211-215. DOI: 10.1016/j.talanta.2016.12.058

[133] Masek A, Chrzescijanska E, Latos M, Kosmalska A. Electrochemical and Spectrophotometric Characterization of the Propolis Antioxidants Properties. International Journal of Electrochemical Science. 2019;14(2):1231-1247. DOI: 10.20964/2019.02.66

[134] Gulaboski R, Mirceski V, Mitrev S. Development of a rapid and simple voltammetric method to determine total antioxidative capacity of edible oils. Food Chemistry. 2013;138(1):116-121. DOI: 10.1016/j.foodchem.2012.10.050

[135] Nikolic MD, Pavlovic AN, Mitic SS, Tosic SB, Mitic MN, Kalicanin BM, et al. Use of cyclic voltammetry to determine the antioxidant capacity of berry fruits: correlation with spectrophotometric assays. European Journal of Horticultural Science. 2019;84(3):152-160. DOI: 10.17660/eJHS.2019/84.3.5

[136] Milardovic S, Ivekovic D, Ruwenjak V, Grabaric BS. Use of DPPH center dot vertical bar DPPH redox couple for biamperometric determination of antioxidant activity. Electroanalysis. 2005;17(20):1847-1853. DOI: 10.1002/elan.200503312

[137] Photinon K, Chalermchart Y, Khanongnuch C, Wang S-H, Liu C-C. A Thick-film Sensor as a Novel Device for Determination of Polyphenols and Their Antioxidant Capacity in White Wine. Sensors. 2010;10(3):1670-1678. DOI: 10.3390/s100301670

[138] Apetrei C, Mirela Apetrei I, Antonio De Saja J, Luz Rodriguez-Mendez M. Carbon Paste Electrodes Made from Different Carbonaceous Materials: Application in the Study of Antioxidants. Sensors. 2011;11(2):1328-1344. DOI: 10.3390/s110201328

[139] Ziyatdinova GK, Nizamova AM, Budnikov HC. Voltammetric determination of curcumin in spices. Journal of Analytical Chemistry. 2012;67(6):591-594. DOI: 10.1134/s1061934812040132

[140] Cardenas A, Frontana C. Evaluation of a carbon ink chemically modified electrode incorporating a copper-neocuproine complex for the quantification of antioxidants. Sensors and Actuators B-Chemical. 2020;313:article number 128070. DOI: 10.1016/j.snb.2020.128070

[141] Ricci A, Parpinello GP, Teslic N, Kilmartin PA, Versari A. Suitability of the Cyclic Voltammetry Measurements and DPPH center dot Spectrophotometric Assay to Determine the Antioxidant Capacity of Food-Grade Oenological Tannins. Molecules. 2019;24(16):article number 2925. DOI: 10.3390/molecules24162925

[142] Pisoschi AM, Pop A, Negulescu GP, Pisoschi A. Determination of Ascorbic Acid Content of Some Fruit Juices and Wine by Voltammetry Performed at Pt and Carbon Paste Electrodes. Molecules. 2011;16(2):1349-1365. DOI: 10.3390/molecules16021349

[143] Yilmaz UT, Kekillioglu A, Mert R. Determination of Gallic acid by differential pulse polarography: Application to fruit juices. Journal of Analytical Chemistry. 2013;68(12):1064-1069. DOI: 10.1134/s1061934813120113

[144] Wang Z, Yang F, Zheng H, Qin X, Luo J, Li Y, et al. Voltammetric determination of TBHQ at a glassy carbon electrode surface activated by in situ chemical oxidation. Analyst. 2014;139(14):3622-3628. DOI: 10.1039/c4an00325j

[145] Silva TR, Westphal E, Gallardo H, Vieira IC. Ionic Organic Film Sensor for Determination of Phenolic Compounds. Electroanalysis. 2014;26(8):1801-1809. DOI: 10.1002/elan.201400197

[146] Tortolini C, Bollella P, Zumpano R, Favero G, Mazzei F, Antiochia R. Metal Oxide Nanoparticle

Based Electrochemical Sensor for Total Antioxidant Capacity (TAC) Detection in Wine Samples. Biosensors-Basel. 2018;8(4): article number 108. DOI: 10.3390/bios8040108

[147] Marcelo Granero A, Fernandez H, Agostini E, Alicia Zon M. An amperometric biosensor based on peroxidases from Brassica napus for the determination of the total polyphenolic content in wine and tea samples. Talanta. 2010;83(1):249-255. DOI: 10.1016/j.talanta.2010.09.016

[148] Amatatongchai M, Laosing S, Chailapakul O, Nacapricha D. Simple flow injection for screening of total antioxidant capacity by amperometric detection of DPPH radical on carbon nanotube modified-glassy carbon electrode. Talanta. 2012;97:267-272. DOI: 10.1016/j.talanta.2012.04.029

[149] Sanchez Arribas A, Martinez-Fernandez M, Moreno M, Bermejo E, Zapardiel A, Chicharro M. Analysis of total polyphenols in wines by FIA with highly stable amperometric detection using carbon nanotube-modified electrodes. Food Chemistry. 2013;136(3-4):1183-1192. DOI: 10.1016/j.foodchem.2012.09.027

[150] Lino FMA, de Sa LZ, Torres IMS, Rocha ML, Dinis TCP, Ghedini PC, et al. Voltammetric and spectrometric determination of antioxidant capacity of selected wines. Electrochimica Acta. 2014;128:25-31. DOI: 10.1016/j.electacta.2013.08.109

[151] Ragubeer N, Beukes DR, Limson JL. Critical assessment of voltammetry for rapid screening of antioxidants in marine algae. Food Chemistry. 2010;121(1):227-232. DOI: 10.1016/j.foodchem.2009.11.076

[152] Santos JS, Alvarenga Brizola VR, Granato D. High-throughput assay comparison and standardization for metal chelating capacity screening: A proposal and application. Food Chemistry. 2017;214:515-522. DOI: 10.1016/j.foodchem.2016.07.091

[153] Singleton VL, Orthofer R, Lamuela-Raventos RM. Analysis of total phenols and other oxidation substrates and antioxidants by means of Folin-Ciocalteu reagent. Oxidants and Antioxidants, Pt A. 1999;299:152-178. DOI:

[154] Magalhaes LM, Segundo MA, Reis S, Lima J. Methodological aspects about in vitro evaluation of antioxidant properties. Analytica Chimica Acta. 2008;613(1):1-19. DOI: 10.1016/j.aca.2008.02.047

[155] Jara-Palacios MJ, Goncalves S, Heredia FJ, Hernanz D, Romano A. Extraction of Antioxidants from Winemaking Byproducts: Effect of the Solvent on Phenolic Composition, Antioxidant and Anti-Cholinesterase Activities, and Electrochemical Behaviour. Antioxidants. 2020;9(8):article number 675. DOI: 10.3390/antiox9080675

[156] Mohtar LG, Messina GA, Bertolino FA, Pereira SV, Raba J, Nazareno MA. Comparative study of different methodologies for the determination the antioxidant activity of Venezuelan propolis. Microchemical Journal. 2020;158:article number 105244. DOI: 10.1016/j.microc.2020.105244

[157] Pico J, Pismag RY, Laudouze M, Martinez MM. Systematic evaluation of the Folin-Ciocalteu and Fast Blue BB reactions during the analysis of total phenolics in legumes, nuts and plant seeds. Food & Function. 2020;11(11):9868-9880. DOI: 10.1039/d0fo01857k

[158] Gao Y, Guo X, Liu Y, Zhang M, Zhang R, Abbasi AM, et al. Comparative assessment of phytochemical profile, antioxidant capacity and anti-proliferative activity in different varieties of brown rice (Oryza sativa L.). Lwt-Food Science and Technology.

2018;96:19-25. DOI: 10.1016/j.lwt.2018.05.002

[159] Wolfe KL, Liu RH. Cellular antioxidant activity (CAA) assay for assessing antioxidants, foods, and dietary supplements. Journal of Agricultural and Food Chemistry. 2007;55(22):8896-8907. DOI: 10.1021/jf0715166

[160] Wang H, Joseph JA. Quantifying cellular oxidative stress by dichlorofluorescein assay using microplate reader. Free Radical Biology and Medicine. 1999;27(5-6):612-616. DOI: 10.1016/s0891-5849(99)00107-0

[161] Sessa M, Tsao R, Liu RH, Ferrari G, Donsi F. Evaluation of the Stability and Antioxidant Activity of Nanoencapsulated Resveratrol during in Vitro Digestion. Journal of Agricultural and Food Chemistry. 2011;59(23):12352-12360. DOI: 10.1021/jf2031346

[162] Kellett ME, Greenspan P, Pegg RB. Modification of the cellular antioxidant activity (CAA) assay to study phenolic antioxidants in a Caco-2 cell line. Food Chemistry. 2018;244:359-363. DOI: 10.1016/j.foodchem.2017.10.035

[163] Guo R, Guo X, Li T, Fu X, Liu RH. Comparative assessment of phytochemical profiles, antioxidant and antiproliferative activities of Sea buckthorn (Hippophae rhamnoides L.) berries. Food Chemistry. 2017;221: 997-1003. DOI: 10.1016/j.foodchem.2016.11.063

[164] Dani C, Bonatto D, Salvador M, Pereira MD, Henriques JAP, Eleutherio E. Antioxidant protection of resveratrol and catechin in Saccharomyces cerevisiae. Journal of Agricultural and Food Chemistry. 2008;56(11):4268-4272. DOI: 10.1021/jf800752s

[165] Baroni MV, Naranjo RDD, Garcia-Ferreyra C, Otaiza S, Wunderlin DA. How good antioxidant is the red wine? Comparison of some in vitro and in vivo methods to assess the antioxidant capacity of Argentinean red wines. Lwt-Food Science and Technology. 2012;47(1):1-7. DOI: 10.1016/j.lwt.2012.01.015

[166] Lv H-p, Zhang Y, Shi J, Lin Z. Phytochemical profiles and antioxidant activities of Chinese dark teas obtained by different processing technologies. Food Research International. 2017;100:486-493. DOI: 10.1016/j.foodres.2016.10.024

[167] Capanoglu E, Beekwilder J, Boyacioglu D, De Vos RCH, Hall RD. The Effect of Industrial Food Processing on Potentially Health-Beneficial Tomato Antioxidants. Critical Reviews in Food Science and Nutrition. 2010;50(10):919-930. DOI: 10.1080/10408390903001503

[168] Granato D, Shahidi F, Wrolstad R, Kilmartin P, Melton LD, Hidalgo FJ, et al. Antioxidant activity, total phenolics and flavonoids contents: Should we ban in vitro screening methods? Food Chemistry. 2018;264:471-475. DOI: 10.1016/j.foodchem.2018.04.012

[169] Nand AV, Swift S, Uy B, Kilmartin PA. Evaluation of antioxidant and antimicrobial properties of biocompatible low density polyethylene/polyaniline blends. Journal of Food Engineering. 2013;116(2):422-429. DOI: 10.1016/j.jfoodeng.2012.11.023

[170] Ferreira FS, Sampaio GR, Keller LM, Sawaya ACHF, Chavez DWH, Torres EAFS, et al. Impact of Air Frying on Cholesterol and Fatty Acids Oxidation in Sardines: Protective Effects of Aromatic Herbs. Journal of Food Science. 2017;82(12):2823-2831. DOI: 10.1111/1750-3841.13967

[171] Yi B, Kim M-J, Lee J. Antioxidant Properties of Astaxanthin in Oil-in-Water Emulsions with Differently-Charged Emulsifiers Under Chlorophyll Photosensitization. Journal of Food Science. 2018;83(3):589-596. DOI: 10.1111/1750-3841.14005